T0298443

Biomedical Image Segmentation
Advances and Trends

edited by
Ayman El-Baz
Xiaoyi Jiang
Jasjit S. Suri

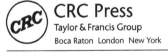

CRC Press
Taylor & Francis Group
Boca Raton London New York

CRC Press is an imprint of the
Taylor & Francis Group, an **informa** business

CRC Press
Taylor & Francis Group
6000 Broken Sound Parkway NW, Suite 300
Boca Raton, FL 33487-2742

First issued in paperback 2019

© 2017 by Taylor & Francis Group, LLC
CRC Press is an imprint of Taylor & Francis Group, an Informa business

No claim to original U.S. Government works

ISBN-13: 978-1-4822-5855-4 (hbk)
ISBN-13: 978-0-367-87086-7 (pbk)

Library of Congress Cataloging-in-Publication Data

Names: El-Baz, Ayman S., editor. | Jiang, Xiaoyi, editor. | Suri, Jasjit S., editor.
Title: Biomedical image segmentation : advances and trends / [edited by] Ayman El-Baz, Xiaoyi Jiang, and Jasjit S. Suri.
Description: Boca Raton : Taylor & Francis, 2017. | Includes bibliographical references and index.
Identifiers: LCCN 2016019546 | ISBN 9781482258554 (hardback : alk. paper)
Subjects: | MESH: Image Interpretation, Computer-Assisted--methods | Image Processing, Computer-Assisted--methods
Classification: LCC RC78.7.D53 | NLM WB 141 | DDC 616.07/54--dc23
LC record available at https://lccn.loc.gov/2016019546

Visit the Taylor & Francis Web site at
http://www.taylorandfrancis.com

and the CRC Press Web site at
http://www.crcpress.com

Contents

Preface

Medical imaging is an indispensable tool for patients' healthcare in modern medicine. It is considered to be one of the basic monitoring tools—today's medical imaging effectively assists clinicians and radiologists in diagnosing diseases, making therapeutic or surgical decisions, and guiding surgery operations. Recent advances in medical imaging modalities provide images with a menagerie of sizes, structures, resolution, and degrees of contrast. A two-dimensional (2D) image is a rectangular array of pixels containing measured scalar or vectorial visual signals (e.g., intensities or colors), which quantify properties of related spatial locations in a whole body or its part. The 2D image of a thin planar cross-section of a 3D object is usually called a *slice*. A collection of successive slices forms a 3D image, which is an array of voxels.

Image segmentation plays an essential role in the medical imaging field, including computer-aided diagnosis (CAD), medical image analysis, image fusion, image-guided therapy, image annotation, and image retrieval. In computer vision, image segmentation is the process of partitioning a 2D/3D image into multiple segments (regions). The goal of segmentation is to simplify or change the representation of an image into something more meaningful and easier to analyze. In the literature, several general approaches have been developed for image segmentation. These approaches can be classified into the following categories: (1) threshold-based segmentation approaches, (2) statistical-based segmentation approaches, (3) deformable model-based segmentation approaches, and (4) graph-based segmentation approaches. This book will cover all these segregation categories with a focus on deformable model-based segmentation approaches.

The target audience for this book includes engineering and medical school professors; graduate and undergraduate college students in engineering and applied science departments; medical students; engineers in medical companies; researchers in industry, academia, and health science; medical doctors such as radiologists and cardiologists; as well as healthcare professionals including radiology technologists and medical physicists.

The book consists of 22 chapters that deal with the segmentation of different problems. A brief summary of each chapter follows.

Chapter 1 focuses on providing a comprehensive survey on deformable-based segmentation methods, specifically, region-based approaches for segmentation which are represented mathematically in partial differential equations. In particular, the mathematical background for such models are detailed whether they are parametric or geometric based. The pros and cons of each type are also discussed, along with future trends. Finally, the chapter summarizes the recent applications of deformable model-based segmentation in medical imaging; and briefly surveys recent work in the segmentation of different tissue types, such as the kidneys, prostate, and lungs.

Chapter 2 reviews recent applications of level set methods to segmentation problems in medical images. The chapter focuses on how treatment domain knowledge about objects and imaging artifacts are represented and integrated into the segmentation solution. The chapter also distinguishes between the means to add this information before, during, and after level set segmentation and discusses the methodology and benefits of each of these different strategies.

Chapter 3 presents a parametric deformable model with energy that tends to approach the learned shapes. Instead of the level set formalism, the target shapes are approximated directly with linear combinations of distance vectors describing positions of the mutually aligned training shapes with respect to their common centroid. Such a vector space is now closed in the matter of linear operations and comprises a smaller dimensionality than the 2D distance maps. Thus, the authors' shape model is easily simplified with principal component analysis (PCA), with the shape-dependent energy terms guiding the boundary evolution to obtain a very simple analytic form. Prior knowledge of the visual appearance of the object is represented by Gibbs energies for the gray levels of the objects. Experiments with natural images confirm the robustness, accuracy, and high speed of this approach.

Chapter 4 introduces 3D active shape models, which perform the estimation of deformable surfaces in 3D volumes using landmark statistics. First, the average shape and deformation modes are obtained from a set of annotated landmarks (training set). These statistics are then used to segment new volumes, involving the estimation of the alignment parameters and deformation coefficients. This approach is well suited to segment the shape of the left ventricle in 3D magnetic resonance imaging (MRI) volumes. In addition, this approach was tested in 20 MRI volumes using a leave-one-out scheme. The results have shown that it achieves good segmentation accuracy in terms of the average Dice coefficient and the average minimum distance to the ground truth.

Chapter 5 presents two different original methodologies designed for segmentation of the myocardium within MRI sequences. The common point between these two techniques is the use of an a priori model to guide and calculate the final segmentation of the epicardial and endocardial walls. These approaches may be related to active contour methodologies, and permit one to precisely extract the geometry of the myocardial walls.

Chapter 6 presents a method for learning and using prior knowledge on shape variability in the implicit template deformation framework. This prior shape is achieved via an original and dedicated process in which both an optimal template and principal modes of variation are estimated from a collection of shapes. This framework maintains the two key properties of implicit template deformation: topology preservation and computational efficiency. This approach can be applied to any organ with a possibly complex shape, yet with fixed topology. This approach has also been validated on myocardium segmentation from cardiac magnetic resonance short-axis images and demonstrates segmentation improvement over standard template deformation.

Chapter 7 presents a method for automatic detection of exudates in digital fundus images using an active contour-based approach. The method can be divided into three main stages: candidate extraction, precise contour segmentation, and the labeling of candidates as true or false exudates. This method has been tested on publicly available databases both to measure the accuracy of the segmentation of exudate regions and for recognizing their presence at an image level.

Chapter 8 presents a preprocessing local feature and fuzzy active contour-based image segmentation technique. Image preprocessing techniques are used to mitigate the effects of different artifacts (noise, contrast degradation, low resolution, etc.). Local features are then computed and assigned weights using fuzzy logic to enhance the segmentation boundaries. A modified active contour-based image segmentation technique has been developed, which provides better accuracy in terms of visual and quantitative analysis.

Chapter 9 presents a recent body of work that provides a complete framework for extracting the geometry and topology of multidimensional curvilinear networks in microscopy images. The proposed multiple Stretching Open Active Contours (SOACs) are automatically initialized and evolve along the network centerlines synergically: they can merge with others, stop upon collision, and reconfigure with others to allow for a smooth continuation across network junctions. This approach is generally applicable to 2D/3D images of curvilinear networks with varying signal-to-noise ratios (SNRs). Qualitative and quantitative evaluations using simulated and experimental images demonstrate its effectiveness and potential.

Chapter 10 presents an approach for segmenting cell nuclei, which is based on level set active contours and convex minimization. This approach employs deferent convex energy functions and uses an efficient numeric scheme for minimization. The performance of this approach has been evaluated using fluorescence microscopy images from deferent experiments comprising deferent cell types. The authors have also performed a quantitative comparison with previous segmentation approaches.

Chapter 11 introduces histogram-based level set methods for medical image segmentation which evolve level set functions by measuring the similarity of histograms. Without preprocessing, a comparable segmentation result on a brain image using a simple gradient descent or gradient ascent method has been demonstrated.

Chapter 12 presents a level set-based deformable model to segment a kidney from diffusion-weighted magnetic resonance imaging (DW-MRI). The proposed deformable model is guided by a stochastic speed relationship based on a prior adaptive shape, which is guided by the visual appearance of the DW-MRI data. The voxel-wise guiding of the level sets is obtained by integrating these three image features into a joint Markov–Gibbs random field (MGRF) model of the kidney and its background. This approach is evaluated and compared against other segmentation methods using three evaluation metrics: the Dice similarity coefficient (DSC), the 95-percentile modified Hausdorff distance, and the absolute kidney volume difference. Experimental result evaluations between manually drawn and automatically segmented contours confirm the robustness and accuracy of the authors' approach.

Chapter 13 focuses on the application of deformable models including both geometric and parametric models, for the prostate segmentation of images acquired from different imaging modalities, such as magnetic resonance imaging, computed tomography (CT), and ultrasound. The clinical data used in these studies are highlighted along with a description of the advantages and limitations in the performance of each segmentation algorithm.

Chapter 14 presents a computer-aided diagnostic (CAD) framework for detecting prostate cancer in DW-MRI data. The proposed CAD method consists of two major steps that use nonnegative matrix factorization (NMF) to find meaningful features from sets of high-dimensional data. The first step is a 3D level set segmentation algorithm guided by a novel probabilistic speed function to segment the prostate region from each 3D DW-MRI for each b-value. The second step is a probabilistic classifier that seeks to label a prostate segmented from 4D DW-MRI data as either malignant (with cancer) or benign (no cancer). Experimental analysis indicates that for both of these frameworks, using NMF produces more accurate segmentation and classification results, respectively, and that combining the information from DWI data at several b-values can assist in detecting prostate cancer.

Chapter 15 presents an active contour method, called the distance regularized two-layer level set (DR2LS) algorithm to automatically segment both the left and right ventricles. In DR2LS, both the 0-level and k-level contours of a level set function are used to mathematically represent the endocardial and epicardial surfaces of both ventricles.

Experimental results have demonstrated the effectiveness of the proposed two-step level set approach to segment cardiac left and right ventricles simultaneously.

Chapter 16 presents a salient object segmentation based on the level set method with shape constraints. Given an image, this method first initializes the curve according to the saliency map, which is subsequently combined into evolution in a multichannel manner, and then rebuilds an energy that is functional with a shape constraint. This proposed method has been applied on synthetic, medical, and natural images that have obtained promising results.

Chapter 17 presents a particle filter-based approach, rooted in Bayesian estimation and Monte Carlo procedures, for tracking and segmenting the left ventricle. Two main ingredients characterize this formalism: the *prediction* that models the dynamic of the object in consecutive frames and *filtering* that collects information in the present frame. The usefulness of the authors' approach is evaluated using a database of disease cases and another dataset of normal cases, where both datasets present long axis views of the left ventricle. Using a training set comprising diseased and healthy cases, the approach produces accurate results for tracking the endocardium.

Chapter 18 discusses the use of a shortest path methodology combined with a region-based selection for a user-assisted segmentation, as either an enclosed object or as an open curve. The segmentation results of generic medical and real-world images have demonstrated that this method is generic and could be utilized in various other types of medical imaging.

Chapter 19 investigates the problem of the estimation of a pixel-dependent and pixel-independent local scale in the context of local parametric region segmentation models. Two main strategies are presented. The first is statistical and is based on a bias-variance trade-off principle. The second is a variational approach. The results of the proposed strategies have been demonstrated on synthetic and realistic simulations of ultrasound images with intensity inhomogeneities of a variable strength.

Chapter 20 discusses typical noise models, which are encountered in biomedical imaging. Additionally, the related algorithmic development, including explicit and implicit physical noise consideration, is briefly reviewed.

Chapter 21 presents an unsupervised segmentation of lung tissues from low-dose computed tomography (LDCT). The CT images and desired maps of regions (lung and other chest tissues) are achieved by a joint MGRF model of independent image signals and interdependent region labels, but focus on the most accurate model identification. Experiments with both the phantom and real datasets confirm high accuracy of the proposed approach.

Chapter 22 presents a fully automatic method for segmenting hip CT images using landmark detection-based atlas selection and optimal graph search-based surface detection. Validation on 30 hip CT images shows that the proposed method achieves high performance in pelvis, left proximal femur, and right proximal segmenting.

MATLAB® is a registered trademark of The MathWorks, Inc. For product information, please contact:

The MathWorks, Inc.
3 Apple Hill Drive
Natick, MA 01760-2098 USA
Tel: 508 647 7000
Fax: 508-647-7001
E-mail: info@mathworks.com
Web: www.mathworks.com

Editors

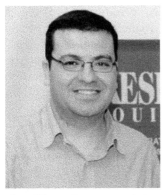

Ayman El-Baz, PhD, is a professor, university scholar, and chair of the Bioengineering Department at the University of Louisville, Kentucky. He earned a bachelor and master's in electrical engineering in 1997 and 2001. He earned a doctorate in electrical engineering from the University of Louisville in 2006. In 2009, Dr. El-Baz was named a Coulter Fellow for his contribution in biomedical translational research. He has 15 years of hands-on experience in the fields of bioimaging modeling and noninvasive computer-assisted diagnosis systems. He has developed new techniques for the accurate identification of probability mixtures for segmenting multimodal images, new probability models, and model-based algorithms for recognizing lung nodules and blood vessels in magnetic resonance and computer tomography imaging systems, as well as new registration techniques based on multiple second-order signal statistics, all of which have been reported at multiple international conferences and journal articles. Dr. El-Baz's work related to novel image analysis techniques for autism, dyslexia, and lung cancer has earned multiple awards, including the Wallace H. Coulter Foundation Early Career Translational Research Award in Biomedical Engineering Phase I & Phase II, a Research Scholar Grant from the American Cancer Society (ACS), 1st place at the Annual Research Louisville 2002, 2005, 2006, 2008, 2009, 2010, 2011, and 2012 meetings, and the Best Paper Award in Medical Image Processing from the prestigious ICGST International Conference on Graphics, Vision and Image Processing (GVIP-2005). He has been invited to present his research on image-based techniques for early diagnosis of lung cancer at the Siemens Research Corporation and Siemens Medical Solutions. He has been the principal investigator (PI) of five research projects that are funded by the Coulter Foundation, PI of a research project funded by the American Cancer Society, and co-PI on two R01 projects awarded by the NIH (National Institutes of Health). Based on these awards, he developed a new CAD system for early diagnosis of lung cancer. PulmoCADx, Inc. (St. Louis, Missouri) has licensed this lung CAD system. Dr. El-Baz has authored or coauthored more than 300 technical articles (87 journals, 9 books, 39 book chapters, 144 refereed-conference papers, 74 abstracts published in proceedings, and 12 U.S. Patents).

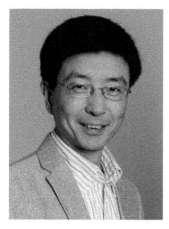

Xiaoyi Jiang, PhD, studied computer science at Peking University and earned a PhD and Venia Docendi (Habilitation) degree in computer science from the University of Bern, Switzerland. He was an associate professor at the Technical University of Berlin, Germany. Since 2002, he has been a full professor of computer science at the University of Münster, Germany. Dr. Jiang is a senior member of IEEE, and since 2006, a Fellow of IAPR (International Association for Pattern Recognition). Currently, he is editor-in-chief of the *International Journal of Pattern Recognition and Artificial Intelligence*. In addition, he serves on the advisory board and editorial board of several journals, including *IEEE Transactions on Medical Imaging*, the *International Journal of Neural Systems*, *Pattern Recognition*, and *Pattern Analysis and Applications*. He is a member of the IEEE-EMBS Technical Committee on Biomedical Imaging and Image Processing (BIIP) and on the Governing Board of IAPR. Dr. Jiang's research interests include biomedical image analysis, 3D image analysis, and structural pattern recognition. He is a principal investigator of the Cluster of Excellence "Cells in Motion" (http://www.uni-muenster.de/CiMIC/) funded by the German Excellence Initiative.

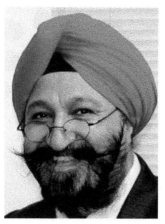

Jasjit S. Suri, PhD, MBA, Fellow AIMBE (American Institute for Medical and Biological Engineering), is an innovator, visionary, scientist, and an internationally known world leader. Dr. Suri was awarded the Director General's gold medal in 1980 and the Fellow of the American Institute of Medical and Biological Engineering, conferred by the National Academy of Sciences in Washington, DC, in 2004. He is currently the chairman of Global Biomedical Technologies, Inc. in Roseville, California. He has published over 500 peer-reviewed articles and book chapters with H-index (~40), and over 100 innovations/trademarks to his credit. He is currently the chairman of AtheroPoint, also in Roseville, California, a company dedicated to atherosclerosis imaging for early screening of stroke and cardiovascular monitoring. Dr. Suri has held positions as chair of IEEE Denver section and advisory board member in healthcare industries and several schools in the United States and abroad.

Contributors

Ahmed Aboulfotouh
Information Systems Department
Mansoura University
Mansoura, Egypt

Roberto Ardon
Philips Research Medisys
Suresnes, France

Souleymane Balla-Arabé
Laboratory of Electronic
    Computing and Imaging
    Science
University of Burgundy
Burgandy, France

Jan-Philip Bergeest
Department of Bioinformatics and
    Functional Genomics
University of Heidelberg
Heidelberg, Germany

Kévin Bianchi
ISIT, UMR CNRS
Université d'Auvergne
Clermont-Ferrand, France

Djamal Boukerroui
Mirada Medical Ltd.
Oxford Centre for Innovation
Oxford, United Kingdom

Gustavo Carneiro
School of Computer Science
Australian Centre for Visual
    Technologies
University of Adelaide
Adelaide, South Australia

Lucie Cassagnes
ISIT, UMR CNRS
Université d'Auvergne
and
CHU Gabriel Montpied
Clermont-Ferrand, France

Guillaume Cerutti
INRIA
Virtual Plants INRIA Team
Montpellier, France

Tanveer Ahmed Cheema
School of Engineering and Applied
    Sciences
Isra University
Islamabad, Pakistan

Chengwen Chu
Institute for Surgical Technology and
    Biomechanics
University of Bern
Bern, Switzerland

Laurent D. Cohen
CEREMADE UMR CNRS
Paris Dauphine University, PSL
Paris, France

Remi Cuingnet
Philips Research Medisys
Suresnes, France

Magdi El-Azab
Department of Mathematics and
    Physical Engineering
Mansoura University
Mansoura, Egypt

Maryam El-Baz
BioImaging Laboratory
Bioengineering Department
University of Louisville
Louisville, Kentucky

Ali Taki Eldeen
BioImaging Laboratory
Bioengineering Department
and
Electrical and Computer Engineering
  Department
University of Louisville
Louisville, Kentucky

Tarek El-Diasty
Department of Radiology
Urology and Nephrology Center
Mansoura University
Mansoura, Egypt

Mohamed Abou El-Ghar
Radiology Department
and
Urology and Nephrology Department
Mansoura University
Mansoura, Egypt

Adel Elmaghraby
Department of Computer Engineering
  and Computer Science
University of Louisville
Louisville, Kentucky

Mohammed Elmogy
Information Technology Department
Mansoura University
Mansoura, Egypt

Ahmed ElTanboly
BioImaging Laboratory
Bioengineering Department
University of Louisville
Louisville, Kentucky
and
Department of Mathematics and Physical
  Engineering
Mansoura University
Mansoura, Egypt

Ehab Essa
Department of Computer Science
Swansea University
Swansea, United Kingdom

António Freitas
Department of Cardiology
Fernando Fonseca Hospital
Lisbon, Portugal

Xinbo Gao
Video and Image Processing
  System Laboratory
School of Electronic Engineering
Xidian University
Shaanxi, China

Abdul Ghafoor
College of Signals
National University of Sciences and
  Technology
Islamabad, Pakistan

Georgy Gimel'farb
Department of Computer Science
University of Auckland
Auckland, New Zealand

Oliver Gloger
Institut für Community Medicine
Universitätsmedizin Greifswald
Abteilung Methoden der Community
  Medicine
Ernst-Moritz-Arndt Universität
  Greifswald
Greifswald, Germany

Andras Hajdu
Faculty of Informatics
University of Debrecen
Debrecen, Hungary

Balazs Harangi
Faculty of Informatics
University of Debrecen
Debrecen, Hungary

Xiaolei Huang
Department of Computer Science and
    Engineering
Lehigh University
Bethlehem, Pennsylvania

Marwa Ismail
BioImaging Laboratory
Bioengineering Department
and
Electrical and Computer Engineering
    Department
University of Louisville
Louisville, Kentucky

Umer Javed
School of Engineering and Applied
    Sciences
Isra University
Islamabad, Pakistan

Jonathan-Lee Jones
Department of Computer Science
Swansea University
Swansea, United Kingdom

Robert Keynton
Bioengineering Department
University of Louisville
Louisville, Kentucky

Fahmi Khalifa
BioImaging Laboratory
Bioengineering Department
and
Electrical and Computer Engineering
    Department
University of Louisville
Louisville, Kentucky

Tim König
Computer Vision Group, ISG
Department of Computer Science
Otto-von-Guericke Universität
    Magdeburg
Magdeburg, Germany

Chunming Li
School of Electronic Engineering
University of Electronic Science and
    Technology of China
Chengdu, China

Xuelong Li
Center for OPTical IMagery Analysis and
    Learning
State Key Laboratory of Transient Optics
    and Photonics
Xi'an Institute of Optics and Precision
    Mechanics
Chinese Academy of Sciences
Shaanxi, China

Yu Liu
College of Electronic Science and
    Engineering
Jilin University
Changchun, China

Jorge S. Marques
Instituto de Sistemas e Robótica
Instituto Superior Técnico
Lisboa, Portugal

Patrick McClure
BioImaging Laboratory
Bioengineering Department
and
Electrical and Computer Engineering
    Department
University of Louisville
Louisville, Kentucky

Benoit Mory
Philips Research Medisys
Suresnes, France

Jacinto C. Nascimento
Institute for Systems and Robotics
and
Informatics and Computer Engineering
    Department
Instituto Superior Técnico
Lisboa, Portugal

Jifeng Ning
College of Information Engineering
Northwest A&F University
Shaanxi, China

Raphael Prevost
Philips Research Medisys
Suresnes, France

Islam Reda
Information Systems Department
Mansoura University
Mansoura, Egypt
and
BioImaging Laboratory
Bioengineering Department
University of Louisville
Louisville, Kentucky

Muhammad Mohsin Riaz
Centre for Advanced Studies in
    Telecommunication, COMSATS
Islamabad, Pakistan

Karl Rohr
Department of Bioinformatics and
    Functional Genomics
University of Heidelberg
Heidelberg, Germany

Carlos Santiago
Instituto de Sistemas e Robótica
Instituto Superior Técnico
Lisboa, Portugal

Laurent Sarry
ISIT, UMR CNRS
Université d'Auvergne
Clermont-Ferrand, France

Mohamed Shehata
BioImaging Laboratory
Bioengineering Department
University of Louisville
Louisville, Kentucky

Ahmed Soliman
BioImaging Laboratory
Bioengineering Department
and
Electrical and Computer Engineering
    Department
University of Louisville
Louisville, Kentucky

Dacheng Tao
Center for Quantum Computation and
    Intelligent Systems
University of Technology
Sydney, New South Wales, Australia

Daniel Tenbrinck
Department of Mathematics and
    Computer Science
University of Münster
and
Cluster of Excellence
Cells in Motion, CiM
Münster, Germany

Klaus D. Toennies
Computer Vision Group, ISG
Department of Computer Science
Otto-von-Guericke Universität
    Magdeburg
Magdeburg, Germany

Laure Tougne
Université de Lyon, CNRS
Lyon, France

Antoine Vacavant
ISIT, UMR CNRS
Université d'Auvergne
Clermont-Ferrand, France

Bin Wang
Video and Image Processing
    System Laboratory
School of Electronic Engineering
Xidian University
Shaanxi, China

Jia Wu
Department of Radiology
University of Pennsylvania
Philadelphia, Pennsylvania

Xianghua Xie
Department of Computer Science
Swansea University
Swansea, United Kingdom

Ting Xu
Department of Computer Science and
  Engineering
Lehigh University
Bethlehem, Pennsylvania

Xiaoping Yang
School of Science
Nanjing University of Science and
  Technology
Nanjing, China

Wei Yu
College of Information Engineering
Northwest A&F University
Shaanxi, China

Shaoxiang Zhang
Institute of Digital Medicine
Third Military Medical University
Chongqing, China

Guoyan Zheng
Institute for Surgical Technology and
  Biomechanics
University of Bern
Bern, Switzerland

Chao Zhou
Department of Electrical and Computer
  Engineering
and
Bioengineering Program
and
Center for Photonics and
  Nanoelectronics
Lehigh University
Bethlehem, Pennsylvania

chapter one

Deformable model-based methods for image segmentation

Marwa Ismail, Ahmed ElTanboly, Magdi El-Azab, Ayman El-Baz, and Robert Keynton

Contents

Abstract

Medical imaging is a rapidly evolving area, where there is a strong need to understand scalar or vector-valued images. The outcome of such processing can have strong diagnostic implications and can be used as an additional tool to detect and treat different diseases in a timely and proper fashion. This chapter targets one of the most popular processes in medical imaging, which is segmentation. Segmentation methods have different classifications; they can be edge-based or region-based, and the process can be manual or fully automated. This chapter focuses on deformable-based methods, specifically, region-based, for segmentation that are mathematically represented in partial differential equations. In particular, the mathematical background for such models is given in terms of parametric- or geometric-based. The pros and cons of each type are also discussed, along with the future trends. Finally, the chapter summarizes the recent applications of deformable model-based segmentation in medical imaging. It briefly surveys recent work in the segmentation of different tissue types, such as the kidney, prostate, and lung.

1.1   Introduction

In computer vision, image segmentation is the process of partitioning an image into multiple segments. In other words, it is the process of labeling every pixel in an image such that pixels with the same label share the same characteristics, such as texture, brightness, or gray level [1]. Segmentation of medical images, in particular, has assumed immense importance as a noninvasive tool that provides physicians with a reliable way of diagnosis of the abnormalities found in different organs.

In the field of medical imaging, accurate segmentation of structures is crucial for detecting lesions and abnormalities. It has recently provided great advances to clinicians in assessing abnormalities through computer-aided diagnostic (CAD) systems. Segmentation, however, is highly challenging due to many factors, such as the low contrast between different tissue types, which makes it difficult to segment the desired object manually, and the motion artifacts associated with the scans which adds noise to images.

In order to formulate the segmentation problem mathematically, consider the finite 2D arithmetic lattice, $\mathbf{R}$, of the size XY supporting pixels, the finite set of intensities $\mathbf{Q}$, and the finite set of region labels $\mathbf{K}$:

$$\mathbf{R} = (r = (x,y): x = 0,1,\ldots,X-1, y = 0,1,\ldots,Y-1)$$

$$\mathbf{Q} = (0,1,\ldots,Q-1)$$

$$\mathbf{K} = (0,1,\ldots,K-1)$$

where x,y denote the Cartesian coordinates of the lattice sites. Let $g\colon \mathbf{R} \to \mathbf{Q}$ and $m\colon \mathbf{R} \to \mathbf{K}$ denote a digital image and a region, respectively. If $H(.)$ is a homogeneity predicate for signals from a connected subset of image pixels, the segmentation divides the image g into K connected subimages, $g_k\colon \mathbf{R}_k \to \mathbf{Q}; k \in \mathbf{K}; \mathbf{R}_k \subset \mathbf{R}$ that cover the whole lattice, $\cup_{k \in \mathbf{K}} \mathbf{R}_k = \mathbf{R}$, without overlaps, $\mathbf{R}_k \cap \mathbf{R}_\mathcal{K} = \emptyset$ for all pairs $(k,\mathcal{K})\colon k \neq \mathcal{K}$, and keep the homogeneity individually, $H(g_k) = true$ for all $k \in \mathbf{K}$, but not in combination with their immediate neighbors, $H(g_k \cup g_k) = false$ for all the pairs of adjacent regions $\mathbf{R}_k$ and $\mathbf{R}_k$ (Figure 1.1).

The segmentation problem has been extensively addressed in literature and can be classified into many categories. One possible classification is methods that are either edge-based or region-based. Edge-based segmentation mainly depends on edge detection, which

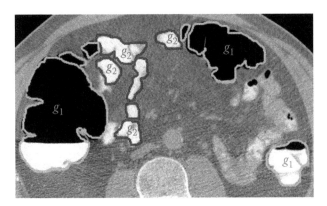

Figure 1.1 Subimages g_1, g_2 under the homogeneity predicate requiring the same gray level for all pixels. g_1 (orange) represents colon segments of a CT slice, whereas g_2 (blue) represent small bowels. The union of any two adjacent regions is inhomogeneous.

is conducted with many algorithms such as edge relaxation methods [2], border detection methods [3–5], and Hough transform-based methods [6,7]. In region-based segmentation, pixels that share the same characteristics, for example, the gray level, are clustered together to form homogeneous regions [8–10]. Segmentation can also be classified with respect to user's intervention. Segmentation could either be manually initialized, semiautomated, or fully automated. Current advances in the field of image processing seek the full automation of segmentation techniques in order to optimize the process and refrain from manual intervention, which is time-consuming and error-prone as well. Segmentation techniques can also be deformable model-based, where a curve is initialized, and then propagates (deforms) according to an energy function to be minimized. Under this category, numerous techniques have been devised that are either parametric, or geometric, also called level set-based, models. In parametric models, Lagrangian methods are used to deform the initial contour according to some external forces along with some internal properties of the image [11]. Geometric models, on the other hand, are capable of handling the topological changes of the object, as it tackles the minimization problem in higher dimensions without the need for parameterization. Osher and Sethian [12] first proposed the evolving curve, which is represented implicitly using a signed distance function, whose zero level represents the original contour.

Although deformable models have been widely used in literature with numerous formulae for the segmentation of different body organs, it is impossible to have a generic framework that is suited for any segmentation problem. The algorithm should also be adapted in order to meet each one's characteristics. This chapter focuses on deformable model-based segmentation, due to the many advances it has recently witnessed in the field of medical imaging analysis, the ease of integrating its concepts in any framework, and the high efficiency it provides in convergence to solutions.

The basics of deformable models with its two major categories, parametric and geometric, are detailed. The chapter also provides an overview of the recent advances in image segmentation using deformable models, which have been extensively used in literature for image segmentation. A variety of energy functions and numerical schemes have been proposed to solve their associated partial differential equations. Some of these major energy functions are provided in detail.

This chapter begins with a review of the parametric deformable models in the literature. It analyzes some of the popular external forces used along with their main drawbacks. It also covers the most widely used numerical schemes for the solution of the energy functions. The geometric deformable models that were designed to overcome the limitations of the classical parametric representation are also discussed. The basics of the level sets method and some of its important concepts are provided in detail. Numerical schemes for solving the level sets equation are provided. The general form, namely, Hamilton–Jacobi is discussed. The popular Euler–Lagrange equation is also provided with its proof as a powerful optimization technique, which is mostly used in many applications. The chapter then goes through some of the popular guiding forces in literature, such as the Chan–Vese model, which is widely applied in image segmentation techniques, along with some of its recent improvements. Finally, a survey on recent medical imaging segmentation techniques using deformable models is conducted.

1.2   Parametric deformable models

A parametric deformable model is represented by a contour that has some criteria for its deformation. These criteria are governed by geometric and image properties. First developed by Kass et al. [11], the contour can either be a collection of discrete points [13–15], Figure 1.2, that are held together by internal forces and guided toward the image boundary by external forces, or it can be parametrically described using basis function such as B-splines [16–19], and Fourier exponentials [20].

The parametric deformable model contour is evolving based on the following energy function:

$$E = E_{\text{internal}} + E_{\text{external}}, \tag{1.1}$$

where the internal energy imposes restrictions to the contour movement by controlling the elasticity and stiffness parameters, while the external energy is responsible for driving the deformable model toward important features in the image [21].

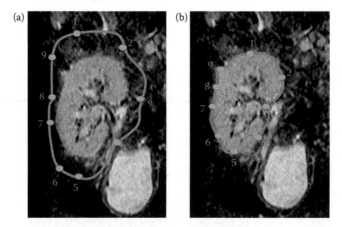

Figure 1.2 Initial contour for (a) a kidney deformable-model based segmentation. The final contour that is attracted to the object's boundaries (b).

Given an image I, and the parametric form of its deforming contour $X(s) = [x(s)y(s)]$, $s \in [0, 1]$, the internal energy can then be formulated as

$$E_{internal} = \frac{1}{2} \int_0^1 \gamma X'(s)^2 + \sigma X''(s)^2 \, ds, \tag{1.2}$$

where γ, σ are the nonnegative weights that control the contour movement [20]. The first term reduces the curve length and removes ripples, while the second controls the contour's smoothness.

The external energy is defined as

$$E_{external} = -\lambda \int_0^1 \nabla(G_\delta(x, y) * (I(x, y))) ds, \tag{1.3}$$

where G is a smoothing filter with width δ, which is applied to improve the edge map of the image and reduce noise. The parameter λ is the magnitude of the external force. As mentioned earlier, the external energy derives the contour toward the object's boundaries [11]. It serves as a potential force that pulls the snake toward the edges of the image.

1.2.1   Solution approaches to the parametric deformable models

Discretization and numerical simulation of parametric deformable models can be conducted using numerous approaches. The finite element and finite difference approaches offer several explicit and implicit direct integration methods, including the central difference, Houbolt, Newmark, or Wilson methods [22]. The literature contains dynamic programming, greedy algorithms, and Lagrangian methods that were used in order to numerically simulate snake models [23–25].

Lagrangian Methods: The Euler–Lagrange equation is a second-order partial differential equation (PDE) whose solutions are the functions for which a given functional is stationary. It is a widely used formula in the literature of deformable models optimization [23,24]. The main problem with Lagrangian methods is the heavy computations requirement until the problem reaches convergence.

Statement. For the functional (function of function) I

$$I[f] = \int_a^b L(s, f(s), f'(s), f''(s), \dots, f^{(n)}) ds;$$

where

L is the Lagrangian function

$f(s)$: is the function to be found (which is a stationary point of I)

Then, The Euler–Lagrange equation, is given by

$$\frac{\partial L}{\partial f} - \frac{d}{ds}\left(\frac{\partial L}{\partial f'}\right) + \frac{d^2}{ds^2}\left(\frac{\partial L}{\partial f''}\right) - \cdots + (-1)^n \frac{d^n}{ds^n}\left(\frac{\partial L}{\partial f^{(n)}}\right) = 0 \tag{1.4}$$

Plenty of numerical approaches have been proposed to solve Equation 1.4 and also various forms for the external energy E_{external}, classified as either edge-based or region-based. The next two sections address both numerical schemes and the guiding forces in detail.

Given the energy function

$$E = \int_0^1 \gamma X'(s)^2 + \sigma X''(s)^2 + E_{\text{external}}(X(s))ds$$

$$= \int_0^1 F(s, X, X', X'')ds$$

(1.5)

The solution to this problem satisfies the following Euler–Lagrange equation:

$$F_X - \frac{d}{ds}F_{X'} + \frac{d^2}{ds^2}F_{X''} = 0$$

(1.6)

Substituting with Equation 1.5 in Equation 1.6:

$$-\gamma'X' - (\gamma + \sigma'')X'' + 2\sigma'X''' + \sigma X^{(4)} + \frac{\partial E_{\text{external}}}{\partial X} = 0,$$

which could be written in a discrete form as:

$$X(s-2) \cdot \sigma + X(s-1) \cdot (\gamma - 4\sigma) + X(s) \cdot (-2\gamma + 6\sigma)$$
$$+ X(s+1) \cdot (\gamma - 4\sigma) + X(s+2) \cdot (\sigma) + f(X(s)) = 0$$

(1.7)

Equation 1.7 produces two independent linear equations for $x(s)$ and $y(s)$ in the form $\mathbf{A}x = f_x$ and $\mathbf{A}y = f_y$, where $\mathbf{A}$ is a circulant pentadiagonal matrix consisting of several combinations of γ and σ. Kass et al. [11] used this approach to minimize the energy function in Equation 1.1, by updating the position of each control point on the contour using an iterative algorithm. The approach reaches convergence when both the internal and external forces balance. The numerical implementation by Kass could be formulated as follows:

$$\mathbf{A}x_t + f_x(x_{t-1}, y_{t-1}) = -\alpha(x_t - x_{t-1})$$
$$\mathbf{A}y_t + f_y(x_{t-1}, y_{t-1}) = -\alpha(y_t - y_{t-1})$$

(1.8)

where $\mathbf{A}x_t$ represents the internal forces, $f_x(x_{t-1}, y_{t-1})$ represents the external forces. The right side is the step size multiplied by a constant α. The position is then updated as follows:

$$(\mathbf{A} + \alpha\mathbf{I})x_t = \alpha x_{t-1} - f_x(x_{t-1}, y_{t-1})$$
$$(\mathbf{A} + \alpha\mathbf{I})y_t = \alpha y_{t-1} - f_y(x_{t-1}, y_{t-1})$$

(1.9)

Dynamic Programming: Dynamic programming is an optimization approach that ensures global optimality of the solution. It embeds the problem of interest as a member of a family of problems to be studied. Dynamic programming allows for hard constraints to be enforced on the behavior of the solution.

The algorithm first discretizes the energy-minimization problem in Equation 1.2 as follows:

$$E_{\text{internal}} = \gamma |X(s) - X(s-1)|^2 + \sigma |X(s+1) - 2X(s) + X(s-1)|^2 \tag{1.10}$$

The total energy in Equation 1.1 is then minimized, which could be obtained from a series of discrete multistage decision processes. A decision is then made from a finite number of possibilities at each stage. This can be formulated as:

$$E(X(1), X(2), \ldots, X(n)) = E_1(X(1), X(2), X(3)) + E_2(X(2), X(3), X(4))$$
$$+ \cdots + E_{n-2}(X(n-2), X(n-1), X(n)) \tag{1.11}$$

where

$$E_{s-1}(X(s-1), X(s), X(s+1)) = E_{\text{external}}(X(s)) + E_{\text{internal}}(X(s-1), X(s), X(s+1)) \tag{1.12}$$

Each control point is allowed to move to only m possible positions, which are its nine nearest neighbors. The solution creates a sequence of functions called the optimal value functions, each obtained by minimizing over one dimension to find the contour with minimum energy. This establishes the new positions of the control points. The whole procedure is then repeated until the minimized energy does not vary with time.

This algorithm was applied on the energy functionals of active contours [23,24], where the optimization problem is setup as a discrete multistage decision process and is solved by a time-delayed discrete dynamic programming algorithm.

One of the major drawbacks of dynamic programming is the extensive computations requirement, which makes it a very slow optimization method. Also the forces on control points act in a perpendicular manner and also along the contour, which results in bunching up the points. A hard constraint is usually added to minimize this effect so that adjacent control points cannot get closer than a certain distance from one another.

Greedy Algorithms: Greedy algorithms have been used with active contours to find convergent solutions [23]. Like dynamic programming, greedy algorithms allow the inclusion of hard constraints. The greedy algorithm is iterative for closed contours, where the neighborhood of each control point is analyzed at each iteration. The pixel with the smallest value in the energy function that belongs to the neighborhood becomes the new position for that control point. The iterations stop when the number of moving points is less than a threshold value.

$$E = \int_s (\gamma E_{\text{elastic}} + \sigma E_{\text{bend}} + \alpha E_{\text{image}}) ds. \tag{1.13}$$

E_{elastic} prevents points from bunching, and is estimated as:

$$E_{\text{elastic}} = d - |X(s) - X(s-1)| \tag{1.14}$$

where d is the distance between two consecutive points.

E_{bend} is the curvature term and is estimated as

$$E_{\text{bend}} = |X(s-1) - 2X(s) + X(s+1)|^2 \tag{1.15}$$

E_{image} is the image energy and is computed as follows:

$$E_{\text{image}} = \frac{\text{min} - \text{mag}}{\text{max} - \text{min}} \tag{1.16}$$

where mag is the magnitude of each point, max, min are the maximum and minimum gradients in each neighborhood, respectively. E_{image} is negative so that points with a large gradient will have smaller energy terms.

Active contours in general suffer from the difficulty in detecting corners and concave edges, which could be improved by adjusting the curvature term E_{bend}, and its parameter σ. Despite being relatively faster than dynamic programming algorithms, greedy algorithms do not guarantee finding a global solution.

1.2.2   Guiding forces

1.2.2.1   Edge-based external force models

Edge-based force models are mainly concerned with detection of boundaries. One of the early proposed models was the distance potential force model [26]. The goal of this model was to widen the range that the deformable model is able to capture. The model is defined as

$$E_{ext}(x,y) = \frac{w\nabla d(x,y)}{\|\nabla d(x,y)\|}, \tag{1.17}$$

where w is a constant, and d is the distance between a point and the nearest edge points in the binary boundary map. The model basically replaces the external force of the deformable model in Equation 1.3 by normalized distance potential force. Although the capture range is high, this model cannot deal with topological changes and sharp corners.

The balloon model was then proposed in Cohen [27] to improve the shortcomings of the original snake model proposed by Kass et al. [11]. The model avoids the traditional snake energy functional's drawback of the sensitivity to initialization by making the curve behave like a balloon, which is inflated by an additional force. The curve also passes over weak edges and is stopped only if the edge is strong.

The external force model has a constant normal force component added to it as follows:

$$F_{ext} = w_1\bar{n}(s) - w\frac{\nabla E_{ext}}{\|E_{ext}\|}, \tag{1.18}$$

where $\bar{n}(s)$ is the normal unit vector with magnitude w_1, w is the external force weight, and the term E_{ext} is defined in Equation 1.3. The model inflates or deflates based on the initialization and the magnitude of the balloon force. The main problem associated with this model is that its performance is not strong with weak edges.

The balloon model was then modified by Chen et al. [28] in order to pull the contour to the desired boundary from both directions. An adaptive pressure force uses the balloon force as an additive one. The model is formulated as follows:

$$E_{ext} = -wF_{ext} + w_p\bar{n}(s), \tag{1.19}$$

where $\bar{n}(s)$ is the normal unit vector with magnitude k_p, k is the external force weight, and the term F_{ext} is defined in Equation 1.18. The contour is pulled at the desired boundary from both directions within a range r that is computed as follows:

$$(x_n - x)^2 + w(y_n - y)^2 \leq r^2, \qquad (1.20)$$

where (x_n, y_n) is a pixel along the normal and w provides the normal direction of the contour at the pixel (x, y).

A major advance with parametric deformable models was achieved by Chenyang et al. [14], where they introduced the so-called gradient vector flow (GVF) model. The GVF model overcame the limitations of the traditional snake model such as the capture range, sensitivity to initialization, and poor convergence in some cases.

A vector field $V(s) = [u(s), v(s)]$ replaces the external force and minimizes the following function:

$$E(V) = \iint \mu \left(u_x^2 + v_x^2 + u_y^2 + u_y^2 \right) + |\nabla f|^2 (V - \nabla f)^2 \, dx \, dy, \qquad (1.21)$$

where u_x, u_y, v_x, v_y are the field's spatial derivatives, μ is the blending parameter, and f is the edge map of the input image, having $|\nabla f|$ as its gradient. The gradient is large at the image boundaries, whereas it tends to zero at areas with constant information.

The main drawback of the GVF model was its poor performance with long and thin boundaries, which motivated the work by Chenyang et al. [29] to generalize their GVF model by replacing the blending parameter μ and the term $|\nabla f|^2$ in Equation 1.21 with varying weight functions $j(.)$ and $h(.)$. This results in the following energy function:

$$E_{GGVF}(u, v) = \iint j(|\nabla f|) \left(u_x^2 + v_x^2 + u_y^2 + u_y^2 \right) + (1 - j(|\nabla f|))(V - \nabla f)^2 \, dx \, dy, \qquad (1.22)$$

where

$$j(|\nabla f|) = \exp \left(- \left(\frac{|\nabla f|}{p} \right) \right), \qquad (1.23)$$

and

$$h(|\nabla f|) = 1 - j(|\nabla f|). \qquad (1.24)$$

The parameter p is user defined and controls the smoothness of the force field. The generalized GVF model converges to very thin boundaries. The boundary information is, however, not exploited directly in the energy function; instead, its gradient is used, which might result in having a similar effect on the flow from both strong and weak edges.

1.2.2.2   *Region-based external force models*

Region-based deformable models are mainly concerned with the image's pixels and their common characteristics. An example of region-based models is the one proposed by El-Baz et al. [30], where it is composed of a parametric deformable model controlled by shape and visual appearance priors that are learned from a training subset of coaligned images. The shape prior is derived from a linear combination of vectors of distances between the training boundaries and their common centroid. The appearance prior considers gray levels within each training boundary as a sample of a Markov–Gibbs random field with pairwise interaction. The evolution of the parametric deformable model is based on solving the Eikonal equation with a force function, which combines the prior shape, prior appearance,

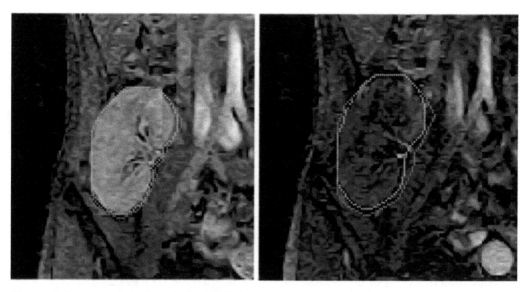

Figure 1.3 Segmentation of two kidney DCE-MR images with the stochastic parametric deformable model proposed in El-Baz and Gimel'farb [30] vs. the ground truth: the final boundaries and the ground truth are in red and green, respectively. (Image is courtesy of A. El-Baz and G. Gimel'farb, Image segmentation with a parametric deformable model using shape and appearance priors, in *IEEE Conference on Computer Vision and Pattern Recognition*, 2008, pp. 1–8.)

and current appearance models. A segmentation example using the parametric deformable model [30] is shown in Figure 1.3.

Figure 1.4 compares the deformable-model based segmentation results of a CT lung image using some of the external forces described above. The stochastic model appears to be better in terms of boundary detection.

1.2.3   Summary on parametric deformable models

To summarize, parametric deformable models achieved a major advance in image processing and its applications when they were first introduced by Kass [11], where several formulae of energy functions had been first integrated in image analysis. The main advantage of them is their fast convergence to the solution as they are mainly formed from a set of points. Parametric deformable models generally suffer from numerous issues though. The major drawbacks are as follows:

1. Models are sensitive to initialization.
2. The performance is significantly affected by the number of control points and data spacing selected.
3. The weighting coefficients that determine the contribution of each one of the energy function terms constantly need to be tuned.
4. There are many problems that arise from topology changes such as merging and splitting.
5. The propagation in one direction is usually restricted by the boundary attraction term, which either expands or shrinks the initial curve. The stopping criteria are also needed [21,31–33].

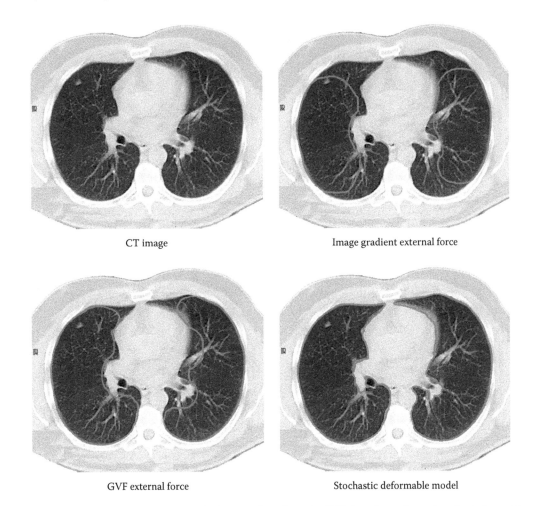

CT image   Image gradient external force

GVF external force   Stochastic deformable model

Figure 1.4   Lung segmentation with the gradient-based, GVF-based, and stochastic deformable models.

The limitations imposed by classical parametric deformable models emerged the need for a better curve representation that handles topological changes, and thus geometric deformable models were introduced.

1.3   Geometric deformable models

In geometric deformable models, the planar curve is implicitly represented by the level set of an appropriate 2D surface [12,31–36]. Due to the limitations of classical deformable models [20,32–34], the level sets were proposed by Osher and Sethian [12], where topological changes were better handled during curve evolution without the need for parameterization (Figure 1.5).

Before deriving the level sets equation, some concepts need to be highlighted.

Level set is a set of points that represents an isocontour of a function mathematically in $\mathbb{R}^n$ space:

$$L(\varphi) = \{(x_1, x_2, \ldots, x_n) \mid f(x_1, \ldots, x_n) = 0\}$$

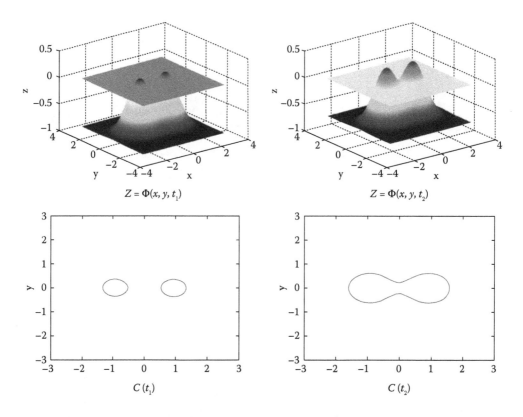

Figure 1.5 Illustration of contour deformation with time using the level set method.

Principal curvatures are the maximum and minimum normal curvatures k_1, k_2 given at any surface point that measure the amount of surface bending at this point [37].

The Gaussian curvature is defined as: $K = k_1 k_2$, while the mean curvature is defined as: $H = 1/2(k_1 + k_2)$. Both can be used to compute both k_1 and k_2, where

$$k_1 = H + \sqrt{H^2 - k},\tag{1.25}$$

and

$$k_2 = H - \sqrt{H^2 - k}.\tag{1.26}$$

Geodesic curvature is another form of curve representation. Given a parametric curve $\mathbf{C(S)}$ embedded into the surface $\mathbf{S}$, this curve will have the following acceleration vector:

$$C_{ss} = k_g \hat{T} + k_n \hat{N}.\tag{1.27}$$

This means that the acceleration vector is represented in terms of the unit normal vector $\hat{N}$ and the unit tangent vector $\hat{T}$, which lie in the same plane with C_{ss} and the surface normal. Geodesics are planar curves with acceleration only in the normal direction, that is, $k_g = 0$ [38].

Level set methods (LSM) are a conceptual framework for using level sets as a tool for numerical analysis of surfaces and shapes. The advantage of the level set model is that one can perform numerical computations involving curves and surfaces on a fixed Cartesian grid without having to parameterize these objects. Also, the level set method makes it very easy to follow shapes that change topology. For example, when a shape splits in two, it develops holes (Figure 1.5) or vice versa. This makes the level set method a powerful tool for modeling time-varying objects. In some image processing applications, the need to manipulate a specific shape inside an image requires deformation of curves. In two dimensions, the level set method amounts to representing a closed curve $\partial\Omega$ using an auxiliary function, φ, called the level set function $\partial\Omega$ is represented as the zero level set of φ by

$$\partial\Omega = \{(x,y) \mid \varphi(x,y) = 0\}, \tag{1.28}$$

and the level set method manipulates $\partial\Omega$ implicitly through the function φ. Level set methods add dynamics to implicit surfaces. The key idea started from the Lagrangian formulation of the interface evolution. Assume a point $\vec{x}$ moves with $\varphi(\vec{x}) = 0$ given the velocity field $\vec{V}(\vec{x})$, then we need to solve the differential equation:

$$\frac{d\vec{x}}{dt} = \vec{V}(\vec{x}) \tag{1.29}$$

The use of the Lagrangian formulation of the interface motion given in the last equation along with numerical techniques for smoothing and regularization are collectively referred to as front tracking methods [39]. In order to avoid problems with instabilities and complicated surgical procedures for topological repair, Osher and Sethian [12] formulate the interface evolution implicitly (from implicit function φ) using the simple convection equation (which defines the evolution of the implicit function φ):

$$\varphi_t + \vec{V} \cdot \nabla\varphi = 0 \tag{1.30}$$

This partial differential equation defines the motion of the interface where $\varphi(\vec{x}) = 0$. The interface here is captured by the implicit function φ as opposed to being tracked by interface elements as was done in the Lagrangian formulation. This last equation is referred to as the level set equation.

Consider the following form for curve propagation:

$$C(p,t) = F(K)\hat{N}, \tag{1.31}$$

where $p = (x,y)$. The level set function represents the curve in the form of an implicit surface as follows:

$$\varphi(x,y,t): \mathcal{R}^2 \times [0,T) \to \mathcal{R}, \tag{1.32}$$

that is derived from the initial contour according to the following condition:

$$C(p,0) = \{(x,y): \varphi(x,y,0) = 0\}. \tag{1.33}$$

Taking the derivative with respect to time:

$$\varphi(C(p,t),t) = 0 \Rightarrow \frac{\partial\varphi}{\partial C} \cdot \frac{\partial C}{\partial t} + \frac{\partial\varphi}{\partial t} = 0. \tag{1.34}$$

The level set function has the following relation with the embedded curve:

$$\varphi(C) = 0 \quad \text{or} \quad C = \varphi^{-1}(0).$$ (1.35)

The curve $\varphi(x, y, t) = 0$ deforms with time, Figure 1.5. Thus, the level set function changes with time as follows:

$$\frac{\partial \varphi}{\partial t} dt + \frac{\partial \varphi}{\partial x} dx + \frac{\partial \varphi}{\partial y} dy = 0.$$ (1.36)

$$\frac{\partial \varphi}{\partial t} + \left(\frac{\partial \varphi}{\partial x}, \frac{\partial \varphi}{\partial y} \right) \cdot \left(\frac{dx}{dt}, \frac{dy}{dt} \right) = 0.$$ (1.37)

This leads to the fundamental level set equation:

$$\frac{\partial \varphi}{\partial t} + \nabla \varphi \cdot \vec{V} = 0.$$ (1.38)

Further analysis may be done to obtain:

$$\frac{\partial \varphi}{\partial t} + |\nabla \varphi| \frac{\nabla \varphi}{|\nabla \varphi|} \cdot \vec{V} = 0.$$ (1.39)

$$\frac{\partial \varphi}{\partial t} + |\nabla \varphi| F = 0.$$ (1.40)

The velocity vector $\vec{V}$ has a component F in the normal direction, whereas the other tangential component has no effect because the gradient works only in the normal direction.

F is called the speed function, and has several forms. One widely used form of F is:

$$F = \pm 1 + \varepsilon K,$$ (1.41)

where the $+$ sign is for expansion and the $-$ sign is for contraction. The coefficient K forces the contour to evolve smoothly, and the bending is controlled by ε [40]. The next two sections address the numerical schemes in detail as well as some of the most popular speed functions proposed in literature.

There are plenty of numerical schemes that can be used for solving the level set equation. The numerical solution of the level set equation, however, requires sophisticated techniques. Simple finite difference methods fail quickly. Upwinding methods, such as the Godunov method, fare better; yet the level set method does not guarantee the conservation of the volume or the shape of the level set in an advection field that does conserve the shape and size, for example, uniform or rotational velocity field. Instead, the shape of the level set may get severely distorted and it may vanish over several time steps. For this reason, high-order finite difference schemes are generally required, such as high-order essentially nonoscillatory (ENO) schemes.

1.3.1   *Numerical approaches solving the level set equation*

As was previously mentioned, the level set equation is:

$$\varphi_t + \vec{V} \cdot \nabla \varphi = 0$$ (1.42)

Once φ and $\vec{V}$ are defined at every grid point (or at least sufficiently close to the interface) on our Cartesian grid, we can apply numerical methods to evolve φ forward in time moving the interface across the grid. At some point in time, say time t^n, let $\varphi^n = \varphi(t^n)$ represent the current values of φ. Updating φ in time consists of finding new values of φ at every grid point after some time increment Δt. We denote these new values of φ by $\varphi^{n+1} = \varphi(t^{n+1})$, where $t^{n+1} = t^n + \Delta t$. Then the time discretization of the above level set equation will be

$$\frac{\varphi^{n+1} - \varphi^n}{\Delta t} + \vec{V}^n \cdot \nabla \varphi^n = 0 \qquad (1.43)$$

where $\vec{V}^n = \langle u^n, v^n, w^n \rangle$ is the given external velocity field at time t^n, and $\nabla \varphi^n$ evaluates the gradient operator using the values of φ at time t^n. One might evaluate the spatial derivatives of φ in a straightforward manner using first-order finite difference formulas. Unfortunately, this straightforward approach will fail [41]. One generally needs to exercise great care when numerically discretizing partial differential equations. We begin by writing this equation in expanded form as

$$\frac{\varphi^{n+1} - \varphi^n}{\Delta t} + (u^n \varphi_x^n + v^n \varphi_y^n + w^n \varphi_z^n) = 0 \qquad (1.44)$$

The techniques used to approximate the term $u^n \varphi_x^n$ can then be applied independently to the $v^n \varphi_y^n$ and $w^n \varphi_z^n$ terms in a dimension-by-dimension manner. For simplicity, consider the one-dimensional ($x, y,$ or z-direction) version of the last equation to be

$$\frac{\varphi^{n+1} - \varphi^n}{\Delta t} + u^n \varphi_x^n = 0, \quad \frac{\varphi^{n+1} - \varphi^n}{\Delta t} + v^n \varphi_y^n = 0 \quad \text{or} \quad \frac{\varphi^{n+1} - \varphi^n}{\Delta t} + w^n \varphi_z^n = 0$$

where the sign of u^n indicates whether the surface point of interest is moving to the right or to the left. Similarly, the sign of v^n and w^n indicate forward or backward and up or down, respectively.

For simplicity in writing, $D^- \varphi$ and $D^+ \varphi$ are used to denote first-order backward and forward differences, respectively as follows: the same abbreviation may be used for y and z dimensions)

$$D^- \varphi = \frac{\partial \varphi}{\partial x} \approx \frac{\varphi_i - \varphi_{i-1}}{\Delta x} \quad \text{and} \quad D^+ \varphi = \frac{\partial \varphi}{\partial x} \approx \frac{\varphi_{i+1} - \varphi_i}{\Delta x} \qquad (1.45)$$

1.3.1.1 Upwind differencing
Considering a specific grid point x_i, then we write the one-dimensional version to be

$$\frac{\varphi_i^{n+1} - \varphi_i^n}{\Delta t} + u_i^n (\varphi_i)_x^n = 0, \qquad (1.46)$$

If $u_i > 0$, the values of φ are moving from left to right, and the method of characteristics tells us to look to the left of x_i to determine what value of φ will land on the point x_i at the end of a time step. Similarly, if $u_i < 0$, the values of φ are moving from right to left, and the method of characteristics implies that we should look to the right to determine an appropriate value of φ_i at time t^{n+1}. Clearly, $D^- \varphi$ from Equation 1.45 should be used to approximate φ when $u_i > 0$. Because $D^+ \varphi$ from Equation 1.45 cannot possibly give a good approximation, since it fails to contain the information to the left of x_i that dictates the new value of φ_i. Similar reasoning indicates $D^+\varphi$ should be used to approximate φ_x when $u_i < 0$. The numerical explicit solution to the one-dimensional version can be rewritten as:

$$\varphi_i^{n+1} = \varphi_i^n - \Delta t \left[\max(0, u_i^n)D^-\varphi_i^n + \min(0, u_i^n)D^+\varphi_i^n\right], \tag{1.47}$$

We summarize the upwind discretization as follows. At each grid point, If $u_i > 0$, approximate φ_x with $D^-\varphi$. If $u_i < 0$, approximate φ_x with $D^+\varphi$. When $u_i = 0$, the $u_i(\varphi_x)_i$ term vanishes, and φ_x does not need to be approximated. This is a first-order accurate discretization of the spatial operator, since $D^-\varphi$ and $D^+\varphi$ are first-order accurate approximations of the derivative; that is, the errors are of order $O(\Delta x)$. The combination of the forward Euler time discretization with the upwind difference scheme is a consistent finite difference approximation to the partial differential equation, since the approximation error converges to zero as $\Delta t \to 0$ and $\Delta x \to 0$. According to the Lax–Richtmyer equivalence theorem a finite difference approximation to a linear partial differential equation is convergent (i.e., the correct solution is obtained) as $\Delta t \to 0$ and $\Delta x \to 0$, if and only if it is both consistent and stable. Stability guarantees that small errors in the approximation are not amplified as the solution is marched forward in time. Stability can be enforced using the Courant–Friedreichs–Lewy (CFL) condition, which asserts that the numerical waves should propagate at least as fast as the physical waves. This means that the numerical wave speed of $\Delta x/\Delta t$ must be at least as fast as the physical wave speed $|u|$. This leads us to the CFL time step restriction of

$$\Delta t < \frac{\Delta x}{\max\{|u|\}}, \tag{1.48}$$

where $\max\{|u|\}$ is chosen to be the largest value of $|u|$ over the entire Cartesian grid. In reality, we only need to choose the largest value of $|u|$ on the interface. This condition is usually enforced by choosing a **CFL** number α, [42] as

$$\Delta t \left(\frac{\max\{|u|\}}{\Delta x}\right) = \alpha \tag{1.49}$$

And $0 < \alpha < 1$. A multidimensional CFL condition can be written as

$$\Delta t \max \left\{\frac{|u|}{\Delta x} + \frac{|v|}{\Delta y} + \frac{|w|}{\Delta z}\right\} = \alpha \quad \text{or} \quad \Delta t \left(\frac{\max\{|\vec{V}|\}}{\min\{\Delta x, \Delta y, \Delta z\}}\right) = \alpha \tag{1.50}$$

Numerical Solution to the Higher-Order Scheme: The numerical solution of the level set equation:

$$\varphi_t + |\nabla\varphi|F = 0$$

can be obtained similar to above, and is as follows:

$$\left(\varphi_{ij}^{n+1}\right) = \left(\varphi_{ij}^n\right) - \Delta t(\nabla^+\nabla^-)\binom{\max(F_{i,j}, 0)}{\min(F_{i,j}, 0)}, \tag{1.51}$$

where

$$\nabla^+ = [\max(A,0)^2 + \min(B,0)^2 + \max(C,0)^2 + \min(D,0)^2]^{0.5}$$

$$\nabla^- = [\min(A,0)^2 + \max(B,0)^2 + \min(C,0)^2 + \max(D,0)^2]^{0.5}$$

$$A = D_{ij}^{-x}\varphi + \frac{\Delta x}{2}m(D_{ij}^{-x-x}\varphi, D_{ij}^{+x-x}\varphi)$$

$$B = D_{ij}^{+x}\varphi - \frac{\Delta x}{2}m(D_{ij}^{+x+x}\varphi, D_{ij}^{+x-x}\varphi)$$

$$C = D_{ij}^{-y}\varphi + \frac{\Delta y}{2}m(D_{ij}^{-y-y}\varphi, D_{ij}^{+y-y}\varphi)$$

$$D = D_{ij}^{+y}\varphi - \frac{\Delta y}{2}m(D_{ij}^{+y+y}\varphi, D_{ij}^{+y-y}\varphi)$$

where the speed function is given by

$$F_{i,j} = \upsilon + \varepsilon K_{ij}, \tag{1.52}$$

and the switching function m is given by:

$$m(a,b) = \begin{cases} aH_\alpha(a,b) & \text{if } |a| \leq |b| \\ bH_\alpha(a,b) & \text{if } |a| > |b| \end{cases}, \tag{1.53}$$

where $H_\alpha(\varphi)$ is the Heaviside function and is defined as:

$$H_\alpha(\varphi) = \begin{cases} 0.5\left(1 + \dfrac{\varphi}{\alpha} + \dfrac{1}{\pi}\sin\left(\dfrac{\pi\varphi}{\alpha}\right)\right), & |\varphi| \leq \alpha \\ 1, & |\varphi| > \alpha \end{cases} \tag{1.54}$$

Instead of upwinding, the spatial derivatives in Equation 1.16 could be approximated with the more accurate central differencing. Unfortunately, simple central differencing is unstable with forward Euler time discretization and the usual **CFL** conditions with $\Delta t \sim \Delta x$. Stability can be achieved by using a much more restrictive **CFL** condition with $\Delta t \sim (\Delta x)^2$, although this is too computationally costly. Stability can also be achieved by using a different temporal discretization, for example, the third-order accurate Runge–Kutta method (discussed later). A third way of achieving stability consists in adding some artificial dissipation to the right-hand side of Equation 1.16 to obtain

$$\varphi_t + \vec{V} \cdot \nabla\varphi = \mu\Delta\varphi \tag{1.55}$$

where the viscosity coefficient μ is chosen proportional to Δx, that is, $\mu \sim \Delta x$, so that the artificial viscosity vanishes as $\Delta x \to 0$, enforcing consistency for this method. While all three of these approaches stabilize central differencing, we instead prefer to use upwind methods, which draw on the highly successful technology developed for the numerical solution of conservation laws.

1.3.1.2   Hamilton–Jacobi

The first-order accurate upwind scheme described in the last section can be improved upon by using a more accurate approximation for φ_x^- and φ_x^+. The velocity u is still used to decide whether φ_x^- or φ_x^+ is used, but the approximations for φ_x^- or φ_x^+ can be improved significantly. Harten et al. [43] introduced the idea of essentially nonoscillatory (ENO) polynomial interpolation of data for the numerical solution of conservation laws. Their basic idea was to compute numerical flux functions using the smoothest possible polynomial interpolants. The actual numerical implementation of this idea was improved considerably by Shu and Osher [44], where the numerical flux functions were constructed directly from a divided difference table of the pointwise data. Osher and Sethian realized that Hamilton–Jacobi equations in one spatial dimension are integrals of conservation laws. They used this fact to extend the ENO method for the numerical discretization of conservation laws to Hamilton–Jacobi equations such as Equation 1.16. This Hamilton–Jacobi with the idea of essentially nonoscillatory (HJ ENO) method allows to extend first-order accurate upwind differencing to higher-order spatial accuracy by providing better numerical approximations to φ_x^- or φ_x^+.

We summarize the idea of (HJ ENO) method as follows. We use the smoothest possible polynomial interpolation (with Newton polynomial interpolation [45]) to find φ and then differentiate to get φ_x. Define $D_i^0 \varphi = \varphi_i$ at each grid node located at x_i. The first divided differences of φ are defined midway between grid nodes as

$$D_{i+1/2}^1 \varphi = \frac{D_{i+1}^0 \varphi - D_i^0 \varphi}{\Delta x} \tag{1.56}$$

Assuming that the mesh spacing uniformly equals Δx. Note that $D_{i+1/2}^1 \varphi = (D^+ \varphi)_i$ and $D_{i-1/2}^1 \varphi = (D^- \varphi)_i$, that is, the first divided differences are the forward and backward difference approximations to the derivatives. The second divided differences are defined at the grid nodes as

$$D_i^2 \varphi = \frac{D_{i+1/2}^1 \varphi - D_{i-1/2}^1 \varphi}{2\Delta x} \tag{1.57}$$

while the third divided differences

$$D_{i+1/2}^3 \varphi = \frac{D_{i+1}^2 \varphi - D_i^2 \varphi}{3\Delta x} \tag{1.58}$$

The divided differences are used to reconstruct a polynomial of the form

$$\varphi(x) = Q_0(x) + Q_1(x) + Q_2(x) + Q_3(x) \tag{1.59}$$

that can be differentiated and evaluated at x_i to find $\left(\varphi_x^+\right)_i$ and $\left(\varphi_x^-\right)_i$. That is,

$$\varphi_x(x_i) = Q_1'(x_i) + Q_2'(x_i) + Q_3'(x_i) \tag{1.60}$$

Note that the constant $Q_0(x)$ vanishes upon differentiation. And to find φ_x^+ we define

$$Q_1(x) = (D_{i+1/2}^1 \varphi)(x - x_i) \quad \text{so that} \quad Q_1'(x_i) = D_{i+1/2}^1 \varphi \tag{1.61}$$

And to define φ_x^-, then we define $Q_1(x) = (D_{i-1/2}^1\varphi)(x - x_{i-1})$ so $Q_1'(x_i) = D_{i-1/2}^1\varphi$. Implying that the contribution from the first-order accurate polynomial interpolation $Q_1'(x_i)$ is exactly first-order upwinding. Improvements are obtained by including the $Q_2'(x_i)$ and $Q_3'(x_i)$ terms, leading to second- and third-order accuracy, respectively.

Looking at the divided difference table, let $j = i$ for φ_x^+ and $j = i - 1$ for φ_x^-. Then we have two choices for the second-order accurate correction. We could include the next point to the left and use $D_j^2\varphi$, or we could include the next point to the right and use $D_{j+1}^2\varphi$. The key observation is that smooth slowly varying data tend to produce small numbers in divided difference tables, while discontinuous or quickly varying data tend to produce large numbers in divided difference tables. This is obvious in the sense that the differences measure variation in the data. Comparing $|D_j^2\varphi|$ to $|D_{j+1}^2\varphi|$ indicates which of the polynomial interpolants has more variation. We would like to avoid interpolating near large variations such as discontinuities or steep gradients, since they cause overshoots in the interpolating function, leading to numerical errors in the approximation of the derivative. Thus, if $|D_j^2\varphi| \leq |D_{j+1}^2\varphi|$, we set $c = D_j^2\varphi$; otherwise, we set $c = D_{j+1}^2\varphi$. Then we define

$$Q_2(x) = c(x - x_j)(x - x_{j+1}) \tag{1.62}$$

So that

$$Q_2'(x_i) = c(2(i - j) - 1)\Delta x$$

Is the second-order accurate correction to the approximation of φ_x in equation (level set). If we stop here, that is, omitting the Q_3 term, we have a second-order accurate method for approximating φ_x^+ and φ_x^-. Similar to the second-order accurate correction, the third-order accurate correction is obtained by comparing $|D_{k+1/2}^3\varphi|$ to $|D_{k+3/2}^3\varphi|$. If $|D_{k+1/2}^3\varphi| \leq |D_{k+3/2}^3\varphi|$, we set $\hat{c} = D_{k+1/2}^3\varphi$; otherwise, we set $\hat{c} = D_{k+3/2}^3\varphi$. Then we define

$$Q_3(x) = \hat{c}(x - x_k)(x - x_{k+1})(x - x_{k+2}) \tag{1.63}$$

So that

$$Q_3'(x_i) = \hat{c}(3(i - k)^2 - 6(i = k) + 2)(\Delta x)^2$$

is the third-order accurate correction to the approximation of φ_x in Equation 1.16.

1.3.1.3 Hamilton–Jacobi WENO

When calculating $(\varphi_x^-)_i$ or $(\varphi_x^+)_i$, the third-order accurate HJ ENO scheme uses a subset of $\{\varphi_{i-3}, \varphi_{i-2}, \varphi_{i-1}, \varphi_i, \varphi_{i+1}, \varphi_{i+2}\}$ or $\{\varphi_{i-2}, \varphi_{i-1}, \varphi_i, \varphi_{i+1}, \varphi_{i+2}, \varphi_{i+3}\}$ respectively. In fact, there are exactly three possible HJ ENO approximations to $(\varphi_x^-)_i$. Defining $v_1 = D^-\varphi_{i-2}$, $v_2 = D^-\varphi_{i-1}$, $v_3 = D^-\varphi_i$, $v_4 = D^-\varphi_{i+1}$ and $v_5 = D^-\varphi_{i+2}$ allows us to write

$$\varphi_x^1 = \frac{v_1}{3} - \frac{7v_2}{6} + \frac{11v_3}{6} \tag{1.64}$$

$$\varphi_x^2 = -\frac{v_2}{6} + \frac{5v_3}{6} + \frac{v_4}{3}$$

and

$$\varphi_x^3 = \frac{v_3}{3} + \frac{5v_4}{6} - \frac{v_5}{6}$$

as the three potential HJ ENO approximations to φ_x^-. The goal of HJ ENO is to choose the single approximation with the least error by choosing the smoothest possible polynomial interpolation of φ.

Liu et al. [46] pointed out that the ENO philosophy of picking exactly one of three candidate stencils is overkill in smooth regions where the data are well behaved. They proposed a weighted ENO (WENO) method, which takes a convex combination of the three ENO approximations. All three approximations are allowed to make a significant contribution in a way that improves the local accuracy from third order to fourth order. Of course, if any of the three approximations interpolates across a discontinuity, it is given minimal weight in the convex combination in order to minimize its contribution and the resulting errors. Later, following the work on HJ ENO by Osher and Shu [47], Jiang and Peng extended WENO to the Hamilton–Jacobi framework. This Hamilton–Jacobi WENO, or HJ WENO, scheme turns out to be very useful for solving Equation 1.42, since it reduces the errors by more than an order of magnitude over the third-order accurate HJ ENO scheme for typical applications.

The HJ WENO approximation of $(\varphi_x^-)_i$ is a convex combination of the three approximations in Equation 1.64 given by

$$\varphi_x = \omega_1 \varphi_x^1 + \omega_2 \varphi_x^2 + \omega_3 \varphi_x^3 \tag{1.65}$$

where the $0 \le \omega_k \le 1$ are the weights with $\omega_1 + \omega_2 + \omega_3 = 1$. The key observation for obtaining high-order accuracy in smooth regions is that weights of $\omega_1 = 0.1$, $\omega_2 = 0.6$ and $\omega_3 = 0.3$ give the optimal fifth-order accurate approximation to φ_x. While this is the optimal approximation, it is valid only in smooth regions. In nonsmooth regions, this optimal weighting can be very inaccurate, and we are better off with digital ($\omega_k = 0$ or $\omega_k = 1$) weights that choose a single approximation to φ_x, that is, the HJ ENO approximation.

In Jiang and Shu [48], it was pointed out that setting $\omega_1 = 0.1 + O((\Delta x)^2)$, $\omega_2 = 0.6 + O((\Delta x)^2)$, and $\omega_3 = 0.3 + O((\Delta x)^2)$ still gives the optimal fifth-order accuracy in smooth regions. In order to see this, we rewrite these as $\omega_1 = 0.1 + C_1(\Delta x)^2$, $\omega_2 = 0.6 + C_2(\Delta x)^2$, and $\omega_3 = 0.3 + C_3(\Delta x)^2$, and plug them into Equation 1.65 to obtain

$$0.1\varphi_x^1 + 0.6\varphi_x^2 + 0.3\varphi_x^3 \tag{1.66}$$

and

$$C_1(\Delta x)^2 \varphi_x^1 + C_2(\Delta x)^2 \varphi_x^2 + C_3(\Delta x)^2 \varphi_x^3 \tag{1.67}$$

as the two terms that are added to give the HJ WENO approximation to φ_x. The term given by Equation 1.66 is the optimal approximation that gives the exact value of φ_x plus an $O((\Delta x)^5)$ error term. Thus, if the term given by Equation 1.67 is $O((\Delta x)^5)$, then the entire HJ WENO approximation is $O((\Delta x)^5)$ in smooth regions. To see that, first note that each of the HJ ENO φ_x^k approximations gives the exact value of φ_x, denoted by φ_x^E, plus an $O((\Delta x)^3)$ error term (in smooth regions). Thus, the term in Equation 1.67 is

$$C_1(\Delta x)^2 \varphi_x^E + C_2(\Delta x)^2 \varphi_x^E + C_3(\Delta x)^2 \varphi_x^E \tag{1.68}$$

Plus, an $O((\Delta x)^2)O((\Delta x)^3) = O((\Delta x)^5)$ term. Since, each of the C_k is $O(1)$, as is φ_x^E, this appears to be an $O((\Delta x)^2)$ term at first glance. However, since $\omega_1 + \omega_2 + \omega_3 = 1$, we have $C_1 + C_2 + C_3 = 0$, implying that the term in Equation 1.68 is identically zero. Thus, the HJ

WENO approximation is $O((\Delta x)^5)$ in smooth regions. Note that Liu et al. [46] obtained only fourth-order accuracy, since they chose $w_1 = 0.1 + O(\Delta x)$, $w_2 = 0.6 + O(\Delta x)$, and $w_3 = 0.3 + O(\Delta x)$.

In order to define the weights w_k, we follow Jiang and Peng [49] and estimate the smoothness of the three stencils in Equation 1.64 as

$$S_1 = \frac{13}{12}(v_1 - 2v_2 + v_3)^2 + \frac{1}{4}(v_1 - 4v_2 + 3v_3)^2$$

$$S_2 = \frac{13}{12}(v_2 - 2v_3 + v_4)^2 + \frac{1}{4}(v_2 - v_4)^2 \quad (1.69)$$

$$S_3 = \frac{13}{12}(v_3 - 2v_3 + v_4)^2 + \frac{1}{4}(3v_1 - 4v_4 + v_5)^2,$$

respectively. Using these smoothness estimates, we define

$$\alpha_1 = \frac{0.1}{(S_1 + \epsilon)^2} \quad \alpha_2 = \frac{0.6}{(S_2 + \epsilon)^2} \quad \alpha_3 = \frac{0.3}{(S_3 + \epsilon)^2}, \quad (1.70)$$

with

$$\epsilon = 10^{-6} \max \left\{ v_1^2, v_2^2, v_3^2, v_4^2, v_5^2 \right\} + 10^{-99}, \quad (1.71)$$

where the 10^{-99} term is set to avoid division by zero in the definition of the α_k. This value for epsilon was first proposed by Fedkiw et al. [50], where the first term is a scaling term that aids in the balance between the optimal fifth-order accurate stencil and the digital HJ ENO weights. In the case that φ is an approximate signed distance function, the v_k that approximate φ_x are approximately equal to one, so that the first term in Equation 1.71 can be set to 10^{-6}. This first term can then absorb the second term, yielding $\epsilon = 10^{-6}$ in place of Equation 1.71 to make this $v_k \approx 1$ estimate in higher dimensions as well.

A smooth solution has small variation leading to small S_k. If they are small enough compared to ϵ, then $\alpha_1 \approx 0.1\epsilon^{-2}$, $\alpha_2 \approx 0.6\epsilon^{-2}$, and $\alpha_3 \approx 0.3\epsilon^{-2}$, exhibiting the proper ratios for the optimal fifth-order accuracy. That is, normalizing the α_k to obtain the weights

$$w_1 = \frac{\alpha_1}{\alpha_1 + \alpha_2 + \alpha_3} \quad w_2 = \frac{\alpha_2}{\alpha_1 + \alpha_2 + \alpha_3} \quad w_3 = \frac{\alpha_3}{\alpha_1 + \alpha_2 + \alpha_3}, \quad (1.72)$$

gives (approximately) the optimal weights of $w_1 = 0.1$, $w_2 = 0.6$, and $w_3 = 0.3$. Nearly optimal weights are also obtained when the S_k are larger than ϵ, as long as all the S_k are approximately the same size, as is the case for sufficiently smooth data. On the other hand, if the data are not smooth as indicated by large S_k, then the corresponding α_k will be small compared to the other α_k's. If two of the S_k are relatively large, then their corresponding α_k's will both be small, and the scheme will rely most heavily on a single stencil similar to the digital behavior of HJ ENO. In the unfortunate instance that all three of the S_k's are large, the data are poorly conditioned, and none of the stencils are particularly useful. This case is problematic for the HJ ENO method as well, but fortunately it usually occurs only locally in space and time, allowing the methods to repair themselves after the situation subsides.

The function $(\varphi_x^+)_i$ is constructed with a subset $\{\varphi_{i-2}, \varphi_{i-1}, \varphi_i, \varphi_{i+1}, \varphi_{i+2}, \varphi_{i+3}\}$. Defining $v_1 = D^+\varphi_{i+2}$, $v_2 = D^+\varphi_{i+1}$, $v_3 = D^+\varphi_i$, and $v_4 = D^+\varphi_{i-1}$ and $v_5 = D^+\varphi_{i-2}$ allows us to use Equations 1.64 as the three HJ ENO approximations to $(\varphi_x^+)_i$. Then the HJ WENO convex combination is given by Equation 1.65 with the weights given by Equation 1.72.

1.3.1.4   TVD Runge–Kutta

Practical experience suggests that level set methods are sensitive to spatial accuracy, implying that the fifth-order accurate HJ WENO method is desirable. On the other hand, temporal truncation errors seem to produce significantly less deterioration of the numerical solution, so one can often use the low-order accurate forward Euler method for discretization in time. There are times when a higher-order temporal discretization is necessary in order to obtain accurate numerical solutions. Shu and Osher [44] proposed total variation diminishing (TVD) Runge–Kutta (RK) methods to increase the accuracy to temporal discretization. The approach assumes that the spatial discretization can be separated from the temporal discretization in a manner that allows the temporal discretization of the PDE to be treated independently as an ODE. While there are numerous RK schemes, these TVD RK schemes guarantee that no spurious oscillations are produced as a consequence of the higher-order accurate temporal discretization. The basic first-order accurate TVD RK scheme is just the forward Euler method. We assume that the forward Euler method is TVD in conjunction with the spatial discretization of the PDE. Then higher-order accurate methods are obtained by sequentially taking Euler steps and combining the results with the initial data using a convex combination. The second-order accurate TVD RK scheme is identical to the standard second-order accurate RK scheme. It is also known as the midpoint rule, as the modified Euler method, and as Heun's predictor-corrector method.

First, a Euler step is taken to advance the solution to time $t^n + \Delta t$,

$$\frac{\varphi^{n+1} - \varphi^n}{\Delta t} + \vec{V}^n \cdot \nabla \varphi^n = 0 \tag{1.73}$$

followed by a second Euler step to advance the solution to time $t^n + 2\Delta t$

$$\frac{\varphi^{n+2} - \varphi^{n+1}}{\Delta t} + \vec{V}^{n+1} \cdot \nabla \varphi^{n+1} = 0, \tag{1.74}$$

followed by an averaging step

$$\varphi^{n+1} = \frac{\varphi^n + \varphi^{n+2}}{2}. \tag{1.75}$$

The final averaging step produces the second-order accurate TVD (for HJ ENO and HJ WENO) approximation to φ at time $t^n + \Delta t$. The third-order accurate TVD RK scheme proposed by Hu and Shu [51] is as follows. First, a Euler step is taken to advance the solution to time $t^n + \Delta t$ in Equations 1.73 and 1.74, followed by an averaging step

$$\varphi^{n+1/2} = \frac{3\varphi^n + \varphi^{n+2}}{4}, \tag{1.76}$$

which produces an approximation to φ at time $t^n + 1/2\Delta t$, then another Euler step is taken to advance the solution to time $t^n + 3/2\Delta t$

$$\frac{\varphi^{n+3/2} - \varphi^{n+1/2}}{\Delta t} + \vec{V}^{n+1/2} \cdot \nabla \varphi^{n+1/2} = 0, \tag{1.77}$$

followed by a second averaging step

$$\varphi^{n+1} = \frac{\varphi^n + 2\varphi^{n+3/2}}{3}. \tag{1.78}$$

which produces a third-order accurate approximation to φ at time $t^n + \Delta t$. This third-order accurate TVD RK method has a stability region that includes part of the imaginary axis. Thus, a stable (although ill-advised) numerical method results from combining third-order accurate TVD RK with central differencing for the spatial discretization. While fourth-order accurate (and higher) TVD RK schemes exist, this improved temporal accuracy does not seem to make a significant difference in practical calculations. Also, the fourth-order accurate (and higher) TVD RK methods require both upwind and downwind differencing approximations, doubling the computational cost of evaluating the spatial operators. See Shu and Osher [44] for fourth- and fifth-order accurate TVD RK schemes. Finally, we note that a rather interesting approach to TVD RK schemes has recently been carried out by Spiteri and Ruuth [52], who proposed increasing the number of internal stages so that this number exceeds the order of the method.

The next section addresses the Hamilton–Jacobi equations, from which the basic level set equation was derived. Numerical solutions to the general form of the Hamilton–Jacobi equations are sought.

1.3.2   Hamilton–Jacobi equations

The level set representation in Equation 1.16 is a simple instance of the general form of the Hamilton–Jacobi equations [41], with numerous numerical methods proposed in literature for solution. Some of these numerical schemes include Lax–Friedrichs scheme [53], the Roe–Fix scheme [54], and Godunov's scheme [55].

Consider the general form of Hamilton–Jacobi equations of the form

$$\varphi_t + H(\nabla\varphi) = 0, \tag{1.79}$$

where H can be a function of both space and time. In three spatial dimensions, we can write

$$\varphi_t + H(\varphi_x, \varphi_y, \varphi_z) = 0$$

as an expanded version of Equation 1.79. Convection in an externally generated velocity field Equation 1.42 is an example of a Hamilton–Jacobi equation where $H(\nabla\varphi) = \vec{V} \cdot \nabla\varphi$. Hamilton–Jacobi equations depend on (at most) the first derivatives of φ, and these equations are hyperbolic.

From first glance Equation 1.79 looks different, however in the next paragraph it will be shown that it is a general form to the convection laws.

Consider the one-dimensional scalar conservation law

$$u_t + F(u)_x = 0; \tag{1.80}$$

where u is the conserved quantity and $F(u)$ is the flux function. A well-known conservation law is the continuity equation for conservation of mass

$$\rho_t + (\rho u)_x = 0 \tag{1.81}$$

where ρ is the density of the material. The continuity equation is combined with equations for conservation of momentum and conservation of energy to obtain the compressible Navier–Stokes equations. When viscous effects are ignored, the Navier–Stokes equations reduce to the compressible inviscid Euler equations. The presence of discontinuities in the Euler equations forces one to consider weak solutions where the derivatives of solution variables can fail to exist. Examples include linear contact discontinuities and nonlinear shock waves. The nonlinear nature of shock waves allows them to develop as the solution progresses forward in time even if the data are initially smooth. The Euler equations may not always have unique solutions, and an entropy condition is used to pick out the physically correct solution.

1.3.2.1 Burgers' equation

$$u_t + \left(\frac{u^2}{2}\right)_x = 0 \qquad (1.82)$$

Is a scalar conservation law that possesses many of the interesting nonlinear properties contained in the more complex Euler equations. It develops discontinuous shock waves from smooth initial data. Many of the numerical methods developed to solve Burgers' equation can be extended to treat both the one-dimensional and the multidimensional Euler equations of gas dynamics.

Consider the one-dimensional Hamilton–Jacobi equation

$$\varphi_t + H(\varphi_x) = 0, \qquad (1.83)$$

which becomes

$$(\varphi_x)_t + H(\varphi_x)_x = 0 \qquad (1.84)$$

after one takes a spatial derivative of the entire equation. Setting $u = \varphi_x$ results in

$$u_t + H(u)_x = 0 \qquad (1.85)$$

which is a scalar conservation law; thus, in one spatial dimension we can draw a direct correspondence between Hamilton–Jacobi equations and conservation laws. The solution u to a conservation law is the derivative of a solution φ to a Hamilton–Jacobi equation. Conversely, the solution φ to a Hamilton–Jacobi equation is the integral of a solution u to a conservation law. This allows us to point out a number of useful facts. For example, since the integral of a discontinuity is a kink, or discontinuity in the first derivative, solutions to Hamilton–Jacobi equations can develop kinks in the solution even if the data are initially smooth. In addition, solutions to Hamilton–Jacobi equations cannot generally develop a discontinuity unless the corresponding conservation law develops a delta function. Thus, solutions φ to Equation 1.79 are typically continuous [41]. Furthermore, since conservation laws can have nonunique solutions, entropy conditions are needed to pick out "physically" relevant solutions to Equation 1.79 as well. Osher and Sethian [12] used the connection between conservation laws and Hamilton–Jacobi equations to construct higher-order accurate numerical methods. Even though the analogy between conservation laws and Hamilton–Jacobi equations fails in multiple spatial dimensions, many Hamilton–Jacobi equations can be discretized in a dimension by dimension fashion. This culminated in a further study [47], in which Osher and Shu proposed a general framework for the numerical solution of Hamilton–Jacobi equations using successful methods from the theory of conservation laws. The next step now is how numerically handling Equation 1.16 in higher dimensions which is as numerical discretization.

A forward Euler time discretization of a Hamilton–Jacobi equation can be written as

$$\frac{\varphi^{n+1} - \varphi^n}{\Delta t} + \hat{H}\left(\varphi_x^-, \varphi_x^+; \varphi_y^-, \varphi_y^+; \varphi_z^-, \varphi_z^+\right) = 0 \qquad (1.86)$$

where $\hat{H}\left(\varphi_x^-, \varphi_x^+; \varphi_y^-, \varphi_y^+; \varphi_z^-, \varphi_z^+\right)$ is a numerical approximation of $H(\varphi_x, \varphi_y, \varphi_z)$. The function $\hat{H}$ is called a numerical Hamiltonian, and it is required to be consistent in the sense that $\hat{H} = H$. Spatial derivatives are discretized with either first-order accurate one-sided differencing or the higher-order accurate HJ ENO or HJ WENO schemes. We will discuss the two-dimensional numerical approximation to $H(\varphi_x, \varphi_y)$, with the ability to extend this analysis to three spatial dimensions. An important class of schemes is that of monotone schemes. A scheme is monotone when φ^{n+1} as defined in Equation 1.86 is a nondecreasing function of all the φ^n. Crandall and Lions proved that these schemes converge to the correct solution, although they are only first-order accurate. The numerical Hamiltonians associated with monotone schemes are important. The forward Euler time discretization also can be extended to higher-order TVD Runge–Kutta in a straightforward manner, as discussed before. The CFL condition for Equation 1.86 is

$$\Delta t \max \left\{ \frac{|H_1|}{\Delta x} + \frac{|H_2|}{\Delta y} + \frac{|H_3|}{\Delta z} \right\} < 1 \tag{1.87}$$

where H_1, H_2, and H_3 are the partial derivatives of H with respect to φ_x, φ_y, and φ_z, respectively. For example, in Equation 1.42, where $H(\nabla\varphi) = V \cdot \nabla\varphi$, the partial derivatives of H are $H_1 = u$, $H_2 = v$, and $H_3 = w$. As another example, consider the level set equation with $H(\nabla\varphi) = V_n|\nabla\varphi|$. Here the partial derivatives are slightly more complicated, with $H_1 = V_n\varphi x/|\nabla\varphi|$, $H_2 = V_n\varphi_y/|\nabla\varphi|$, and $H_3 = V_n\varphi_z/|\nabla\varphi|$, assuming that Vn does not depend on φ_x, φ_y, or φ_z otherwise, the partial derivatives can be substantially more complicated.

1.3.2.2 The Lax–Friedrichs scheme

The first approximation to $\hat{H}$ that we consider is the Lax–Friedrichs (LF) scheme from Crandall and Lions [53] given by

$$\hat{H} = H\left(\frac{\varphi_x^- + \varphi_x^+}{2}, \frac{\varphi_y^- + \varphi_y^+}{2}\right) - \alpha^x\left(\frac{\varphi_x^+ - \varphi_x^-}{2}\right) - \alpha^y\left(\frac{\varphi_y^+ - \varphi_y^-}{2}\right), \tag{1.88}$$

where α^x and α^y are dissipation coefficients that control the amount of numerical viscosity,

$$\alpha^x = \max|H_1(\varphi_x, \varphi_y)|, \alpha^y = \max|H_2(\varphi_x, \varphi_y)| \tag{1.89}$$

These dissipation coefficients are chosen based on the partial derivatives of H. The choice of these dissipation coefficients can be rather subtle. In the traditional implementation of the LF scheme, the maximum is chosen over the entire computational domain. First, the maximum and minimum values of φ_x are identified by considering all the values of φ_x^- and φ_x^+ on the Cartesian mesh. Then one can identify the interval $I^x = [\varphi_x^{min}, \varphi_x^{max}]$. A similar procedure is used to define $I^y = [\varphi_y^{min}, \varphi_x^{max}]$. The coefficients α^x and α^y are set to the maximum possible values of $|H_1(\varphi_x, \varphi_y)|$ and $|H_2(\varphi_x, \varphi_y)|$, respectively, with $\varphi_x \in I^x$ and $\varphi_y \in I^y$. Although it is occasionally difficult to evaluate the maximum values of $|H_1|$ and $|H_2|$, it is straightforward to do so in many instances. For example, in Equation 1.42, both $H_1 = u$ and $H_2 = v$ are independent of φ_x and φ_y, so α^x and α^y can be set to the maximum values of $|u|$ and $|v|$ on the Cartesian mesh. The price we pay for using bounds to choose α larger than it should be is increased numerical dissipation. That is, while the numerical method will be stable and give an accurate solution as the mesh is refined, some details of this solution may be smeared out and lost on a coarser mesh.

Since increasing α increases the amount of artificial dissipation, decreasing the quality of the solution, it is beneficial to choose α as small as possible without inducing oscillations or other nonphysical phenomena into the solution. In approximating $\hat{H}_{i,j}$ at a grid point $\vec{x}_{i,j}$ on a Cartesian mesh, it then makes little sense to do a global search to define the intervals I^x and I^y. In particular, consider the simple convection Equation 1.42 where $\alpha^x = \max|u|$ and $\alpha^y = \max|v|$. Suppose that some region had relatively small values of $|u|$ and $|v|$, while another region had relatively large values. Since the LF method chooses α^x as the largest value of $|u|$ and α^y as the largest value of $|v|$, the same values of α will be used in the region where the velocities are small as is used in the region where the velocities are large. In the region where the velocities are large, the large values of α are required to obtain a good solution. But in the region where the velocities are small, these large values of α produce too much numerical dissipation, wiping out small features of the solution. Thus, it is advantageous to use only the grid points sufficiently close to $\vec{x}_{i,j}$ in determining α. A rule of thumb is to include the grid points from $\vec{x}_{i-3,j}$ to $\vec{x}_{i+3,j}$ in the x-direction and from $\vec{x}_{i,j-3}$ to $\vec{x}_{i,j+3}$ in the y-direction in the local search neighborhood for determining α. This includes all the grid nodes that are used to evaluate $\varphi_x^{\pm}$ and $\varphi_y^{\pm}$ at $\vec{x}_{i,j}$ using the HJ WENO scheme. This type of scheme has been referred to as a Stencil Lax–Friedrichs (SLF) scheme, since it determines the dissipation coefficient using only the neighboring grid points that are part of the stencil used to determine φ_x and φ_y. An alternative to the dimension-by-dimension neighborhoods is to use the 49 grid points in the rectangle with diagonal corners at $\vec{x}_{i-3,j-3}$ and $\vec{x}_{i+3,j+3}$ to determine α. This idea of searching only locally to determine the dissipation coefficients can be taken a step further. The local Lax–Friedrichs (LLF) scheme proposed for conservation laws by Shu and Osher [44] does not look at any neighboring grid points when calculating the dissipation coefficients in a given direction. Osher and Shu [47] interpreted this to mean that α^x is determined at each grid point using only the values of φ_x^- and φ_x^+ at that specific grid point to determine the interval I^x. The interval I^y is still determined in the LF or SLF manner (in the SLF case we rename LLF as SLLF). Similarly, α^y uses an interval I^y, defined using only the values of φ_y^- and φ_y^+ at the grid point in question while I^x is still determined in the LF or SLF fashion. Osher and Shu [47] also proposed the local local Lax–Friedrichs (LLLF) scheme with even less numerical dissipation. At each grid point I^x is determined using the values of φ_x^- and φ_x^+ at that grid point; I^y is determined using the values of φ_y^- and φ_y^+ at that grid point; and then these intervals are used to determine both α^x and α^y. When H is separable, that is, $H(\varphi_x, \varphi_y) = H_x(\varphi_x) + H_y(\varphi_y)$, LLLF reduces to LLF, since α^x is independent of φ_y and α^y is independent of φ_x. When H not separable, LLF and LLLF are truly distinct schemes. In practice, LLF seems to work better than any of the other options. LF and SLF are usually too dissipative, while LLLF is usually not dissipative enough to overcome the problems introduced by using the centrally averaged approximation to φ_x and φ_y in evaluating H in Equation 1.88. Note that LLF is a monotone scheme.

1.3.2.3 *The Roe–Fix scheme*

As discussed above, choosing the appropriate amount of artificial dissipation to add to the centrally evaluated H in Equation 1.88 can be problematic. Therefore, it is often desirable to use upwind-based methods with built-in artificial dissipation. For conservation laws, Shu and Osher [44] proposed using Roe's upwind method along with an LLF entropy correction at sonic points where entropy-violating expansion shocks might form. The added dissipation from the LLF entropy correction forces the expansion shocks to develop into continuous rarefaction waves. The method was named Roe–Fix (RF) and it can be written for Hamilton–Jacobi equations (see Osher and Shu [47]) as

$$\hat{H} = H\left(\varphi_x^*, \varphi_y^*\right) - \alpha^x \left(\frac{\varphi_x^+ - \varphi_x^-}{2}\right) - \alpha^y \left(\frac{\varphi_y^+ - \varphi_y^-}{2}\right) \tag{1.90}$$

In the RF scheme, I^x and I^y are initially determined using only the nodal values for $\varphi_x^\pm$ and $\varphi_y^\pm$ as in the LLLF scheme. In order to estimate the potential for upwinding, we look at the partial derivatives H_1 and H_2. If $H_1(\varphi_x, \varphi_y)$ has the same sign (either always positive or always negative) for all $\varphi_x \in I^x$ and all $\varphi_y \in I^y$, we know which way information flows and can apply upwinding. Similarly, if $H_2(\varphi_x, \varphi_y)$ has the same sign for all $\varphi_x \in I^x$ and $\varphi_y \in I^y$, we can upwind this term as well. If both H_1 and H_2 do not change sign, we upwind completely, setting both α^x and α^y to zero. If $H_1 > 0$, information is flowing from left to right, then we set $\varphi_x^* = \varphi_x^-$. Otherwise, $H_1 < 0$ and we set $\varphi_x^* = \varphi_x^+$. Similarly, $H_2 > 0$ indicates $\varphi_y^* = \varphi_y^-$, and $H_2 < 0$ indicates $\varphi_y^* = \varphi_y^+$.

If either H_1 or H_2 changes sign, we are in the vicinity of a sonic point where the eigenvalue (in this case H_1 or H_2) is identically zero. This signifies a potential difficulty with nonunique solutions, and artificial dissipation is needed to pick out the physically correct vanishing viscosity solution. We switch from the RF scheme to the LLF scheme to obtain the needed artificial viscosity. If there is a sonic point in only one direction, that is, x or y, it makes little sense to add damping in both directions. Therefore, we look for sonic points in each direction and add damping only to the directions that have sonic points. This is done using the I^x and I^y defined as in the LLF method.

With the RF scheme, upwinding in the x-direction dictates that either φ_x^- or φ_x^+ be used, but not both. Similarly, upwinding in the y-direction uses either φ_y^- or φ_y^+, but not both. Since evaluating $\varphi_x^\pm$ and $\varphi_y^\pm$ using high-order accurate HJ ENO or HJ WENO schemes is rather costly, it seems wasteful to do twice as much work in these instances. Unfortunately, one cannot determine whether upwinding can be used (as opposed to LLF) without computing $\varphi_x^\pm$ and $\varphi_y^\pm$. In order to minimize CPU time, one can compute $\varphi_x^\pm$ and $\varphi_y^\pm$ using the first-order accurate forward and backward difference formulas and use these cheaper approximations to decide whether or not upwinding or LLF will be used. After making this decision, the higher-order accurate HJ ENO or HJ WENO method can be used to compute the necessary values of $\varphi_x^\pm$ and $\varphi_y^\pm$ used in the numerical discretization, obtaining the usual high-order accuracy. Sonic points rarely occur in practice, and this strategy reduces the use of the costly HJ WENO method by approximately a factor of two.

1.3.2.4 *Godunov's scheme*

Godunov [55] proposed a numerical method that gives the exact solution to the Riemann problem for one-dimensional conservation laws with piecewise constant initial data. The multidimensional Hamilton–Jacobi formulation of this scheme can be written as

$$\hat{H} = ext_x \, ext_y H(\varphi_x, \varphi_y) \tag{1.91}$$

as was pointed out by Bardi and Osher [56]. This is the canonical monotone scheme. Defining our intervals I^x and I^y in the LLLF manner using only the values of $\varphi_x^\pm$ and $\varphi_y^\pm$ y at the grid node under consideration, we define ext_x and ext_y as follows. If $\varphi_x^- < \varphi_x^+$, then $ext_x H$ takes on the minimum value of H for all $\varphi_x \in I^x$. If $\varphi_x^- > \varphi_x^+$, then $ext_x H$ takes on the maximum value of H for all $\varphi_x \in I^x$. Otherwise, if $\varphi_x^- = \varphi_x^+$, then ext_xH simply plugs $\varphi_x^- \left(= \varphi_x^+\right)$ into H for φ_x. Similarly, If $\varphi_y^- < \varphi_y^+$, then ext_yH takes on the minimum value of H for all $\varphi_y \in I^y$. If $\varphi_y^- > \varphi_y^+$, then ext_yH takes on the maximum value of H for all $\varphi_y \in I^y$. Otherwise, if $\varphi_y^- = \varphi_y^+$, then ext_yH simply plugs $\varphi_y^- \left(= \varphi_y^+\right)$ into H for φ_y. In general, $ext_xext_yH \neq ext_yext_xH$, so different versions of Godunov's method are obtained depending on the order of operations. Although Godunov's method can sometimes be difficult to implement, there are times when it is straightforward. Consider Equation 1.42 for motion in an externally generated velocity field. Here, we can consider the x and y directions independently, since H is separable with $ext_xext_yH = ext_x(u\varphi_x) + ext_y(v\varphi_y)$ If $\varphi_x^- < \varphi_x^+$, we want the minimum value of $u\varphi_x$. Thus, if $u > 0$, we use φ_x^-, and if $u < 0$, we use φ_x^+. If $u = 0$, we obtain $u\varphi_x = 0$ regardless of the choice of φ_x. On the other hand, If $\varphi_x^- > \varphi_x^+$, we want the maximum value of $u\varphi_x$. Thus, if $u > 0$, we use φ_x^-, and if $u < 0$, we use φ_x^+. Again $u = 0$, gives $u\varphi_x = 0$. Finally, if $\varphi_x^- = \varphi_x^+$, then $u\varphi_x$ is uniquely determined. This can be summarized as follows. If $u > 0$, use φ_x^-; if $u < 0$, use φ_x^+; and if $u = 0$, set $u\varphi_x = 0$. This is identical to the standard upwind differencing method described in solving basic level set method, Equation 1.42. That is, for motion in an externally generated velocity field, Godunov's method is identical to simple upwind differencing.

1.3.3   Optimization schemes

In this section, the minimization technique followed is the Euler–Lagrange equation [57], and the gradient descent technique [58] that gives the flow that minimizes the energy functions. Light is shed on the basics of Euler–Lagrange equation and the gradient descent technique in the following section.

1.3.3.1   Euler–Lagrange equation

Consider the following problem from calculus of variation: minimize an integral of a twice differentiable Lagrangian $q(x, b, \nabla b)$ over a regular bounded domain Ω with a smooth boundary $\partial\Omega$. q mainly depends on the minimizer b and its gradient ∇b. The minimization problem can thus be formulated as

$$\min_{b:b|\partial\Omega=b_0} E(b), E(b) = \int_\Omega q(x, b, \nabla b)\, dx \tag{1.92}$$

Because a differentiable functional is stationary at its local maxima and minima, the Euler–Lagrange equation is useful for solving optimization problems in which, given some functional, one seeks the function b which minimizes the functional $E(b)$.

In order to derive the Euler equation, consider the variation δb of the minimizer b and the difference $\delta E = E(b + \delta b) - E(b)$. Assuming that this variation is small and twice differentiable, then:

$$\delta b(x + t) = 0, \quad \forall t : |t| > \epsilon, \quad |\nabla(\delta b)| < C_\epsilon \cdot \forall x, \tag{1.93}$$

where $\epsilon \to 0$.

When q is twice differentiable, the Lagrangian can be linearized as follows:

$$q(x, b + \delta b, \nabla(b + \delta b)) = q(x, b, \nabla b) + \frac{\partial q(x, b, \nabla b)}{\partial b}\delta b + \frac{\partial q(x, b, \nabla b)}{\partial \nabla b}\delta \nabla b + O(\|\delta b\|, \|\nabla \delta b\|),$$

$$\tag{1.94}$$

where $\partial q(x, b, \nabla b/\partial \nabla b)$ represents the vector of partial derivatives of q with respect to the partial derivatives of b,

$$\frac{\partial q(x, b, \nabla b)}{\partial \nabla b} \left[\frac{\partial q(x, b, \nabla b)}{\partial(\partial b/\partial x_1)}, \ldots, \frac{\partial q(x, b, \nabla b)}{\partial(\partial b/\partial x_n)} \right]. \tag{1.95}$$

The substitution of the linearized Lagrangian into the formula for δE results in

$$\delta E = \int_{\Omega} \left(\frac{\partial q}{\partial b} \delta b + \frac{\partial q}{\partial \nabla b} . \delta \nabla b \right) dx + O(||\delta b||, ||\nabla \delta b||) \tag{1.96}$$

Simplifying Equation 1.96, performing integration by parts, and interchanging the two linear operators of variation and differentiation leads to

$$\int_{\Omega} \left(\frac{\partial q}{\partial \nabla b} \cdot \nabla(\delta b) \right) dx = - \int_{\Omega} \delta b \left(\nabla \cdot \frac{\partial q}{\partial \nabla b} \right) dx + \int_{\partial \Omega} \delta b \left(\frac{\partial q}{\partial \nabla b} \cdot n \right) ds, \tag{1.97}$$

so that

$$\delta E = \int_{\Omega} \left(\frac{\partial q}{\partial b} - \nabla \cdot \frac{\partial q}{\partial \nabla b} \right) \delta b \, dx + \int_{\partial \Omega} \delta b \left(\frac{\partial q}{\partial \nabla b} \cdot n \right) ds, \tag{1.98}$$

where n is the normal vector. The coefficient by δb in the first integral of Equation 1.98 is called the variational derivative in Ω, and is called the Euler–Lagrange equation:

$$\frac{\partial q}{\partial b} - \nabla \cdot \left(\frac{\partial q}{\partial \nabla b} \right) = 0. \tag{1.99}$$

When b is a function of more than one independent variable; for example, when q has the form

$$q = q \left(x_i, b, b_{x_i}, b_{x_i x_j} \right), \quad \forall i, \quad j \in [1, L], \tag{1.100}$$

and following the same strategy when having one variable, the following Euler–Lagrange equation can be obtained:

$$\frac{\partial q}{\partial b} - \sum_{i=1}^{L} \frac{d}{dx_i} \frac{\partial q}{\partial b_{x_i}} + \sum_{i=1}^{L} \sum_{j=1}^{L} \frac{d^2}{dx_i dx_j} \frac{\partial q}{\partial b_{x_i x_j}} = 0 \tag{1.101}$$

Euler–Lagrange and the Gradient Descent: The gradient descent technique helps in solving for the function E and its derivative with respect to a set of variables $\mathbf{S} = [S_1 \ldots S_m]^T$:

$$\frac{\partial E}{\partial \mathbf{S}} = 0, \tag{1.102}$$

using the following formula:

$$\frac{\partial S}{\partial t} = -\frac{\partial E}{\partial S}, \tag{1.103}$$

where the minus sign denoted that it is a minimization problem, where variables change with time until reaching the steady state at $\partial E/\partial \mathbf{S} = 0$.

The need for reinitialization: The signed distance function for the level sets equation is

$$\varphi(X) = \begin{cases} +D(x) & \text{if point is inside the contour} \\ 0 & \text{if point is on the boundary} \\ -D(x) & \text{if point is outside the contour} \end{cases} \tag{1.104}$$

where $D(x)$ is the minimum Euclidean distance between the point x and the contour. The distance function needs to be frequently reinitialized after solving the level set PDE. This helps maintaining the smoothness of the evolution [59]. Reinitialization of the level set equation can be handled using the following formula:

$$\frac{\partial}{\partial t}\varphi = sgn(\varphi^0)(1 - |\nabla\varphi|) \tag{1.105}$$

The solution of this equation keeps the function close to the signed distance function if it is conducted in parallel with the main equation, Equation 1.16.

The solution of the reinitialization equation is

$$\varphi_{i,j}^{n+1} = \varphi_{i,j}^n - \Delta t S\left(\varphi_{i,j}^0\right) G(\varphi)_{i,j}, \tag{1.106}$$

where

$$G(\varphi)_{i,j} = \begin{cases} \sqrt{\max\left(a_+^2, b_-^2\right) + \max\left(c_+^2, d_-^2\right)} & -1 \quad \text{if } \varphi_{i,j}^0 > 0 \\ \sqrt{\max\left(a_-^2, b_+^2\right) + \max\left(c_-^2, d_+^2\right)} & -1 \quad \text{if } \varphi_{i,j}^0 < 0 \end{cases}$$

$$a = D^{x-}\varphi_{i,j} = \varphi_{i,j} - \varphi_{i-1,j}/\Delta x$$
$$b = D^{x+}\varphi_{i,j} = \varphi_{i+1,j} - \varphi_{i,j}/\Delta x$$
$$c = D^{y-}\varphi_{i,j} = \varphi_{i,j} - \varphi_{i,j-1}/\Delta y$$
$$d = D^{y+}\varphi_{i,j} = \varphi_{i,j+1} - \varphi_{i,j}/\Delta y$$
$$a_+ = \max(a, 0)$$
$$a_- = \max(a, 0)$$

$$S(\varphi) = 2 * \left(H_\alpha(\varphi) - \frac{1}{2}\right),$$

where $H_\alpha(\varphi)$ is the Heaviside function.

A major drawback of the level set method is the extensive computation time. This motivated researchers to speed up its algorithms for convergence. One of these notable ideas is narrow banding. The narrow banding theory was first introduced by Chopp [60], and was later developed by Adalsteinsson and Sethian [61]. The idea of narrow banding is that the interest is mainly in the motion of the zero level set, and other points are not considered, Figure 1.6. Instead, they are assigned either large positive or large negative values. This limits the computation to fewer points that are around the zero level set, whereas the rest of the domain is considered to be only a sign holder [62]. Narrow banding significantly decreases the computational complexity. The narrow banding algorithm is summarized in Algorithm 1.1.

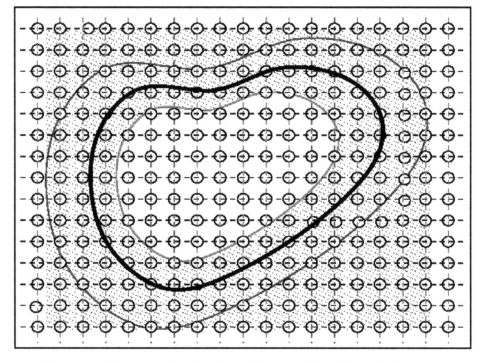

Figure 1.6 Illustration of the narrow banding theory. The inward band (red), the front position (black), and the outward band (blue) are the interest in the image. All other points are of no importance.

ALGORITHM 1.1   Steps of the Narrow Banding Algorithm

1: Extract the latest position.
2: Define a band within a certain distance.
3: Update the level set function.
4: Check the new position with respect to the limits of the band.
5: Update the position of the band regularly and reinitialize the implicit function.

1.3.4   Guiding forces

Like parametric deformable models, geometric models can also be either region-based or edge-based. There have been numerous forms for the speed function F proposed in literature, Equation 1.41, which can be roughly categorized into either region-based or edge-based functions. Some of the most popular forms for F in both categories are outlined below.

1.3.4.1   Edge-based forces
Geodesic Active Contour (GAC) Model: This can be alternatively referred to as variational edge-based segmentation and is considered to be a geometric alternative for the snake model. This model is known to be geometrically intrinsic because the energy function is invariant with respect to the curve parameterization [31,63]. The model is defined by the

following minimization problem:

$$\min_C \left\{ E_{GAC}(C) = \int_0^{L(C)} g(|\nabla I_0(C(s))|) \, ds \right\}, \tag{1.107}$$

where ds is the Euclidean element of length and $L(C)$ is the length of the curve C defined by $L(C) = \int_0^{L(C)} ds$. The function g is an edge indicator function that does not exist at object boundaries and is given by:

$$g(|\nabla I_0|) = \frac{1}{1 + \beta |\nabla I_0|^2}, \tag{1.108}$$

where I_0 is the original image and β is an arbitrary positive constant.

Although this model provides good results, it is highly sensitive to the initial condition [64,65]. This is due to the non-convex nature of the energy functional to be minimized, E_{GAC}, which leads to the existence of local minima (Figure 1.7). This drawback is not specific to this model because variational models in image processing often suffer from local minima.

Gradient Vector Flow Fast GAC: Paragios et al. [65] proposed a fast evolution model where boundaries are extracted using a front propagation flow that combines GAC [31] and GVF [14] models and is implemented using a level set approach. It is thus capable of dealing with topological changes, along with shape deformations. Paragios et al. [65] modified the GVF energy function slightly as follows:

$$E(V) = \iint \mu \left(u_x^2 + v_x^2 + u_y^2 + u_y^2 \right) + f |\nabla f|^2 |(V - \nabla f)|^2 \, dx \, dy. \tag{1.109}$$

The only difference between Equations 1.109 and 1.21 is that image boundaries as well as the gradients are involved, thus enabling the strong edges to overcome the flow generated by weak edges.

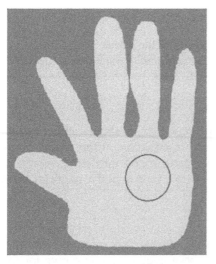 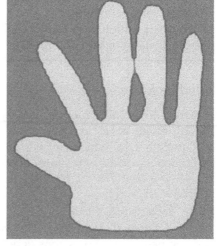

Figure 1.7 Initialization of the standard snake model in Caselles et al. [31] and Liu et al. [46] fails to segment the image (left) into its two objects and considers them as one object instead.

The flow in Paragios et al. [65] was then determined by obtaining the inner product of the modified GVF $\hat{v}$ and the unit normal $\mathcal{N}$ as follows:

$$C_t = (\hat{v} \cdot \mathcal{N})\mathcal{N}. \tag{1.110}$$

Inspired by the work of Osher et al. [12], the front in Equation 1.110 evolves according to the following level set implicit representation:

$$C_t(p,t) = F(p)\mathcal{N}(p), \tag{1.111}$$

given that the implicit level set function deforms according to:

$$\varphi_t(p,t) = F(p)|\nabla \varphi(p,t)|. \tag{1.112}$$

1.3.4.2   Region-based forces

Chan–Vese Model (Active Contour without Edges) for Image Segmentation: An example of a segmentation model is the well-known Chan–Vese model, also known as the active contour without edges (ACWE) [66], which is based on the Mumford–Shah model [67]. The energy function for ACWE comes in the following form:

$$\min_{\Omega_c,c_1,c_2} \left\{ E_{ACWE}(\Omega_c,c_1,c_2,\lambda) = \text{per}(\Omega_c)\lambda \int_{\Omega_c} (c_1 - f(x))^2\, dx + \lambda \int_{\Omega \backslash \Omega_c} (c_2 - f(x))^2\, dx \right\}, \tag{1.113}$$

This model finds two regions in the image domain Ω. These two regions are designated as object and background, where mean intensities are as disjoint as possible. The first term is the length of the boundary of Σ, where $\Sigma \subset \Omega$. c_{in} and c_{out} are the mean intensities in $\Omega \backslash \Sigma$ and Σ respectively, Figure 1.8.

The minimization in Equation 1.113 does not enable the solution to assume continuous values, lending itself to a non-convex formulation.

For the limitation above, there have been various recent attempts in literature to obtain global solutions from such non-convex energy functions by integrating edge-based

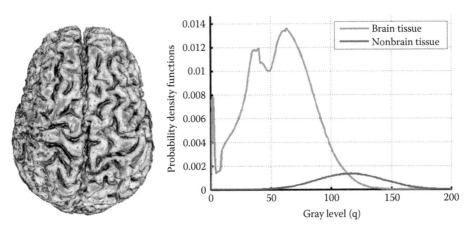

Figure 1.8 A human brain (left), with intensity distribution of the two terms c_{in} (brain tissue) and c_{out} (nonbrain tissue) in Equation 1.113.

methods such as the GAC model [31]. One example is given by Bresson et al. [64], where global minimization of the active contour model is obtained based on the Mumford–Shah model [67] and the active contours without edges model by Chan and Vese [66]. Details of this global energy function are outlined below.

Chan and Vese represent the regions Ω, Ω_c with the Heaviside of the level sets function; hence the energy function in Equation 1.113 can be rewritten as:

$$E^2_{ACWE}(\Phi, c_1, c_2, \lambda) = \int_\Omega |\nabla H_\epsilon(\Phi)| \, dx + \lambda \int_\Omega (H_\epsilon(\Phi)(c_1 - f(x))^2 + H_\epsilon(-\Phi)(c_2 - f(x))^2) \, dx,$$

(1.114)

where $H_\epsilon(\Phi)$ is the regularization of the Heaviside function. The steady-state solution of the gradient flow becomes:

$$\partial_t \varphi = div \left(\frac{\nabla \varphi}{|\nabla \varphi|} \right) - \lambda r_1(x, c_1, c_2),$$

(1.115)

where $r_1(x, c_1, c_2) = ((c_1 - f(x))^2 - (c_2 - f(x))^2)$. Equation 1.115 is the gradient descent flow of the following energy:

$$E^3_{ACWE}(\varphi, c_1, c_2, \lambda) = \int_\Omega |\nabla \varphi| \, dx + \lambda \int_\Omega r_1(x, c_1, c_2) \varphi \, dx.$$

(1.116)

Based on this, Bresson et al. [64] proposed to minimize the following energy function to obtain the global minimum solution for any parameter >0:

$$E_1(u, c_1, c_2, \lambda) = TV_g(u) + \lambda \int r_1(x, c_1, c_2) u \, dx,$$

(1.117)

where the difference between Equations 1.116 and 1.117 is based on the weighted total variation (TV) of a function u [68], with a weight function g, that contains information concerning the boundaries of an image I_0 [31] and is given by Equation 1.108.

Equation 1.117 provides the link between ACWE and GAC when g is an edge indicator function and u is a characteristic function, 1_{Ω_c}. The following relation thus stands:

$$TV_g\left(u = 1_{\Omega_c}\right) = \int_\Omega g(x) \left|\nabla 1_{\Omega_c}\right| \, dx = \int_C g(s) \, ds = E_{GAC}(C).$$

(1.118)

Equation 1.117 could thus be rewritten as

$$E_2\left(u = 1_{\Omega_c}, c_1, c_2, \lambda\right) = TV_g\left(1_{\Omega_c}\right) + \lambda \int r_1(x, c_1, c_2) 1_{\Omega_c} \, dx,$$

(1.119)

where E_2 is homogeneous of degree 1 in u. This means that for any minimizer u of E_2 got with any minimization framework, the set of points in the function u such that u is a positive constant, defines a set whose boundary is a global minimum of the snake model. The constrained minimization problem for the segmentation problem is then

$$\min_{0 \leq u \leq 1} = \left\{ E_2(u, c_1, c_2, \lambda) = TV_g(u) + \lambda \int r_1(x, c_1, c_2) u \, dx \right\}.$$

(1.120)

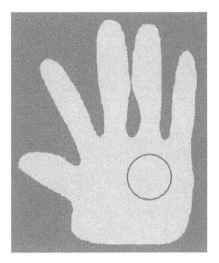 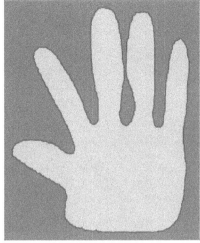

Figure 1.9 The proposed deformable model-based segmentation model in Bresson et al. [64], which provides a global solution to the standard snake model segments—the image on the left into two objects.

which has the same set of minimizers as the following convex, unconstrained minimization problem:

$$\min_{u} \left\{ TV_g(u) + \lambda \int r_1(x, c_1, c_2)u + \alpha v(u)\, dx \right\}. \tag{1.121}$$

where $v(\xi) = \max\{0, 2|\xi{,}1/2|1\}$ is an exact penalty function provided that α is large enough compared to λ. The function in Equation 1.121 is not strictly convex, thus does not possess local minima that are not global. Now the convex formulation for Equation 1.121 guarantees the segmentation framework to have a global minimizer [64], Figure 1.9.

The global solution obtained for the convex formulation of the GAC model by Bresson et al. [64] using region-based functions such as the ACWE model [66] and the Mumford–Shah model [67] does not guarantee good segmentation however. Such models are not mainly concerned with feature detection unlike the segmentation models based on shape priors as in El-Baz and Gimel'farb [30] and El-Baz et al. [69].

Level Set Segmentation Using Statistical Shape Priors: The work by El Baz et al. [69] proposed the use of level sets with shape constraints for 3D segmentation. The approach uses prior shape information from a set of training images. A signed distance function is assigned to each shape, and the signed distance values are formed in a histogram. Probability density functions (PDFs) of the object and background are then determined based on both signed distance function and gray level values. Details of this approach are outlined in the following.

Given a curve/surface M that represents boundaries of a certain shape, the following level set function can be defined:

$$\varphi(x, y, z) = \begin{cases} 0 & (x, y, z) \in M \\ d((x, y, z), M) & (x, y, z) \in R_M \\ -d((x, y, z), M) & \text{otherwise} \end{cases} \tag{1.122}$$

where R_M is the region defined by the shape and $d((x, y, z), M)$ is the minimum Euclidean distance between the image location (x, y, z) and the curve/surface M.

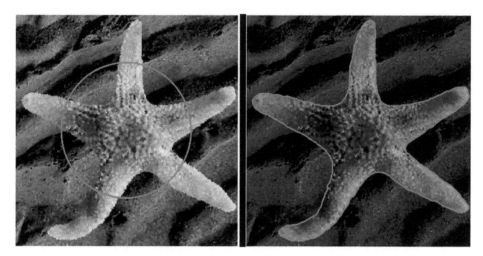

Figure 1.10 The proposed geometric deformable segmentation model in El-Baz et al. [69] showing the initial segmentation on the left and the final segmentation on the right. (Image is courtesy of A. El-Baz and G. Gimel'farb, Image segmentation with a parametric deformable model using shape and appearance priors, in *IEEE Conference on Computer Vision and Pattern Recognition*, 2008, pp. 1–8.)

Using Equation 1.122, a database of curves and signed distance functions can be constructed, representing shape variations. From this information, a histogram of the occurrences of signed distance values which characterizes the shape and its local variations can be extracted.

The evolving surface is a propagating front embedded as the zero level of a scalar function $\varphi(x, y, z, t)$. The continuous change of $\varphi(x, y, z, t)$ can be described by the partial differential equation:

$$\frac{\partial \varphi(x, y, z, t)}{\partial t} + F(x, y, z)|\nabla \varphi(x, y, z, t)| = 0, \qquad (1.123)$$

where $F(x, y, z)$ is a velocity function and $\nabla = [\partial/\partial x, \partial/\partial y, \partial/\partial z]^T$.

The function $\Phi(x, y, z, t)$ deforms iteratively according to $F(x, y, z)$ and the position of the 2D/3D front is given at each iteration by solving the equation $\Phi(x, y, z, t)$. Finally, the speed function $F(x, y, z)$ is formulated as:

$$F(x, y, z) = \upsilon - \epsilon k(x, y, z), \qquad (1.124)$$

where $\upsilon = 1$ or -1 for the contracting or expanding front respectively, ϵ is a smoothing coefficient which is always small with respect to 1, and $k(x, y, z)$ is the local curvature of the front. The latter parameter acts as a regularization term. A segmentation example is shown in Figure 1.10.

1.3.4.3 *Summary on geometric deformable models*

This section addressed the geometric deformable models that emerged in the late 1980s to overcome the limitations of the parametric deformation, which does not have the ability to handle topological changes of the evolving contour such as merging and splitting. The basic level set, its numerical schemes, and some of its popular guiding forces in literature were provided in detail.

The extensive computations required for the convergence of the level set equation could be partially remedied by applying the narrow banding theorem. However, there is no guarantee for finding a global solution with level set evolution, and there is a high tendency to get stuck in local minima.

1.4   Applications in medical imaging

This section surveys the recent work in medical image deformable model-based segmentation. A countless number of research studies have exploited the deformable models, whether geometric or parametric, in segmenting different body structures such as the brain, heart, kidney, colon, lung, and prostate. As mentioned earlier, it is very hard to generalize a segmentation framework for all medical imaging segmentation problems. There would be different stopping criteria and guiding forces on the evolving contour in order to converge to the desired solution at each case [70]. For example, He et al. [71] conducted a comparative study reviewing eight parametric and geometric deformable models and applying them to different structures such as the knee, brain, blood cells, kidney, and brain's corpus callosum and sulci. The key was to select the appropriate approach for each application. The study highlighted the advantages and disadvantages of each one of the eight deformable models. Tsai et al. [72] proposed a shape-based approach for the segmentation of medical images. A parametric model for an implicit representation of the segmenting curve was derived by applying principal component analysis to a collection of signed distance representations of the training data. The parameters of this representation were then used to minimize the segmentation objective function.

Heart: Segmentation of cardiac images was heavily conducted in literature using deformable models. For example, Pluempitiwiriyawej et al. [73] proposed a stochastic active contour model for the segmentation of cardiac MR images to overcome the limitations of boundary of topology and extensive computations. Montagnat et al. [74] proposed a 4D deformable model for heart segmentation, where simplex meshes were constructed and the mean curvature at each vertex was estimated. In Khalifa et al. [75–77], the heart was segmented using a level set-based deformable model where evolution is controlled by a stochastic speed function.

A framework that combines the benefits of both the deformable models and graph cuts was constructed by Uzunbas et al. [78] to segment the epicardium and the myocardium of the left ventricle of the heart from magnetic resonance images. A good initialization scheme for the deformable model was exploited, which resulted in smooth segmentation results with lower interaction costs than using only graph cut segmentation. The deformable model was defined as a region defined by two nested contours in order to segment the epicardium and endocardium by optimizing a single energy functional. Khaifa et al. [79] proposed an automated framework for analyzing the wall thickness and thickening function on cine cardiac magnetic resonance images, which included the segmentation as a first step. The inner and outer wall borders were segmented using a geometric deformable model guided by a special stochastic speed relationship. Gopal et al. [80] segmented the left ventricle (LV) from cardiac MR images using an approach that combined statistical and deterministic deformable models. A 3D active appearance model (AAM) was also incorporated. Cardiac first-pass MR images were analyzed in Khalifa et al. [81–83] and Beache et al. [84], where the left ventricle (LV) was segmented using a level set-based function. A shape-based framework for the segmentation of the left ventricle (LV) wall on cardiac first-pass magnetic resonance imaging (FP-MRI) using level sets was proposed. The level set evolution was constrained using three features: a weighted probabilistic shape prior, the first-order pixelwise image intensities, and a second-order Markov–Gibbs random field (MGRF) spatial interaction model. The left ventricle was also segmented using level set-based functions in Sliman et al. [85–88] for the assessment of myocardium function.

Brain: As far as brain segmentation is concerned, numerous researchers have made use of deformable models. Ho et al., for example, segmented the brain tumors using level set evolution with region competition [89]. A signed local statistical force that replaced the constant propagation term was proposed to avoid boundary leakage problems. The probabilities for background and tumor regions were computed from a pre- and postcontrast image and mixture-modeling of the histogram. Goldenberg et al. [90] used a shape-based level set approach that exploited the coupled surfaces model to segment the brain cortex. A neonatal image segmentation method was proposed [91], where local intensity information, atlas spatial prior, and cortical thickness constraint were combined in a single level set framework. A longitudinally guided level sets method for neonatal image segmentation was done by the same group [92], combining local intensity information, atlas spatial prior, cortical thickness constraint, and longitudinal information into a variational framework. A novel patch-driven level set method for the segmentation of neonatal brain MR images using sparse representation techniques was later proposed by the same group [93]. After building an atlas, the probability maps were integrated into a coupled level set framework. In Casanova et al. [94] and Alansary et al. [95,96], the brain was extracted using a hybrid approach that integrates geometrical and statistical models. The brain is parceled to a set of nested isosurfaces using the fast marching level set method in order to accurately discriminate between brain and nonbrain tissues.

Colon: Colon segmentation using deformable models was also addressed in the literature. A hybrid segmentation procedure, which can handle both air- and fluid-filled parts of the colon, was adopted [97]. The proposed hybrid algorithm uses modified region growing, fuzzy connectedness, and level set segmentation as key components. A level set approach was also developed [98] for automatic segmentation of the colon's haustral folds based on their boundaries.

Kidney: Kidney segmentation has also been conducted using deformable models [99–108]. The kidney borders were extracted using a geometric deformable model guided by a special stochastic speed relationship. This accounts for a shape prior and appearance features in terms of voxel-wise image intensities and their pairwise spatial interactions integrated into a two-level joint Markov–Gibbs random field (MGRF) model of the kidney and its background. Kidney segmentation was also conducted using an evolving deformable model that is based on two density functions [109–118]; the first function describes the distribution of the gray level inside and outside the kidney region, and the second function describes the prior shape of the kidney. The gray level density is calculated for a given kidney image using a modified expectation maximization (EM) algorithm.

In order to get the kidney's shape prior, an average kidney shape is constructed from a dataset of previously segmented kidneys, and an average signed distance map density is then obtained.

Liver: As far as the liver segmentation is concerned, Cvancarova et al. [119] modified the original GVF algorithm for segmenting ultrasound images of liver tumors by coupling the smoothness of the edge map to the contour's initial size. The tuning parameters of the GVF model were also adjusted, and the numerical discretization was improved as well. An automated liver segmentation method was proposed [120], where the level set-based contour evolution from T2 weighted magnetic resonance datasets was approximated. The method avoided solving partial differential equations and was applied to all slices with a constant number of iterations. The method also did not require any manual initialization.

A level set model was also proposed [121] to integrate image gradient, region competition, and prior information for CT liver tumor segmentation. The probabilistic distribution of liver tumors was used to enhance the object indication function, formulate the directional balloon force, and regulate region competition.

Lung: Lung segmentation was also heavily considered in literature using deformable models. A segmentation framework was developed [122] to capture the high curvature features of the lung cavities from the magnetic resonance images. It computed an external force field based on the solution of partial differential equations with boundary condition defined by the initial positions of the evolving contours. An algorithm for isolating lung nodules from spiral CT scans was proposed [123]. The proposed algorithm exploited four different types of deformable templates describing typical geometry and gray level distribution of lung nodules. These four types are (i) a solid spherical model of large-size calcified and noncalcified nodules appearing in several successive slices; (ii) a hollow spherical model of large lung cavity nodules; (iii) a circular model of small nodules appearing in only a single slice; and (iv) a semicircular model of lung wall nodules. Each template had a specific gray level pattern, which was analytically estimated in order to fit the available empirical data. Finally, the detection combined the normalized cross-correlation template matching by genetic optimization and Bayesian postclassification. A level set-based method for automatic medical image segmentation was adopted [124]. The intensity distribution of the organic structures was investigated, and a calibrating mechanism was conducted in order to automatically weight image intensity and gradient information in the level set speed function. Lung segmentation was also conducted [125], where two adaptive probability models of visual appearance of small 2D and large 3D pulmonary nodules were used to control the evolution of deformable boundaries. An algorithm for unsupervised segmentation of the lung tissues from low-dose computed tomography (LDCT) was adopted [126,127]. It used a joint Markov–Gibbs random field model (MGRF) of independent image signals and interdependent region labels. Lung segmentation was performed [128] using a 3D generalized Gauss–Markov random field (GGMRF) model of voxel intensities with pairwise interaction to model the 3D appearance of the lung tissues. Segmentation of lung was also conducted using deformable models [129–136]. In order to isolate pulmonary nodules from background in chest images, adaptive probability models of the visual appearance of small 2D and large 3D pulmonary nodules have been jointly incorporated to control the evolution of the deformable model. The appearance prior was modeled with a translation and rotation invariant Markov–Gibbs random field (MGRF) of voxel intensities with pairwise interaction. The model was then analytically identified from a set of training nodule images with normalized intensity ranges.

Prostate: Prostate segmentation techniques using deformable models have also been addressed. A deformable model for automatic segmentation of prostate from three-dimensional ultrasound images was proposed [137]. A set of Gabor-support vector machines (G-SVMs) was positioned on different patches of the model surface and trained to capture texture priors of ultrasound images in order to classify tissues as prostate or nonprostate. These G-SVMs were used to label voxels around the surface of deformable model as prostate or nonprostate tissues using a statistical texture matching. This resulted in driving the surface of deformable model to the boundary between the prostate and nonprostate tissues. An automatic method for the coupled 3D localization and segmentation of lower abdomen structures was proposed [138]. The approach allowed for easily adapting to high shape variation and to intensity inhomogeneities. Also, a statistical shape prior was enforced on the prostate. A statistical shape model was used as prior information for the segmentation of prostate [139], and gray level distribution was modeled by fitting histogram modes with a Gaussian mixture. Markov fields were used to introduce contextual information for the voxels' neighborhoods. Final labeling optimization was conducted based on Bayesian a-posteriori classification. An approach for segmenting the prostate region from dynamic contrast enhancement magnetic resonance images (DCE-MRI) based on using deformable models was adopted [140–146]. They combined three descriptors: (i) First-order visual appearance descriptors of the DCE-MRI; (ii) a spatially invariant second-order homogeneity descriptor, and (iii) a prostate shape descriptor. In McClure et al. [147,148], prostate segmentation was conducted using a level set deformable model and nonnegative matrix factorization (NMF) techniques. In the proposed framework, the level set was guided by a novel speed function that was derived using NMF, which extracts meaningful features from a large dimensional feature space.

To summarize, pattern recognition in image processing was the origin of the exploration of the space of images. Simplistic digital techniques used at the beginning of the sixties for gray image processing operations have been now replaced with complex mathematical frameworks that aim to exploit and understand images in two and three dimensions. The medical sector is also a major area for the use of images. The evolution of the acquisition devices led to new ways of capturing information not visible to the human eye. Medical imaging is probably the most established market for processing visual information. Visualization of complex structures and automated processing of computer aided diagnosis is used more and more by physicians in the diagnostic process. Image segmentation is perhaps the most well-studied topic in image processing and computer vision. Evolving an initial curve toward the boundaries of the structure of interest is a method that can be used to deal with this problem.

Deformable models have been widely used in the literature for a vast majority of medical imaging problems. The introduction of the snake model presented by Kass et al. aimed at evolving an initial curve toward the lowest potential of a cost function. Level set techniques have proved to be the most suitable method to track moving interfaces. Being implicit, intrinsic, and parametric free, level sets can deal with topological changes while for tracking moving interfaces. Recent work in the literature aims at combining level set method with other techniques to better manipulate it. Li et al. [149], for example, proposed a fuzzy level set algorithm that is able to evolve from the initial segmentation by spatial fuzzy clustering. The controlling parameters of the level set evolution are also estimated from the results of fuzzy clustering. Also, the fuzzy level set algorithm is enhanced with locally regularized evolution. Topological graph prior information was considered [150], in order to evolve the contour within a multi-level set formulation. The use of graph priors allowed for segmenting adjacent objects with similar intensity levels that were impossible to segment with the ordinary level set formulation.

1.5   Conclusion and future trends

This chapter discussed the deformable models with their explicit and implicit representations in detail. It started with the parametric deformable models, which were introduced in late eighties and showed many advances in the field of image processing. Due to their poor performance in some aspects, geometric deformable models were later introduced that could successfully handle most of these problems.

Future work includes many promising aspects. The combination of the benefits of both parametric and geometric deformable models in a hybrid framework can be useful with certain problems which require the speed of the parametric models as well as the capabilities of the implicit representation of the geometric ones. Also, one of the useful trends could be obtaining the convex formulation of complex level set-based functions. Another useful trend can be integrating the spatial, intensity, and shape models. This would solve the drawbacks of getting stuck in local minima and obtaining global solutions to the problem. The shift toward parallel programming and cloud computing of level set methods has also been rapidly growing in the 2000 s in order to speed up the convergence and optimize solutions, especially when dealing with large volumes in medical imaging problems. Also, recent work in the literature is aiming at improving and easily manipulating level sets, which could eventually lead to more robust segmentation, such as the integration with fuzzy clustering and topological prior information.

References

1. N. Sharma and L. M. Aggarwal, Automated medical image segmentation techniques, *Journal of Medical Physics*, vol. 35, no. 1, pp. 3–14, 2010.
2. E. R. Hancock and J. Kittler, Edge-labeling using dictionary-based relaxation, *IEEE Transactions on Pattern Analysis and Machine Intelligence*, vol. 12, no. 2, pp. 165–181, 1990.
3. Y. T. Liow, A contour tracing algorithm that preserves common boundaries between regions, *CVGIP: Image Understanding*, vol. 53, no. 3, pp. 313–321, 1991.
4. T. Law, H. Itoh, and H. Seki, Image filtering, edge detection, and edge tracing using fuzzy reasoning, *IEEE Transactions on Pattern Analysis and Machine Intelligence*, vol. 18, no. 5, pp. 481–491, 1996.
5. H. Ney, A comparative study of two search strategies for connected word recognition: Dynamic programming and heuristic search, *IEEE Transactions on Pattern Analysis and Machine Intelligence*, vol. 14, no. 5, pp. 586–595, 1992.
6. L. Xu and E. Oja, Randomized Hough transform (RHT): Basic mechanisms, algorithms, and computational complexities, *CVGIP: Image Understanding*, vol. 57, no. 2, pp. 131–154, 1993.
7. H. Kälviäinen, P. Hirvonen, L. Xu, and E. Oja, Probabilistic and non-probabilistic Hough transforms: Overview and comparisons, *Image and Vision Computing*, vol. 13, no. 4, pp. 239–252, 1995.
8. H. T. Nguyen, M. Worring, and R. Boomgaard, Watersnakes: Energy-driven watershed segmentation, *IEEE Transactions on Pattern Analysis and Machine Intelligence*, vol. 25, no. 3, pp. 330–342, 2003.
9. L. Najman and M. Schmitt, Geodesic saliency of watershed contours and hierarchical segmentation, *IEEE Transactions on Pattern Analysis and Machine Intelligence*, vol. 18, no. 12, pp. 1163–1173, 1996.
10. A. M. López, F. Lumbreras, J. Serrat, and J. J. Villanueva, Evaluation of methods for ridge and valley detection, *IEEE Transactions on Pattern Analysis and Machine Intelligence*, vol. 21, no. 4, pp. 327–335, 1999.
11. M. Kass, A. Witkin, and D. Terzopoulos, Snakes: Active contour models, *International Journal of Computer Vision*, vol. 1, pp. 321–331, 1987.
12. S. Osher and J. A. Sethian, Fronts propagating with curvature-dependent speed: Algorithms based on Hamilton–Jacobi formulations, *Journal of Computational Physics*, vol. 79, no. 1, pp. 12–49, 1988.
13. M. Jacob, T. Blu, and M. User, Efficient energies and algorithms for parametric snakes, *IEEE Transactions on Image Processing*, vol. 13, no. 9, pp. 1231–1244, 2004.
14. C. Xu and J. L. Prince, Generalized gradient vector flow external force for active contours, *Signal Processing*, vol. 71, no. 2, pp. 131–139, 1998.
15. J. Gao, A. Kosaka, and A. Kak, A deformable model for human organ extraction, in *Proceedings of the IEEE International Conference on Image Processing (ICIP)*, 1998, pp. 323–327.
16. S. Menet, P. Saint-Marc, and G. Medioni, B-snakes: Implementation and application to stereo, in *Proceedings DARPA*, 1990, pp. 720–726.

17. M. Gebhard, J. Mattes, and R. Eils, An active contour model for segmentation based on cubic B-splines and gradient vector flow, in *Medical Image Computing and Computer-Assisted Intervention–MICCAI*, 2001, pp. 1373–1375.

18. M. A. Figueiredo and J. M. N. Letao, Unsupervised contour representation and estimation using B-splines and minimum description length criteria, *IEEE Transaction on Image Processing*, vol. 9, no. 6, pp. 1075–1087, 2000.

19. P. Brigger, J. Hoeg, and M. User, B-splines snakes: A flexible tool for parametric contour detection, *IEEE Transaction on Image Processing*, vol. 9, no. 9, pp. 1484–1496, 2000.

20. L. H. Staib and J. S. Duncan, Boundary fitting with parametrically deformable model, *IEEE Transactions on Machine Intelligence*, vol. 14, no. 11, pp. 1061–1075, 1992.

21. B. Amarapur and P. K. Kulkarni, External force for deformable models in medical image segmentation: A survey, *Signal Image Process*, vol. 2, no. 2, pp. 82–101, 2011.

22. K.-J. Bathe and E.L. Wilson, *Numerical Methods in Finite Element Analysis*. Englewood Cliffs, NJ: Prentice–Hall, 1976.

23. T. McInerney and D. Terzopoulos, Deformable models in medical image analysis: A survey, *Medical Image Analysis*, vol. 1, no. 2, pp. 91–108, 1996.

24. A. A. Amini, T. E. Weymouth, and R. C. Jain, Using dynamic programming for solving variational problems in vision, *IEEE Transactions on Pattern Analysis and Machine Intelligence*, vol. 12, no. 9, pp. 855–867, 1990.

25. D. Terzopoulos, Deformable models: Classic, topology-adaptive and generalized formulations, in *Geometric Level Set Methods in Imaging, Vision, and Graphics*, pp. 21–40, 2003.

26. L. D. Cohen and I. Cohen, Finite-element methods for active contour models and balloons for 2-D and 3-D images, *IEEE Transactions on Pattern Analysis and Machine Intelligence*, vol. 15, no. 11, pp. 1131–1147, 1993.

27. L. D. Cohen, On active contour models and balloons, *CVGIP: Image Understanding*, vol. 53, no. 2, pp. 211–218, 1991.

28. C. Chen, T. L. Poepping, J. J. Beech-Brandt, S. J. Hammer, R. Baldock, B. Hill, P. Allan, W. J. Easson, and P. R. Hoskins, Segmentation of arterial geometry from ultrasound images using balloon models, in *Proceedings of IEEE International Symposium on Biomedical Imaging: Nano to Macro*, 2004, pp. 1319–1322.

29. C. Xu and J. L. Prince, Snakes, shapes, and gradient vector flow, *IEEE Transactions on Image Processing*, vol. 7, no. 3, pp. 359–369, 1998.

30. A. El-Baz and G. Gimel'farb, Image segmentation with a parametric deformable model using shape and appearance priors, in *IEEE Conference on Computer Vision and Pattern Recognition*, 2008, pp. 1–8.

31. V. Caselles, R. Kimmel, and G. Sapiro, Geodesic active contours, in *Fifth International Conference on Computer Vision*, 1995, pp. 694–699.

32. R. Mallabadi, J. A. Sethian, and B. C. Vemuri, Shape modeling with front propagation: A level set approach, *IEEE Transactions on Pattern Annual, Machine Intelligence*, vol. 17, no. 2, pp. 158–175, 1995.

33. A. Chakkraborthy, L. H. Staib, and J. S. Duncan, Deformable boundary finding in medical images by integrating gradient and region information, *IEEE Transaction on Medical Imaging*, vol. 15, no 6, pp. 859–870, 1996.

34. J. A. Sethian, *Level Set Methods and Fast Marching Methods: Evolving Interfaces in Computational Geometry, Fluid Mechanics, Computer Vision and Material Science*, vol. 3. Cambridge: Cambridge University Press, 1999.

35. G. Sapiro, *Geometric Partial Differential Equation and Image Analysis*. Cambridge: Cambridge University Press, 2006.

36. C. Xu, A. Yezzi Jr, and J. L. Prince, On the relationship between parametric and geometric active contours, in *Conference Record of the 34th Asilomar Conference on Signals, Systems and Computers*, vol. 1, 2000, pp. 483–489.

37. J. J. Koenderink and A. J. van Doorn, Surface shape and curvature scales, *Image and Vision Computing*, vol. 10, no. 8, pp. 557–564, 1992.

38. R. Kimmel, Intrinsic scale space for images on surfaces: The geodesic curvature flow, in *Scale-Space Theory in Computer Vision*, pp. 212–223, 1997.
39. G. Tryggvason, B. Bunner, D. Juric, W. Tauber, S. Nas, J. Han, N. Al-Rawahi, and Y.-J. Jan, A front tracking method for the computations of multiphase flow, *Journal of Computational Physics*, vol. 169, no. 2, pp. 708–759, 2001.
40. S. Osher, Stanley, and N. Paragios, (Eds.), *Geometric Level Set Methods in Imaging, Vision, and Graphics*. Berlin: Springer Science & Business Media, 2003.
41. S. Osher and R. Fedkiw, *Level Set Methods and Dynamic Implicit Surfaces*. Berlin: Springer Science & Business Media, vol. 153, 2003.
42. J. Strikwerda, *Finite Difference Schemes and Partial Differential Equations*. Pacific Grove, CA: Wadsworth & Brooks/Cole Advanced Books and Software, 1989.
43. A. Harten, B. Engquist, S. Osher, and S. Chakravarthy, Uniformly high-order accurate essentially non-oscillatory schemes III, *Journal of Computational Physics*, vol. 71, no. 2, pp. 231–303, 1987.
44. C. W. Shu and S. Osher, Efficient implementation of essentially non-oscillatory shock capturing schemes, *Journal of Computational Physics*, vol. 77, no. 2, pp. 439–471, 1988.
45. L. M. Milne-Thomson. *The Calculus of Finite Differences*, American Mathematical Society, 2000.
46. X. D. Liu, S. Osher, and T. Chan, Weighted essentially non-oscillatory schemes, *Journal of Computational Physics*, vol. 115, no. 1, pp. 202–212, 1994.
47. S. Osher and C. W. Shu, High order essentially non-oscillatory schemes for Hamilton–Jacobi equations, *SIAM Journal on Numerical Analysis*, vol. 28, no. 4, pp. 902–921, 1991.
48. G. S. Jiang and C. W. Shu, Efficient implementation of weighted ENO schemes, *Journal of Computational Physics*, vol. 126, pp. 202–228, 1996.
49. G. S. Jiang and D. Peng, Weighted ENO schemes for Hamilton–Jacobi equations, *SIAM Journal on Scientific Computing*, vol. 21, no. 6, pp. 2126–2143, 2000.
50. R. Fedkiw, B. Merriman, and S. Osher, Simplified upwind discretization of systems of hyperbolic conservation laws containing advection equations, with applications to compressible flows of multiphase, chemically reacting and explosive materials, UCLA CAM Report 98–16, *Journal of Computational Physics*, 1998.
51. C. Hu and C. W. Shu, Weighted essentially non-oscillatory schemes on triangular meshes, *Journal of Computational Physics*, vol. 150, no. 1, pp. 97–127, 1999.
52. R. J. Spiteri and S. J. Ruuth, A new class of optimal high-order strong-stability-preserving time discretization methods, *SIAM Journal on Numerical Analysis*, vol. 40, no. 2, pp. 469–491, 2002.
53. M. G. Crandall and P.-L. Lions, Two approximations of solutions of Hamilton–Jacobi equations, *Mathematics of Computation*, vol. 43, no. 167, pp. 1–19, 1984.
54. S. Osher and C-W. Shu, High-order essentially nonoscillatory schemes for Hamilton–Jacobi equations, *SIAM Journal on Numerical Analysis*, vol. 28, no. 4, pp. 907–922, 1991.
55. S. K. Godunov, A finite difference method for the computation of discontinuous solutions of the equations of fluid dynamics, *Sbornik Mathematics*, vol. 47, 1959, pp. 357–393.
56. M. Bardi and S. Osher, The non-convex multidimensional riemann problem for Hamilton–Jacobi equations, *SIAM Journal on Mathematical Analysis*, vol. 22, no. 2, pp. 344–351, 1991.
57. O. P. Agrawal, Formulation of Euler–Lagrange equations for fractional variational problems, *Journal of Mathematical Analysis and Applications*, vol. 272, no. 1, pp. 368–379, 2002.
58. R. Fletcher and M. J. D. Powell, A rapidly convergent descent method for minimization, *The Computer Journal*, vol. 6, no. 2, pp. 163–168, 1963.
59. M. Sussman, P. Smereka, and S. Osher, A level set approach for computing solutions to incompressible two-phase flow, *Journal of Computational Physics*, vol. 114, no. 1, pp. 146–159, 1994.
60. D. L. Chopp, Computing minimal surfaces via level set curvature flow, *Journal of Computational Physics*, vol. 106, no. 1, pp. 77–91, 1993.
61. D. Adalsteinsson and J. A. Sethian, A fast level set method for propagating interfaces, *Journal of Computational Physics*, vol. 118, no. 2, pp. 269–277, 1995.

62. R. Goldenberg, R. Kimmel, E. Rivlin, and M. Rudzsky, Fast geodesic active contours, *IEEE Transactions on Image Processing*, vol. 10, no. 10, pp. 1467–1475, 2001.
63. S. Kichenassamy, A. Kumar, P. Olver, A. Tannenbaum, and A. Yezzi, Conformal curvature flows: From phase transitions to active vision, *Archive for Rational Mechanics and Analysis*, vol. 134, no. 3 pp. 275–301, 1996.
64. X. Bresson, S. Esedoğlu, P. Vandergheynst, J. P. Thiran, and S. Osher, Fast global minimization of the active contour/snake model, *Journal of Mathematical Imaging and Vision*, vol. 28, no. 2, pp. 151–167, 2007.
65. N. Paragios, O. Mellina-Gottardo, and V. Ramesh, Gradient vector flow fast geodesic active contours, in *Eighth IEEE International Conference on Computer Vision*, vol. 1, 2001, pp. 67–73.
66. T., Chan and L. Vese, Active contours without edges, *IEEE Transactions on Image Processing*, vol. 10, no. 2, pp. 266–277, 2001.
67. D. Mumford and J. Shah, Optimal approximations of piecewise smooth functions and associated variational problems, *Communications in Pure and Applied Mathematics*, vol. 42, no. 5, pp. 577–685, 1989.
68. A. Chambolle, An algorithm for total variation minimization and applications, *Journal of Mathematical Imaging and Vision*, vol. 20, no. 1–2, pp. 89–97, 2004.
69. A. El-Baz, A. Farag, H. Abd El Munim, and S. E. Yuksel, Level set segmentation using statistical shape priors, in *IEEE Conference on Computer Vision and Pattern Recognition Workshop*, 2006, pp. 78–85.
70. D. Jayadevappa, S. S. Kumar, and D. S. Murty, Medical image segmentation algorithms using deformable models: A review, *IETE Technical Review*, vol. 28, no. 3, pp. 248–255, 2011.
71. L. He, Z. Peng, B. Everding, X. Wang, C. Y. Han, K. L. Weiss, and W. G. Wee, A comparative study of deformable contour methods on medical image segmentation, *Image and Vision Computing*, vol. 26, no. 2, pp. 141–163, 2008.
72. A. Tsai, A. Yezzi Jr, W. Wells, C. Tempany, D. Tucker, A. Fan, W. Eric Grimson, and Alan Willsky. A shape-based approach to the segmentation of medical imagery using level sets, *IEEE Transactions on Medical Imaging*, vol. 22, no. 2, pp. 137–154, 2003.
73. C. Pluempitiwiriyawej, J. M. F. Moura, Y.-J. Lin Wu, and C. Ho, STACS: New active contour scheme for cardiac MR image segmentation, *IEEE Transactions on Medical Imaging*, vol. 24, no. 5, pp. 593–603, 2005.
74. J. Montagnat and H. Delingette, 4D deformable models with temporal constraints: Application to 4D cardiac image segmentation, *Medical Image Analysis*, vol. 9, no. 1, pp. 87–100, 2005.
75. F. Khalifa, G. Beache, A. El-Baz, and G. Gimel'farb, Deformable model guided by stochastic speed with application in cine image segmentation, in *International Conference on Image Processing (ICIP)*, 2010, pp. 1725–1728.
76. F. Khalifa, G. M. Beache, G. Gimel'farb, and A. El-Baz, A novel approach for accurate estimation of left ventricle global indexes from short-axis cine MRI, in *International Conference on Image Processing (ICIP)*, 2011, pp. 2697–2700.
77. F. Khalifa, G. M. Beache, M. Nitzken, G. Gimel'farb, G. Giridharan, and A. El-Baz, Automatic analysis of left ventricle wall thickness using short-axis cine CMR images, in *International Symposium on Biomedical Imaging: From Nano to Macro (ISBI)*, 2011, pp. 1306–1309.
78. M. G. Uzunbas, S. Zhang, K. M. Pohl, D. Metaxas, and L. Axel, Segmentation of myocardium using deformable regions and graph cuts, in *IEEE International Symposium on Biomedical Imaging (ISBI)*, 2012, pp. 254–257.
79. F. Khalifa, G. M. Beache, G. Gimel'farb, G. A. Giridharan, and A. El-Baz, Accurate automatic analysis of cardiac cine images, *IEEE Transactions on Biomedical Engineering*, vol. 59, no. 2 pp. 445–455, 2012.
80. S. Gopal, Y. Otaki, R. Arsanjani, D. Berman, D. Terzopoulos, and P. Slomka, Combining active appearance and deformable superquadric models for LV segmentation in cardiac MRI, *SPIE Medical Imaging*, 2013, vol. 4, pp. 86690G–86690G-8.

81. F. Khalifa, G. M. Beache, G. Gimel'farb, and A. El-Baz, A novel CAD system for analyzing cardiac first-pass MR images, in *IEEE International Conference on Pattern Recognition (ICPR)*, 2012, pp. 77–80.
82. F. Khalifa, G. Beache, A. Firjani, K. Welch, G. Gimel'farb, and A. El-Baz, A new non-rigid registration approach for motion correction of cardiac first-pass perfusion MRI, in *International Conference on Image Processing (ICIP'12)*, 2012, pp. 1665–1668.
83. F. Khalifa, G. M. Beache, A. Elnakib, H. Sliman, G. Gimel'farb, K. Conn Welch, and A. El-Baz, A new shape-based framework for the left ventricle wall segmentation from cardiac first-pass perfusion MRI, in *International Symposium on Biomedical Imaging (ISBI)*, 2013, pp. 41–44.
84. G. M. Beache, F. Khalifa, G. Gimel'farb, and A. El-Baz, Fully automated framework for the analysis of myocardial first-pass perfusion MR images, *Medical Physics*, vol. 41, no. 10, 2014.
85. H. Sliman, F. Khalifa, A. Elnakib, A. Soliman, G. Beache, A. Elmaghraby, G. Gimel'farb, and A. El-Baz, Myocardial borders segmentation from cine MR images using bi-directional coupled parametric deformable models, *Medical Physics*, vol. 40, no. 9, pp. 1–13, 2013.
86. H. Sliman, F. Khalifa, A. Elnakib, A. Soliman, G. Beache, A. Elmaghraby, and A. El-Baz, A new segmentation-based tracking framework for extracting the left ventricle cavity from cine cardiac MRI, in *IEEE International Conference on Image Processing (ICIP'13)*, 2013, pp. 685–689.
87. H. Sliman, F. Khalifa, A. Elnakib, A. Soliman, G. Beache, G. Gimel'Farb, A. Emam, A. Elmaghraby, and A. El-Baz, Accurate segmentation framework for the left ventricle wall from cardiac cine MRI, in *Proceedings of the International Symposium on Computational Models for Life Science*, vol. 1559, no. 1, 2013, pp. 287–296.
88. H. Sliman, A. Elnakib, G. M. Beache, A. Soliman, F. Khalifa, G. Gimel'farb, A. Elmaghraby, and A. El-Baz, A novel 4D PDE-based approach for accurate assessment of myocardium function using cine cardiac magnetic resonance images, in *IEEE International Conference on Image Processing (ICIP)*, 2014, pp. 3537–3541.
89. S. Ho, E. Bullitt, and G. Gerig, Level-set evolution with region competition: Automatic 3-D segmentation of brain tumors, in *International Conference on Pattern Recognition*, vol. 1, 2002, pp. 532–535.
90. R. Goldenberg, R. Kimmel, E. Rivlin, and M. Rudzsky, Cortex segmentation: A fast variational geometric approach, *IEEE Transactions on Medical Imaging*, vol. 21, no. 12, pp. 1544–1551, 2002.
91. L. Wang, F. Shi, W. Lin, J. H. Gilmore, and D. Shen, Automatic segmentation of neonatal images using convex optimization and coupled level sets, *NeuroImage*, vol. 58, no. 3, pp. 805–817, 2011.
92. L. Wang, F. Shi, P-T Yap, W. Lin, J. H. Gilmore, and D. Shen, Longitudinally guided level sets for consistent tissue segmentation of neonates, *Human Brain Mapping*, vol. 34, no. 4, pp. 956–972, 2013.
93. L. Wang, F. Shi, G. Li, Y. Gao, W. Lin, J. H. Gilmore, and D. Shen, Segmentation of neonatal brain MR images using patch-driven level sets, *NeuroImage*, vol. 84, pp. 141–158, 2014.
94. M. Casanova, A. El-Baz, and J. Suri, Editors, *Imaging the Brain in Autism*. New York: Springer-Verlag, 2013.
95. A. Alansary, M. Ismail, A. Soliman, F. Khalifa, M. Nitzken, A. Elnakib, M. F. Casanova, and A. El-Baz, Infant brain extraction in T1-weighted MR images using BET and refinement using LCDG and MGRF models, *IEEE Journal of Biomedical and Health Informatics*, vol. 20, no. 3, pp. 925–935, 2015.
96. A. Alansary, A. Soliman, M. Nitzken, F. Khalifa, A. Elnakib, M. F. Casanova, and A. El-Baz, An integrated geometrical and stochastic approach for accurate infant brain extraction, in *International Conference on Image Processing (ICIP)*, 2014, pp. 3542–3546.
97. M. Franaszek, R. M. Summers, P. J. Pickhardt, and J. R. Choi, Hybrid segmentation of colon filled with air and opacified fluid for CT colonography, *IEEE Transactions on Medical Imaging*, vol. 25, no. 3, pp. 358–368, 2006.
98. H. Zhu, M. Barish, P. Pickhardt, and Z. Liang, Haustral fold segmentation with curvature-guided level set evolution, *IEEE Transactions on Biomedical Engineering*, vol. 60, no. 2, pp. 321–331, 2013.

99. F. Khalifa, A. El-Baz, G. Gimel'farb, and M. Abu El-Ghar, Non-invasive image-based approach for early detection of acute renal rejection, in *Medical Image Computing and Computer-Assisted Intervention–MICCAI*, 2010, pp. 10–18.

100. F. Khalifa, A. Elnakib, G. M. Beache, G. Gimel'farb, M. Abo El-Ghar, R. Ouseph, G. Sokhadze, S. Manning, P. McClure, and A. El-Baz, 3D kidney segmentation from CT images using a level set approach guided by a novel stochastic speed function, in *Medical Image Computing and Computer-Assisted Intervention–MICCAI*, 2011, pp. 587–594.

101. F. Khalifa, G. Beache, M. Abou El-Ghar, T. El-Diasty, G. Gimel'farb, M. Kong, and A. El-Baz, Dynamic contrast-enhanced MRI-based early detection of acute renal transplant rejection, *IEEE Transactions on Medical Imaging*, vol. 32, no. 10, pp. 1910–1927, 2013.

102. F. Khalifa, A. Soliman, M. Abou El-Ghar, G. Gimel'farb, R. Ouseph, A. C. Dwyer, T. El-Diasty, and A. El-Baz, Models and methods for analyzing DCE MRI: A review, *Medical Physics*, vol. 41, no. 12, 2014.

103. F. Khalifa, M. Abou El-Ghar, B. Abdollahi, H. Frieboes, T. El-Diasty, and A. El-Baz, A comprehensive non-invasive framework for automated evaluation of acute renal transplant rejection using DCE-MRI, *NMR in Biomedicine*, vol. 26, no. 11, pp. 1460–1470, 2013.

104. F. Khalifa, G. Gimel'farb, M. Abo El-Ghar, G. Sokhadze, S. Manning, P. McClure, R. Ouseph, and A. El-Baz, A new deformable model-based segmentation approach for accurate extraction of the kidney from abdominal CT images, in *International Conference on Image Processing (ICIP)*, 2011, pp. 3454–3457.

105. F. Khalifa, A. El-Baz, G. Gimel'farb, R. Ouseph, and M. Abo El-Ghar, Shape-appearance guided level-set deformable model for image segmentation, in *International Conference on Pattern Recognition (ICPR)*, 2010, pp. 4581–4584.

106. M. Shehata, F. Khalifa, A. Soliman, R. Alrefai, M. Abou El-Ghar, and A. Dwyer, R. Ouseph, and A. El-Baz, A novel framework for automatic segmentation of kidney from DW-MRI, in *International Symposium on Biomedical Imaging: From Nano to Macro (ISBI)*, 2015, pp. 951–954.

107. M. Mostapha, F. Khalifa, A. Alansary, A. Soliman, G. Gimel'farb, and A. El-Baz, Dynamic MRI-based computer aided diagnostic system for early detection of kidney transplant rejection: A survey, in *International Symposium on Computational Models for Life Science*, vol. 1559, no. 1, pp. 297–306, 2013.

108. M. Mostapha, F. Khalifa, A. Alansary, A. Soliman, J. Suri, and A. El-Baz, Computer aided diagnosis systems for acute renal transplant rejection: Challenges and methodologies, in *Handbook Abdomen and Thoracic Imaging: An Engineering and Clinical Perspective*, A. El-Baz, L. Saba, and J. Suri, Eds. New York: Springer-Verlag, 2014, ch. 1, pp. 1–36.

109. S. Yuksel, A. El-Baz, and A. Farag, A kidney segmentation framework for dynamic contrast enhanced magnetic resonance imaging, *Journal of Vibration and Control*, vol. 13, no. 5, pp. 1505–1516, 2007.

110. A. El-Baz, A. Farag, S. Yuksel, M. Abou El-Ghar, T. Eldiasty, and M. Ghoneim, Application of deformable models for the detection of acute renal rejection, in *Handbook of Parametric and Geometric Deformable Models: An Application in Biomaterials and Medical Imagery*, J. S. Suri and A. Farag, Eds. Berlin: Springer, August, 2007, Volume. 2, Chapter 10, pp. 293–334.

111. A. El-Baz, G. Gimel'farb, and M. Abou El-Ghar, Image analysis approach for identification of renal transplant rejection, in *International Conference on Pattern Recognition (ICPR)*, 2008, pp. 1–4.99,102,103,107–110,114–123

112. A. El-Baz, G. Gimel'farb, and M. El-Ghar, A novel image analysis approach for accurate identification of acute renal rejection, in *IEEE International Conference on Image Processing (ICIP)*, 2008, pp. 1812–1815.

113. A. El-Baz, G. Gimel'farb, and M. Abou El-Ghar, New motion correction models for automatic identification of renal transplant rejection, in *International Conference on Medical Image Computing and Computer-Assisted Intervention (MICCAI)*, 2007, pp. 235–243.

114. A. Farag, A. El-Baz, S. Yuksel, T. El-Diasty, and M. Ghoneim, A framework for the detection of acute rejection with dynamic contrast enhanced magnetic resonance imaging, in *International Symposium on Biomedical Imaging: From Nano to Macro (ISBI)*, 2006, pp. 418–421.

115. E. Yuksel, A. El-Baz, and A. Farag, A kidney segmentation framework for dynamic contrast enhanced magnetic resonance imaging, in *International Symposium on Mathematical Methods in Engineering (MME'06)*, 2006, pp. 55–64.
116. A. El-Baz, A. Farag, R. Fahmi, S. Yuksel, M. Abou El-Ghar, and T. Eldiasty, Image analysis of renal DCE MRI for the detection of acute renal rejection, in *International Conference on Pattern Recognition (ICPR)*, vol. 3, 2006, pp. 822–825.
117. A. El-Baz, A. Farag, R. Fahmi, S. Yuksel, W. Miller, M. Abou El-Ghar, T. El-Diasty, and M. Ghoneim, A new CAD system for the evaluation of kidney diseases using DCE-MRI, in *International Conference on Medical Image Computing and Computer-Assisted Intervention (MICCAI)*, vol. 2, 2006, pp. 446–453.
118. S. Yuksel, A. El-Baz, A. Farag, M. Abou El-Ghar, T. Eldiasty, and M. Ghoneim, Automatic detection of renal rejection after kidney transplantation, in *Proceedings of Computer Assisted Radiology and Surgery (CARS)*, 2005, pp. 773–778.
119. M. Cvancarova, F. Albregtsen, K. Brabrand, and E. Samset, Segmentation of ultrasound images of liver tumors applying snake algorithms and GVF, in *International Congress Series*, vol. 1281, 2005, pp. 218–223.
120. E. Goceri, M. Z. Unlu, C. Guzelis, and O. Dicle, An automatic level set-based liver segmentation from MRI data sets, in *International Conference on Image Processing Theory, Tools and Applications (IPTA)*, 2012, pp. 192–197.
121. B. N. Li, C. K. Chui, S. Chang, and S. H. Ong, A new unified level set method for semiautomatic liver tumor segmentation on contrast-enhanced CT images, *Expert Systems with Applications*, vol. 39, no. 10, pp. 9661–9668, 2012.
122. N. Ray, S. T. Acton, T. Altes, E. E. De Lange, and J. R. Brookeman, Merging parametric active contours within homogeneous image regions for MRI-based lung segmentation, in *IEEE Transactions on Medical Imaging*, vol. 22, no. 2, pp. 189–199, 2003.
123. A. A. Farag, A. El-Baz, G. G. Gimel'farb, R. Falk, and S. G. Hushek, Automatic detection and recognition of lung abnormalities in helical CT images using deformable templates, in *Medical Image Computing and Computer-Assisted Intervention–MICCAI*, 2004, pp. 856–864.
124. S. Liu and J. Li, Automatic medical image segmentation using gradient and intensity combined level set method, in *International Conference of the Engineering in Medicine and Biology Society*, 2006, pp. 3118–3121.
125. A. A. Farag, A. El-Baz, G. Gimel'farb, R. Falk, M. A. El-Ghar, T. Eldiasty, and S. Elshazly, Appearance models for robust segmentation of pulmonary nodules in 3D LDCT chest images, in *Medical Image Computing and Computer-Assisted Intervention–MICCAI*, 2006, pp. 662–670.
126. A. El-Baz, G. Gimel'farb, R. Falk, T. Holland, and T. Shaffer, A new stochastic framework for accurate lung segmentation, in *Medical Image Computing and Computer-Assisted Intervention–MICCAI*, 2008, pp. 322–330.
127. A. El-Baz, G. Gimel'farb, R. Falk, and M. Abo El-Ghar, Automatic analysis of 3D low dose CT images for early diagnosis of lung cancer, *Pattern Recognition*, vol. 42, no. 6, pp. 1041–1051, 2009.
128. A. Soliman, F. Khalifa, A. Alansary, G. Gimel'farb, and A. El-Baz, Segmentation of lung region based on using parallel implementation of joint MGRF: Validation on 3D realistic lung phantoms, in *International Symposium on Biomedical Imaging (ISBI)*, 2013, pp. 864–867.
129. A. El-Baz, G. Beache, G. Gimel'farb, K. Suzuki, and K. Okada, Lung imaging data analysis, *International Journal of Biomedical Imaging*, vol. 2013, pp. 1–2, 2013.
130. A. El-Baz, P. Sethu, G. Gimel'farb, F. Khalifa, A. Elnakib, R. Falk, and M. Abo El-Ghar, Elastic phantoms generated by microfluidics technology: Validation of an imaged-based approach for accurate measurement of the growth rate of lung nodules, *Biotechnology Journal*, vol. 6, no. 2, pp. 195–203, February 2011.
131. A. El-Baz, G. Gimel'farb, R. Falk, and M. Abo El-Ghar, 3D MGRF-based appearance modeling for robust segmentation of pulmonary nodules in 3D LDCT chest images, in *Handbook of Lung Imaging and Computer Aided Diagnosis*, A. El-Baz and J. Suri, Eds. Boca Raton, FL: Taylor & Francis, October 2011, ch. 3.

132. A. El-Baz, G. Gimel'farb, R. Falk, and M. Abo El-Ghar, A novel level set-based CAD system for automatic detection of lung nodules in low dose chest CT scans, in *Handbook of Lung Imaging and Computer Aided Diagnosis*, A. El-Baz and J. Suri, Eds. Boca Raton, FL: Taylor & Francis, October 2011, ch. 10.

133. A. El-Baz, G. Gimel'farb, R. Falk, M. Abo El-Ghar, and J. Suri, Appearance analysis for the early assessment of detected lung nodules, in *Handbook of Lung Imaging and Computer Aided Diagnosis*, A. El-Baz and J. Suri, Eds. Boca Raton, FL: Taylor & Francis, October 2011, ch. 17.

134. A. El-Baz, P. Sethu, G. Gimel'farb, F. Khalifa, A. Elnakib, R. Falk, M. Abo El-Ghar, and J. Suri, Validation of a new imaged-based approach for the accurate estimating of the growth rate of detected lung nodules using real CT images and elastic phantoms generated by state-of-the-art microfluidics technology, in *Handbook of Lung Imaging and Computer Aided Diagnosis*, A. El-Baz and J. Suri, Eds. Boca Raton, FL: Taylor & Francis, October 2011, ch. 18.

135. A. El-Baz, A. Farag, G. Gimel'farb, R. Falk, M. Abou El-Ghar, and T. Eldiasty, A framework for automatic segmentation of lung nodules from low dose chest CT scans, in *Proc. of International Conference on Pattern Recognition (ICPR'06)*, Hong Kong, August 20–24, 2006, vol. 3, pp. 611–614.

136. A. El-Baz, A. Ali, A. Farag, and G. Gimel'farb, A novel approach for image alignment using a Markov-Gibbs appearance model, in *Proc. of International Conference on Medical Image Computing and Computer-Assisted Intervention (MICCAI'06)*, Copenhagen, Denmark, October 1–6, 2006, vol. 2, pp. 734–741.

137. Y. Zhan and D. Shen, Deformable segmentation of 3-D ultrasound prostate images using statistical texture matching method, in *IEEE Transactions on Medical Imaging*, vol. 25, no. 3, pp. 256–272, 2006.

138. M. J. Costa, H. Delingette, S. Novellas, and N. Ayache, Automatic segmentation of bladder and prostate using coupled 3D deformable models, in *Medical Image Computing and Computer-Assisted Intervention–MICCAI*, pp. 252–260. Springer Berlin, Heidelberg, 2007.

139. N. Makni, P. Puech, R. Lopes, A-S Dewalle, O. Colot, and N. Betrouni, Combining a deformable model and a probabilistic framework for an automatic 3D segmentation of prostate on MRI, *International Journal of Computer Assisted Radiology and Surgery*, vol. 4, no. 2, pp. 181–188, 2009.

140. A. Firjany, A. Elnakib, A. El-Baz, G. Gimel'farb, M. Abo El-Ghar, and A. Elmagharby, Novel stochastic framework for accurate segmentation of prostate in dynamic contrast enhanced MRI, *Prostate Cancer Imaging. Computer-Aided Diagnosis, Prognosis, and Intervention*, 2010, pp. 121–130.

141. A. Firjani, A. Elnakib, F. Khalifa, G. Gimel'farb, M. Abo El-Ghar, A. Elmaghraby, and A. El-Baz, A new 3D automatic segmentation framework for accurate extraction of prostate from diffusion imaging, in *Biomedical Sciences and Engineering Conference (BSEC)*, 2011, pp. 1–4.

142. A. Firjani, A. Elnakib, F. Khalifa, G. Gimel'farb, M. Abo El-Ghar, J. Suri, A. Elmaghraby, and A. El-Baz, A new 3D automatic segmentation framework for accurate segmentation of prostate from DCE-MRI, in *International Symposium on Biomedical Imaging: From Nano to Macro*, 2011, pp. 1476–1479.

143. A. Firjani, A. Elnakib, F. Khalifa, G. Gimel'farb, M. Abou El-Ghar, A. Elmaghraby, and A. El-Baz, A diffusion-weighted imaging based diagnostic system for early detection of prostate cancer, *Journal of Biomedical Science and Engineering*, vol. 6, no. 3, pp. 346–356, 2013.

144. A. Firjani, F. Khalifa, A. Elnakib, G. Gimel'farb, M. Abou El-Ghar, A. Elmaghraby, and A. El-Baz, A novel image-based approach for early detection of prostate cancer using DCE-MRI, in *Handbook of Computational Intelligence in Biomedical Imaging*, K. Suzuki Ed. New York: Springer-Verlag, 2014, ch. 1, pp. 55–82.

145. A. Firjani, A. Elmaghraby, and A. El-Baz, MRI-based diagnostic system for early detection of prostate cancer, in *Biomedical Sciences and Engineering Conference (BSEC)*, 2013, pp. 1–4.

146. A. Firjani, F. Khalifa, A. Elnakib, G. Gimel'farb, M. Abo El-Ghar, A. Elmaghraby, and A. El-Baz, 3D automatic approach for precise segmentation of the prostate from diffusion-weighted magnetic resonance imaging, in *Proc. IEEE International Conference on Image Processing (ICIP'11)*, pp. 2333–2337, 2011.

147. P. McClure, F. Khalifa, A. Soliman, M. Abou El-Ghar, G. Gimelfarb, A. Elmagraby, and A. El-Baz, A novel NMF guided level-set for DWI prostate segmentation, *Journal of Computer Science & System Biology*, vol. 7, no. 6, pp. 209–216, 2014.

148. P. McClure, A. Elnakib, M. Abou El-Ghar, F. Khalifa, A. Soliman, T. El-Diasty, J. S. Suri, Adel Elmaghraby, and A. El-Baz, In vitro and in vivo diagnostic techniques for prostate cancer: A review, *Journal of Biomedical Nanotechnology*, vol. 10, pp. 2747–2777, 2014.

149. B. N. Li, C. K. Chui, S. Chang, and S. H. Ong, Integrating spatial fuzzy clustering with level set methods for automated medical image segmentation, *Computers in Biology and Medicine*, vol. 41, no. 1, pp. 1–10, 2011.

150. S. D. S. Al-Shaikhli, M. Y. Yang, and B. Rosenhahn, Medical image segmentation using multi-level set partitioning with topological graph prior, in *Image and Video Technology–PSIVT Workshops*, Berlin: Springer, 2014, pp. 157–168.

chapter two

Domain knowledge for level set segmentation in medical imaging
A review

Klaus D. Toennies, Tim König, and Oliver Gloger

Contents

Abstract

The level set framework is a very variable concept for specifying an optimal function for some purpose and one of the ways to arrive at this function given an initialization. If used for segmentation, the function assigns a label to each pixel or voxel. Optimality is defined based on desired segmentation properties. In medical images, segmentation often includes a detection step to extract some specific object via segmentation. This requires segmentation criteria that account for unique attributes of the object to be extracted (such as a characteristic shape), generic attributes (such as smooth boundaries), and potentially also attributes that allow to suppress influences from artifacts.

In this chapter, we review recent applications of level set methods to segmentation problems in medical images. We concentrate on a treatment of how domain knowledge about objects and imaging artifacts is represented and integrated into the segmentation solution. We will distinguish between means to add this information before, during, and after level set segmentation and discuss methodology and benefits of each of these different strategies.

2.1   Introduction

A T-level set of a function f is the set of all locations $\mathbf{x}$ where the function has a specific value $f(\mathbf{x}) = T$. If f is continuous, each of its level sets is a set of closed hypersurfaces (curves, surfaces, etc.) separating the interior from the exterior. Used for segmentation, level sets represent segment boundaries. A simple example would be the 0-level set of the Laplace operator. Assuming that intensity values are samples of a continuous, twice-differentiable function, the 0-level set, that is, the zero-crossings of the Laplacian, represents a segmentation of an image with homogeneity of the intensity function being the segmentation criterion.

However, the level set model, as it is commonly used for segmentation, is more. It provides a mechanism to find a separation under a great variety of segmentation conditions. It integrates model and data terms with schemes to evolve the level set function from an initial level set function toward the desired result.

The level set function is defined as an implicit function of image space $\mathbf{x} = (x_1\ x_2 \dots x_N)$ of arbitrary dimension N. Two approaches exist to evolve an initial level set to the desired segmentation. The front propagation of Sethian [1] and Osher and Fedkiw [2] embeds the N-dimensional level set function into $(N + 1)$-dimensional space with an artificial time t as additional dimension. A wide variety of so-called speed functions may be defined that specify how the level set function evolves in time. Level set evolution may also be derived from the derivative of a functional describing the desired optimal solution. The derivative has a similar semantic than the speed function specifying how the level set function evolves toward the optimum. Different from front propagation, such a variational level set defines the searched optimum and moves toward it by gradient descent on the functional, whereas it is not always easy to derive a definition of an optimal level set if only the speed function is given. The variational approach has been applied, for example, by Caselles et al. [3] in their introduction of geodesic active contours and by Chan and Vese [4] for their active contours without edges.

Using *front propagation*, the desired segmentation is achieved by specifying constraints that let the initial wave propagate toward its final result. Hence, level set propagation reduces to an initial value problem where values (in this case, level set functions) of a differential equation are estimated from finite difference given the initial level set. The change ϕ_t of ϕ in time t is given by

$$\phi_t = -F|\nabla\phi| \tag{2.1}$$

where the speed function F determines wave propagation based on local and global properties of ϕ itself (the model terms) and on image-related terms (the data terms). The function ϕ may be chosen arbitrarily, but assuming it to be a signed distance function ($|\nabla(\phi)| = 1$)

avoids numerical problems when computing level set propagation. If used for segmentation, data terms of F are usually decrease with the length of the intensity gradient. It causes the propagation to slow down near the edges. The global and local properties of the level set function are set in a way to expand (or shrink) the level set and to prefer smooth boundaries (e.g., by using curvature of the level set as criterion). As mentioned above, the front propagation method does not describe a priori what minimum should be found and may not even possess a nontrivial minimum. Thus, a criterion is needed to define when to stop wave propagation. This is usually related to the speed of propagation (e.g., propagation is terminated when for a certain time the 0-level set did change by less than a prespecified rate).

The data and model terms are separated from the propagation method. Hence, computation is independent of these terms, although choosing the speed function has a substantial influence on the convergence speed. Front propagation is attractive since the developer can chose among a variety of different speed functions without having to reparameterize or reformulate the wave evolution method.

Front propagation methods often employ the narrow band technique for speeding up convergence of the level set. This implicitly adds a localization prior since the level set is evolved only in the vicinity of the 0-level set. Hence, if the user places an initial 0-level set, the final segmentation will prefer segment boundaries that are close to this initial level set. Although this is often advantageous, parts of an object may not be found because the 0-level set never moved close enough for including this part of the image into the level set computation.

The evolution of the level set function deforms the signed distance wave. Since this may lead to artifacts, it requires frequent reinitialization of the wave form.

Variational level set evolution is derived from the direct specification of a condition for an optimal level set function. An initial guess is evolved toward this function along the gradient of the functional using variational techniques. Optimality is defined as minimization of energy functional from integrating a function f of ϕ over the domain Ω of the level set function:

$$E(\phi) = \int_\Omega f(\phi(\mathbf{x}), \nabla\phi(\mathbf{x}))d\mathbf{x} \qquad (2.2)$$

Given an initial level set $\phi^{(0)}$, the functional is minimized by evolving ϕ in the direction of its derivative (the Euler–Lagrange derivative, e.g., in Chan and Vese [4] or the Gateaux derivative as generalized directional derivative, e.g., in Cremers et al. [5]). The derivative has to be computed based on the specific constraint f. Since the energy is integrated over the complete region, region-based terms are possible as part of the functional. An example is the active contours without edges approach presented by Chan and Vese [4]. The (regularized) Heaviside function H defines two different regions based on the sign of the level set function. The energy is given by the difference of the intensity function I from an expected value c_1 and c_2, respectively. The gradient of the Heaviside function, that is, the Dirac function δ, penalizes long boundaries between the two regions. The minimization of this functional

$$E(\phi) = \int_\Omega \alpha_1 H(\phi(\mathbf{x}))[I(\mathbf{x}) - c_1] + \alpha_2[1 - H(\phi(\mathbf{x}))][I(\mathbf{x}) - c_2] + \alpha_3\delta(\phi(\mathbf{x}))d\mathbf{x} \qquad (2.3)$$

over region Ω optimizes a specialization of the Mumford–Shah functional. It assumes that segments have a constant intensity and that segments of two different kinds, that is, with

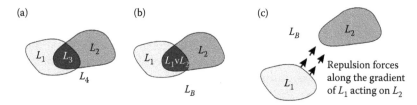

Figure 2.1 (a) If multiphase level sets are used, n level sets define 2^n different segments. For $n = 2$, this results in four different segments. (b) If each segment L_i is represented by its own level set functions, then a background region L_B is defined as a set of all pixels or voxels where all level set functions are negative. It is possible that segments overlap. (c) Repulsion forces along the gradient of the level set function may be used to avoid overlapping segments.

two different intensities, have to be separated. The weights α_1, α_2, and α_3 depend on the importance and/or reliability of the three constraints.

The formulation has later been extended to separate multiple objects by combining several level set functions. For instance, four different regions can be separated, if two level set functions ϕ_1 and ϕ_2 are defined (see Figure 2.1a). The regions are then given by

$$H(\phi_1(\mathbf{x}))H(\phi_2(\mathbf{x})),$$

$$H(\phi_1(\mathbf{x}))(1 - H(\phi_2(\mathbf{x}))),$$

$$(1 - H(\phi_1(\mathbf{x})))H(\phi_2(\mathbf{x})),$$

$$(1 - H(\phi_1(\mathbf{x})))(1 - H(\phi_2(\mathbf{x}))).$$

An alternative for multiple segments is to assign $r = 1, \ldots, R - 1$ level set functions to segment an object into $R - 1$ regions plus a background region (e.g., the work of Yazdanpanah et al. [6]). A pixel belongs to region r if it has a positive distance to the r-th 0-level set. Different from the above case, this strategy allows segments to overlap and therefore requires defining the semantics of overlapping segments (see Figure 2.1b,c).

If the functional is convex (this would be, for instance, the case if the two intensities c_1 and c_2 were fixed and known), fast schemes exist that produce the optimal result independent of initialization. If functionals are non-convex, the final segmentation will depend on the initial level set function. This dependence is often desired to add a position constraint to the segmentation.

The level set formulation above may also be used to define more complex homogeneity constraints. Chan et al. [7] already extended it to define homogeneity between vectors of function values.

An example for using multiple input channels in medical imaging is the work of Klann et al. [8] to reconstruct single photon emission computed tomography (SPECT) images. Here, two independent types of information, the attenuation of γ-rays in tissue, and the activity distribution of the tracer are jointly computed by maximizing local contrast and searching for short segment boundaries.

Different from front propagation, iterative evolution is not separated from the evolution constraints (as in the speed function). Each new energy formulation requires computation of its own derivative. Regularization techniques are often used to overcome singularities for nonlinear inverse problems.

As in front propagation, the level set function is assumed to be a signed distance function. This requires again either frequent reinitialization or the inclusion of an extra term into the energy functional that penalizes deviation from a signed distance function. Also, the narrow band technique for speeding up computation may be used, since, for example, the optimization of Equation 2.3 results in an iterative scheme that requires updates only in the vicinity of the current 0-level set.

Level set segmentation has been used for numerous applications in medical imaging. This often includes the extraction of a specific object. Segmentation criteria, such as the ones defined by the Mumford–Shah functional, need to be supplemented by information that identifies this object. Integrating this information into the level set function may become difficult as level sets are defined in the 2D or 3D image domain, whereas many of the conditions are invariant w.r.t. transformations (such as rotations, translations, scaling) in just this domain.

2.2 Domain knowledge in medical image segmentation

Domain knowledge is used to separate the object from other objects with similar appearance and also to account for artifacts in the image that alter the expected appearance of an object (such as noise or shading). Since the choice of a medical imaging device is intentional, the object of interest (organ, pathological process, etc.) is expected to be discernible in the image. Hence, expected intensity is often part of the domain knowledge. It may simply be given by the expected value of intensity in the segment but may also contain more information of the distribution characteristics, such as the parameterization of a normal distribution, a Gaussian mixture model, or an arbitrary distribution function. In this case, the domain knowledge implicitly encompasses also information about artifacts, such as noise or shading, which are source of intensity variation in the object and the background. Parameters of these distribution characteristics are estimated from training data.

Texture may be used as well to describe the appearance of objects [9,10]. Paragios and Deriche [9] use a set of filter responses—containing Gaussian, Laplacian, and Gabor filters—to derive probabilistic texture descriptors, which are then integrated into a Bayesian probabilistic framework. An energy functional containing a level set function is derived, which is minimized by using variational methods.

However, texture is not often used for the segmentation of medical images, since the spatial resolution of medical images is usually insufficient to reveal textures of tissues (with the exception of microscopic images). One of the few examples is Wang et al. [11], who extend the work of Vemuri et al. [12] on diffusion tensor imaging level sets. Wang et al. [11] use Gabor wavelets of Paragios and Deriche [9] to compute texture features for each pixel that are represented by rank-3 tensors. They are then segmented by an extension defined by Chan and Vese [4], which accepts tensors in the regional terms. In Olveres et al. [13], texture descriptors based on the Hermite transform are incorporated in a vector-valued and region-based level set segmentation to quantify left ventricular blood flow in computed tomography (CT) images.

Instead of using region intensity, the intensity difference between the object and background may be used as part of the boundary characteristics. Since the object of interest may not be the one with highest contrast in the image, the expected gradient length may be used to represent this information. Parameterization may be derived from training or set a priori by the user. Furthermore, most medical objects do not possess sharp corners. Hence, boundary smoothness is also part of the domain knowledge.

Low-level local domain knowledge such as that presented above may be insufficient to extract an object of interest, since other objects may have similar appearance. Furthermore, no boundary may be visible if two such similar objects touch each other. In such a case, the expected shape of the object is needed to complete the segment boundary in regions of insufficient contrast. If shape is sufficiently characteristic of the object, it may also be used for its detection. The shape representation has then to be able to distinguish between acceptable within-class shape variation and between-class variation.

An average shape may be useful for detecting an object, but is not sufficient for guiding the boundary search at locations with nonexisting contrast between object and background. Shape and shape variation may either be trained from representative sample shapes (statistical shape models [14], possibly also including shape-dependent appearance information [15]) or be predefined as elastic deformation of an average shape (e.g., in atlas-based segmentation).

Location and orientation are also important to detect objects in medical images. For many medical imaging devices, the positioning of the patient in the device is highly restricted. Hence, a weak relationship exists between the known device coordinate system and an unknown patient coordinate system. If the object of interest has a preferred location and orientation in the patient coordinate system, this knowledge can be applied to the location in image device coordinates. Since the information is not exact, it is more useful for detecting an object than for delineating the object's boundary.

Detection may also be supported by information about the expected spatial configuration of the searched object with respect to other objects. Again, atlases may be used to represent this knowledge. Alternatively, a part model may be constructed, consisting of the object of interest and all spatially related objects as its parts. The shape and appearance of the parts as well as the specific configuration serve to identify the correct object location. An acceptable variation of part relationships may be trained from examples or prespecified via a deformable atlas or a deformable part model.

2.3   Integration of domain knowledge into level set segmentation

Domain knowledge for object detection and segmentation may be applied prior to level set segmentation, integrated into the level set model, or used to postprocess results from level set segmentation. If used in preprocessing, it maps domain knowledge into the image domain. Hence, it can be treated as part of the data terms. If, on the other hand, domain knowledge is integrated into the level set function, it is part of the model terms. Then, potential dependencies between domain knowledge and data terms can be accommodated as the domain knowledge and not its mapping onto image space is optimized. Sometimes, level set segmentation is corrected by a postprocessing step. This is particularly suitable if properties of segments from the level set step can be used for selecting a subset from the segments that actually represent the object of interest. The three different strategies will be discussed in the following sections.

2.3.1   Preprocessing

The purpose of preprocessing is either to map image intensities to a function to which applying the data term of the level set model is easier, or to map additional information to the image domain so that it can be used as additional data term.

2.3.1.1   Noise reduction and boundary enhancement

An often used preprocessing step is edge-preserving noise reduction, for example, by anisotropic diffusion. Boundary-based level sets, such as most front propagation methods or geodesic active contours [3], indirectly take care of influences from noise by linear

filtering the gradient information and by enforcing smooth boundaries. It requires a sufficiently strong signal so that smoothing does not reduce local contrast too much. Methods
based on region terms [4] enforce boundary smoothness indirectly by searching for short
object boundaries. However, if the noise level is too high compared to the local contrast or
if local intensity variation is present but has not been accounted for, the computed object
boundary may become too ragged. Edge-preserving smoothing then uses a simple edge
model for removing noise and creating smooth boundaries prior to level set segmentation.
Examples for such preprocessing are soft tissue segmentation in CT [16] or liver segmentation in MRI [17]. A more elaborate approach was presented by Lee et al. [18]. The authors
compute gradient vector flow from gradients. Gradient vector flow optimizes flow at each
point in the scene to a possible edge subject to smoothness and distance constraints. It has
originally been presented by Xu and Prince [19] to guide an explicit active contour and has
been shown to allow a contour to evolve into concavities (which is otherwise hindered by
the constraint of finding short boundaries).

Successful noise reduction may even allow removing the smoothness term from the
level set equation. This was done in Shyu et al. [20] in their variational formulation of a
fuzzy clustering-based segmentation. It resulted in a greatly simplified update rule for the
level set function as the model term on the boundary length is removed from Equation 2.3.
If the average values c_1 and c_2 in Equation 2.3 are known and constant, optimization can
be done in a single step based on the histogram of data values $I(\mathbf{x})$. The optimal 0-level set
would consist of all locations $\mathbf{x}$ with

$$I(\mathbf{x}) = \frac{1}{2}(\alpha_1 c_1 + \alpha_2 c_2) \tag{2.4}$$

and the level set function would be generated from this equation. If c_1 and c_2 represent
average values of the current foreground and background segments, optimization reduces
to computation of current averages:

$$c_1 = \frac{\int_\Omega H(\phi(\mathbf{x}))I(\mathbf{x})d\mathbf{x}}{\int_\Omega H(\phi(\mathbf{x}))d\mathbf{x}} \quad \text{and} \quad c_2 = \frac{\int_\Omega (1 - H(\phi(\mathbf{x})))I(\mathbf{x})d\mathbf{x}}{\int_\Omega (1 - H(\phi(\mathbf{x})))d\mathbf{x}}, \tag{2.5}$$

followed by computing a new 0-level set using Equation 2.4, which is then used to build
the new level set function.

The approach does not require ϕ to be a signed distance function. Hence, ϕ may be as
in Equation 2.3 or it may depend on fuzzy membership as in Shyu et al. [20]. The authors
computed the new fuzzy membership in a single step instead of first finding the 0-level
set and then extending it to the full level set function. It may also be any other function
of the data, of which level sets are meaningful segment boundaries. A similar method was
previously presented by Kiridis and Chatzis [21] who also used a local variation term to
deal with shading in the image.

It should be noted, however, that decoupling the constraint for short boundaries from
the remainder of the level set equation will result in a different segmentation. For instance,
edge-preserving smoothing may retain small connected components in foreground or
background that would be removed if the short boundary constraint is part of the level
set optimization.

2.3.1.2   Defining initial level sets

Preprocessing may also be used to define an initial level set function. Since many level set
formulations do not guarantee that a global minimum is reached, the final result depends

on the initialization. This is often wanted in medical imaging because the information represented by the level set model does not uniquely specify the object to be searched (for instance, if the data term is not unique to a specific organ). The search is then guided by the location, orientation, and possibly even shape of the initial level set.

Initial 0-level sets can be defined manually by the user. Because of the locality of the many non-convex level set formulations, this is a direct means to introduce domain knowledge without having to formalize it. However, there are a number of disadvantages. If the noise level is high or if objects have a low contrast to the background, initial level sets have to be positioned close to the true boundary (see for instance Li et al. [22] for a comparison between manual and automatic initialization). The same is true when the boundary is long and convoluted such as in gray and white matter segmentation in brain MRI. In this case, the smoothness constraint cannot be enforced strongly enough to evolve a roughly defined initial level set into the true boundary.

Furthermore, many medical images come as a sequence of 2D slices where interaction would be required in many slices. To avoid this, some 2D segmentation techniques have been extended to 3D by using a segmentation result from the previous slice to initialize segmentation of the current slice. This strategy has been followed by Gao and Chae [23] for segmenting teeth in CT images. Shape information using this strategy has been introduced by the method of Qiu et al. [24] who segment the prostate in 3D ultrasound images. The result from the previous slice serves as shape constraint for the segmentation in the current slice. It should be noted, however, that the transfer of information between slices makes the result dependent on the segmentation of the first slice. In Qiu et al. [24], this has been dealt with by expecting the user to specify a number of boundary points in the first slice that roughly represent the initial shape so that the initial level set segmentation starts with a very good guess for the segment in this slice.

Fully automatic initialization schemes often make the assumption that object and background have homogeneous and distinct intensity or color. These level set methods are often variants of the Chan–Vese algorithm [4] using homogeneity and distinctiveness in the level set function. Initial level sets are generated from clustering in feature space. An example that not only introduces location information but also a part of the knowledge about the spatial configuration of the different segments is the work of Qi et al. [25] to segment cells in histopathological specimen microscopies. Since stained cells are darker than the background, cell centers are found by a mean-shift-like procedure where votes are transported along intensity gradients. According to the authors, all centers are found. Subsequent segmentation evolves separate level sets from each center letting level sets compete for the free space.

The work of Duan et al. [26] implicitly integrates some shape knowledge in the initialization step. They estimate expected gray level distributions from a clustering step to define segment and background probabilities for segmenting cysts in MR images. The probability distributions for foreground and background then define an initial 0-level set, which is extended to an initial level set function by applying the distance transform. Local refinement in the subsequent level set segmentation then determines the final boundary. Since the initial 0-level set can already be assumed to be close to the boundary, its shape has influence on the specification of the segment.

Clustering has also been extended to include local smoothness of the intensity function for defining the initial level set function. Bunyak et al. [27] separate color images from cell microscopy into several different regions represented by different clusters. They use an adaptation of the fuzzy c-means algorithm that enforces spatial clustering. The standard objective function of the fuzzy c-means algorithms is complemented by a weighted neighborhood term N that penalizes differences in membership degree u_{ik} to cluster i of pixels p_k in a neighborhood Ω around pixel p_j (m is the fuzzification):

$$N_\Omega(i,j) = (u_{ij})^m \exp\left(-\sum_{k\in\Omega}(u_{ik})^m\right) \tag{2.6}$$

Initial 0-level sets are given by the cluster boundaries. Similar to Qi et al. [25], these images show fairly homogeneous foreground and background regions although in this case, three different structures are separated (nucleus, pseudo-lumen, epithelial cytoplasm) from the background using multiphase level sets. The approach succeeds because the objects to be segmented have a similar appearance inside and outside of the 0-level sets.

Another interesting example is Li et al. [22] who employ spatially constrained fuzzy clustering (similar to Bunyak et al. [27]) to define a smooth transition at potential segment boundaries that depends on fuzzy membership. Instead of generating the level set function from an initial 0-level set by computing a signed distance function, the binarized membership function itself is the level set function. The subsequent level set segmentation of Li et al. [22] includes a distance transform constraint, which deforms the initial function into the distance transform during level set evolution. The authors compare their approach with a manual initialization and with a threshold initialization on ultrasound images of the carotid artery, on CT images of the liver and on MR images of the brain. Manual initialization only roughly sketches the shape of the object of interest whereas thresholding and fuzzy clustering produce initial level sets that represent the shapes of the objects already pretty well. The difference between the two is that clustering is less susceptible to noise leading to smoother boundaries. Again, this approach lives from the fact that optimization of the level set function is only local. The results improved with the accuracy with which the initial level set function represents the segment boundary. Hence, fuzzy classification produced the best results.

Finally, a good model that represents intensity variation in the different segments may also lead to a good initialization. An example is the work of Park et al. [28] who train a Gaussian mixture model to represent variable foreground and background and use the probabilities to initialize a geodesic active contour. Although they did not apply their method to medical images, it seems to be a good strategy to deal with the variability of the background, which is caused by the fact that it usually consists of several different anatomic structures that shall be separated from the object of interest via segmentation.

2.3.1.3 Finding initial regions of interest

If several structures have a similar appearance than the object of interest, the clustering methods described above will not allow their unique separation, since 0-level sets will be generated for all objects with the same appearance. The problem becomes worse when the homogeneity assumption that underlies the clustering strategy presented in the previous section is not true and feature values of different clusters become too similar.

If high-level knowledge such as the expected shape cannot be generated from the image data, an intermediate step is to single out a region of interest (ROI). The goal is to remove similar looking parts of the image from further consideration. Hence, the ROI avoids leaking of the 0-level set into similar objects and reduces the room for error when computing the initial 0-level set (which becomes easier after reducing the search to the ROI).

An example is the work of Lin et al. [29] that segments lesions in dental x-rays. First, teeth are found in noise-reduced contrast-enhanced images by thresholding followed by connected component analysis. The level set method is then initialized using trained thresholds on the result. Level set segmentation is needed to introduce an indirect smoothness constraint via the level set equation.

A similar strategy was followed by Gloger et al. [30] for kidney segmentation. They applied shape constraints on threshold-segmented MR images to find an initial kidney region. Thresholds were determined from training sets. It was further extended by Gloger et al. [31] to compute subject-specific intensity distributions to account for intersubject variation. Level set segmentation is carried out only in the initial kidney region. An additional shape constraint is then applied to generate the final result.

Multiple organs were searched by Kohlberger et al. [32] and resulted in an ROI that approximately delineated the segment boundary. This extensive preprocessing step for abdominal organs in MRI—described by Ling et al. [33] for liver segmentation—is based on trained knowledge about the expected shape and appearance of each organ of interest as well as on the relative position of each organ w.r.t. other organs. The initial segmentation is used to define the number of necessary level sets (one for each organ) for the final level set evolution. The final step just resolves small inaccuracies such as overlapping boundaries of different segments. Similar to Qi et al. [27], the level sets then compete for space, as segments should fill the space but not overlap.

2.3.1.4   Using atlases and shape models

Shape may be defined by initial 0-level sets or by initially determined regions of interest generated from the data (such as in Gao and Chae [23] described above). If the data itself is not rich enough for generating such initial shape with sufficient accuracy, a shape prior is needed to distinguish the object of interest from other structures. A digital anatomic atlas is particularly suitable for this purpose. It contains information about the shape of depicted organs and about spatial relations between organs.

The atlas needs to be registered with the image prior to level set segmentation [26,34–38]. As an atlas contains a wealth of information about the scene to be segmented, there is often sufficient redundancy between atlas and data to allow constrained deformation apart from rotation and translation in the registration process. Hence, segment labels of the atlas are—within the degrees of freedom of the deformation transformation—individualized for the particular image. After registration, the labels can be used as additional data term. The purpose is similar to slice-sequential approaches using shapes from previous slices to initialize the current slice, however, with the difference that initialization is automatic and driven by prior information about the shape.

The original image data is still necessary besides the atlas labels since nonrigid registration will not exactly map atlas boundaries to image boundaries. Subsequent level set segmentation will generate a compromise between mapped atlas labels, image appearance, and external smoothness constraints.

If only a single structure needs to be described, shape variation may also be trained from samples. If the training data base is sufficiently large and representative for the object shape, it produces a representation that discriminates better between the target object and other objects than an elastically deforming atlas. The spatial relationship to neighboring structures, which is present in atlases and which may be an even better discriminator, is not present in most shape models. An example for the use of a trained shape model is Hu et al. [36] where segmentation takes place in registered eigenshape space. Although registration of this kind of shape model could be integrated into the level set formulation

([5], see Section 2.3.2.5), it is sometimes easier to find the registration transformation in preprocessing, apply it to the shape representation, and map it onto image space as presented in Hu et al. [36]. The authors compute an active appearance model from training data to segment hippocampus and amygdala in brain MRI. The appearance terms are then used in the data term predicting the expected intensity while the shape terms constrain the propagation of the level set.

2.3.1.5　Concluding remarks

Preprocessing for level set segmentation ranges from image enhancement to the inclusion of complex domain knowledge. Doing the latter prior to level set segmentation has the advantage that all of this information may be formulated as part of the data terms. It also reduces the complex task to find and delineate a specific organ to a sequence of simpler subtasks. This is not just a kind of divide-and-conquer strategy, but it also has the potential for reusing modules for different but similar segmentation tasks. Examples for this method are the work of Gloger et al. [30,32], who defined between four and eight subtasks to generate the final result.

The disadvantage is that the knowledge is applied separately and independently to the constraints that are part of the level set model. Hence, the result can no longer be seen as the minimization based on a single constraint system but as a sequence of minimizations where some of the constraints (for instance, those based on object appearance) may be used differently during preprocessing and subsequent level set segmentation.

2.3.2　Integration of domain knowledge into the level set equation

Integration of domain knowledge into the level set model ensures a unified treatment of all aspects that extract an object from image data. Such knowledge is easily integrated if it is defined in the domain of the level set (such as curvature of the 0-level set or expected intensity inside the 0-level set). The speed function in front propagation, for instance, drives the level set front by a combination of independent, external and internal components toward the segment boundary. Each of the components is defined in the domain of the level set function. Internal components ensure smoothness of the boundary, which is appropriate for most anatomical or pathological structures and counteracts influences from noise. External terms depend on the image gradient and let the level set slow down at object boundaries since high gradients between object and background can often be assumed. The independent term is a driving force similar to the balloon forces in active contours and helps to overcome local minima, hence relieving the user to initialize the 0-level set close to the final boundary.

The front propagation method sketched above is an example for a boundary-based level set segmentation. Region attributes, defined in the level set function domain, are used by a variational level set-based on the initial work of Chan and Vese [4]. Separate regions with different average intensities are searched. Noise is accounted for indirectly by searching for short boundaries. Different from the front propagation algorithm sketched above, the searched level set is defined by a functional that integrates image properties over the complete domain. Several publications extend the data term to accommodate feature vectors instead of scalar values. Usually, this is just a vector norm between expected and present feature values (e.g., Joshi et al. [39] for the segmentation of color images of the retina).

Region-based segmentation is often more robust w.r.t. noise and other image artifacts that may cause a boundary-based front propagation to bleed into the background or to stop early before reaching the true boundary. However, if shading defies the homogeneity assumption, region-based segmentation may fail unless shading is added as part of the domain knowledge (see below).

An alternative minimization formulation, which is boundary-based but uses a variational formulation, are geodesic active contours [3]. Boundary smoothness is ensured by a curvature term while the gradient term separates different homogenous regions. Different from Chan and Vese [4], homogeneity is only indirectly enforced by searching boundaries with high gradient whereas smoothness of the boundary is explicitly integrated via a curvature term of the boundary. Since homogeneity is not defined by deviation from some average intensity, geodesic active contours should be less sensitive to shading artifacts as they are frequently found, for example, in magnetic resonance (MR) images.

A hybrid approach combining region- and boundary-based constraints has been presented by Lee et al. [18]. The authors derive three different derivatives for a boundary term (similar to Caselles et al. [3]), a region term (similar to Chan and Vese [4]), and a smoothness term. The weighted combination of these terms is used for the level set evolution to segment brain tumors in MRI.

The methods described above are basic building blocks of most level set methods applied in medical image analysis. However, a number of extensions have been suggested to counteract image artifacts, to improve the iterative minimization, and to add knowledge that allows distinguishing between different objects that are similar based on the features mentioned above. These will be presented and discussed in the following sections.

2.3.2.1 *Avoiding reinitialization*

Most but not all formulations of the evolution of the level set function require it to be a signed distance function in order to avoid numerical problems during level set evolution. An exemption is, for instance, the simple level set of Shyu et al. [20]. Level set functions requiring a normalized gradient are initialized as signed distance function (e.g., by fast marching [1]) given the initial 0-level set. Evolutions using the narrow band technique of Malladi et al. [40] require reinitialization at the latest when the 0-level set hits the boundary of the narrow band, since everything outside the band is not updated at all. However, even if the level set function is updated everywhere, it will lead to its deformation with time. Hence, a distance transform needs to be carried out at regular time intervals (see, for example, the efficient scheme in Sussman and Fatemi [41]).

Since the deformed level set function has a different behavior than the original distance function, each reinitialization changes the evolution behavior. Furthermore, frequent reinitialization costs time. Hence, an additional internal constraint on the level set function may be included that enforces unit length of the gradient of the level set function everywhere. Reinitialization is avoided and the constraint may even be used to deform an arbitrary function into a distance transform. The latter is important if initialization does not only produce a 0-level set but an arbitrary, but differentiable function of which the 0-level set is the first approximation of the segment boundary. This was proposed by Li et al. [42] for a variational formulation. The following additional term, properly weighted, was added to the evolution:

$$\zeta(\phi) = \Delta\varphi - div\left(\frac{\nabla\phi}{|\nabla\phi|}\right). \tag{2.7}$$

It penalizes the deviation of the level set function ϕ from a signed distance function with $|\nabla\phi| = 1$ everywhere. It has been used by Li et al. [22] to let the level set function start from a regularized version of a binary function that has the value $-C$ outside the segment and

C inside of it. Li et al. [42] later extended their approach to achieve a more stable behavior. Instead of requiring a level set function with $|\nabla\phi| = 1$ everywhere, Li et al. [43] suggested a function that has gradient length $|\nabla\phi| = 1$ away from the 0-level set and unit length gradients only in the vicinity of the 0-level set.

A similar strategy was followed by Estellers et al. [44], whose main contribution, however, was to present a variant of the Split–Bregman method to decouple the two different norms used in their optimization term (L1- and L2-norm) by variable substitution for which efficient solution schemes exist.

The approach of Zhang et al. [45] is different, as they vary the regularization concept, which is the reason for requiring the level set function to be a signed distance function. Their method evolves the level set-based on repulsion forces that depend on the intensity of each pixel compared to the expected foreground and background intensity. They showed that the computation of the Laplacian (which is the result of taking the derivative of the level set equation) is equivalent to a Gaussian smoothing. Hence, their regularization consists of evolving a binary level set function by repulsion forces and regularizing the result by Gaussian smoothing at each step of the evolution.

2.3.2.2 Inclusion of noise models

The data term of a region-based level set function can be seen as the logarithm of an exponential function that measures the deviation of image intensity from the mean. Hence, minimizing the energy translates into maximizing the likelihood of segment membership given the data and assuming Gaussian noise. If the latter is not true, the resulting segmentation may contain errors because of the inappropriate noise model. This was addressed by Ben Salah et al. [46] who use a two-step procedure where the expected gray value distribution is estimated from the first segmentation and then used in repetition. It uses kernels on intensities instead of the intensities themselves to account for noise.

Another solution is the replacement of the intensity value by a pixel classification based on local features. This has been applied as speed term in front propagation level sets by Smeets et al. [47], therefore empowering these kinds of evolution schemes to include regional information. Intensity-based probability distributions were also used by Chen [48] to minimize the risk of misclassification.

2.3.2.3 Accounting for intensity variations

Many objects in medical images should have a homogeneous intensity because the imaging procedure has been chosen to discriminate a specific object by its intensity. Ideally, the only sources of intensity variation should be zero-mean noise and partial volume effects at the boundary between objects. The former is automatically dealt with in region-based level set methods if the object contrast is higher than the noise level. In boundary-based level set methods, it is only indirectly accounted for because the noise gradients are assumed to be smaller than boundary gradients and the curvature terms counteract potential boundary errors from noise close to the object boundary.

Partial volume effects may impact a region-based level set method if the intensity variation in the background is higher than for the foreground object. Such case frequently arises because the background contains many different objects, each of which has a different average intensity. In this case, the variation due to the partial volume effect may be attributed to the permissible background intensity variation, causing an underestimation of the extent of the foreground object. This can be avoided by explicitly accounting for the nonhomogeneous background instead of treating it as a kind of super-noise (see Section 2.3.2.4).

Boundary-based level sets should not be affected by partial volume effects unless the effect is so strong with respect to the object contrast that it overly reduces gradient strength.

Some imaging devices are also subjected to a third source for intensity variation. Measured signal strength varies because the signal-exciting source varies locally—an example is shading in MR imaging—or because the sent signal is varied depending on the location—examples are ultrasound images and again MR images. The image can be assumed to be overlaid with a bias field that represents object-independent signal variation. The bias field varies usually slowly. Hence, its major components in the frequency domain are found in the low frequency range.

For boundary-based level sets, bias field variation should have little to no influence on the image gradient because of this low-pass characteristic. The existence of a bias field is more critical for region-based level set functions as it adds to the intensity variation across the segments.

Several different ways exist to deal with bias fields in such case, mainly by localizing the intensity term in the region-based Chan–Vese model. The original method of Chan and Vese [4] iteratively updates the average value in the foreground and background region followed by gradient descent on a functional combining a data term that penalized deviation of the image intensity from these averages with a model term that emphasizes short boundaries. The method works well in cases where gradient strength varies (e.g., if partial volume effects cause weak gradients), but relies on constant intensity in the segments.

A simple way to account for intensity variation is to partition the space so that in each partition the intensity can be assumed to be approximately constant. This has been done by Sokoll et al. [49] for segmentation of gray matter, white matter, and cerebrospinal fluid (csf) in MR brain images. They subdivided the data into $20 \times 20 \times 20$ voxel partitions and estimated the evolution in each partition separately. In order to guarantee smooth evolution at partition boundaries, they used weighted features from a six-neighborhood of each partition for feature computation.

A smoothly varying shading function has been presented by Li et al. [50], who define a data term for the energy functional of the level set function that computes a difference between image intensity and the product of the expected average intensity and a local bias field. Level set function, local bias field, and bias-corrected average values in the segment are iteratively updated. Compared to the Chan–Vese model, which updates two independent variables (level set function and average value), iteratively. Li et al. [50] compute three variables by this process iterating through the variables keeping all but one variable constant. The bias field is computed from local averages and the extent of this local neighborhood is to be parameterized. The optimization assumes that the bias field is almost constant in this neighborhood, which is an adequate assumption for their application on MR images.

Wang et al. [51] extend the Chan–Vese model by a local intensity term again assuming a slowly changing bias field. It minimizes differences of the original function from a smoothed version of it. Similar solutions have been presented by Wang et al. [52], who modeled the bias field by a locally varying Gaussian function, and Zhang et al. [53], who considered segment-dependent noise variances.

The local binary fitting energy of Li et al. [54] does not attempt to model a bias field but instead assumes that the local neighborhood at the object boundary is always representable by a binary function. The local binary fitting energy is a term that integrates for each point $\mathbf{x}$ in the image a difference between functions $f_1(\mathbf{x})$ and $f_2(\mathbf{x})$ and the intensities in the neighborhood of $\mathbf{x}$. The neighborhood is defined by a kernel function that decreases with distance to $\mathbf{x}$. Li et al. [54] use a Gaussian kernel. Optimization repeatedly updates

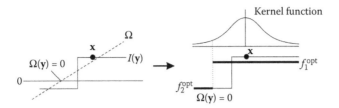

Figure 2.2 The 0-level set $\Omega(\mathbf{x}) = 0$ of a level set function Ω defines a current segmentation. The local binary fitting energy is a constraint to the level set function that attempts to minimize a weighted difference between optimal average foreground and background intensities f_1^{opt} and f_2^{opt} and actual intensity $I(\mathbf{y})$. Weighting is given by a decreasing kernel function around $\mathbf{x}$.

the current level set function given f_1^{opt} and f_2^{opt} as local intensity models for foreground and background and then finds new optimal values f_1^{opt} and f_2^{opt} for a given level set (see Figure 2.2). Since, different from the original formulation of Chan and Vese [4], the model intensities vary locally (f_1 and f_2 are functions of $\mathbf{x}$), the method will find boundaries even if the local contrast between foreground and background varies. The method has been applied to vessel segmentation in MR angiography and to the segmentation of white matter and gray matter in MRI. A variant that can be computed more efficiently is the method of Zhang et al. [55], who use a truncated Gaussian kernel.

2.3.2.4 Accounting for nonhomogeneous background
The expected average intensity of foreground and background is estimated continuously in the Chan–Vese model from the current foreground and background. Background, however, is often inhomogeneous and implicitly assumed homogeneity may be an inappropriate representation (see Figure 2.3).

The simplest way to deal with this is to ignore the background altogether. Hence, Kosic et al. [56] optimize homogeneity only in the foreground constrained by short segment boundaries. Normally, this approach would result in a trivial minimum and only succeeds here because the optimization in Kosic et al. [56] is intentionally made local using a narrow band strategy. A similar method to base level set evolution mainly on foreground characteristics has been presented by Jimenez-Carretero et al. [57]. They suggested a heuristic variation of the Euler–Lagrange derivative of Chan and Vese [4], which does not use the

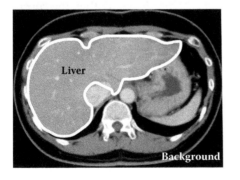

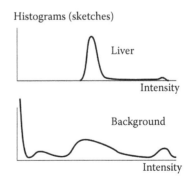

Figure 2.3 The background in a two-label segmentation is often much less homogeneous than the foreground.

background homogeneity constraint. Several additional steps are introduced to improve on this result. The method was applied to liver segmentation in CT images. Unfortunately, due to the heuristic nature of the propagation, little can be said about the functional, which is optimized by this strategy.

Another option is to use a multiphase model that assigns a separate segment to each structure in the background, as it has been presented by Yazdanpanah et al. [6] to segment the retina in OCT images. In this case, the assumed intensity homogeneity of segments is appropriate in the foreground as well as in the background. However, it does make the segmentation overly complicated if this separation of the background into several segments is not required.

A third option is to model the background as an inhomogeneous structure and compute membership values for each pixel to belong to the foreground or the background based on this model. This has been suggested by Lee et al. [18], who acknowledges that background consisting of several anatomic objects would best be modeled by a Gaussian mixture model although they finally decided to approximate the background by a single Gaussian. The weighting of foreground and background terms can be used to account for the different accuracy of the homogeneity assumption in the foreground and in the background. The disadvantage here is that the constraint given by the background model becomes weak compared to the foreground. It may be inappropriate since deviations from the assumed average intensity are mainly meant to account for the influence from 0-mean noise. Modeling the background really as Gaussian mixture has been used in Park et al. [28] for initializing a geodesic active contour. However, it has been applied to color photos of flowers where the constituting Gaussians of the mixture are probably easier found than in medical images since the noise in photos is low and the contrast between different segments is high.

2.3.2.5   *Integrating shape and appearance information*

Shape (and partially also appearance) information is used in medical image segmentation for two different purposes and these should not be confused. First, shape may be used to add uniqueness to the searched object. If—as it is often the case—the intensity distributions of different organs overlap, a purely intensity-driven search will not succeed. Pose information (location, orientation, and size) introduced by an initial level set may resolve the problem, but if this information cannot be given or is too inaccurate, a shape model will help to distinguish between objects of similar appearance but with different shape. Hence, shape information is used to aid object detection. Shape may also help to determine object boundaries. If objects of similar appearance are adjacent to each other, the contrast of this part of the boundary may be insufficient to determine the object border. Smoothness constraints on the object boundary may help if these parts are small, but otherwise a shape model is required to hypothesize the course of the boundary from boundary information in the vicinity.

Several existing approaches encode prior shape information via signed distance maps of trained shape boundaries that are then incorporated into a level set framework taking different strategies for level set evolution, minimization, and pose invariance into account. Paragios [58] integrates shape priors in a level set framework to segment and track the left ventricle in cardiac MR as well as ultrasound images. Signed distance maps of trained prior shape models are used to build a pixelwise stochastic level set representation that describes local shape variability by using a maximum likelihood criterion between shape model and training set. The stochastic level set representation is embedded in a global registration model. Boundary-based as well as region-based terms are combined in the energy functional. Leventon et al. [59] apply principal component analysis (PCA) to signed distance maps of trained shape examples to determine lower-dimensional shape representations. Gaussian probability distributions are then calculated in this space and used in a Bayesian probabilistic approach. The maximum a posteriori shape is determined in each level set iteration step and combined with an image gradient and curvature term to propagate the level set evolution. Rousson and Cremers [60] use the PCA-based lower-dimensional shape representation in an infinite-dimensional Bayesian inference approach that incorporates translation and rotation of the respective shapes. In contrast to Leventon et al. [59], the shape probabilities are computed with a nonparametric kernel density estimator that adapts the training data more flexible than parametric Gaussian distributions. Bayesian inference is reformulated as an energy minimization problem, which is solved in a coupled gradient descent equation system to segment the heart in 2D ultrasound images and the prostate from 3D CT images.

The model of Yazdanpanah et al. [6] incorporates shape knowledge by introducing an implicit registration constraint that causes the shape part to adapt its pose w.r.t. rotation and translation. The shape prior probability is given by a shape space that is defined by a finite number of sample shape level sets. These span a finite subspace in the infinite-dimensional shape space. Shape variation in this subspace is given by kernel density estimates as this better captures the true shape variation than assuming a Gaussian distribution such as in Cootes et al. [14] and Leventon et al. [59] (see Figure 2.4). The authors optimize the logarithm of the a posteriori probability of the shape and pose parameters given the image. This results in an energy term where the shape parameters (the a priori probability) are simply an additional summand that replaces the regularizer of the Chan–Vese model [4]. The variational derivatives of the pose parameters only depend on the image data while the prior term influences the shape parameters of the level set function.

For simpler shapes, the integration becomes simpler as well, since the shape can be represented in terms of local attributes of the level set. For segmenting sphere-like structures, Lim et al. [61] introduced Willmore flow as (indirect) shape prior. They use a shape prior based on Cremers et al. [5] to represent the shape of the vertebra. The prior is complemented by introducing Willmore flow to replace the usual curvature-dependent smoothness constraint. Willmore energy of a surface is minimal when its average curvature is minimal. Hence, minimizing Willmore energy would prefer sphere-like structures. The authors integrate this into the level set equation to achieve a smooth sphere-like boundary in regions where the contrast in the image does not suffice for defining the surface.

Using Willmore energy would not be necessary if the shape models were sufficiently accurate to predict the individual shape in such case, but—as usual—the shape model is

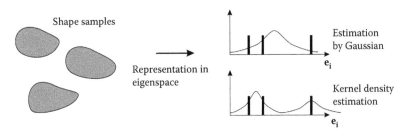

Figure 2.4 Using kernel density estimates may better represent the true shape distribution in shape space.

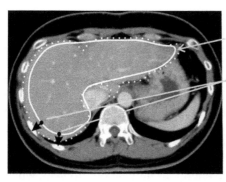

Approximately
aligned liver shape

Different key points may
carry different expected features

Figure 2.5 The front propagation of Kohlberger et al. [62] tracks key points on an approximately aligned liver shape and controls propagation speed by expected local features for these key points.

not based on sufficient samples to make such accurate predictions. In other words, either the finite-dimensional shape subspace of Cremers et al. [5] has too few dimensions or the kernel density estimate is too inaccurate. Hence, the shape model locks in the level set at places where boundary information is sufficient, whereas the Willmore flow helps at locations where neither data information nor the shape model can make a prediction as where to find the boundary.

The work of Kohlberger et al. [62] is another example of adding local knowledge to a global shape prior. The authors train expected local features, such as intensities at the organ boundary and curvature of the boundary, from livers and kidney in CT images. The key points on an approximately aligned reference shape are tracked in a front propagation approach and local features associated to these key points are then used to control the evolution of the level set (see Figure 2.5). The local features are combined with a global explicitly defined shape prior, which is integrated with the implicit level set representation using the method presented by Farzinfa et al. [63].

Another simple shape prior has been presented by Yazdanpanah et al. [6]. They introduce a circular shape prior parameterized by center and radius for segmenting retina structures in OCT. Since their segmentation goal was to separate the different layers of the retina, they defined as many level sets as they have layers to segment. This way of defining a multiple segment level set solution may cause segments to overlap, which must be prevented. In their application, the layers form concentric circles in the 2D image domain. Defining shape priors of all level sets to have the same center not only further constrains the shape (by determining a common location of all centers) but also resolves the overlap issue as the shape prior leads to segment boundaries that are nonoverlapping concentric circle-like shapes. Segments can then be ordered by the size of the radius and the region for each segment is defined by the inside of the respective level set that is outside of all segments with smaller radius.

Another way to introduce a shape constraint is to use shape similarities that exist, for instance, between consecutive slices of a 3D dataset or between consecutive frames of a 4D dataset. An example is the work of Riklin-Raviv et al. [64], who segment several images simultaneously that are aligned and then segmented. An implicit shape prior is given by the assumption that images contain spatially aligned similar structures. Hence, homogeneity represented by potential functions of a Markov random field enforces shape similarity between segments of the different images.

Qiu et al. [65] propose an energy functional in which a shape prior is incorporated to penalize the difference between the evolving contour and the shape prior. The shape prior is activated if a certain predefined distance between shape prior and evolving contour is exceeded. Their approach is applied to delineate the prostate in transrectal ultrasound images.

A completely different way to use shape information is presented by Kosic et al. [56]. They do not use shapes to constrain the image data but want to segment the shape space itself. Their shape space represents the population variation of femur shapes and they want to optimize the implant design. Hence, they map shape space to some constraint defined from implant design (in their case the average error of fitting the implant to the bone) and find the space of bone shapes for a given implant that is appropriate for this particular implant.

2.3.2.6 Integrating relative and absolute localization information

The simplest way to integrate high-level domain knowledge about the location of an object is by interactive specification of the initial 0-level set. Since most level set methods do not guarantee to find an optimal solution, the results are dependent on the initialization (see also Section 2.3.1.2). This disadvantage is used to remedy another disadvantage, which is the fact that the level set model is usually insufficient for uniquely defining the object and its appearance in the image. This makes also the narrow band technique for front propagation algorithms advantageous, as it reduces level sets to a kind of advanced region growing from user-specified start locations. An example that derives location and appearance information from initialization is Taheri et al. [66] on tumor segmentation. They let the 0-level set propagate from an initial position fully inside the tumor. The evolution is driven by intensity-based tumor probabilities of the voxels. Parameters of a Gaussian distribution are estimated from the region inside the initial 0-level set and updated during level set evolution.

The work of Rink and Toennies [67] is an example of using information about the current shape of the 0-level set to guide its evolution. Their bridging force to segment dendritic spines in electron microscopy is based on the current evolution direction and speeds up evolution at high curvature locations when another part of the 0-level set is sufficiently close. Hence, it is able to bridge small gaps in longish structures, which are due to insufficient support by the data.

The work of Zhang et al. [45] describes a level set that may either use or not use the localization information from the initial 0-level set. Their level set function is not a signed distance function but a smoothed binary function that is positive inside and negative outside of the 0-level set. The function is evolved according to a region-based pressure force that expands the 0-level set if it is within an object and shrinks it otherwise. The pressure force at each location depends on the intensity of this location w.r.t. the average of the two average intensities in the foreground and in the background. By reinitializing the level set function to a binary function after each iteration, the 0-level set is hindered to evolve in locations that are not close to the initial 0-level set. How far it evolves depends on the amount of smoothing and a moment force that drives the level set further in the preferred direction depending on the level set gradient. If the level set function is not reinitialized to a binary function, it behaves similar to the Chan–Vese method but will produce smoother boundaries since boundary smoothness in the Chan–Vese method is only indirectly enforced by searching for short boundaries.

Spatial relationships between different segments are included if coupled level sets are used, that is, level sets where evolution of the one level set influences that of the other.

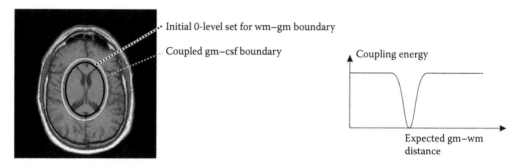

Figure 2.6 The coupling energy in Sokoll et al. [49] penalizes deviations from the expected thickness of the gray matter.

This has been presented by Zeng et al. [68], who use two active surfaces for the segmentation of the cortex into white matter (wm), gray matter (gm), and cerebrospinal fluid (csf). While each of the surfaces may evolve according to different features within the data, they have to stay in a predefined normal range to each other given by the estimated cortical thickness. A similar technique has also been used by Sokoll et al. [49], who derived and adapted features during level set evolution (see Figure 2.6). Similarly, Wang et al. [37,38] introduce a distance term between csf–gm interface and gm–wm interface that penalizes deviations from the acceptable thickness range of gray matter. Another example is the already mentioned work of Yazdanpanah et al. [6], where different segments form a sequence of concentric rings and each ring is represented by its own level set.

An example that uses coupling in different ways at several steps of a multistep segmentation is Duan et al. [26]. Their goal is to segment the inner and outer walls of the bladder in MR images. Since the inner wall is much better visible, it is segmented in the first step and serves as the initialization for the level set function representing the outer wall. Since the appearance of the bladder wall is different from the background, the authors modify the formulation of the data term in the Chan–Vese model so that only a small ring outside of the inner wall is evaluated for computing the difference between average intensity in the background and the pixel intensity. After having an indirect definition of the outer wall based on the current estimate for the inner wall, a new level set function is defined that includes both walls that are then evolved together.

Another example is Dzyubachyk et al. [69] to segment cells in microscopy. The coupling term is designed such that overlap is avoided. This is similar to Kohlberger et al. [32], who also use coupling to avoid overlaps between level sets representing different segments. A semiautomatic approach is designed by Ma et al. [70] in which three level set functions are used to segment bladder, vagina, and rectum simultaneously. Since these organs are located near to each other and MR intensities of same organs can vary, initial contours must be placed manually. For multiphase organ segmentation a region competition model [71] is used that avoids overlaps between regions of different organs. Since bladder shape variability is high, prior shape knowledge is incorporated only for vagina and rectum by using the approach of Cremers et al. [5].

2.3.2.7 Concluding remarks

A wide range of different kinds of domain knowledge can be included directly into the level set formulation. The majority of approaches model either local attributes or they represent global attributes (e.g., a shading bias field, preferred shapes, or preferred topology) by local features of the underlying space Ω, which can be easily introduced into the level set formulation. Introducing global attributes as global features is more difficult. An example is the work of Cremers et al. [5] who integrated the registration of a position- and orientation-independent shape constraint into a variational level set optimization.

2.3.3 Postprocessing

Level set segmentation should not contain too much postprocessing, since it changes the optimal result according to the level set formulation completely independent of it. Hence, postprocessing takes place only in cases where some of the necessary information has not been part of the level set constraints. Sometimes, this is rather far-reaching, such as in Rajpoot et al. [72], who use interactive input and smoothing to correct a level set segmentation on ultrasound images of the heart. It was necessary in this case as the authors used simple geodesic active contours that—without specific regularizers—perform badly on these images because the noise level is too high for the smoothness regularizer used in Caselles et al. [3] and a shape constraint has not been included. In most cases, however, postprocessing either corrects for boundary details or is used to select searched segments from a list of segments produced by the level set segmentation.

Examples for the former are mentioned in Jimenez-Carretero et al. [57], who remove voxels from their multiresolution liver segmentation in which their intensity differs from the average intensity in the region by some threshold. It is not a true postprocessing as it is not done at the highest resolution. Hence, this correction may be achieved again by the next higher resolution level set. Another example is Wang et al. [37], who employ a local smoothness constraint to correct for falsely labeled voxels due to insufficient contrast and partial volume effects in MR neonatal brain segmentation. Boundary smoothness is, of course, part of most level set formulations and could probably be integrated into this level set solution as well. However, it seems that sometimes users are more comfortable with the level set segmentation producing a "raw" result more or less following the information in the data, which is then explicitly smoothed with standard filtering techniques.

Selection of segments becomes necessary when the level set segmentation does not include enough discriminating information to separate wanted structures from other similarly looking segments. This does not necessarily mean that the segmentation and hence the formulation of the energy function has been incomplete. Segmentation in its original sense just meant to partition a scene into meaningful subsets. Although in medical imaging the assignment of a class membership to segments is often part of the process segmentation may as well follow the original paradigm in image understanding where first segments are created that are then further analyzed based on segment attributes. An example is the work of Antunes et al. [73], who remove small regions after applying level set segmentation to ultrasound images of the heart in order to identify the four chambers among the segments. Another example is Bunyak et al. [27], where the level set result is an intermediate step to detect nuclei in histopathological cell images. Postprocessing combines shape-based selection and rule-based decision based on segment characteristics for arriving at the final decision.

2.4 Conclusions

The efficiency of the level set framework in medical image analysis has been demonstrated by the relative ease by which necessary domain knowledge can be integrated into a level set equation. Object-specific knowledge such as shape, appearance, or pose as well as image acquisition-specific knowledge such as noise characteristics or spatial bias on the intensity can be included into the energy functional. If it is included into the data term, it requires a preprocessing step for turning the domain knowledge into data. If it is included into the model term, it requires appropriate modeling of the domain knowledge. Although sometimes level sets are evolved based on some not very well justified heuristics most cited papers stay within the framework of optimizing an energy functional or tracking the evolution of the level set function. Often, however, domain knowledge has been turned into an additional data term prior to level set segmentation instead of modeling it within the level set framework. This is probably due to the fact that the general framework of modeling and optimizing level set functionals is not very accessible to developers in the application field. However, the general idea of defining a segmentation as an optimal level set function seems to be attractive enough for research in a large number of application papers.

Acknowledgments

The work presented in this paper has been funded by DFG priority program 1335: Scalable Visual Analytics (TO 166/13-2) and by DFG grant GL 785/1-1.

References

1. J. A. Sethian, A fast marching level set method for monotonically advancing fronts, *Proceedings of the National Academy of Sciences*, vol. 93, no. 4, pp. 1591–1595, 1996.
2. S. Osher and R. P. Fedkiw, Level set methods: An overview and some recent results, *Journal of Computational Physics*, vol. 169, no. 2, pp. 463–502, 2001.
3. V. Caselles, R. Kimmel, and G. Sapiro, Geodesic active contours, *International Journal of Computer Vision*, vol. 22, no. 1, pp. 61–79, 1997.
4. T. F. Chan and L. A. Vese, Active contours without edges, *IEEE Transactions on Image Processing*, vol. 10, no. 2, pp. 266–277, 2001.
5. D. Cremers, S. J. Osher, and S. Soatto, Kernel density estimation and intrinsic alignment for shape priors in level set segmentation, *International Journal of Computer Vision*, vol. 69, no. 3, pp. 335–351, 2006.
6. A. Yazdanpanah, G. Hamarneh, B. R. Smith, and M. V. Sarunic, Segmentation of intra-retinal layers from optical coherence tomography images using an active contour approach, *IEEE Transactions on Medical Imaging*, vol. 30, no. 2, pp. 484–496, 2011.
7. T. F. Chan, B. Y. Sandberg, and L. A. Vese, Active contours without edges for vector-valued images, *Journal of Visual Communication and Image Representation*, vol. 11, no. 2, pp. 130–141, 2000.
8. E. Klann, R. Ramlau, and W. Ring, A Mumford-Shah level-set approach for the inversion and segmentation of SPECT/CT data, *Inverse Problem Imaging*, vol. 5, no. 1, pp. 137–166, 2011.
9. N. Paragios and R. Deriche, Geodesic active regions and level set methods for supervised texture segmentation, *International Journal of Computer Vision*, vol. 46, no. 3, pp. 223–247, 2002.
10. T. Brox, M. Rousson, R. Deriche, and J. Weickert, Colour, texture, and motion in level set-based segmentation and tracking, *Image and Vision Computing*, vol. 28, no. 3, pp. 367–390, 2010.
11. B. Wang, X. Gao, D. Tao, and X. Li, A unified tensor level set for image segmentation, *IEEE Transactions on Systems, Man, and Cybernetics*, vol. 40, no. 3, pp. 857–867, 2010.
12. B.C. Vemuri, Y. Chen, M. Rao, T. McGraw, Z. Wang, and T. Mareci, Fiber tract mapping from diffusion tensor MRI, in *IEEE Workshop on Variational and Level Set Methods in Computer Vision*, Vancouver, Canada, pp. 81–88, 2001.
13. J. Olveres, R. Nava, E. Moya-Albor, B. Escalante-Ramírez, J. Brieva, G. Cristóbal, and E. Vallejo, Texture descriptor approaches to level set segmentation in medical images, in *Proc. SPIE 9138. Optics, Photonics, and Digital Technologies for Multimedia Applications III*, Brussels, Belgium, 91380J, 2014.

14. T. F. Cootes, C. J. Taylor, D. H. Cooper, and J. Graham, Active shape models—their training and application, *Computer Vision and Image Understanding*, vol. 61, no. 1, pp. 38–59, 1995.

15. T. F. Cootes, G. J. Edwards, and C. J. Taylor, Active appearance models, *IEEE Transactions on Pattern Analysis and Machine Intelligence*, vol. 23, no. 6, pp. 681–685, 2001.

16. K. Suzuki, R. Kohlbrenner, M. L. Epstein, A. M. Obajuluwa, J. Xu, and M. Hori, Computer-aided measurement of liver volumes in CT by means of geodesic active contour segmentation coupled with level-set algorithm, *Medical Physics*, vol. 37, no. 5, pp. 2159–2166, 2010.

17. O. Gloger, J. Kühn, A. Stanski, H. Völzke, and R. Puls, A fully automatic three-step liver segmentation method on LDA-based probability maps for multiple contrast MR images, *Magnetic Resonance Imaging*, vol. 28, no. 6, pp. 882–897, 2010.

18. M. Lee, W. Cho, S. Kim, S. Park, and J. H. Kim, Segmentation of interest region in medical volume images using geometric deformable model, *Computers in Biology and Medicine*, vol. 42, no. 5, pp. 523–537, 2012.

19. C. Xu and J. L. Prince, Snakes, shapes, and gradient vector flow, *IEEE Transactions on Image Processing*, vol. 7, no. 3, pp. 359–369, 1998.

20. K.-K. Shyu, V.-T. Pham, T.-T. Tran, and P.-L. Lee, Global and local fuzzy energy-based active contours for image segmentation, *Nonlinear Dynamics*, vol. 67, pp. 1559–1578, 2012.

21. S. Kiridis and V. Chatzis, Fuzzy energy-based active contour, *IEEE Transactions on Image Processing*, vol. 18, no. 12, pp. 2747–2755, 2009.

22. B. N. Li, C. K. Chui, S. Chang, and S. H. Ong, Integrating spatial fuzzy clustering with level set methods for automated medical image segmentation, *Computers in Biology and Medicine*, vol. 41, pp. 1–10, 2011.

23. H. Gao and O. Chae, Individual tooth segmentation from CT images using level set method with shape and intensity prior, *Pattern Recognition*, vol. 43, no. 7, pp. 2406–2417, 2010.

24. W. Qiu, J. Yuan, E. Ukwatta, D. Tessier, and A. Fenster, Rotational-slice-based prostate segmentation using level sets with shape constraint for 3D end-firing TRUS guided biopsy, in *Medical Image Computing and Computer-Assisted Intervention–MICCAI 2011*. Berlin: Springer, 2012, pp. 537–544.

25. X. Qi, F. Xing, D. J. Foran, and L. Yang, Robust segmentation of overlapping cells in histopathology specimens using parallel seed detection and repulsive level set, *IEEE Transactions on Biomedical Engineering*, vol. 59, no. 3, pp. 754–765, 2012.

26. C. Duan, Z. Liang, S. Bao, H. Zhu, S. Wang, G. Zhang, J. J. Chen, and H. Lu, A coupled level set framework for bladder wall segmentation with application to MR cystography, *IEEE Transactions on Medical Imaging*, vol. 29, no. 3, pp. 903–915, 2010.

27. F. Bunyak, A. Hafiane, and K. Palaniappan, Histopathology tissue segmentation by combining fuzzy clustering with multiphase vector level sets, in *Software Tools and Algorithms for Biological Systems*, H. R. Arabnia and Q.-N. Tran, Eds. Berlin: Springer, 2011, pp. 413–424.

28. S.C. Park, S. H. Kim, G. S. Lee, C. W. Lee, I. S. Na, A. V. H. Le, and T. Y. Do, Flower area segmentation by a level set-based on GMM initialization, in *KSII: The 3rd International Conference on Internet (ICONI) 2011*, Sepang, Malaysia, pp. 17–21, 2011.

29. P.-L. Lin, P.-Y. Huang, and P.-W. Huang, An automatic lesion detection method for dental x-ray images by segmentation using variational level set, in *International Conference on Machine Learning and Cybernetics (ICMLC)*, Xian, China, vol. 5. pp. 1821–1825, 2012.

30. O. Gloger, K. D. Toennies, V. Liebscher, B. Kugelmann, R. Laqua, and H. Völzke, Prior shape level set segmentation on multistep generated probability maps of MR datasets for fully automatic kidney parenchyma volumetry, *IEEE Transactions on Medical Imaging*, vol. 31, no. 2, pp. 312–325, 2012.

31. O. Gloger, K. D. Toennies, R. Laqua, and H. Völzke, Fully automated renal tissue volumetry in MR volume data using prior shape based segmentation in proband-specific probability maps, *IEEE Transactions on Biomedical Engineering*, vol. 62, no. 10, pp. 2338–2351, 2015.

32. T. Kohlberger, M. Sofka, J. Zhang, N. Birkbeck, J. Wetzl, J. Kaftan, J. Declerck, and S. K. Zhou, Automatic multi-organ segmentation using learning-based segmentation and level set

optimization, in: *Medical Image Computing and Computer-Assisted Intervention–MICCAI 2011*. Berlin: Springer, 2011, pp. 338–345.

33. H. Ling, S. K. Zhou, Y. Zheng, B. Georgescu, M. Suehling, and D. Comaniciu, Hierarchical, learning-based automatic liver segmentation, in *IEEE Conference on Computer Vision and Pattern Recognition CVPR 2008*, Anchorage, USA, pp. 1–8, 2008.

34. A. Akhond-Asl, K. Jafari-Khousani, K. Elisevich, and H. Soltanian-Zadeh, Hippocampal volumetry for lateralization of temporal lobe epilepsy: Automated versus manual methods, *NeuroImage*, vol. 54, pp. 218–226, 2011.

35. M. Cabezas, A. Oliver, X. Llado, J. Freixenet, and M. B. Cuada, A review of atlas-based segmentation for magnetic resonace brain images, *Computer Methods and Programs in Biomedicine*, vol. 104, pp. 158–177, 2011.

36. S. Hu, P. Coupé, J.S. Pruessner, and D. L. Collins, Appearance-based modeling for segmentation of hippocampus and amygdala using mult-contrast MR imaging, *NeuroImage*, vol. 58, no. 2, pp. 549–559, 2011.

37. L. Wang, F. Shi, W. Lin, J. H. Gilmore, and D. Shen, Automatic segmentation of neonatal images using convex optimization and coupled level sets, *NeuroImage*, vol. 58, pp. 805–817, 2011.

38. L. Wang, F. Shi, G. Li, Y. Gao, W. Lin, J. H. Gilmore, and D. Shen, Segmentation of neonatal brain MR images using patch-driven level sets, *NeuroImage*, vol. 84, pp. 141–158, 2014.

39. G. D. Joshi, J. Sivaswamy, and S. R. Krishnadas, Optic disk and cup segmentation from monocular colour retinal images for glaucoma assessment, *IEEE Transactions on Medical Imaging*, vol. 30, no. 6, pp. 1192–1205, 2011.

40. R. Malladi, J. A. Sethian, and B. C. Vemuri, Shape modeling with front propagation: A level set approach, *IEEE Transactions on Pattern Analysis and Machine Intelligence*, vol. 17, no. 2, pp. 158–175, 1995.

41. M. Sussman and E. Fatemi, An efficient, interface-preserving level set redistancing algorithm and its application to interfacial incompressible fluid flow, *SIAM Journal on Scientific Computing*, vol. 20, no. 4, pp. 1165–1191, 1999.

42. C. Li, C. Xu, C. Gui, and M. D. Fox, Level set evolution without re-initialization: A new variational formulation, in *IEEE Conference on Computer Vision and Pattern Recognition CVPR 2005*, vol. 1, pp. 430–436, 2005.

43. C. Li, C. Xu, C. Gui, and M. D. Fox, Distance regularized level set evolution and its application to image segmentation, *IEEE Transactions on Image Processing*, vol. 19, no. 12, pp. 3243–3254, 2010.

44. V. Estellers, D. Zosso, R. Lai, J.-P. Thiran, S. Osher, and X. Bresson, Efficient algorithm for level set method preserving distance function, *IEEE Transactions on Image Processing*, vol. 21, no. 12, pp. 4722–4734, 2012.

45. K. Zhang, L. Zhang, H. Song, and W. Zhou, Active contours with selective local or global segmentation: A new formulation and level set method, *Image and Vision Computing*, vol. 28, pp. 668–676, 2010.

46. M. Ben Salah, A. Mitiche, and I. Ben Ayed, Effective level set image segmentation with a kernel induced data term, *IEEE Transactions on Image Processing*, vol. 19, no. 1, pp. 220–232, 2010.

47. D. Smeets, D. Loeckx, B. Stijnen, B. de Dobbelaer, D. Vandermeulen, and P. Suetens, Semi-automatic level set segmentation of liver tumors combining a spiral-scanning technique with supervised fuzzy pixel classification, *Medical Image Analysis*, vol. 14, no. 1, pp. 13–20, 2010.

48. Y.-T. Chen, A level set method based on the Bayesian risk for medical image segmentation, *Pattern Recognition*, vol. 43, no. 11, pp. 3699–3711, 2010.

49. S. Sokoll, K. Rink, K. D. Toennies, and A. Brechmann, Dynamic segmentation of the cerebral cortex in MR data using implicit active contours, In: *12th Annual Conference on Medical Image Understanding and Analysis MIUA 2008*, Dundee, UK, pp. 184–188, 2008.

50. C. Li, R. Huang, J. C. Gatenby, D. N. Metaxas, and J. C. Gore, A level set method for image segmentation in the presence on intensity inhomogeneities with applications to MRI, *IEEE Transactions on Image Processing*, vol. 20, no. 7, pp. 2007–2016, 2011.

51. X.-F. Wang, D.-S. Huang, and H. Xu, An efficient local Chan–Vese model for image segmentation, *Pattern Recognition*, vol. 43, no. 3, pp. 603–618, 2010.

52. L. Wang, Y. Chen, X. Pan, X. Hong, and D. Xia, Level set segmentation of brain magnetic resonance images based on local Gaussian distribution fitting energy, *Journal of Neuroscience Methods*, vol. 188, pp. 316–352, 2010.

53. K. Zhang, L. Zhang, and S. Zhang, A variational mulitphase level set approach to simultaneous segmentation and bias correction, in *17th IEEE International Conference on Image Processing ICIP 2010*, Hongkong, China, pp. 4105–4108, 2010.

54. C. M. Li, C. Kao, J. Gore, and Z. Ding, Implicit active contours driven by local binary fitting energy, in *IEEE Conf Computer Vision and Pattern Recognition CVPR 2007*, Minneapolis, USA, pp. 1–7, 2007.

55. K. Zhang, H. Song, and L. Zhang, Active contours driven by local image fitting energy, *Pattern Recognition*, vol. 43, no. 4, pp. 1199–1206, 2010.

56. N. Kosic, S. Weber, P. Büchler, C. Lutz, N. Reimers, M. A. Gonzales Ballester, and M. Reyes, Optimisation of orthopaedic implant design using statistical shape analysis based on level set, *Medical Image Analysis*, vol. 14, no. 3, pp. 265–275, 2010.

57. D. Jimenez-Carretero, L. Fernandez-de-Manuel, J. Pascau, J. M. Tellado, E. Ramon, M. Desco, A. Santos, and M. J. Ledesma-Carbayo, Optimal multiresolution 3D level-set method for liver segmentation incorporating local curvature constraints, in *Annual International Conference on IEEE Engineering in Medicine and Biology Society, EMBC 2011*, Boston, USA, pp. 3419–3422, 2011.

58. N. Paragios, A level set approach for shape-driven segmentation and tracking of the left ventricle, *IEEE Transactions on Medical Imaging*, vol. 22, no. 6, pp. 773–776, 2003.

59. M. E. Leventon, W. E. L. Grimson, and O. Faugeras, Statistical shape influence in geodesic active contours, in *IEEE Conference on Computer Vision and Pattern Recognition CVPR 2000*, Hilton Head, USA, vol. 1. pp. 316–323, 2000.

60. M. Rousson and D. Cremers, Efficient kernel density estimation of shape and intensity priors for level set segmentation, in *Medical Image Computing and Computer-Assisted Intervention–MICCAI 2005*. Berlin: Springer, 2005, pp. 757–764.

61. P. H. Lim, U. Bagci, and L. Bai, Introducing Willmore flow into level set segmentation of spinal vertebrae, *IEEE Transactions on Biomedical Engineering*, vol. 60, no. 1, pp. 115–122, 2013.

62. T. Kohlberger, M. G. Uzubas, C. Alvino, T. Kadir, D. Slosman, and G. Funka-Lea, Organ segmentation with level sets using local shape and appearance priors, in *Medical Image Computing and Computer-Assisted Intervention–MICCAI 2009*. Berlin: Springer, 2009, pp. 34–42.

63. M. Farzinfar, Z. Xue, and E. K. Teoh, Joint parametric and non-parametric curve evolution for medical image segmentation, on: *European Conference on Computer Vision ECCV 2008*, Marseille, France, pp. 167–178, 2008.

64. T. Riklin-Raviv, K. van Leemput, B. H. Menze, W. W. Wells III, and P. Golland, Segmentation of image ensembles via latent atlases, *Medical Image Analysis*, vol. 14, no. 5, pp. 654–665, 2010.

65. W. Qiu, J. Yuan, E. Ukwatta, D. Tessier, and A. Fenster, Three-dimensional prostate segmentation using level set with shape constraint based on rotational slices for 3D end-firing TRUS guided biopsy, *Medical Physics*, vol. 40, no. 7, p. 072903, 2013.

66. S. Taheri, S. H. Ong, and V. F. H. Chong, Level-set segmentation of brain tumors using a threshold-based speed function, *Image and Vision Computing*, vol. 28, no 1, pp. 26–37, 2010.

67. K. Rink and K. D. Toennies, A level set bridging force for the segmentation of dendritic spines, in *Computer Analysis of Images and Patterns CAIP 2007*. Berlin: Springer, 2007, pp. 571–578.

68. X. Zeng, L. H. Staib, R. T. Schultz, and J. S. Duncan, Segmentation and measurements of the cortex from 3-D MR images using coupled-surfaces propagation, *IEEE Transactions on Medical Imaging*, vol. 18, no. 10, pp. 927–937, 1999.

69. O. Dzyubachyk, W. A. van Cappellen, J. Essers, W. J. Niessen, and E. Meijering, Advanced level set-based cell tracking in time-lapse fluorescence microspcopy, *IEEE Transactions on Medical Imaging*, vol. 29, no. 3, pp. 852–867, 2010.

70. Z. Ma, R. M. N. Jorge, T. Mascarenhas, and J. M. R. Tavares, Segmentation of female pelvic organs in axial magnetic resonance images using coupled geometric deformable models, *Computers in Biology and Medicine*, vol. 43, no. 4, pp. 248–258, 2013.

71. T. Brox and J. Weickert, Level set segmentation with multiple regions, *IEEE Transactions on Image Processing*, vol. 15, no. 10, pp. 3213–3218, 2006.

72. K Rajpoot, V. Grau, J. A. Noble, H. Becher, and C. Szmigielski, The evaluation of single-view and multi-view fusion 3D echocardiography using image-driven segmentation and tracking, *Medical Image Analysis*, vol. 15, no. 4, pp. 514–528, 2011.

73. S. G. Antunes, J. S. Silva, and J. B. Santos, A level set segmentation method of the four heart cavities in pediatric ultrasound images, in *Image Analysis and Recognition*. Berlin: Springer, 2010, pp. 99–107.

chapter three

Robust image segmentation with a parametric deformable model using learned shape priors

Ahmed Soliman, Marwa Ismail, Ali Taki Eldeen, Georgy Gimel'farb, Ayman El-Baz, and Robert Keynton

Contents

Abstract

Objects of specific shapes in an image are typically segmented with a deformable model, starting at a zero level for a geometric level set function specifying sign-alternate shortest distances to the object boundary from each pixel. The targeted shapes are approximated by a linear combination of 2D distance maps built from mutually aligned images for given training objects. Unfortunately, the approximate shapes may deviate from the training shapes because the space of the distance maps is not closed with respect to linear operations and the map for the zero level of a particular linear combination need not coincide with the shape. To avoid this drawback, we propose a parametric deformable model with the energy tending to approach the learned shapes. Instead of the level sets formalism, the target shapes are approximated directly with linear combinations of distance vectors describing positions of the mutually aligned training shapes with respect to their common centroid. Such a vector space is now closed with respect to the linear operations and it comprises a smaller dimensionality than the 2D distance maps. Thus our shape model is easily simplified with the principal component analysis (PCA) with the shape-dependent energy terms guiding the boundary evolution to obtain a very simple analytic form. Prior knowledge of the visual appearance of the object is represented by Gibbs energies for the objects gray levels. To accurately separate the object from its background, each current empirical marginal probability distribution of gray values within a deformable boundary is also approximated with an adaptive linear combination of discrete Gaussians. Both the shape and appearance priors and the current probabilistic appearance description control the boundary evolution with the appearance-dependent energy terms also having simple forms due to analytical estimates of the Gibbs energy. Experiments with natural images confirm the robustness, accuracy, and high speed of the proposed approach (3.1).

3.1   Introduction

Parametric and geometric deformable models (based on level set techniques) are widely used for image segmentation. However, in many applications, especially in medical image analysis, accurate segmentation with these models is a challenging problem due to (1) noisy or low-contrast 2D/3D images with fuzzy boundaries between goal objects (e.g., anatomical structures); (2) both the objects of interest and multiple background objects consist of small areas or volumes in a typical image; (3) objects have almost the same shape, but different visual appearance (grayscale or color pattern); and (4) the boundaries are frequently discontinuous due to occlusions of the other objects or very similar visual appearance of adjacent parts of different shaped objects [1,2]. This is why prior knowledge about the targeted shape and/or visual appearance may help in its solution [2].

3.1.1   Relationship to the prior works

Traditional deformable models (active contours or "snakes") proposed initially by Kass et al. [3] account for not having prior shape constraints and search for strong signal discontinuities, or grayscale/color edges in an image. Further modifications to this model [4] focus on a numerically stable model evolution process to identify intricate object boundaries by using level set techniques [5]. But, the evolution method of the deformable model is guided by signal edges and general continuity or curvature limitations encounters difficulties when the targeted object is not clearly separated from the background. More accurate and robust results are obtained by evolving a deformable surface under more detailed limitations of the interior grayscale or color pattern, but at the expense of a considerably reduced speed [6].

   Today's image analysis actively explores 2D/3D deformable models based on learning the prior shape and/or appearance constraints from a given training set of manually segmented images. Most of the known approaches make use of only the targeted shapes. Leventon et al. [7] and Shen et al. [8] augment a level set-based energy function to guide the model evolution with statistical and geometrical information enabling their deformable model to generate shapes more like those produced with principal component analysis (PCA) of the training set. Chen et al. [9] use a prior "average shape" in the geometric active contour, while Cootes et al. [10] develop a parametric point distribution model to describe the evolving curve. The latter model describe variations from the average shape with a linear combination of eigenvectors. The points are matched to strong image gradients by determining the shape and pose parameters of the point distribution. Another modified version of this approach is proposed by Pentland and Sclaroff [11].

Staib and Duncan [12] introduced a parametric point model based on an elliptic Fourier decomposition of landmark points, with the model parameters ensuring the best match between the evolving curve and the points of high signal gradient. Chakraborty et al. [13] extend this approach to a hybrid model incorporating information about both the gradient and the appearance homogeneity of the region.

Pizer et al. [14] and Styner et al. [15] segment 3D medical images using coarse-to-fine voxel deformation of a shape-based medial representation ("m-rep"). A geometric deformable contour model proposed by Tsai et al. [1] evolves a zero level of a level set function by generating the 2D map of the signed (positive/negative) shortest distances between each pixel and the contour. The targeted shapes are approximated by a linear combination of the training distance maps for a set of mutually aligned training images. To simplify the model, only a few top-ranked principal components are included in the linear combination. Unfortunately, the approximate shapes may differ from the training shapes because the distance maps space is not closed with respect to the linear operations, so that the map for zero level of a particular linear combination need not coincide with the prior shape. The deformable model of Huang et al. [16] integrates region, shape, and interior signal features assuming an approximate region shape is a priori known and is aligned with the image to initialize the model.

Typically, the total energy function in all these models is based on a simple predefined appearance model that assume significantly different means or variances of the gray values in the object and background (see e.g. Tsai and Yezzi [1] and Tsai et al. [17]). A more promising approach is to also learn the appearance model, although the segmentation in this case is typically based on a pixel- or voxel-wise classification [18]. An alternative approach of Joshi [19] performs nonparametric warping of a targeted surface to a deformable atlas. The atlas contours are then transferred to the targeted volume, but due to lack of shape prior information in guiding the contour evolution, the resulting boundaries may not approach the actual ones. Additionally, the speed for calculating the iterative warpings for a whole image volume is also quite slow.

To overcome these problems, some active contour models, for example, the models of Paragios and Deriche [20] and Cootes et al. [21], assume that the prior probabilistic appearance characteristics have to be learned in order to jointly model both the shape and appearance of a targeted object using PCA. These shape or appearance models have been successfully applied to segment complex 3D medical images, for example, brain, heart, and articular cartilage MRI [21–24]; however, because establishing the pixel- or voxel-wise correspondences between the model and the image is computationally intensive, this segmentation method becomes extremely slow.

3.1.2   Our approach

The approach presented in this chapter involves both the prior shape and appearance knowledge approaches. But instead of using the level set formalism, which runs into problems when combining the training 2D distance maps, we control the evolution of a simple parametric deformable model with energy functions that directly use both the learned shape and appearance data in order to approach the targeted shapes.

Specifically, each targeted shape is represented as a piecewise-linear boundary having a predefined number of control points. These control points are positioned along a number of equiangular rays projection from a common center acting as the centroid of the control points. The boundary is described with a vector of square distances from the center to the circularly ordered control points. All the targeted shapes are represented with a linear combination of the training distance vectors with the training boundaries being mutually aligned to have a common centroid and similar sets as its components.

Given the same center and the same equiangular system of rays, the space of the distance vectors is closed with respect to linear operations, and its dimensionality is considerably smaller than the space of the conventional 2D distance maps. Thus the previously mentioned shape representation is easily simplified using the PCA and excluding the noisy bottom-ranked eigenvectors with small eigenvalues. An evolving boundary is analytically approximated with the closest shape prior and the evolution is controlled by simple energy terms attempting to decrease the approximation errors.

Grayscale patterns that manifest as visual appearance of the training objects are roughly described by Gibbs energies for a spatially homogeneous central-symmetric Markov–Gibbs random field (MGRF) model. The model involves only first-order and central-symmetric second-order statistics of gray levels. Because Gibbs potentials are analytically estimated from the training set of images, the energy terms depending on the appearance prior are also simplified. Simultaneously, the object and background patterns in an image to be segmented are specified with the marginal gray value probability distributions learned by approximating the mixed empirical gray value distribution for the image with a linear combination of discrete Gaussians (LCDG). The LCDG models of the current object and background also are taken into account in the energy terms controlling the model evolution.

This chapter is organized as follows. Section 3.2 describes the proposed shape priors and discusses briefly how the robust scale invariant feature transform (SIFT) by Lowe [25,26] is used to affinely align the images to either build the priors or segment them. Sections 3.3 and 3.4 introduce the MGRF-based appearance prior and the LCDG models of a current image to be segmented, respectively. Section 3.5 presents with full details the evolution of the parametric model guided by the learned shape/appearance priors and the current image appearance. Several experimental results and conclusions are given in Section 3.6.

3.1.3 Basic notation

- (x, y)—Cartesian coordinates of points in the image plane.
- $\mathbf{R} = [(x, y) : x = 0, \ldots, X - 1; y = 0, \ldots, Y - 1]$—A finite arithmetic lattice supporting digital images and their region maps.
- $\mathbf{g} = [g_{x,y} : (x, y) \in \mathbf{R}; g_{x,y} \in \mathbf{Q}]$—A grayscale digital image taking gray values from a finite set $\mathbf{Q} = \{0, \ldots, Q - 1\}$.
- $\mathbf{m} = [m_{x,y} : (x, y) \in \mathbf{R}; m_{x,y} \in \mathbf{L}]$—A region map taking region labels from a finite set $\mathbf{L} = \{\text{ob}, \text{bg}\}$; each label $m_{x,y}$ indicates whether the pixel (x, y) in the corresponding image $\mathbf{g}$ belongs to the targeted object ($m_{x,y} = \text{ob}$) or to the background ($m_{x,y} = \text{bg}$).
- $\mathbf{b} = [\mathbf{p}_k : k = 1, \ldots, K]$—A deformable piecewise-linear boundary with the K control points $\mathbf{p}_k = (x_k, y_k)$ forming a circularly connected chain of line segments $(\mathbf{p}_1, \mathbf{p}_2), \ldots, (\mathbf{p}_{K-1}, \mathbf{p}_K), (\mathbf{p}_K, \mathbf{p}_1)$.
- $\mathbf{d} = [d_k^2 : k = 1, \ldots, K]$—A vector description of the boundary $\mathbf{b}$ in terms of the square distances $d_k^2 = (x_k - x_0)^2 + (y_k - y_0)^2$ from the control points to the model centroid

$\mathbf{p}_0 = (x_0 = \frac{1}{K}\sum_{k=1}^{K} x_k, y_0 = \frac{1}{K}\sum_{k=1}^{K} y_k)$, that is, to the point at the minimum mean square distance from all the control points.

- $\mathbf{S} = \{(\mathbf{g}_t, \mathbf{m}_t, \mathbf{b}_t, \mathbf{d}_t) : t = 1, T\}$—A training set of grayscale images of the targeted objects with manually prepared region maps and boundary models.
- $|\mathbf{A}|$—The cardinality of a finite set $\mathbf{A}$.

3.2   Shape prior to control a parametric model

Attractive and repulsive forces that cause a deformable model to evolve from an initial form to the targeted object boundary have to account for the learned prior knowledge of the shape and visual appearance (grayscale or color pattern) of the targeted object. To build a shape prior, all the training objects in $\mathbf{S}$ are mutually aligned to have the same centroid and unified orientations and scales of all the objects boundaries (see, e.g. Figure 3.1). For the definiteness, each training boundary $\mathbf{b}_t \in \mathbf{S}$ is described with the K control points positioned on the same polar system of $K°$ equiangular rays emitted from the common centroid $\mathbf{p}_0$. The rays are enumerated clockwise and have the angular pitch $2\pi/K°$ and zero angle for the first position $\mathbf{p}_{t,1}$ of each boundary. We assume the alignment centers and uniquely orients each boundary with respect to that polar system. Generally, there may be rays with no or more than one intersection of a particular boundary, so that the number of the control points K may differ from the number of the rays $K°$. For simplicity, it is assumed that $K = K°$, although the model holds for the general case, too.

Because the training boundaries $\mathbf{b}_t \in \mathbf{S}$; $t = 1, \ldots, T$, share the same centroid $\mathbf{p}_0$, any linear combination $\mathbf{d} = \sum_{t=1}^{T} w_t \mathbf{d}_t$ of the training distance vectors defines a unique new boundary $\mathbf{b}$ with the same centroid. Typically, shapes of the training objects are very similar, and their linear combinations should be simplified by the PCA to escape singularities when adjusting to a given boundary.

Let $\mathbf{D} = [\mathbf{d}_1 \, \mathbf{d}_2 \, \cdots \, \mathbf{d}_T]$ and $\mathbf{U} = \mathbf{D}\mathbf{D}^\mathsf{T}$ denote the $K \times T$ matrix with the training distance vectors as columns and the symmetric $K \times K$ Gram matrix of sums of squares and pair products $\sum_{t=1}^{T} d_{t,k}d_{t,k'}$; $k, k' = 1, \ldots, K$ of their components, respectively. The PCA of the matrix $\mathbf{U}$ produces K eigen-vectors $[\mathbf{e}_i : i = 1, \ldots, K]$ sorted by their eigenvalues $\lambda_1 \geq \lambda_2 \geq \cdots \geq \lambda_K \geq 0$. Due to identical or very similar training shapes, most of the bottom-rank eigenvalues are zero or very small, so that the corresponding "noise" eigenvectors are discarded. Only a few top-rank eigenvectors actually represent the training shapes, the

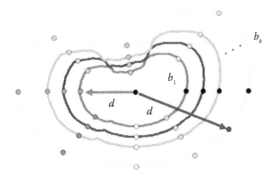

Figure 3.1 Mutually aligned training boundaries.

top distance eigenvector $\mathbf{e}_1$ corresponding to an "average" shape and several others determining its basic variability. For simplicity, we select the top-rank subset of the eigenvectors $(\mathbf{e}_i : i = 1, \ldots, K')$; $K' < K$ by thresholding: $\sum_{i=1}^{K'} \lambda_i \approx \theta \sum_{i=1}^{K} \lambda_i$ with an empirical threshold $\theta = 0.8 \ldots 0.9$.

Let an arbitrary boundary $\mathbf{b}_c$ be aligned with the training set to get the vector description $\mathbf{d}_c$ with the square distances of its control points from the centroid along the same K equiangular rays. Then the prior shape closely approximating this boundary is specified by the following linear combination of the training distance vectors:

$$\mathbf{d}^* = \sum_{i=1}^{K'} w_i^* \mathbf{e}_i \equiv \sum_{i=1}^{K'} \left(\mathbf{e}_i^\mathsf{T} \mathbf{d}_c \right) \mathbf{e}_i \tag{3.1}$$

The signed differences $\Delta_k = d_k^* - d_{c,k}$ determine the directions and forces to control the evolution of the boundary $\mathbf{b}_c$ toward the closest shape prior $\mathbf{b}^*$ specified by the distance vector $\mathbf{d}^*$ in Equation 3.1.

Just as the more conventional geometric (level set-based) deformable models with the shape priors, for example, Tsai and Yezzi [1], our approach depends essentially on a proper mutual alignment of the objects of similar shapes at both the training and segmentation stages. In the latter case, to initialize the deformable model, an image $\mathbf{g}$ to be segmented is to be aligned with one of the training images, say, $\mathbf{g}_1$, arbitrarily chosen in $\mathbf{S}$ as a reference image.

We establish first a number of point-wise correspondences between the two images assuming affine relative geometric distortions and limited contrast/offset signal distortions. Then an affine transform aligning $\mathbf{g}$ most closely to $\mathbf{g}_1$ is determined by minimizing the mean squared positional error between the corresponding points with the gradient descent method. To reliably determine image correspondences, we use the scale invariant feature transform (SIFT) proposed by Lowe [25,26]. Comparisons to several other approaches in Mikolajczyk and Schmidi [27] confirm its higher robustness with the affine geometric distortions present. SIFT determines the correspondences in the three main steps: (i) detection of interest points, (ii) descriptor building, and (iii) descriptor matching.

The interest points are located at the extrema in a difference-of-Gaussian (DOG) image pyramid. The points are localized with subpixel accuracy to have more stable local features [28,29]. The key elements of the SIFT descriptor are local gradient-orientation histograms in the neighbors of an interest point at the same pyramidal level. The orientations are relative to a canonical orientation of the interest point to make the descriptor invariant to the global object orientation. The translation invariance follows directly from the locality of the features, and the DOG pyramid decreases the scale changes of the descriptors.

After the closest SIFT descriptors of the image $\mathbf{g}$ and the reference $\mathbf{g}_1$ are determined, the global 2D affine transform giving the best alignment of these images is estimated using the locations, scales, and canonical orientations of each corresponding pixel pair. Figure 3.2 shows the corresponding points obtained by SIFT for two types of natural images: digital images of starfishes and dynamic magnetic resonance images (DMRI) of human kidneys. The corresponding affinely aligned images in Figure 3.3 have roughly the same center, similar orientation, and approximately equal sizes. Figure 3.3 evaluates quality of the SIFT-based affine alignment with the region maps and grayscale images being the pixelwise averages of all the training maps $\mathbf{m}_t$ and images $\mathbf{g}_t$; $t = 1, \ldots, T$, respectively, before and after the mutual alignment of the training set $\mathbf{S}$. The similar shapes overlap more significantly after the alignment as shown in Figure 3.4.

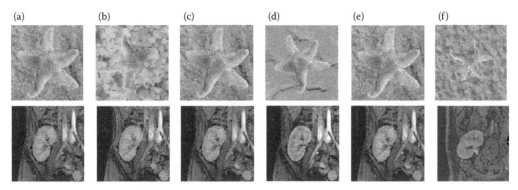

Figure 3.2 Corresponding points found by SIFT in each image pair (a,b), (c,d), and (e,f) (shown in red, green, and yellow, respectively).

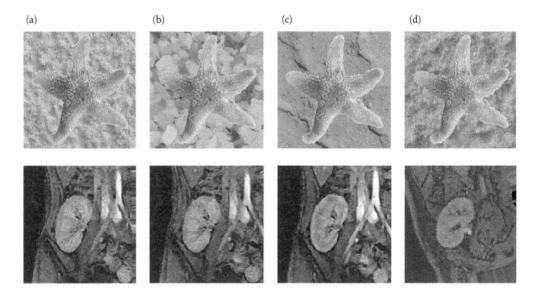

Figure 3.3 Alignment of the images shown in Figure 3.2a–d.

3.3   MGRF image model as an appearance prior

Although mutually aligned training images make it possible, in principle, to construct the appearance priors, typical complex grayscale or color patterns of the targeted objects force to use only rough image descriptors, for example, based on first and second-order grayscale statistics. The latter implicitly "homogenize" each image, that is, substitute certain spatially homogeneous patterns with the same statistics for the actual object. Nonetheless, even such limited prior knowledge is useful in many practical cases to segment the initial complex images.

We describe the aligned training objects as samples of a generic piecewise homogeneous Markov–Gibbs random field (MGRF) with pixelwise and central-symmetric pairwise pixel interactions. Let $\mathbf{N} = \{1, 2, 3, \ldots\}$, $\mathbf{n}_\nu$, and $\mathbf{V}$ denote an index set for successive semi open intervals of characteristic interpixel distances $(d_{\nu,\min}, d_{\nu,\max}]$ specifying central-symmetric pixel neighborhoods, the latter neighborhood as a set of (x, y)-coordinate offsets

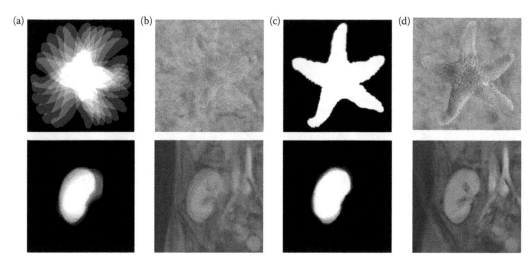

Figure 3.4 Comparison of the shape overlaps in the training datasets: (a,c) region maps and (b,d) grayscale images before (a,b) and after (c,d) the alignment.

between each pixel (x, y) and its neighbor (x', y') such that $d_{\nu,\min} < \sqrt{(x - x')^2 + (y - y')^2} \leq d_{\nu,\max}$, and a set of Gibbs potential functions of gray values in individual pixels and gray value co-occurrences in the neighboring pixel pairs, respectively:

$$\mathbf{V} = \left[\mathbf{V}_{\mathrm{pix}}; \{\mathbf{V}_\nu : \nu \in \mathbf{N}\}\right] \equiv \left[\left[V_{\mathrm{pix}}(q) : q \in \mathbf{Q}\right]; \left\{\left[V_\nu(q, q') : \nu \in \mathbf{N}; (q, q') \in \mathbf{Q}^2\right]\right\}\right]$$

The neighborhood sets $\mathbf{n}_\nu$ corresponding to the uniform distance ranges $(\nu - 0.5, \nu + 0.5]$; $\nu = 1, \ldots, 8$, respectively, are shown in Figure 3.5.

Let $\mathbf{R}_t = \{(x, y) : (x, y) \in \mathbf{R} \wedge m_{t;x,y} = \mathrm{ob}\}$ and $\mathbf{C}_{\nu,t}$ denote the part of the lattice $\mathbf{R}$ supporting the training object in the image–map pair $(\mathbf{g}_t, \mathbf{m}_t) \in \mathbf{S}$ and the family of all pixel pairs in $\mathbf{R}_t^2$ such that each pair has the co ordinate offset $(\xi, \eta) \in \mathbf{n}_\nu$, respectively. Let $\mathbf{F}_{\mathrm{pix},t}$ and $\mathbf{F}_{\nu,t}$ denote joint empirical probability distributions of gray values and gray value

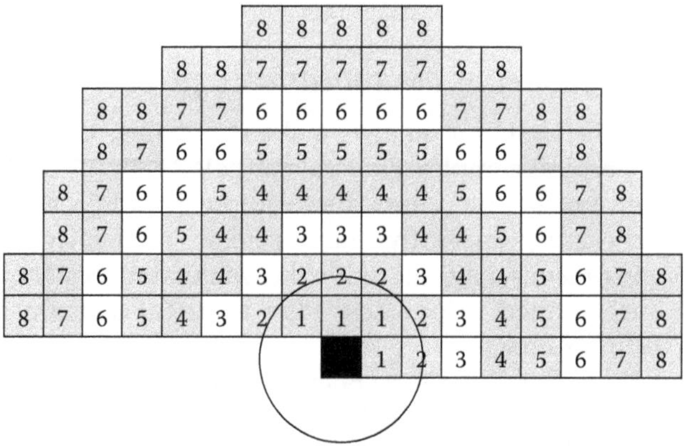

Figure 3.5 Central-symmetric neighborhood sets for the eight distance ranges $(\nu - 0.5, \nu + 0.5)$; $\nu = 1, \ldots, 8$.

co-occurrences in the training object from the image $\mathbf{g}_t$, respectively:

$$\mathbf{F}_{\text{pix},t} = \left[f_{\text{pix},t}(q) = \frac{|\mathbf{R}_{t,q}|}{|\mathbf{R}_t|}; \sum_{q \in \mathbf{Q}} f_{\text{pix},t}(q) = 1 \right]$$

$$\mathbf{F}_{\nu,t} = \left[f_{\nu,t}(q,q') = \frac{|\mathbf{C}_{\nu,t;q,q'}|}{|\mathbf{C}_{\nu,t}|}; \sum_{(q,q') \in \mathbf{Q}^2} f_{\nu,t}(q,q') = 1 \right]$$

where $\mathbf{R}_{t,q} = \{(x,y) : (x,y) \in \mathbf{R}_t \wedge g_{x,y} = q\}$ is a subset of pixels supporting the object's gray value q in the training image $\mathbf{g}_t$ and $\mathbf{C}_{\nu,t;q,q'}$ is a subfamily of all the pixel pairs $\mathbf{c}_{\xi,\eta}(x,y) = ((x,y),(x+\xi,y+\eta)) \in \mathbf{R}_t^2$ supporting the object's gray value co-occurrence (q,q') in the same image, respectively.

The MGRF model of the t-th object is specified by the joint Gibbs probability distribution on the sublattice $\mathbf{R}_t$:

$$P_t = \frac{1}{Z_t} \exp \left(\sum_{(x,y) \in \mathbf{R}_t} \left(V_{\text{pix}}(g_{x,y}) + \sum_{\nu \in \mathbf{N}} \sum_{\mathbf{c}_{\xi,\eta}(x,y) \in \mathbf{C}_{\nu,t}} V_\nu(g_{x,y}, g_{x+\xi,y+\eta}) \right) \right)$$

$$= \frac{1}{Z_t} \exp \left(|\mathbf{R}_t| \left(\mathbf{V}_{\text{pix}}^\top \mathbf{F}_{\text{pix},t} + \sum_{\nu \in \mathbf{N}} \rho_{\nu,t} \mathbf{V}_{\nu,t}^\top \mathbf{F}_{\nu,t} \right) \right) \tag{3.2}$$

where $\rho_{\nu,t} = |\mathbf{C}_{\nu,t}|/|\mathbf{R}_t|$ is an average cardinality of $\mathbf{n}_\nu$ over the sublattice $\mathbf{R}_t$.

Because the areas and shapes of the aligned training objects are similar, then $|\mathbf{R}_t| \approx R_{\text{ob}}$ and $|\mathbf{C}_{\nu,t}| \approx C_{\nu,\text{ob}}$ for $t = 1, \ldots, T$, where R_{ob} and $C_{\nu,\text{ob}}$ are the average cardinalities over the training set $\mathbf{S}$. Assuming the independent samples, the joint probability distribution of gray values for all the training objects has the similar form

$$P_{\mathbf{S}} = \frac{1}{Z} \exp \left(T R_{\text{ob}} \left(\mathbf{V}_{\text{pix}}^\top \mathbf{F}_{\text{pix}} + \sum_{\nu \in \mathbf{N}} \rho_\nu \mathbf{V}_\nu^\top \mathbf{F}_\nu \right) \right)$$

Here, $\rho_\nu = C_{\nu,\text{ob}}/R_{\text{ob}}$, and the empirical probability distributions $\mathbf{F}_{\text{pix,ob}}$ and $\mathbf{F}_{\nu,\text{ob}}$ describe now the gray values and the gray value co-occurrences in all the objects from the training set. Zero empirical probabilities caused by a relatively small volume of the training data available to identify the above mentioned MGRF model are eliminated if fractions defining the empirical probabilities in terms of cardinalities of the related sublattices or subfamilies are modified as follows: $(\langle \text{nominator} \rangle + \varepsilon)/(\langle \text{denominator} \rangle + S\varepsilon)$. The Bayesian quadratic loss estimate suggests the offset $\varepsilon = 1$ and $S = Q$ for the first-order or $S = Q^2$ for the second-order interactions. More conservative approach in Titterington et al. [30] suggests $\varepsilon = 1/S$.

Using the same analytical approach as in Gimel'farb et al. [31], the Gibbs potentials are approximated with the scaled centered empirical probability distributions:

$$V_{\text{pix,ob}}(q) = \lambda \left(f_{\text{pix,ob}}(q) - \frac{1}{Q} \right); \quad (q) \in \mathbf{Q};$$

$$V_{\nu,\text{ob}}(q,q') = \lambda \left(f_{\nu,\text{ob}}(q,q') - \frac{1}{Q^2} \right); \quad (q,q') \in \mathbf{Q}^2; \nu \in \mathbf{N} \tag{3.3}$$

where the common scaling factor λ is also computed analytically. It can be omitted ($\lambda = 1$) when only relative potential values are involved, for example, for relative energies $E_{v,\text{rel}}$ of the central-symmetric pairwise pixel interactions in the training objects. These latter energies are equal to the variances of the co-occurrence distributions:

$$E_{v,\text{rel}} = \sum_{q,q' \in \mathbf{Q}^2} f_{v,\text{ob}}(q,q') \left(f_{v,\text{ob}}(q,q') - \frac{1}{Q^2} \right)$$

and rank the neighborhoods $\mathbf{n}_v$ for choosing most characteristic top-rank prior appearance descriptors $\mathbf{N}' \subset \mathbf{N}$ specifying the central-symmetric neighborhoods of Equation 3.3. Under these priors, a grayscale pattern within a deformable boundary $\mathbf{b}$ in an image $\mathbf{g}$ is described by its Gibbs energy

$$E(\mathbf{g},\mathbf{b}) = \mathbf{V}_{\text{pix,ob}}^{\mathsf{T}} \mathbf{F}_{\text{pix,ob}}(\mathbf{g};\mathbf{b}) + \sum_{v \in \mathbf{N}'} \mathbf{V}_{v,\text{ob}}^{\mathsf{T}} \mathbf{F}_{v,\text{ob}}(\mathbf{g},\mathbf{b})$$

Here, $\mathbf{N}'$ is a selected top-rank index subset of the neighborhoods and the empirical probability distributions are collected within the boundary $\mathbf{b}$ in $\mathbf{g}$.

3.4   LCDG probability model of a current appearance

To account for a current image appearance in addition to the learned shape and appearance priors, the gray level distribution within the evolving boundary $\mathbf{b}$ in an image $\mathbf{g}$ is described with a dynamic mixture of the object and background distributions. To identify the latter, it is closely approximated with a bi-modal linear combination of discrete Gaussians (LCDG) and then split into the object and background LCDG submodels. The approximation is performed with our expectation maximization (EM)-based techniques previously introduced in Gimel'farb et al. [32] and adapted in El-Baz et al. [33] to the DGs.

The DG $\Psi_\theta = (\psi(q|\theta) : q \in \mathbf{Q})$ integrates the continuous Gaussian density over the successive intervals related to the discrete gray values in $\mathbf{Q}$, that is, $\psi(0|\theta) = \Phi_\theta(0.5)$, $\psi(q|\theta) = \Phi_\theta(q+0.5) - \Phi_\theta(q-0.5)$ for $q = 1, \ldots, Q-2$, and $\psi(Q-1|\theta) = 1 - \Phi_\theta(Q-1.5)$ where $\Phi_\theta(q)$ is the cumulative Gaussian probability function with a shorthand notation $\theta = (\mu, \sigma^2)$ for its mean, μ, and variance, σ^2.

Each current appearance is represented with the bi modal LCDG having two dominant positive components that approximate the marginal empirical probability distribution of gray values within the evolving boundary and a number of subordinate positive and negative DGs describing deviations of the empirical distribution from the dominant mixture. Let C_p and C_n such that $C_p \geq 2$ denote the total numbers of the positive and negative components. Then the LCDG model is as follows:

$$p_{\mathbf{w},\Theta}(q) = \sum_{r=1}^{C_p} w_{p,r} \psi(q|\theta_{p,r}) - \sum_{l=1}^{C_n} w_{n,l} \psi(q|\theta_{n,l}) \tag{3.4}$$

where the nonnegative weights $\mathbf{w} = [w_{p,.}, w_{n,.}]$ meet the obvious restriction $\sum_{r=1}^{C_p} w_{p,r} - \sum_{l=1}^{C_n} w_{n,l} = 1$. To identify the model of Equation 3.4, the numbers C_p and C_n of its positive and negative components and the parameters $\mathbf{w}$, Θ (weights, means, and variances) of the positive and negative DGs are estimated first with a sequential EM-based initializing algorithm producing a close initial LCDG approximation of the empirical distribution. Then under the fixed numbers C_p and C_n, all other parameters are refined with an modified EM algorithm that accounts for the alternating components. The final LCDG model is partitioned into the two LCDG submodels $\mathbf{p}_{\text{pix},l} = [p_{\text{pix},l}(q) : q \in \mathbf{Q}]$, one per class $l \in \mathbf{L}$, by associating the subordinate DGs with the dominant terms such that the misclassification rate is minimal. The complete process is detailed in Gimel'farb et al. [32] and El-Baz et al. [33].

3.5   Model evolution

The evolution $\mathbf{b}_\tau \to \mathbf{b}_{\tau+1}$ of the deformable boundary $\mathbf{b}$ in discrete time, $\tau = 0, 1, \ldots$, is specified by the following difference equations system:

$$\mathbf{p}_{k,\tau+1} = \mathbf{p}_{k,\tau} + F(\mathbf{p}_{k,\tau})\mathbf{u}_{k,\tau}; \quad k = 1, \ldots, K \tag{3.5}$$

where $F(\mathbf{p})$ is a velocity function for the control point $\mathbf{p}$ and $\mathbf{u}_{k,\tau}$ is the unit vector along the k-th ray from the centroid to the control point $\mathbf{p}$ of the current boundary. Our velocity function depends on the shape prior, the current appearance evaluated with the LCDG model, and the appearance prior based on the MGRF model as follows:

$$F(\mathbf{p} = (x,y)) = \begin{cases} e^{-\beta\Delta} p_{\text{pix,ob}}(g_{x,y}) \pi_\mathbf{p}(g_{x,y}|\mathbf{S}) & \text{if } \Delta \geq 0 \\ -e^{\beta\Delta} p_{\text{pix,bg}}(g_{x,y}) \pi_\mathbf{p}(g_{x,y}|\mathbf{S}) & \text{if } \Delta < 0 \end{cases} \tag{3.6}$$

Here, Δ is the signed distance between the current control point $\mathbf{p} \in \mathbf{b}_\tau$ and the like one in the closest shape prior along the ray from the current boundary centroid. The constant factor β determines the evolution speed ($0 < \beta < 1$ for a smooth propagation). The marginal probabilities $p_{\text{pix,ob}}(q)$ and $p_{\text{pix,bg}}(q)$ of the gray value q are estimated with the LCDG submodels for the object and its background, respectively, specified in Section 3.4. The prior conditional probability $\pi_\mathbf{p}(q|\mathbf{S})$ of the gray value q in the pixel $\mathbf{p}$, given the current gray values in its particular central-symmetric neighborhood, is estimated in line with the MGRF model of the object appearance in Section 3.3:

$$\pi_\mathbf{p}(g_{x,y}|\mathbf{S}) = \frac{\exp\left(E_\mathbf{p}(g_{x,y}|\mathbf{S})\right)}{\sum\limits_{q \in \mathbf{Q}} \exp\left(E_\mathbf{p}(q|\mathbf{S})\right)}$$

where $E_\mathbf{p}(q|\mathbf{S})$ is the pixelwise Gibbs energy for the gray value q in the pixel $\mathbf{p}$, given the fixed gray values in its neighborhood:

$$E_\mathbf{p}(q|\mathbf{S}) = V_{\text{pix,ob}}(q) + \sum_{\nu \in \mathbf{N}'} \sum_{(\xi,\eta) \in \mathbf{n}_\nu} \left(V_{\nu,\text{ob}}(g_{x-\xi,y-\eta}, q) + V_{\nu,\text{ob}}(q, g_{x+\xi,y+\eta})\right)$$

In total, the proposed segmentation algorithm is summarized as follows:

1. Initializing stage ($\tau = 0$):
   a. Find the mutually matching pixel pairs in a given image $\mathbf{g}$ and one of the aligned training images $\mathbf{g}_{\text{tr}} \in \mathbf{S}$ using the SIFT technique.
   b. Find the affine alignment of $\mathbf{g}$ to $\mathbf{g}_{\text{tr}}$ with the gradient descent technique.

   c. Initialize the deformable boundary with the training one $\mathbf{b}_{tr}$ for $\mathbf{g}_{tr}$.

   d. Initialize the two dominant DGs representing the object and the background with the mean gray values for the arbitrarily selected pixels within and outside the deformable boundary, respectively.

   e. Use the modified EM algorithm in Gimel'farb et al. [32] and El-Baz et al. [33] to estimate the LCDG submodels $\mathbf{p}_{pix,ob}$ and $\mathbf{p}_{pix,bg}$ representing the current object and its background.

2. Evolution stage ($\tau \leftarrow \tau + 1$):

   a. Evolve the deformable boundary in accord with Equation 3.6.

   b. If the overall absolute deformation $\sum_{k=1}^{K} |d_{k,\tau+1} - d_{k,\tau}| \leq \alpha$ (a small predefined threshold), terminate the process; otherwise return to Step 2(a).

3. Segmentation stage: The final boundary is transferred to the initial (nonaligned) image $\mathbf{g}$ by the inverse affine transform.

3.6 Experimental results and conclusions

The performance of the proposed parametric deformable model is evaluated below on two different types of images: the digitized photos of a starfish with the known ground truth (actual object boundaries) and the dynamic contrast-enhanced magnetic resonance imaging (DCE-MRI) of human kidneys. The latter images have been acquired with a Signa Horizon GE 1.5T scanner using a Gadolinium-DTPA contrast agent. After injecting the agent, the abdomen is scanned rapidly and repeatedly, with the fast image acquisition resulting in the high image noise. Moreover, the kidney contrast is continuously changing in the images in accord with perfusion of the contrast agent into the kidney and becomes very low at some perfusion stages. This necessitates the use of the shape priors for segmentation.

Basic stages of segmenting a starfish image are shown in Figures 3.6 through 3.9. In particular, Figure 3.6 demonstrates one of the aligned training images of a starfish, an image to segment, and the SIFT-based alignment of the latter to the former. Figure 3.7 illustrates the initialization of our deformable model with a training boundary and shows the LCDG estimates of the marginal probability distributions over the object (starfish) and background. The resulting segmentation in Figure 3.8 has the error of 0.008% with respect to the ground truth. Figure 3.9 demonstrates the robustness of our segmentation in the case when the same starfish is placed to the uniform background and the whole image is distorted by the uniform independent random noise. When the signal-to-noise ratio (SNR) changes from 20 dB to -1.5 dB, the segmentation error increases from 0.00013% to only 2.9%.

(a) (b) (c)

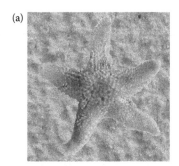 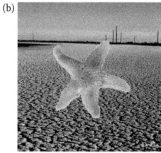 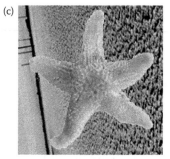

Figure 3.6 One of the mutually aligned training starfish images (a), an image to be segmented (b), and its alignment to the training set (c).

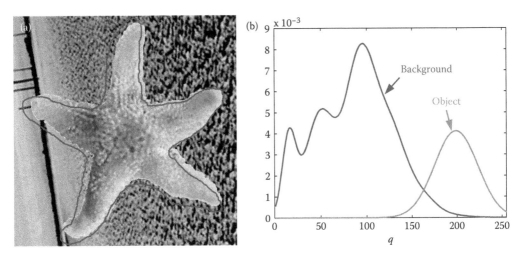

Figure 3.7 Initialization of the deformable model (a) shown in blue, and the LCDG estimates of the marginal gray value distributions $\mathbf{p}_{\text{pix,ob}}$ and $\mathbf{p}_{\text{pix,bg}}$ (b).

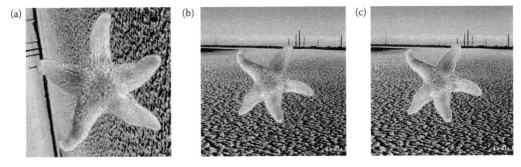

Figure 3.8 Final segmentation of the image aligned to the training set (a) and the same result (b) after its inverse affine transform to the initial image in Figure 3.6b in comparison to the ground truth (c); the total error 0.008% (our boundaries and the ground truth are in red and green, respectively).

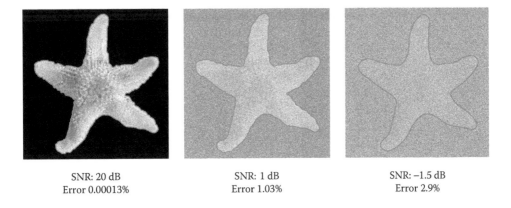

SNR: 20 dB   SNR: 1 dB   SNR: −1.5 dB
Error 0.00013%   Error 1.03%   Error 2.9%

Figure 3.9 Segmentation errors vs. the SNR (our boundaries are in red).

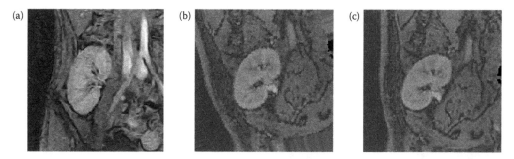

Figure 3.10 One of the mutually aligned training kidney images (a), an image to be segmented (b), and its alignment to the training set (c).

The same segmentation stages for the typical DCE-MRI kidney images are shown in Figures 3.10 through 3.12. Here, the total error of our segmentation is 0.63% with respect to the ground truth provided by a radiologist. Figure 3.13 shows more experimental results for the DCE-MRI with the different kidney contrast. The geometric deformable models with the level set shape priors in Tsai and Yezzi [1] and Tsai et al. [17] produce the like accurate results on the contrast images such as the 11 top images in Figure 3.13, but degrade with the decreasing contrast, for example, on the nine bottom images there.

These and other experiments with various natural images confirm the promising potential of embedding the shape and appearance priors to the parametric deformable models. Our approach assumes the boundaries of the training and targeted objects are similar under the affine transform and the SIFT technique reliably detects the matching points to automatically align the images of the goal objects in spite of their different backgrounds. While the assumptions restrict the application area to comparing to more conventional parametric deformable models, the latter totally fail on the above and similar images. By comparing to more accurate geometric models with linear combinations of the training distance maps as the shape priors, our approach avoids theoretical inconsistencies of the latter, is computationally much simpler and faster, has a similar performance on the contrast images but outperforms on the low-contrast ones.

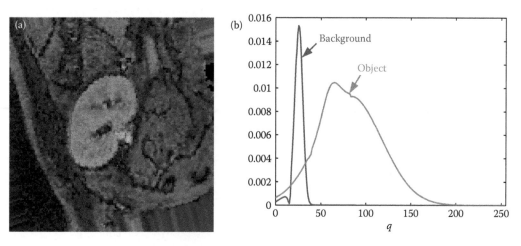

Figure 3.11 Initialization of the deformable model (a) shown in blue, and the LCDG estimates of the marginal gray value distributions $\mathbf{p}_{\text{pix,ob}}$ and $\mathbf{p}_{\text{pix,bg}}$ (b).

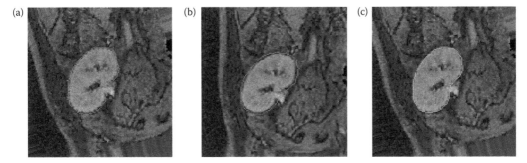

Figure 3.12 Final segmentation of the image aligned to the training set (a) and the same result (b) after its inverse affine transform to the initial image in Figure 3.10b in comparison to the ground truth (c); the total error 0.63% (our boundaries and the ground truth are in red and green, respectively).

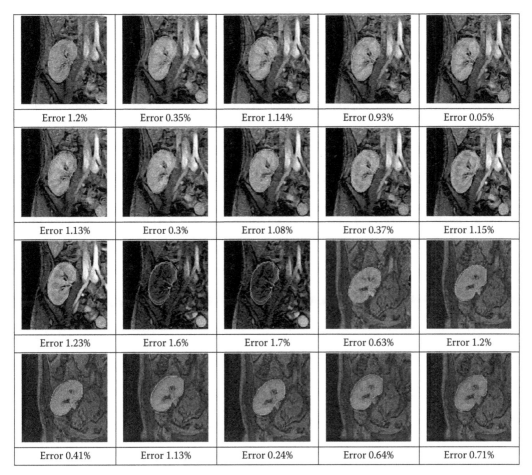

Figure 3.13 Segmentation of 20 other kidney DCE-MRIs: Our final boundaries and the radiologist ground truth are shown in red and green, respectively.

3.7   Conclusions and future work

These and other experiments with various natural images confirm the promising potential of embedding the shape and appearance priors to the parametric deformable models.
Our approach assumes the boundaries of the training and targeted objects are similar
under the affine transform and the SIFT technique reliably detects the matching points
to automatically align the images of the targeted objects in spite of their different backgrounds. By comparing to more accurate geometric models with linear combinations of
the training distance maps as the shape priors, our approach avoids the theoretical inconsistencies of these shape priors, is computationally much simpler and faster, and has a
similar performance on the contrast images, but outperforms on the low-contrast ones.

In addition, several possibilities exist for future work by relating and/or extending this
work to segment 3D medical images such as MR-brain images dyslexia [34–54], DW/MR
kidney images [55–75], and CT chest images [76–105].

References

1. W. W. e. a. A. Tsai and A. Yezzi, A shape based approach to the segmentation of medical imagery
   using level sets, *IEEE Transactions on Medical Imaging*, vol. 22, pp. 137–154, 2003.
2. M. Rousson and N. Paragios, Accurate automatic analysis of cardiac cine images, in *European
   Conference on Computer Vision*, Copenhagen, Denmark, 2002, pp. 78–92.
3. A. W. M. Kass and D. Terzopoulos, Snakes: Active contour models, *International Journal of
   Computer Vision*, vol. 1, pp. 321–331, 1987.
4. R. K. V. Caselles and G. Sapiro, On geodesic active contours, *International Journal of Computer
   Vision*, vol. 22, pp. 61–79, 1997.
5. S. Osher and J. Sethian, Fronts propagating with curvature-dependent speed: Algorithms
   based on Hamilton–Jacobi formulation, *Journal of Computational Physics*, vol. 79, pp. 12–49,
   1988.
6. T. Chan and L. Vese, Active contours without edges, *IEEE Transaction on Image Processing*, vol. 10,
   pp. 266–277, 2001.
7. E. G. M. Leventon and O. Faugeras, Statistical shape influence in geodesic active contours, in
   Proceedings of the IEEE Conf. Computer Vision Pattern Recognition, Hilton Head, SC, June 13–15,
   2000, pp. 316–323.
8. D. Shen and C. Davatzikos, An adaptive-focus deformable model using statistical and geometric information, *IEEE Transaction on Pattern Analysis and Machine Intelligence*, vol. 22, pp. 906–913,
   2000.
9. H. T. E. A. Y. Chen and S. Thiruenkadam, On the incorporation of shape priors into geometric
   active contours, in *Proceedings of the IEEE Workshop Variational and Level Set Methods*, Vancouver,
   Canada, July 13, 2001, pp. 145–152.
10. D. C. T. Cootes, C. Taylor, and J. Graham, Active shape models: Their training and application,
    Computer Vision Image Understanding, vol. 61, pp. 38–59, 1995.
11. A. Pentland and S. Sclaroff, Closed-form solutions for physically based shape modeling and
    recognition, *IEEE Transaction on Pattern Analysis and Machine Intelligence*, vol. 13, pp. 715–729,
    1991.
12. L. Staib and J. Duncan, Boundary finding with parametrically deformable contour models, *IEEE
    Transaction on Pattern Analysis and Machine Intelligence*, vol. 14, pp. 1061–1075, 1992.
13. L. S. A. Chakraborty and J. Duncan, An integrated approach to boundary finding in medical
    images, in *Proceedings of the IEEE Workshop on Biomedical Image Analysis*, Seattle, WA, June 24–25,
    1994, pp. 13–22.
14. S. M. Pizer, G. Gerig, S. Joshi, and S. R. Aylward, Multiscale medial shape-based analysis of
    image objects, *Proceedings of the IEEE*, vol. 91, no. 10, pp. 1670–1679, 2003.

15. M. Styner, G. Gerig, S. Joshi, and S. Pizer, Automatic and robust computation of 3D medial models incorporating object variability, *International Journal of Computer Vision*, vol. 55, no. 2–3, pp. 107–122, 2003.

16. X. Huang, D. Metaxas, and T. Chen, Metamorphs: Deformable shape and texture models, in *Proceedings of the IEEE Conference on Computer Vision Pattern Recognition, 2004*, vol. 1. IEEE, 2004, pp. 1–496.

17. A. Tsai, W. M. Wells, C. Tempany, E. Grimson, and A. S. Willsky, Coupled multi-shape model and mutual information for medical image segmentation, in *Information Processing in Medical Imaging*. Berlin: Springer, 2003, pp. 185–197.

18. K. Van Leemput, F. Maes, D. Vandermeulen, and P. Suetens, A unifying framework for partial volume segmentation of brain MR images, *IEEE Transaction on Medical Imaging*, vol. 22, no. 1, pp. 105–119, 2003.

19. S. Joshi, Large deformation diffeomorphisms and Gaussian random fields for statistical characterization of brain submanifolds, Doctoral thesis., St. Louis, MO: Department of Electrical Engineering, Sever Institute of Technology, Washington University, 1998.

20. N. Paragios and R. Deriche, Geodesic active contours and level sets for the detection and tracking of moving objects, *IEEE Transaction on Pattern Analysis and Machine Intelligence*, vol. 22, no. 3, pp. 266–280, 2000.

21. T. F. Cootes and C. J. Taylor, Statistical models of appearance for medical image analysis and computer vision, in *Medical Imaging 2001*, International Society for Optics and Photonics, 2001, pp. 236–248.

22. A. Hill, A. Thornham, and C. J. Taylor, Model-based interpretation of 3D medical images, in *Proc. 4th British Machine Vision Conference*, Citeseer, 1993, pp. 1–10.

23. A. Kelemen, G. Székely, and G. Gerig, Elastic model-based segmentation of 3-D neuroradiological data sets, *IEEE Transaction on Medical Imaging*, vol. 18, no. 10, pp. 828–839, 1999.

24. Y. Wang and L. H. Staib, Integrated approaches to non-rigid registration in medical images, in *Proceedings of the Applications of Computer Vision, 1998*, IEEE, Princeton, NJ, October 19–21, 1998, pp. 102–108.

25. D. G. Lowe, Object recognition from local scale-invariant features, in *Proceedings of the International Conference on Computer Vision*, vol. 2, IEEE, Kerkyra, Corfu, Greece, September 20–25: 1999, pp. 1150–1157.

26. D. G. Lowe, Distinctive image features from scale-invariant keypoints, *International Journal of Computer Vision*, vol. 60, no. 2, pp. 91–110, 2004.

27. K. Mikolajczyk and C. Schmid, A performance evaluation of local descriptors, *IEEE Transaction on Pattern Analysis and Machine Intelligence*, vol. 27, no. 10, pp. 1615–1630, 2005.

28. M. Brown and D. G. Lowe, Invariant features from interest point groups. in *BMVC*, no. s1, 2002.

29. B. Johansson and R. Söderberg, A repeatability test for two orientation based interest point detectors, 2004.

30. D. Titterington, G. Murray, L. Murray, D. Spiegelhalter, A. Skene, J. Habbema, and G. Gelpke, Comparison of discrimination techniques applied to a complex data set of head injured patients, *Journal of Royal Statistical Society Series A (General)*, pp. 145–175, 1981.

31. G. Gimel'farb, *Image Textures and Gibbs Random Fields*, Dordrecht: Kluwer Academic, 1999.

32. G. Gimel'farb, A. Farag, and A. El-Baz, Expectation–maximization for a linear combination of Gaussians, in *Proceedings of the International Conference on Pattern Recognition (ICPR'2004)*, Cambridge, UK, August 23–26: 2004, pp. 422–425.

33. A. El-Baz, R. M. Mohamed, A. Farag, G. Gimel'farb et al., Unsupervised segmentation of multimodal images by a precise approximation of individual modes with linear combinations of discrete Gaussians, in *Proceedings of Computer Vision and Pattern Recognition Workshops*, IEEE, 2005, pp. 54–54.

34. A. El-Baz, M. Casanova, G. Gimel'farb, M. Mott, A. Switala, E. Vanbogaert, and R. McCracken, Dyslexia diagnostics by 3D texture analysis of cerebral white matter gyrifications, in *Proceedings*

of the International Conference on Pattern Recognition (ICPR'08), IEEE, Tampa, FL, December 8–11: 2008, pp. 1–4.

35. A. El-Baz, M. Casanova, G. Gimel'farb, M. Mott, and A. Switala, An MRI-based diagnostic framework for early diagnosis of dyslexia, *International Journal of Computer Assisted Radiological Surgery*, vol. 3, no. 3–4, pp. 181–189, 2008.

36. A. Elnakib, M. F. Casanova, G. Gimelrfarb, A. E. Switala, and A. El-Baz, Dyslexia diagnostics by 3-D shape analysis of the corpus callosum, *IEEE Transactions on Information Technology in Biomedicine*, vol. 16, no. 4, pp. 700–708, 2012.

37. E. L. Williams, A. El-Baz, M. Nitzken, A. E. Switala, and M. F. Casanova, Spherical harmonic analysis of cortical complexity in autism and dyslexia, *Translat. Neurosci*, vol. 3, no. 1, pp. 36–40, 2012.

38. M. Nitzken, M. F. Casanova, G. Gimel'farb, A. Elnakib, F. Khalifa, A. Switala, and A. El-Baz, 3D shape analysis of the brain cortex with application to dyslexia, in *Proceedings of the IEEE International Conference on Image Processing (ICIP'11)*, 2011, pp. 2657–2660.

39. M. F. Casanova, A. El-Baz, A. Elnakib, J. Giedd, J. M. Rumsey, E. L. Williams, and A. E. Switala, Corpus callosum shape analysis with application to dyslexia, *Translational Neuroscience*, vol. 1, no. 2, pp. 124–130, 2010.

40. A. Elnakib, A. El-Baz, M. F. Casanova, G. Gimel'farb, and A. E. Switala, Image-based detection of corpus callosum variability for more accurate discrimination between dyslexic and normal brains, in *Proceedings of the IEEE International Symposium on Biomedical Imaging: From Nano to Macro, (ISBI'10)*, 2010, pp. 109–112.

41. A. Elnakib, A. El-Baz, M. F. Casanova, and A. E. Switala, Dyslexia diagnostics by centerline-based shape analysis of the corpus callosum, in *Proceedings of the International Conference on Pattern Recognition (ICPR'10)*, 2010, pp. 261–264.

42. A. El-Baz, M. Casanova, G. Gimel'farb, M. Mott, A. Switala, E. Vanbogaert, and R. McCracken, Dyslexia diagnostics by 3D texture analysis of cerebral white matter gyrifications, in *Proceedings of the International Conference on Pattern Recognition (ICPR'08)*, 2008, pp. 1–4.

43. A. El-Baz, M. F. Casanova, G. Gimelfarb, M. Mott, and A. E. Switala, Autism diagnostics by 3D texture analysis of cerebral white matter gyrifications, in *Proceedings of the International Conference on Medical Image Computing and Computer-Assisted Intervention (MICCAI'07)*, Brisbane, Australia, October 29 to November 2: 2007, pp. 882–890.

44. A. El-Baz, A. Elnakib, M. F. Casanova, G. Gimelfarb, A. E. Switala, D. Jordan, and S. Rainey, Accurate automated detection of autism related corpus callosum abnormalities, *Journal of Medical Systems*, vol. 35, no. 5, pp. 929–939, 2011.

45. M. Nitzken, M. F. Casanova, F. Khalifa, G. Sokhadze, and A. El-Baz, Shape-based detection of cortex variability for more accurate discrimination between autistic and normal brains, in *Handbook of Multi Modality State-of-the-Art Medical Image Segmentation and Registration Methodologies*, A. El-Baz, R. Acharya, A. Laine, and J. Suri, Eds. Berlin: Springer, 2011, ch. 7, pp. 161–185.

46. A. Elnakib, M. F. Casanova, G. Gimel'farb, A. E. Switala, and A. El-Baz, Autism diagnostics by centerline-based shape analysis of the corpus callosum, in *Proceedings of the IEEE International Symposium on Biomedical Imaging: From Nano to Macro, (ISBI'11)*, 2011, pp. 1843–1846.

47. A. El-Baz, A. Elnakib, M. F. Casanova, G. Gimel'farb, A. E. Switala, D. Jordan, and S. Rainey, Accurate automated detection of autism related corpus callosum abnormalities, *Journal of Medical Systems*, vol. 35, no. 5, pp. 929–939, 2011.

48. M. F. Casanova, A. El-Baz, A. Elnakib, A. E. Switala, E. L. Williams, D. L. Williams, N. J. Minshew, and T. E. Conturo, Quantitative analysis of the shape of the corpus callosum in patients with autism and comparison individuals, *Autism*, vol. 15, no. 2, pp. 223–238, 2011.

49. M. Nitzken, M. F. Casanova, G. Gimel'farb, F. Khalifa, A. Elnakib, A. E. Switala, and A. El-Baz, 3D shape analysis of the brain cortex with application to autism, in *Proceedings of the IEEE International Symposium on Biomedical Imaging: From Nano to Macro, (ISBI'11)*, 2011, pp. 1847–1850.

50. M. F. Casanova, B. Dombroski, and A. E. Switala, *Imaging and the Corpus Callosum in Patients with Autism*. Berlin: Springer, 2014.

51. M. F. Casanova, A. S. El-Baz, and J. S. Suri, *Imaging the Brain in Autism*. Berlin: Springer.
52. B. Dombroski, M. Nitzken, A. Elnakib, F. Khalifa, A. El-Baz, and M. F. Casanova, Cortical surface complexity in a population-based normative sample, *Translational Neuroscience*, vol. 5, no. 1, pp. 1–8, 2014.
53. M. F. Casanova, A. El-Baz, S. S. Kamat, B. A. Dombroski, F. Khalifa, A. Elnakib, A. Soliman, A. Allison-McNutt, and A. E. Switala, Focal cortical dysplasias in autism spectrum disorders, *Acta Neuropathologica Communications*, vol. 1, no. 1, p. 67, 2013.
54. A. Elnakib, M. F. Casanova, G. Gimel'farb, and A. El-Baz, Autism diagnostics by 3D shape analysis of the corpus callosum, in *Machine Learning in Computer-aided Diagnosis: Medical Imaging Intelligence and Analysis*, K. Suzuki, Ed. Berlin: IGI Global, 2012, ch. 15, pp. 315–335.
55. F. Khalifa, G. M. Beache, M. A. El-Ghar, T. El-Diasty, G. Gimel'farb, M. Kong, and A. El-Baz, Dynamic contrast-enhanced MRI- based early detection of acute renal transplant rejection, *IEEE Transactions on Medical Imaging*, vol. 32, no. 10, pp. 1910–1927, 2013.
56. M. Mostapha, F. Khalifa, A. Alansary, A. Soliman, J. Suri, and A. El-Baz, Computer-aided diagnosis systems for acute renal transplant rejection: Challenges and methodologies, in *Abdomen and Thoracic Imaging*, A. El-Baz and L. Saba J. Suri, Eds. Berlin: Springer, 2014, pp. 1–35.
57. F. Khalifa, M. A. El-Ghar, B. Abdollahi, H. Frieboes, T. El-Diasty, and A. El-Baz, A comprehensive non-invasive framework for automated evaluation of acute renal transplant rejection using DCE-MRI, *NMR Biomedicine*, vol. 26, no. 11, pp. 1460–1470, 2013.
58. S. E. Yuksel, A. El-Baz, A. A. Farag, M. El-Ghar, T. Eldiasty, and M. A. Ghoneim, A kidney segmentation framework for dynamic contrast enhanced magnetic resonance imaging, *Journal of Vibration Control*, vol. 13, no. 9–10, pp. 1505–1516, 2007.
59. F. Khalifa, G. Gimel'farb, M. El-Ghar, G. Sokhadze, S. Manning, P. McClure, R. Ouseph, and A. El-Baz, A new deformable model-based segmentation approach for accurate extraction of the kidney from abdominal CT images, in *Proceedings of the IEEE International Conference on Image Processing (ICIP'11)*, Brussels, Belgium, September 11–14, 2011, pp. 3393–3396.
60. A. Rudra, A. Chowdhury, A. Elnakib, F. Khalifa, A. Soliman, G. M. Beache, and A. El-Baz, Kidney segmentation using graph cuts and pixel connectivity, *Pattern Recognition Letters*, vol. 34, no. 13, pp. 1470–1475, 2013.
61. F. Khalifa, A. Elnakib, G. M. Beache, G. Gimel'farb, M. A. El-Ghar, G. Sokhadze, S. Manning, P. McClure, and A. El-Baz, 3D kidney segmentation from CT images using a level set approach guided by a novel stochastic speed function, in *Proceedings of the Medical Image Computing and Computer-Assisted Intervention (MICCAI'11)*, Toronto, Canada, September 18–22, 2011, pp. 587–594.
62. F. Khalifa, A. El-Baz, G. Gimel'farb, and M. Abo El-Ghar, Non-invasive image-based approach for early detection of acute renal rejection, in *Proceedings of the Medical Image Computing and Computer-Assisted Intervention (MICCAI'10)*, 2010, pp. 10–18.
63. F. Khalifa, A. El-Baz, G. Gimel'farb, R. Ouseph, and M. A. El-Ghar, Shape-appearance guided level-set deformable model for image segmentation, in *Proceedings of the International Conference on Pattern Recognition (ICPR'10)*, 2010, pp. 4581–4584.
64. A. El-Baz and G. Gimel'farb, Robust medical images segmentation using learned shape and appearance models, in *Proceedings of the Medical Image Computing and Computer-Assisted Intervention (MICCAI'09)*, 2009, pp. 281–288.
65. A. El-Baz, G. Gimel'farb, and M. Abo El-Ghar, A novel image analysis approach for accurate identification of acute renal rejection, in *Proceedings of the IEEE International Conference on Image Processing (ICIP'08)*, San Diego, CA, October 12–15, 2008, pp. 1812–1815.
66. A. El-Baz, G. Gimel'farb, and M. A. El-Ghar, Image analysis approach for identification of renal transplant rejection, in *Proceedings of the IEEE International Conference on Pattern Recognition (ICPR'08)*, San Diego, CA, October 12–15, 2008, pp. 1–4.

67. A. El-Baz and G. Gimel'farb, Image segmentation with a parametric deformable model using shape and appearance priors, in *Proceedings of the IEEE International Conference on Computer Vision and Pattern Recognition (CVPR'08)*, Anchorage, AK, June 24–26, 2008, pp. 1–8.

68. A. El-Baz, A. A. Farag, S. E. Yuksel, M. E. A. El-Ghar, T. A. Eldiasty, and M. A. Ghoneim, Application of deformable models for the detection of acute renal rejection, in *Deformable Models*, A. A. Farag and J. S. Suri, Eds. 2007, vol. 1, ch. 10, pp. 293–333.

69. A. El-Baz, G. Gimel'farb, and M. Abou El-Ghar, New motion correction models for automatic identification of renal transplant rejection, in *Proceedings of the Medical Image Computing and Computer-Assisted Intervention (MICCAI'07)*, Brisbane, Australia, October 29 to November 2, 2007, pp. 235–243.

70. A. M. Ali, A. A. Farag, and A. El-Baz, Graph cuts framework for kidney segmentation with prior shape constraints, in *Proceedings of the Medical Image Computing and Computer-Assisted Intervention (MICCAI'07)*, vol. 1, Brisbane, Australia, October 29 to November 2, 2007, pp. 384–392.

71. A. El-Baz, A. Farag, R. Fahmi, S. Yuksel, W. Miller, M. Abou El-Ghar, T. El-Diasty, and M. Ghoneim, A new CAD system for the evaluation of kidney diseases using DCE-MRI, in *Proceedings of the Medical Image Computing and Computer-Assisted Intervention (MICCAI'08)*, New York, NY, September 6–10, 2006, pp. 446–453.

72. A. El-Baz, A. Farag, R. Fahmi, S. Yuksel, M. Abo El-Ghar, and T. Eldiasty, Image analysis of renal DCE MRI for the detection of acute renal rejection, in *Proceedings of the IEEE International Conference on Pattern Recognition (ICPR'06)*, Arlington, VA, April 6–9, 2006, pp. 822–825.

73. A. Farag, A. El-Baz, S. Yuksel, M. Abou El-Ghar, and T. Eldiasty, A framework for the detection of acute rejection with dynamic contrast enhanced magnetic resonance imaging, in *Proceedings of the IEEE International Symposium on Biomedical Imaging: From Nano to Macro (ISBI'06)*, Arlington, VA, April 6–9, 2006, pp. 418–421.

74. S. E. Yuksel, A. El-Baz, and A. A. Farag, A kidney segmentation framework for dynamic contrast enhanced magnetic resonance imaging, in *Proceedings of the International Symposium on Mathmatical Methods in Engineering, (MME'06)*, 2006, pp. 55–64.

75. S. E. Yuksel, A. El-Baz, A. A. Farag, M. E. Abo El-Ghar, T. A. Eldiasty, and M. A. Ghoneim, Automatic detection of renal rejection after kidney transplantation, in *International Congress Series*, vol. 1281, 2005, pp. 773–778.

76. A. El-Baz, A. A. Farag, R. Falk, and R. La Rocca, Automatic identification of lung abnormalities in chest spiral CT scans, in *Proceedings of the IEEE International Conference on Acoustic, Speech, and Signal Processing (ICASSP'03)*, vol. 2, Hong Kong, April 6–10, 2003, pp. 261–264.

77. A. El-Baz, A. A. Farag, R. Falk, and R. L. Rocca, A unified approach for detection, visualization, and identification of lung abnormalities in chest spiral CT scans, in *International Congress Series*, vol. 1256, 2003, pp. 998–1004.

78. A. El-Baz, A. A. Farag, R. Falk, and R. La Rocca, Detection, visualization and identification of lung abnormalities in chest spiral CT scan: Phase-I, in *Proceedings of the International Conference on Biomedical Engineering*, 2002, pp. 38–42.

79. A. A. Farag, A. El-Baz, G. Gimel'farb, and R. Falk, Detection and recognition of lung abnormalities using deformable templates, in *Proceedings of the International Conference on Pattern Recognition (ICPR'04)*, vol. 3, Cambridge, UK, August 23–26, 2004, pp. 738–741.

80. A. A. Farag, A. El-Baz, G. G. Gimelfarb, R. Falk, and S. G. Hushek, Automatic detection and recognition of lung abnormalities in helical CT images using deformable templates, in *Proceedings of the Medical Image Computing and Computer-Assisted Intervention (MICCAI'04)*, Sint-Malo, France, September 26–29, 2004, pp. 856–864.

81. A. El-Baz, S. E. Yuksel, S. Elshazly, and A. A. Farag, Non-rigid registration techniques for automatic follow-up of lung nodules, in *Proceedings of the Conference on Computer Assisted Radiology and Surgery (CARS'05)*, vol. 1281, Berlin, Germany, June 22–25, 2005, pp. 1115–1120.

82. A. A. Farag, A. El-Baz, G. Gimelfarb, M. A. El-Ghar, and T. Eldiasty, Quantitative nodule detection in low dose chest CT scans: new template modeling and evaluation for CAD system design,

in *Proceedings of the Medical Image Computing and Computer-Assisted Intervention (MICCAI'05)*, Palm Springs, CA, October 26–29, 2005, pp. 720–728.

83. A. El-Baz, A. Farag, G. Gimel'farb, R. Falk, M. A. El-Ghar, and T. Eldiasty, A framework for automatic segmentation of lung nodules from low dose chest CT scans, in *Proceedings of the International Conference on Pattern Recognition (ICPR'06)*, 2006, pp. 611–614.

84. A. M. Ali, A. S. El-Baz, and A. A. Farag, A novel framework for accurate lung segmentation using graph cuts, in *Proceedings of the IEEE International Symposium on Biomedical Imaging: From Nano to Macro (ISBI'07)*, Washington, DC, April 12–15, 2007, pp. 908–911.

85. A. El-Baz, G. Gimel'farb, R. Falk, and M. A. El-Ghar, A novel approach for automatic follow-up of detected lung nodules, in *Proceedings of the IEEE International Conference on Image Processing (ICIP'07)*, vol. 5, San Antonio, TX, September 16–19, 2007, pp. 501–504.

86. A. A. Farag, A. El-Baz, G. Gimelfarb, R. Falk, M. A. El-Ghar, T. Eldiasty, and S. Elshazly, Appearance models for robust segmentation of pulmonary nodules in 3D LDCT chest images, in *Proceedings of the International Conference on Medical Image Computing and Computer-Assisted Intervention (MICCAI'06)*, Copenhagen, Denmark, October 1–6, 2006, pp. 662–670.

87. A. M. Ali and A. A. Farag, Automatic lung segmentation of volumetric low-dose CT scans using graph cuts, *Advances in Visual Computing*, 2008, pp. 258–267.

88. A. El-Baz, G. L. Gimel'farb, R. Falk, M. Abou El-Ghar, T. Holland, and T. Shaffer, A new stochastic framework for accurate lung segmentation, in *Proceedings of the Medical Image Computing and Computer-Assisted Intervention (MICCAI'08)*, 2008, pp. 322–330.

89. A. El-Baz, G. L. Gimel'farb, R. Falk, D. Heredis, and M. Abou El-Ghar, A novel approach for accurate estimation of the growth rate of the detected lung nodules, in *Proceedings of the International Workshop on Pulmonary Image Analysis*, 2008, pp. 33–42.

90. A. El-Baz, G. L. Gimel'farb, R. Falk, T. Holland, and T. Shaffer, A framework for unsupervised segmentation of lung tissues from low dose computed tomography images. in *Proceedings of the British Machine Vision Conference (BMVC'08)*, M. Everingham, C. J. Needham, and R. Fraile, Eds. Leeds, UK: British Machine Vision Association, September 1–4, 2008.

91. A. El-Baz, G. Gimel'farb, R. Falk, T. Holland, and T. Shaffer, A new stochastic framework for accurate lung segmentation, in *Proceedings of the International Conference on Medical Image Computing and Computer-Assisted Intervention (MICCAI'08)*, New York, NY, September 6–10, 2008.

92. A. El-Baz, G. Gimel'farb, R. Falk, M. A. El-Ghar, and H. Refaie, Promising results for early diagnosis of lung cancer, in *Proceedings of the IEEE International Symposium on Biomedical Imaging: From Nano to Macro (ISBI'08)*, Paris, France, May 14–17, 2008, pp. 1151–1154.

93. A. El-Baz, G. Gimel'farb, R. Falk, and M. Abo El-Ghar, Automatic analysis of 3D low dose CT images for early diagnosis of lung cancer, *Pattern Recognition*, vol. 42, no. 6, pp. 1041–1051, 2009.

94. A. El-Baz, G. Gimel'farb, R. Falk, M. A. El-Ghar, S. Rainey, D. Heredia, and T. Shaffer, Toward early diagnosis of lung cancer, in *Proceedings of the International Conference on Medical Image Computing and Computer-Assisted Intervention (MICCAI'09)*, London, UK, September 20–24, 2009, pp. 682–689.

95. A. El-Baz, G. Gimel'farb, R. Falk, and M. El-Ghar, Appearance analysis for diagnosing malignant lung nodules, in *Proceedings of the IEEE International Symposium on Biomedical Imaging: From Nano to Macro (ISBI'10)*, Rotterdam, The Netherlands, April 14–17, 2010, pp. 193–196.

96. A. El-Baz, P. Sethu, G. Gimel'farb, F. Khalifa, A. Elnakib, R. Falk, and M. A. El-Ghar, Elastic phantoms generated by microfluidics technology: Validation of an imaged-based approach for accurate measurement of the growth rate of lung nodules, *Biotechnology Journal*, vol. 6, no. 2, pp. 195–203, 2011.

97. A. El-Baz, G. Gimel'farb, R. Falk, M. A. El-Ghar, and J. Suri, Appearance analysis for the early assessment of detected lung nodules, in *Lung Imaging and Computer-Aided Diagnosis*, 2011, ch. 17, pp. 395–404.

98. A. El-Baz, P. Sethu, G. Gimelfarb, F. Khalifa, A. Elnakib, R. Falk, M. A. El-Ghar, and J. Suri, Validation of a new imaged-based approach for the accurate estimating of the growth rate of

detected lung nodules using real computed tomography images and elastic phantoms generated by state-of-theart microfluidics technology, in *Lung Imaging and Computer Aided Diagnosis*, 2011, ch. 18, pp. 405–420.

99. A. El-Baz, M. Nitzken, G. Gimelfarb, E. Van Bogaert, R. Falk, M. A. El-Ghar, and J. Suri, Three-dimensional shape analysis using spherical harmonics for early assessment of detected lung nodules, in *Lung Imaging and Computer Aided Diagnosis*, 2011, ch. 19, pp. 421–438.

100. A. El-Baz, M. Nitzken, F. Khalifa, A. Elnakib, G. Gimel'farb, R. Falk, and M. A. El-Ghar, 3D shape analysis for early diagnosis of malignant lung nodules, in *Proceedings of the Conference on Information Processing in Medical Imaging, (IPMI'11)*, 2011, pp. 772–783.

101. B. Abdollahi, A. Soliman, A. Civelek, X.-F. Li, G. Gimelfarb, and A. El-Baz, A novel 3D joint MGRF framework for precise lung segmentation, *Machine Learning in Medical Imaging*, 2012, pp. 86–93.

102. A. El-Baz, F. Khalifa, A. Elnakib, M. Nitzken, A. Soliman, P. McClure, M. A. El-Ghar, and G. Gimelfarb, A novel approach for global lung registration using 3D Markov–Gibbs appearance model, in *Proceedings of the International Conference on Medical Image Computing and Computer-Assisted Intervention (MICCAI'12)*, Nice, France, October 1–5, 2012, pp. 114–121.

103. A. El-Baz, A. Soliman, P. McClure, G. Gimel'farb, M. A. El-Ghar, and R. Falk, Early assessment of malignant lung nodules based on the spatial analysis of detected lung nodules, in *Proceedings of the IEEE International Symposium on Biomedical Imaging: From Nana to Macro (ISBI'12)*. IEEE, 2012, pp. 1463–1466.

104. A. El-Baz, A. Elnakib, M. Abou El-Ghar, G. Gimel'farb, R. Falk, and A. Farag, Automatic detection of 2D and 3D lung nodules in chest spiral CT scans, *International Journal of Biomedical Imaging*, vol. 2013, 2013.

105. A. Elnakib, G. Gimelfarb, J. S. Suri, and A. El-Baz, Medical image segmentation: A brief survey, in *Multi Modality State-of-the-Art Medical Image Segmentation and Registration Methodologies*. Springer, 2011, pp. 1–39.

chapter four

A 3D active shape model for left ventricle segmentation in MRI

Carlos Santiago, Jacinto C. Nascimento, and Jorge S. Marques

Contents

Abstract

3D active shape models perform the estimation of deformable surfaces in 3D volumes using landmark statistics. First, the average shape and deformation modes are obtained from a set of annotated landmarks (training set). Then, these statistics are used to segment new volumes, involving the estimation of the alignment parameters and deformation coefficients. This approach is well suited to segment the shape of the left ventricle in 3D MRI volumes. However, there are several challenging issues since each MRI volume has a different number of slices, which means that it is difficult to establish correspondences between landmarks of different volumes. This leads to the main question: how can we learn a shape model from volumes with a variable number of slices? Motion artifacts and the large distance between slices make interpolation of voxel intensities a bad choice. The question can, thus, be reformulated: how can we use active shape models without interpolating voxel intensities between slices? This chapter provides an answer to these questions.

We propose an interpolated model that allows the landmarks of each training volume to be resampled. Then, we propose a resampling method for the learned shape model (mean shape and main modes of deformation), in order to ensure that it matches the slices of the test volume without requiring voxel interpolation. The proposed algorithm was tested in 20 MRI volumes using a leave-one-out scheme. The results show that it achieves good segmentation accuracy, with an average Dice coefficient of 0.88 ± 0.06 and an average minimum distance to the ground truth of 1.2 ± 0.7 mm.

4.1   Introduction

Active shape models (ASMs) have been widely used in medical image analysis for their ability to include shape information in the segmentation process. Over the past decade, several ASM-based methods have been proposed to address the 3D segmentation of medical images [1]. Most of them use the point distribution model (PDM) [2] to learn the shape statistics from a set of annotated volumes (training set). The PDM defines the surface of an object using a set of labeled landmarks. These landmarks correspond to specific locations such that there is a correspondence between the i-th landmark on one surface and the i-th landmark on another surface. This allows the computation of shape statistics (mean shape and modes of deformation). However, it requires that all the surfaces are described by the same landmarks.

The previous assumption is not always true. For instance, consider the left ventricle (LV) in 3D cardiac magnetic resonance (MR) volumes. An MR volume consists of a set of 2D images orthogonal to the LV axis and equally spaced. The surface of the LV is often defined by the 2D contours on each volume slice. However, the dimensions of the heart depend on the person and on the cardiac phase, which means the number of slices required to cover the heart varies. This leads to the following question: how can we learn the shape statistics of the LV surface from volumes with a variable number of slices?

This chapter addresses this problem by normalizing the surfaces of the volumes in the training phase, with respect to the number of slices. The normalization is achieved by modeling the position of each landmark (surface point) along the LV axis through interpolation. This allows the surface to be resampled at a set of predefined slices, which guarantees that the surface models in the training set have the same number of landmarks. A schematic illustration of this approach is shown in Figure 4.1 (learning phase). Once the landmark correspondences have been established, we learn a shape model for each volume slice.

After computing the shape statistics (mean shape and main modes of deformation), we use them to segment a new volume, as shown in Figure 4.1 (test phase). However, as before, this new volume may have a different number of slices, which means that the 2D contours of the learned model may not match the volume slices. In most 3D segmentation problems, this is not an issue because the interpolation of voxel intensities provides reliable data. This is not the case in cardiac MR volumes due to the low resolution along the LV axis (e.g., the spacing between slices is typically 1 cm) and to motion artifacts [3]. Interpolating the voxel intensities in this scenario often leads to a loss of contrast between the blood pool (inside the endocardium of the LV) and the myocardium (outside the endocardium of the LV), making the segmentation task very difficult (see Section 4.5 for an example). This leads to a second question: how can we segment a test volume without interpolating voxel intensities between slices? We propose to interpolate the shape model instead, which means resampling the shape statistics (mean shape and the main modes of deformation).

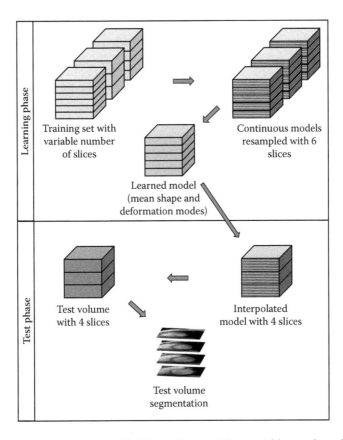

Figure 4.1 Learning and test phases of ASM for volumes with a variable number of slices.

This way, the contours of the shape model are located at the same axial position as the volume slices, which means there is no need to interpolate voxel intensities.

The next section provides an overview of the state of the art for 3D segmentation using shape models. Sections 4.3 and 4.4 describe the proposed shape representation and how it is used to resample the training surfaces. Section 4.5 explains the interpolation of the learned shape model and describes the estimation of the shape model parameters that segment the LV in a test volume. Section 4.6 describes the experimental setup used to evaluate the proposed method and Section 4.7 shows the results obtained. Final conclusions are presented in Section 4.8.

4.2   State of the art

Learning 3D shape models, defined by landmarks is not a simple task [1]. In some problems, such as in cardiac MR volumes, there are no salient features in the volume and it is difficult to obtain unique landmark positions. Consequently, establishing correspondences between landmarks of two objects is not trivial. A popular approach [4–6] to overcome this issue is based the iterative closest point (ICP) algorithm [7]. This algorithm registers two shapes by iteratively establishing landmark correspondences between the two shapes using the best pose estimate and aligning the shapes based on those correspondences.

Several variants of the ICP algorithm have been proposed to improve its results and to allow the use of different numbers of landmarks [8–10].

In the case of the LV segmentation problem, where the LV surface is defined by a set of contours (one per slice), the ICP would be unable to effectively align two LV surfaces with a different number of slices. That is why many works in the 3D LV segmentation problem use other approaches. Mitchell et al. [11], for example, propose the use of a normalized cylindrical coordinate system to define the position of the landmarks. First, they resample each contour at predefined angle intervals around the LV axis, which guarantees that all the 2D contours have the same number of landmarks. It also guarantees that there is a correspondence between the landmarks in consecutive slices. Then, they interpolate the position of the landmarks along the LV axis using linear interpolation. This allows them to resample the number of slices in a volume. Finally, by assuming a fixed position for the basal and axial slices in all the volumes, landmark correspondences between different volumes are easily established. A similar approach is also used by Andreopoulos et al. [3].

Another work [12] performs a preliminary step to establish the position and correspondences of landmarks, based on volumetric registration. Frangi et al. [13] also proposed an automatic method to determine the position of landmarks using this approach. They use a volumetric mesh, in which voxels are labeled based on the type of structure they belong to. These labeled voxels allow the alignment of the volume to a reference one using a non-rigid registration algorithm [14]. After the two volumes have been aligned, the reference landmarks are used to establish the position of the landmarks in the other volume.

As an alternative, the level set method [15] has also been used. For instance, Tsai et al. [16] learned the shape statistics using the signed distance maps in the training set, instead of the landmark's positions. This approach has the advantage of not requiring landmark correspondences between shapes, as well as the advantage of being able to change the topology of the segmentation. The latter is not of particular interest for the problem of segmentation of the LV in MRI, since the LV does not change topology, but may be useful in other applications such as the segmentation of brain structures [17].

As previously mentioned, there is also an additional problem when applying a learned shape model to 3D cardiac (MRI): the interpolation of voxel intensities located between two slices may not provide reliable data due to the large distance between slices and to motion artifacts. To overcome this problem, Andreopoulos et al. [3] proposed using a preprocessing step that corrects misalignments between consecutive slices using an image registration procedure (translation only). Correcting the misalignments increases the reliability of the interpolated voxel intensities. A different approach was also introduced by Van Assen et al. [12,18]. They start by building a triangular mesh using the landmarks of the learned model. This mesh has edges that intersect the volume slices. In an initial step, the set of points that intersect the volume slices are the ones used to obtain the necessary displacement vectors that segment the volume. Then, the displacement vectors are propagated to the corresponding landmarks in the shape model and used to update the model parameters. In this way, they are able to use the available intensity information in the volume without having to interpolated voxel intensities. Nonetheless, some works have used trilinear interpolation to obtain the intensity values at any position within the limits of the volume [11,19].

In the proposed method, landmark correspondences are obtained in a way that is similar to the approach used in Andreopoulos and Tsotsos [3] and Mitchell et al. [11]. However, instead of using a linear interpolation to resample the number of slices, which may create sharp edges in the surface of the LV (due to the large distance between the volume slices), we use a polynomial interpolation of the landmarks' position along the LV axis (see Figure 4.2 for an illustration). In addition, our method is different in the test phase. First, we do not interpolate voxel intensities between slices; instead, we resample the shape model so that it fits the test volume. Second, we use the robust estimation method proposed in Santiago et al. [20] to obtain the shape parameters that segment that volume.

4.3 Interpolation of surface models with a variable number of slices

The PDM approach requires that all surfaces in the training set have the same number of landmarks. As discussed before, in cardiac MRI, this poses a problem because the volumes have a variable number of slices. For a specific volume, v, the slices are located at equally spaced axial positions

$$s_m = \frac{m-1}{S^v - 1},\tag{4.1}$$

where $m = 1, \ldots, S^v$ and S^v is the total number of slices in volume v. We assume that the basal slice is located at $s_1 = 0$ and that the apical slice is located at $s_{S^v} = 1$. The shape model is learned based on medical segmentations, which correspond to the 2D contour of the LV on each slice. This means that the LV surface of volume v in the training set is defined by a set of S^v contours located at the axial positions defined by Equation 4.1.

In order to learn the shape model, the surface models in the training set must have the landmarks at corresponding positions. This can be achieved by (1) using specific landmarks to define each slice contour and (2) using a fix number of slices in all volumes.

Regarding the first step, we resample the contours in arc length at N points, starting at a specific anatomical landmark. Let $x_v(s_m) \in \mathbb{R}^{2N \times 1}$ be the left ventricle contour on the m-th slice of volume v

$$x_v(s_m) = \begin{bmatrix} x^1(s_m) \\ x^2(s_m) \\ \vdots \\ x^N(s_m) \end{bmatrix} = \begin{bmatrix} x_1^1(s_m) \\ x_2^1(s_m) \\ x_1^2(s_m) \\ x_2^2(s_m) \\ \vdots \\ x_1^N(s_m) \\ x_2^N(s_m) \end{bmatrix},\tag{4.2}$$

where $x^i(s_m) = \left[x_1^i(s_m), x_2^i(s_m) \right]^\top \in \mathbb{R}^{2 \times 1}$ is the position of the i-th point. This guarantees that there is a correspondence between the i-th point of one contour and the i-th point of another contour, that is, they represent the same landmark. Concerning the second step, we use an interpolated or approximate model of the landmark positions along the LV axis, defined by $\hat{x}_v(s)$. We wish to model the slice contour as a function of the axial position $s \in [0, 1]$. This is done using a combination of K polynomial basis functions, $\psi(s) \in \mathbb{R}^{K \times 1}$,

$$\hat{x}_v(s) = C_v \psi(s),\tag{4.3}$$

where $C_v \in \mathbb{R}^{2N \times K}$ is the coefficient matrix associated to volume v, defined by

$$C_v = \begin{bmatrix} c_1^1 \\ c_2^1 \\ c_1^2 \\ c_2^2 \\ \vdots \\ c_1^N \\ c_2^N \end{bmatrix}, \tag{4.4}$$

and where the line vector, $c_j^i \in \mathbb{R}^{1 \times K}$, contains the K coefficients associated to the j-th coordinate of the i-th contour point. This coefficient matrix is specific of volume v, that is, each surface is interpolated using a different coefficient matrix. On the other hand, the polynomial basis, $\psi(s) = [1, s, \ldots, s^{K-1}]^\top$, depend only on the slice position, s.

This representation provides an estimate of the LV contour for any position $s \in [0, 1]$ along the LV axis. Ultimately, this means that we are able to redefine the surface of any volume using a predefined number of slices, as shown in Figure 4.2. This approach is used to resample the surface models in the training set. However, the coefficient matrix, C_v, associated to the surface in volume, v, has to be estimated from the corresponding annotations. This problem is addressed in the following section.

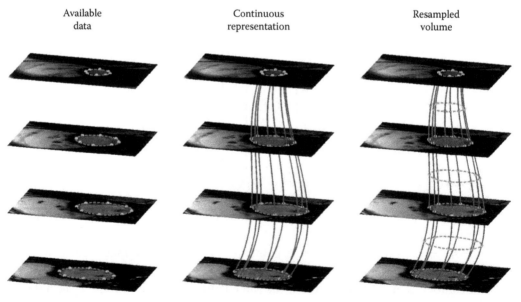

Available data   Continuous representation   Resampled volume

Figure 4.2 Illustration of the resampling process. In this example, the available data (left) consists of an MR volume with four slices and respective contours in red. The blue lines (middle and right) show the interpolated model for a subset of the contour points (green dots), obtained using the four contours, which allows us to obtain the contour at any axial location between the basal and apical slices (right).

4.4 Learning the shape model

We use the interpolation method described in the previous section to resample the surfaces of the training set. This section explains the computation of the coefficient matrix, C_v, for each volume v in the training set and the computation of the shape model.

4.4.1 Resampling the surface models in the training set

The surface of the LV of a particular volume v is represented by a matrix $X_v \in \mathbb{R}^{2N \times S^v}$, given by the concatenation of the slice contours,

$$X_v = [x_v(s_1), x_v(s_2), \ldots, x_v(s_{S^v})]. \tag{4.5}$$

Each pair of lines in X_v, denoted by $X_v^i \in \mathbb{R}^{2 \times S^v}$, can be regarded as samples of the trajectory of the i-th contour point as a function of the slice position, s_m (see the green dots along each blue line in Figure 4.2). Specifically, the trajectory samples are given by

$$X_v^i = \begin{bmatrix} x_1^i(s_1), \ldots, x_1^i(s_{S^v}) \\ x_2^i(s_1), \ldots, x_2^i(s_{S^v}) \end{bmatrix} = \begin{bmatrix} X_{1v}^i \\ X_{2v}^i \end{bmatrix}, \tag{4.6}$$

where X_{jv}^i, $j = 1, 2$, corresponds to a coefficient line vector $c_j^i \in \mathbb{R}^{1 \times K}$, which is a line from matrix C_v (recall Equation 4.4).

The trajectory sample points are used to estimate c_j^i by computing

$$c_j^i = \arg \min_c \| {X_{jv}^i}^\top - \Psi c^\top \|^2 + \gamma \| c \|^2, \tag{4.7}$$

where $\Psi = [\psi(s_1), \ldots, \psi(s_{S^v})]^\top \in \mathbb{R}^{S^v \times K}$ is the concatenation of the polynomial basis $\psi(s_m)$ for $m = 1 \ldots, S^v$, and γ is a regularization constant. This is a ridge regression problem [21] with the following solution

$$c_j^i = X_{jv}^i \Psi \left(\Psi^\top \Psi + \gamma I \right)^{-1}, \tag{4.8}$$

where I is the $K \times K$ identity matrix. Setting $\gamma = 0$ would lead to the ordinary least squares (OLS) solution. A regularization term is used ($\gamma > 0$) because the OLS solution can only be computed for $K \leq S^v$, which means it requires at least the same number of sample points, S^v, as the number of basis functions, K. Since our goal is to use a sufficiently large K ($K = 6$ was the value used in our tests) and to use the same K for all volumes, the OLS would not be suitable. The solution (4.8) can be computed for all the lines in C_v, leading to

$$C_v = X_v \Psi \left(\Psi^\top \Psi + \gamma I \right)^{-1}. \tag{4.9}$$

Now, the contour, $\hat{x}_v(s)$, can be obtained for any position $s \in [0, 1]$ using Equation 4.3.

This approach is used to resample all the surface models included in the training set at $s_m = \frac{m-1}{S^r-1}$, $m = 1, \ldots, S^r$, where S^r is the desired number of slices. This guarantees that all volumes have the same number of landmarks.

4.4.2 Learning the shape statistics

Once all the surface models in the training volumes have been resampled, it is possible to learn a shape model. We assume a surface model results from deforming the mean shape and applying a transformation associated to the pose of the LV [1]. Therefore, in order to compute the shape statistics, all the surface models have to be aligned. This is done by finding, for each surface, a global (pose) transformation T_θ that minimizes the following sum of squared errors

$$E(\theta) = \sum_{m=1}^{S^r} \sum_{i=1}^{N} \left\| T_\theta \left(\widehat{x}^i(s_m) \right) - x_{\text{ref}}^i(s_m) \right\|^2, \tag{4.10}$$

where x_{ref} is a reference shape (for instance, one of the training shapes randomly selected), and $T_\theta(\cdot)$ is a 2D similarity transformation with parameters $\theta = \{a, t\}$, applied to all slices, such that

$$T_\theta \left(\widehat{x}^i(s_m) \right) = \widehat{X}^i(s_m)a + t, \tag{4.11}$$

where

$$\widehat{X}^i(s_m) = \begin{bmatrix} \widehat{x}_1^i(s_m) & -\widehat{x}_2^i(s_m) \\ \widehat{x}_2^i(s_m) & \widehat{x}_1^i(s_m) \end{bmatrix}, \quad a = \begin{bmatrix} a_1 \\ a_2 \end{bmatrix}, \quad t = \begin{bmatrix} t_1 \\ t_2 \end{bmatrix}.$$

We are only interested in the translation, rotation, and scaling within the axial (slice) plane to guarantee that the slice contours remain orthogonal to the LV axis. The minimization of Equation 4.10 leads to a standard least squares solution similar to the alignment algorithm presented in Cootes et al. [2].

After the training surfaces have been aligned, the mean shape of each slice, $\bar{x}(s_m)$, is computed as the average slice contour over all the volumes in the training set. The main modes of deformation, $D(s_m) = [d_1(s_m), \ldots, d_L(s_m)] \in \mathbb{R}^{2N \times L}$, and the corresponding eigenvalues, $\lambda(s_m) = [\lambda_1(s_m), \ldots, \lambda_L(s_m)]^\top \in \mathbb{R}^{L \times 1}$, are obtained by applying principal component analysis (PCA) [1], where $d_l(s_m) \in \mathbb{R}^{2N \times 1}$ and $\lambda_i(s_m) \in \mathbb{R}$ are the l-th main mode of deformation at the m-th slice and corresponding eigenvalue, respectively, and $L \leq 2N$ is the number of main deformation modes that are used.

4.5 ASM for 3D data

After the training phase, the learned shape model can then be used to segment a new MR volume—the test phase. However, the number of slices in the new volume, which we denote as S^t, may not be the same as the learned shape model, S^r. In case $S^t \neq S^r$, one possible approach would be to interpolate the test volume to determine the intensity values at the axial positions of the shape model contours. This would require computing interpolated images. However, the spatial resolution of MRI between axial slices is very low, that is, the distance between two consecutive slices is very large, and significantly larger than the distance between two consecutive pixels in a slice. Typical values for the distance between slices is 10 mm, whereas the distance between two pixels in a slice is approximately 1 mm. Furthermore, motion artifacts can cause significant displacement between the location of the LV contour in consecutive slices. Therefore, interpolating images often leads to the loss of contrast between the blood pool and the myocardium, which determines

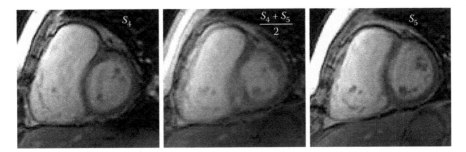

Figure 4.3 Slice interpolation. Example of an interpolated image (middle), located at $s = \frac{s_4 + s_5}{2}$, obtained by linear interpolation between slices s_4 and s_5.

the location of the LV boundary. The images in Figure 4.3 show the result of computing an interpolated image on a slice located between two consecutive slices, using trilinear interpolation. The edges in the new image are blurred and, therefore, it is difficult to accurately determine the location of the LV contour. This means that this approach is a bad choice for 3D segmentation of cardiac MRI.

We use a different approach that consists in resampling the learned shape model, that is, the mean shape and the main modes of deformation. This guarantees that the shape model contours are located at the same axial positions as the volume slices, and thus voxel interpolation is no longer required. The following sections address (i) the interpolation of the learned shape model and (ii) the estimation of the model parameters that segment the LV in a test volume.

4.5.1 Interpolation of shape statistics

In the learning phase, we obtained the mean shape, $\bar{x}(s_m)$, and the main modes of deformation, $D(s_m)$, and their corresponding eigenvalues, $\lambda(s_m)$. These shape statistics were computed for the axial positions $s_m = \frac{m-1}{S^r-1}$, $m = 1, \ldots, S^r$. Now, given a test volume with S^t slices, we wish to obtain the shape statistics for new slice positions $s_m = \frac{m-1}{S^t-1}$, $m = 1, \ldots, S^t$, where $S^t \neq S^r$.

The mean shape in the new slice positions is computed using the same strategy described in the previous sections, that is, by computing the corresponding coefficient matrix, $\bar{C}$, and resampling at the new slice positions. Formally, let $\bar{X} = [\bar{x}(0), \ldots, \bar{x}(1)] \in \mathbb{R}^{2N \times S^t}$ be the concatenation of all the S^t slices of the mean shape. The corresponding coefficient matrix, $\bar{C}$, is computed using Equation 4.9, where the trajectory samples are now given by $\bar{X}$. Then, the mean shape is resampled at S^t slices using Equation 4.3.

On the other hand, resampling the main modes of deformation at intermediate slices is not straightforward, since we need to match deformation modes of different slices. In fact, the modes of deformation are sorted according to the value of the corresponding eigenvalues. Since eigenvalues are learned independently for each slice, it is not easy to find corresponding deformation modes in different slices. In this chapter, we adopt a simple approach that consists of finding the nearest correspondence between deformation modes in consecutive slices and use them to perform a linear interpolation.

Consider a slice position, $s \in [s_m, s_{m+1}]$, located between slices s_m and s_{m+1}. The deformation modes at this slice, $D(s) = [d_1(s), \ldots, d_L(s)]$, are determined using linear interpolation between corresponding deformation modes in s_m and s_{m+1}. Let $\alpha \in [0, 1]$ be the relative distance of slice $s \in [s_m, s_{m+1}]$ to s_m,

$$\alpha = \frac{s - s_m}{s_{m+1} - s_m}. \qquad (4.12)$$

Without loss of generality, we assume that s_m is the closest slice (i.e., $\alpha \leq 0.5$). The l-th deformation mode and corresponding eigenvalue are given by

$$d_l(s) = (1 - \alpha)d_l(s_m) + \alpha d_{F(l)}(s_{m+1}) \qquad (4.13)$$

$$\lambda_l(s) = (1 - \alpha)\lambda_l(s_m) + \alpha \lambda_{F(l)}(s_{m+1}), \qquad (4.14)$$

where $F(\cdot)$ defines the correspondence between the deformation modes in s_m and s_{m+1},

$$F(l) = \arg \min_n \| d_l(s_m) - d_n(s_{m+1}) \|. \qquad (4.15)$$

This interpolation process is repeated for all the deformation modes at all the required slices, that is, for $l = 1, \ldots, L$ and for $s = \frac{m-1}{S^t - 1}$, with $m = 1, \ldots, S^t$.

Once all the deformation modes and eigenvalues have been computed, we define the LV surface as

$$x(s) = T_\theta \left(\bar{x}(s) + D(s)b(s) \right), \qquad (4.16)$$

where $b(s)$ are the deformation coefficients. This means that the segmentation of the test volume is obtained by finding the parameters for the pose transformation, $\theta = \{a, t\}$, and the deformation coefficients, $b(s)$.

The following section describes the estimation of the pose and shape parameters for a new test volume using a robust estimation method.

4.5.2   Automatic surface estimation

Given the test volume, the segmentation of the LV is obtained by estimating the pose, defined by a similarity transformation T_θ with parameters $\theta = \{a, t\}$, and deformation coefficients of the shape model, $b(s)$. However, automatically obtaining these parameters is difficult due to the presence of other structures in the images, such as the epicardium, papillary muscles, and trabeculations [22], which should be considered as noise or outliers.

In this work, the automatic segmentation of the LV is achieved by using the expectation–maximization robust ASM (EM-RASM) estimation method [20], which is robust in the presence of outliers. An overview of the estimation method is shown in Figure 4.4.

First, an initial guess of the pose parameters is required—a rough location of the LV center in the basal slice (first block in Figure 4.4). We assume that the initial values for the

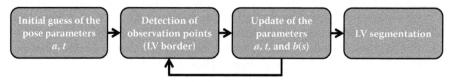

Figure 4.4 Block diagram of the automatic segmentation process using the EM-RASM algorithm [20]. The observation points include outliers that should be rejected by the update block.

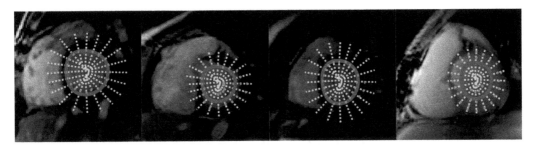

Figure 4.5 Detection of observation points. In each example, the slice contour is shown in blue, the search lines in dashed cyan, and the red dots represent the detected observation points.

deformation coefficients are $b(s) = 0$, that is, that the mean shape is a good initialization. With these parameters, we can determine the location of the slice contours. Then, observation points, corresponding to the LV border, are detected in the vicinity of the model (second block in Figure 4.4). These observation points are searched in each slice, along lines orthogonal to the contour model, as shown in Figure 4.5. The LV border is detected along the search lines by applying an edge detector (see Section 5.2 in Blake and Isard [23] for details). This approach often leads to the detection of outliers, that is, observation points that do not belong to the LV border (see Figure 4.5). These outliers should not be taken into account in the update of the pose and deformation parameters. The EM-RASM is able to handle the outliers by assuming that each observation point may be either an outlier or a valid point. It assigns a weight to each observation point proportional to the probability that the point belongs to the LV border. The weights determine their influence in the estimation of the model parameters, θ and $b(s)$. Since outliers typically get lower weights, their influence in the estimation procedure is reduced and the results are more robust. The final update equations correspond to the weighted least squares solution to the problem of minimizing the distance between each observation point and the corresponding model point (see Santiago et al. [20] for further details), computed over all the slice contours simultaneously (third block in Figure 4.4).

Once the parameters have been updated, the slice contours are updated and new observation points are extracted from the volume. This process iterates until no significant changes in the parameters occur. The final position of the slice contours determines the segmentation of the LV in the MR volume (fourth block in Figure 4.4).

4.6   Experimental setup

The proposed method was evaluated on a set of 20 volumes extracted from a publicly available dataset provided by Andreopoulos and Tsotsos [3]. These volumes consist of end-diastolic short axis cardiac MR volumes, acquired from 20 different subjects at the Department of Diagnostic Imaging of the Hospital for Sick Children in Toronto, Canada. They were acquired using the fast imaging employing steady-state acquisition (FIESTA) scan protocol and a GE Genesis Signa MR scanner. The age of the subjects ranged between 8 and 15 and they displayed not only healthy hearts but also heart abnormalities, such as enlarged right ventricles and ischemia. The image slices were acquired with 256×256 pixels, with a resolution of 0.93–1.64 mm. The number of slices in the volumes ranged from 5 to 10 (recall that we are only interested in the slices depicting the endocardial border of the LV) and the spacing between consecutive slices range from 6 to 13 mm. The dataset also provided the endocardial contour of the LV, which was considered as ground truth (GT). The segmentations obtained using the proposed method were evaluated by comparison with the GT.

The segmentation obtained with the proposed approach was quantitatively evaluated using two metrics: (1) the average Dice similarity coefficient [24] and (2) the average minimum distance between the surface points and the GT. These metrics were computed as follows. Let $z(s) \in \mathbb{R}^{2M \times 1}$ be the GT contour at slice s, defined by M points (the GT and the contour model may have a different number of points). Also, let $R_{x(s)}$ and $R_{z(s)}$ be the regions delimited by the obtained slice contour, $x(s)$, and by the corresponding GT contour, $z(s)$, respectively. The average Dice similarity coefficient is given by

$$d_{\text{Dice}} = \frac{1}{S^t} \sum_{m=1}^{S^t} 2 \frac{A\left(R_{x(s_m)} \cap R_{z(s_m)}\right)}{A\left(R_{x(s_m)}\right) + A\left(R_{z(s_m)}\right)}, \tag{4.17}$$

where $A(\cdot)$ denotes the area of a region. The average minimum distance is given by

$$d_{\text{AV}} = \frac{1}{NS^t} \sum_{m=1}^{S^t} \sum_{i=1}^{N} \min_{j} \|x^i(s_m) - z^j(s_m)\|, \tag{4.18}$$

and was measured in mm.

The results were obtained using a leave-one-out scheme, where the shape model was trained using 19 volumes and then the model was applied to segment the remaining volume. This process was repeated for each test volume. In all the tests, the contours in the training surface models were resampled in arc length to have $N = 40$ points, and the surface model was resampled to have $S^r = 8$ slices (regardless of the number of slices of the test volume). This means that the shape model was learned using a total number of points of $N \times S^r = 320$. Then, the shape model was resampled to have the same number of slices as the test volume, S^t, which means the total number of points in the test phase was $N \times S^t$ (it depends on the test volume).

The interpolation models were computed using the parameters $K = 6$ and $\gamma = 10^{-4}$. These values were empirically chosen by comparing the interpolated model with the corresponding training surface models for different values of K and γ. Figure 4.6 (left) shows the error obtained for different values of K (using $\gamma = 10^{-4}$), and Figure 4.6 (right) shows the error for different values of γ (using $K = 6$). It is possible to see that for values of $K > 6$, the average error does not justify the increase in computational complexity of using larger values of K. Regarding the regularization parameter γ, it is concluded that, for values of $\gamma < 10^{-4}$, the average error does not significantly change. This parameter can be interpreted as a confidence degree of a prior over the coefficients in matrix C_v. By decreasing the value of γ, the influence of the prior over the estimation of C_v is reduced, and the estimation is primarily influenced by the observed data (the trajectories X_v). On the other hand, a higher value of γ helps the estimation of C_v when the number of slices is smaller than K. For this reason, we chose $\gamma = 10^{-4}$ for the following tests.

The obtained shape statistics are exemplified in Figure 4.7. The figure shows the mean shape and the variation introduced by the two first modes of deformation. It is possible to see that, besides local (2D) deformation, these modes also capture the 3D shape variation, caused by misalignments between consecutive slices. In order to determine the influence of the number of deformation modes, L, used in the shape model (recall that we use $L \leq 2N$ modes of the deformation), we compute the error of approximating the contours of the

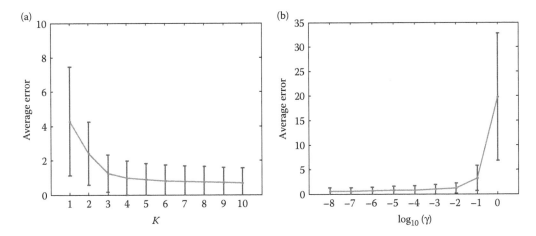

Figure 4.6 Average error (in pixels) of the interpolated model for: (a) different number of polynomial basis functions, K (using $\gamma = 10^{-4}$), and (b) different values of the regularization coefficient, γ (using $K = 6$).

training surfaces by Equation 4.16, that is, a linear combination of the mean shape and the main modes of deformation. The results are shown in Figure 4.8. The plot shows that using more modes of deformation than $L = 10$ does not significantly improve the accuracy of the approximation. Again, choosing a larger value of L would only lead to an increase of the computational complexity of the algorithm. Furthermore, $L = 10$ corresponds to approximately 90% of the variation shown in the training set, which is also a common criterion to select the number of deformation modes used in the shape model [1].

First Deformation Mode

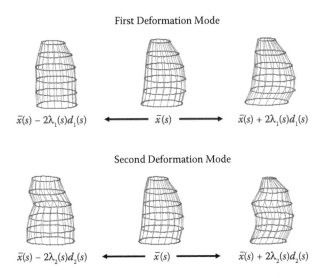

$\bar{x}(s) - 2\lambda_1(s)d_1(s)$ $\longleftarrow$ $\bar{x}(s)$ $\longrightarrow$ $\bar{x}(s) + 2\lambda_1(s)d_1(s)$

Second Deformation Mode

$\bar{x}(s) - 2\lambda_2(s)d_2(s)$ $\longleftarrow$ $\bar{x}(s)$ $\longrightarrow$ $\bar{x}(s) + 2\lambda_2(s)d_2(s)$

Figure 4.7 Shape statistics for the LV. The top row shows the shape variation along the first mode of deformation and the bottom row shows the same for the second mode of deformation. The shape in the middle column corresponds to the mean shape $\bar{x}(s)$. These contours were computed for all the slice positions, $s = s_1, s_2, \ldots, s_6$.

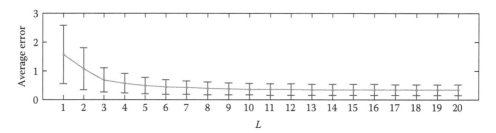

Figure 4.8 Average error (in pixels) of the shape model approximation for different values of the number of deformation modes, L.

4.7 Results

This section shows the evaluation of the segmentations obtained using the proposed method. Some examples of the segmentations are shown in Figure 4.9. It is possible to see that the obtained segmentations are close to the GT. However, in some cases (e.g., the second row), the algorithm is not able to accuracy segment both the apical and basal slices. This is because it is not always possible to find a proper pose transformation that fits all slices, particularly in volumes where there is significant misalignment between slices. The statistics for the two metrics are shown in Figure 4.10 for each test volume. The overall results achieved in these tests were $d_{\text{Dice}} = 0.88 \pm 0.06$ and $d_{\text{AV}} = 1.2 \pm 0.7$ mm.

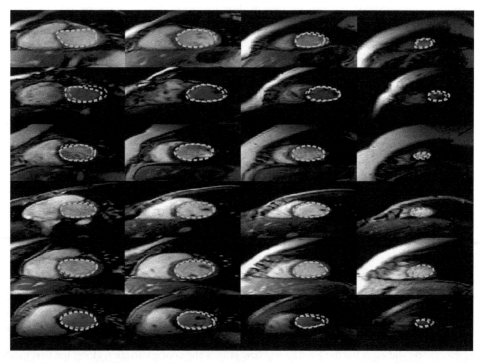

Figure 4.9 Examples of the obtained segmentations. Each line shows a different volume and each row shows a different slice: the left column corresponds to the basal slice and the right column to the apex slice. The red contour is the obtained segmentation and the dashed green is the ground truth.

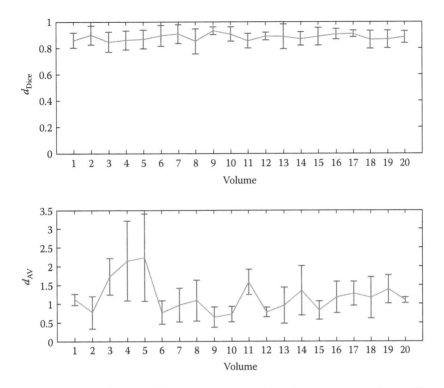

Figure 4.10 Statistical results for all the test volumes using a leave-one-out scheme. The top row shows the Dice coefficient and the bottom row shows the average minimum distance metric (in mm).

Although the proposed method is able to accurately segment the LV, the apical slice remains the most difficult part of the volume to segment. This is due to the fact that the LV chamber is very small in these slices, its borders are often irregular and this makes it difficult to detect the endocardium. This can be verified by the results in Figure 4.11, which shows a 3D representation of the LV surface, as well as a color-coded representation of each slice contours, where the color depends on the corresponding Dice coefficient (green corresponds to a good segmentation and red corresponds to a poor segmentation). In this figure, it is possible to see that most apical slices have poorer accuracy that the basal slices. Nonetheless, the segmentation accuracy is still high, with Dice coefficients of approximately $d_{\text{Dice}} \approx 0.7$.

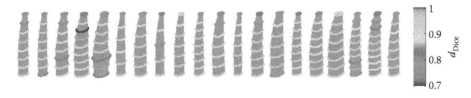

Figure 4.11 Segmentations obtained using the proposed method. The color code shows the accuracy of the segmentation in each slice and for each volume (according to the Dice coefficient).

4.8   Conclusion

Many medical image problems use an active shape model (ASM) based approach to include shape constraints into the segmentation process. However, obtaining the 3D segmentation of cardiac MR volumes has additional difficulties due to the variable number of slices.

Learning a 3D shape model based on a training set of surfaces with a variable number of slices is not easy. We propose to deal with this issue by using a continuous (interpolated) representation for the surface. With this representation, we are able to obtain a smooth continuous surface that can be resampled to have a predefined number of slices. By resampling all the surfaces in the training set, we establish a one-to-one correspondence between the landmarks (surface points) of all the training surfaces. Then, the shape model can be easily learned by aligning the surfaces and applying PCA to determine the shape statistics.

On the other hand, in order to use the learned shape model in a test volume, one has to be careful in case the number of slices of the shape model is different from the number of slices of the test volume. In this case, carelessly applying trilinear interpolation to obtain the intensities of locations in between slices may result in the appearance of dubious edges, due to the large distance between consecutive slices and by the misalignment caused by motion artifacts. We address this issue by resampling the learned model so that it has the same number of slices as the test volume, noting that this involves resampling the mean shape as well as the main modes of deformation. Only then we apply the model to the test volume and estimate the parameters that best segment the volume. This means finding the pose and deformation of the LV. We restrict the possible transformations to rotation, scaling, and translation in 2D, to ensure the surface points remain within the volume slices. The model parameters are obtained using a robust estimation technique, based on the EM algorithm [20].

The proposed approach was tested using 20 volumes from the Andreopoulos and Tsotsos dataset [3]. The shape model was learned using a leave-one-out scheme and the segmentations were evaluated using the Dice similarity coefficient and the average minimum distance metric. The results show that the proposed method is able to accurately segment the LV. However, further improvements may still be achieved. For instance, when the volume slices are misaligned, finding a proper similarity transformation to fit the learned model to the volume is nearly impossible. In these cases, a preprocessing step may be required to correct the misalignment as proposed in Andreopoulos and Tsotsos [3]. Alternatively, one could allow the possibility of having minor independent translations associated to each slice, allowing the model to correct the misalignment of the slices.

Acknowledgments

This work was supported by FCT (SFRH/BD/87347/2012) and (PEst-OE/EEI/LA0009/2013).

References

1. T. Heimann and H. Meinzer, Statistical shape models for 3D medical image segmentation: A review, *Medical Image Analysis*, vol. 13, no. 4, pp. 543–563, 2009.
2. T. F. Cootes, C. J. Taylor, D. H. Cooper, and J. Graham, Active shape models—their training and application, *Computer Vision and Image Understanding*, vol. 61, no. 1, pp. 38–59, 1995.
3. A. Andreopoulos and J. K. Tsotsos, Efficient and generalizable statistical models of shape and appearance for analysis of cardiac MRI, *Medical Image Analysis*, vol. 12, no. 3, pp. 335–357, 2008.

4. A. Caunce and C. J. Taylor, Building 3D sulcal models using local geometry, *Medical Image Analysis*, vol. 5, no. 1, pp. 69–80, 2001.

5. H. Chen and B. Bhanu, Shape model-based 3D ear detection from side face range images, in *Computer Vision and Pattern Recognition Workshops, 2005, CVPR Workshops, IEEE Computer Society Conference on*. IEEE, 2005, pp. 122–122.

6. D. Fritz, D. Rinck, R. Dillmann, and M. Scheuering, Segmentation of the left and right cardiac ventricle using a combined bi-temporal statistical model, in *Medical Imaging*, International Society for Optics and Photonics, 2006, pp. 614 121–614 121.

7. P. J. Besl and N. D. McKay, Method for registration of 3-D shapes, in *Robotics—DL Tentative*. International Society for Optics and Photonics, 1992, pp. 586–606.

8. D. Chetverikov, D. Stepanov, and P. Krsek, Robust euclidean alignment of 3D point sets: The trimmed iterative closest point algorithm, *Image and Vision Computing*, vol. 23, no. 3, pp. 299–309, 2005.

9. B. Jian and B. C. Vemuri, Robust point set registration using Gaussian mixture models, *Pattern Analysis and Machine Intelligence, IEEE Transactions on*, vol. 33, no. 8, pp. 1633–1645, 2011.

10. F. Pomerleau, F. Colas, R. Siegwart, and S. Magnenat, Comparing ICP variants on real-world data sets, *Autonomous Robots*, vol. 34, no. 3, pp. 133–148, 2013.

11. S. C. Mitchell, J. G. Bosch, B. P. Lelieveldt, R. J. van der Geest, J. H. Reiber, and M. Sonka, 3-D active appearance models: segmentation of cardiac mr and ultrasound images, *Medical Imaging, IEEE Transactions on*, vol. 21, no. 9, pp. 1167–1178, 2002.

12. H. C. Van Assen, M. G. Danilouchkine, A. F. Frangi, S. Ordas, J. J. Westenberg, J. H. Reiber, and B. P. Lelieveldt, Spasm: A 3D-ASM for segmentation of sparse and arbitrarily oriented cardiac MRI data, *Medical Image Analysis*, vol. 10, no. 2, pp. 286–303, 2006.

13. A. F. Frangi, D. Rueckert, J. A. Schnabel, and W. J. Niessen, Automatic construction of multiple-object three-dimensional statistical shape models: Application to cardiac modeling, *Medical Imaging, IEEE Transactions on*, vol. 21, no. 9, pp. 1151–1166, 2002.

14. D. Rueckert, L. I. Sonoda, C. Hayes, D. L. Hill, M. O. Leach, and D. J. Hawkes, Nonrigid registration using free-form deformations: Application to breast MR images, *Medical Imaging, IEEE Transactions on*, vol. 18, no. 8, pp. 712–721, 1999.

15. S. Osher and J. A. Sethian, Fronts propagating with curvature-dependent speed: Algorithms based on Hamilton–Jacobi formulations, *Journal of Computational Physics*, vol. 79, no. 1, pp. 12–49, 1988.

16. A. Tsai, A. Yezzi Jr, W. Wells, C. Tempany, D. Tucker, A. Fan, W. E. Grimson, and A. Willsky, A shape-based approach to the segmentation of medical imagery using level sets, *Medical Imaging, IEEE Transactions on*, vol. 22, no. 2, pp. 137–154, 2003.

17. A. Tsai, W. Wells, C. Tempany, E. Grimson, and A. Willsky, Mutual information in coupled multi-shape model for medical image segmentation, *Medical Image Analysis*, vol. 8, no. 4, pp. 429–445, 2004.

18. H. C. Van Assen, M. G. Danilouchkine, M. S. Dirksen, J. Reiber, and B. P. Lelieveldt, A 3-D active shape model driven by fuzzy inference: Application to cardiac CT and MR, *Information Technology in Biomedicine, IEEE Transactions on*, vol. 12, no. 5, pp. 595–605, 2008.

19. M. R. Kaus, J. v. Berg, J. Weese, W. Niessen, and V. Pekar, Automated segmentation of the left ventricle in cardiac MRI, *Medical Image Analysis*, vol. 8, no. 3, pp. 245–254, 2004.

20. C. Santiago, J. C. Nascimento, and J. S. Marques, A robust active shape model using an expectation-maximization framework, in *Image Processing (ICIP), 2014 21th IEEE International Conference on*. IEEE, 2014, pp. 6076–6080.

21. A. E. Hoerl and R. W. Kennard, Ridge regression: Biased estimation for nonorthogonal problems, *Technometrics*, vol. 12, no. 1, pp. 55–67, 1970.

22. C. Petitjean and J. Dacher, A review of segmentation methods in short axis cardiac MR images, *Medical image analysis*, vol. 15, no. 2, pp. 169–184, 2011.

23. A. Blake and M. Isard, *Active Shape Models*. Berlin: Springer, 1998.

24. L. R. Dice, Measures of the amount of ecologic association between species, *Ecology*, vol. 26, no. 3, pp. 297–302, 1945.

chapter five

Model-based segmentation algorithms for myocardial magnetic resonance imaging sequences

Antoine Vacavant, Kévin Bianchi, Guillaume Cerutti, Lucie Cassagnes, Laurent Sarry, and Laure Tougne

Contents

Abstract

This chapter deals with the segmentation of the myocardium from sequences acquired by magnetic resonance imaging (MRI). This muscle surrounds the left ventricle of the heart, and its structure has been well established by the American Heart Association (AHA). The computerized segmentation of the myocardium can lead to several computer-aided diagnosis applications, and in particular the calculation of the myocardial strain, which helps afterwards in diagnosing cardiomyopathies. We describe in detail two different original methodologies designed for the segmentation of the myocardium within short-axis MRI slices of the cardiac sequences.

These approaches have the common point to use an a priori model, related to AHA convention, to guide the calculation of the final segmentation. The first one employs a couple of polygonal contours, while the second is based on a dual B-spline model. We finally show the application of both approaches on samples of MRI sequences extracted from MICCAI 2009 challenge and discuss their extensions and applications.

5.1   Introduction

The heart is a deep, muscular organ ensuring blood flow in the organism [1]. It is decomposed in four parts: left and right auricles (LA, RA) and the left and right ventricles (LV, RV). The right and left cavities are completely separated by walls called the interatrial and interventricular septums, and surrounded by a muscle: the myocardium. Two walls border this organ: the endocardium (interior) and the epicardium (exterior), as depicted in Figure 5.1. As a general viewpoint, the role of the ventricles is to pump the blood to the body or to the lungs. For the LV, the deformation induced by this pumping activity is correlated to the structures of the muscular fibers of the myocardium. To define the structure of the LV and thus be able to study its deformations, the American Heart Association has established a decomposition of this organ into the 17 segments illustrated in Figure 5.2 [2]. This model helps in evaluating myocardial functions in a reproducible and standardized manner. Moreover, it is applicable to every imaging modalities (magnetic resonance imaging, x-ray computed tomography, ultrasound, etc.).

Studying myocardium's activity is an important task for the diagnosis of cardiomyopathies (as ischemic, restrictive, hypertrophic, or dilated cardiomyopathies, for example), and may be based on several imaging modalities. Amongst these modalities, magnetic resonance imaging (MRI) is acknowledged as the reference imaging modality for noninvasive assessment of LV function. MRI allows to acquire diagnostic images for all patients, whatever their morphology is (this is not the case for ultrasound, which is not applicable for 10% of patients). Furthermore, this modality can be employed to obtain images in every anatomic planes (median, frontal, axial planes). Even if the slices of the MRI may be spaced

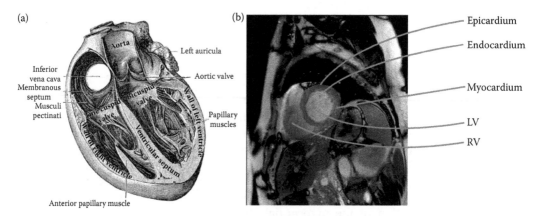

Figure 5.1   (a) Illustration of the components of the heart. (From Wikipedia, Ventricle [heart]— Wikdipedia, the free encyclopedia, 2014. Online. Available: http://en.wikipedia.org/wiki/ Ventricle.) (b) Names of the regions focused on in this chapter, within an MR image (short axis).

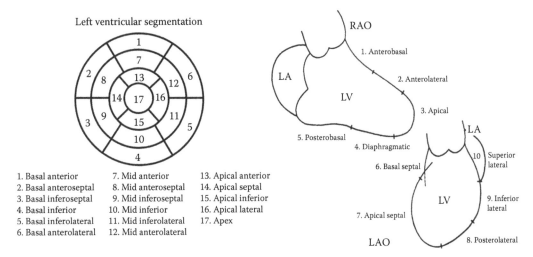

1. Basal anterior	7. Mid anterior	13. Apical anterior
2. Basal anteroseptal	8. Mid anteroseptal	14. Apical septal
3. Basal inferoseptal	9. Mid inferoseptal	15. Apical inferior
4. Basal inferior	10. Mid inferior	16. Apical lateral
5. Basal inferolateral	11. Mid inferolateral	17. Apex
6. Basal anterolateral	12. Mid anterolateral	

Figure 5.2 Standardization of segmentation of the heart by the American Heart Association (AHA). (Images from W. C. Members et al., ACC/AHA/ACR/ASE/ASNC/HRS/NASCI/RSNA/SAIP/SCAI/ SCCT/SCMR/SIR 2008 key data elements and definitions for cardiac imaging: A report of the American College of Cardiology/American Heart Association Task Force on Clinical Data Standards [Writing Committee to Develop Clinical Data Standards for Cardiac Imaging], *Circulation*, vol. 119, no. 1, pp. 154–186, 2009.)

too much to reconstruct an isotropic 3D volume of the heart, MRI is a modality completely adapted to the complex anatomy of this organ. In the cardiac anatomy, two planes are defined: the short and the long axes. In particular, the first one has a key role in the quantification of LV function, imaging all the cardiac cycle with cine MRI (see an example of short axis MRI slice in Figure 5.1). The results obtained in this plane can be directly linked and compared to those from other imaging modalities. This orientation allows to acquire images of LV from the heart's base to its peak (or apex). To acquire all the volume of the LV during the cardiac cycle, the MRI is synchronized with an ECG (electrocardiogram) for a period of 15–20 seconds (to comply with any patient's apnea), depending on the patient's (BPM).

MR images may be altered by a kinetic blurring effect due to the movement of the rib cage of a patient not able to hold his breath correctly. This noise can also be generated by a wrong synchronization with the ECG. Furthermore, since the resolution in the Z-axis is low, a partial volume may happen, which is the consequence of an average of several signals from different tissues on a single pixel.

Computing global or segmental functional indexes as ejection fraction, ventricular mass or wall motion score require to segment and to track myocardium walls. Another challenging application of myocardium's segmentation is the estimation of the myocardial strain. This deformation has been originally introduced in echo-cardiography [3,4], and corresponds to the relative length of a LV segment:

$$E = \frac{(L - L_0)}{L_0},$$

(5.1)

where L_0 is the initial length of a segment and L the one after deformation. This scalar value (commonly represented as a percentage) is positive (resp. negative) when the heart lengthens (resp. reduces) w.r.t. one of the following axes, represented in Figure 5.3:

- The longitudinal strain, representing the deformation between base and apex.
- The radial strain corresponds to the centripetal deformation to the center of the cavity.
- The circumferential strain expresses the decrease of the perimeter of LV.

As a clinical point of view, the diagnosis of cardiomyopathies is generally focused on the value of the peak of strain, at the late systolic time (i.e. at the end of the systole, when the LV is contracted and with its lowest blood volume). In this case, the strain is positive along circumferential and longitudinal axes, and negative in the radial direction.

The segmentation of the myocardium is done within short-axis MRI slices, which allows to directly calculate the radial component of the strain, andthe thickening of the myocardium. To obtain the complete decomposition of the strain, the deformations must be computed for the LV's segments along the circumferential, longitudinal, and radial axes, based on the segmentations on the whole volume of the LV. This extraction of the myocardium implies that the algorithms developed in this context have to track endocardial and/or epicardial walls, during a whole sequence of cardiac MRI.

In this chapter, we propose to present two different original methodologies designed for this segmentation of the myocardium within MRI sequences. The common point between these two techniques is the use of an a priori model to guide and calculate the final segmentation of the epicardial and endocardial walls. These approaches may be related to active contour methodologies, and permit to extract precisely the geometry of the myocardial walls.

The remainder of the chapter covers the following. In Section 5.2, we present a wide state of the art of the segmentation algorithms designed for myocardium segmentation, and we focus on the methods based on active contours and related models. Then, the two algorithms are explained in the two next sections: in Section 5.4, a model composed of two B-spline contours [5]; in Section 5.3, a structure containing two polygonal contours inspired

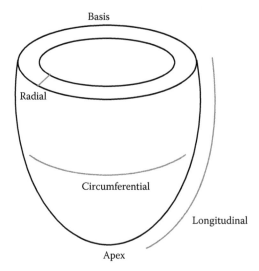

Figure 5.3 The three main possible deformations of the myocardial muscle.

by Cerutti et al. [6]. We end this chapter by showing some illustrations of the results obtained with both approaches for samples of MRI sequences extracted from the MICCAI 2009 challenge [7] before concluding about the added value of this kind of methods in the clinical study of LV.

5.2   State of the art

Generally, the segmentation of epicardium is more difficult than the one of endocardiums, due to the similarity of pixel intensities between external tissues and the heart (see Figure 5.4). This fact implies a very low contrast at the epicardium wall, making it disappear partially. The endocardium separates two homogeneous regions containing different intensities, with a good contrast. In the rest of this section, we present the segmentation methods devoted to extract epicardial and endocardial walls, taking into account these properties observed in cardiac MRI sequences. This nonexhaustive state of the art, which may be completed by the recent reviews [8,9] is decomposed into three categories: The approaches based only on image features, the classification-based algorithms, and the methods applying a statistical shape model.

5.2.1   Image-based approaches

The first articles of the literature dealing with our problem consist in localizing the contour of endocardium, generally by applying a thresholding process [10–12] and/or by dynamic programming (DP) [13–15]. The epicardium is then searched in a second step by using the endocardial contour computed previously and by creating geometric models that take into account the thickness of the myocardium. More recently, we can cite for example the work of Lu et al. [16], who present an automatic segmentation method based on the computation of the convex hull of the cavity, automatically detected in a first phase by mathematical morphology operators. The result is filtered by a 1D Fourier transform to obtain a smooth contour. In this approach, endocardium and epicardium are segmented separately. In Huang et al. [17], is proposed a technique that combines several operations: a detection of image contours with a Canny filter, mathematical morphology operators, and a radial region growing. Once again, the segmentation of epicardium employs the result of

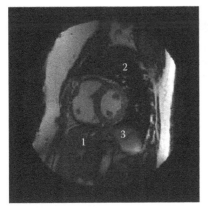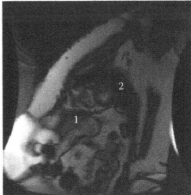

Figure 5.4 Organs surrounding the heart (slide of MRI along short axis): (1) liver, (2) left lung, (3) stomach.

endocardium extraction and the thickness of myocardium. In these kind of methodologies, the user may interact during the initialization of the algorithms, by indicating the center of LV, or by drawing a region of interest (ROI) around the myocardium.

5.2.2 Classification-based approaches

The methods based on the fuzzy connectedness [18] associate seed points (selected in a supervised manner) to the object to segment. They build, for each seed point, a connectedness map by aggregating pixels. This map represents the connectedness between each image point and each seed. A thresholding operation, whose value is determined by the user, is applied on the map so that the structures of interest are conserved. In the approaches based on graph-cuts [19], the user has to select two regions (one for the object of interest and one for the background) to initialize the energy minimization process that uses an algorithm of graph-cut. As an example, this framework has been employed for myocardium segmentation in Kedenburg et al. [20] and Mahapatra [21]. In Marak et al. [22], the authors propose a segmentation 4D (3D+t) method, based on mathematical morphology operators, to segment endocardial and epicardial walls. First, the endocardium is extracted by a geodesic reconstruction depending on several markers. For epicardium, an Euclidean distance transform is calculated to take into account its geometry, and homotopic transformations to guarantee its topology. Finally, a binarization phase is conducted by a watershed cut algorithm [23]. In Jolly [24] is presented an approach that uses a histogram built from a fuzzy connectivity and multi-criteria algorithm. It provides the histograms of lung, myocardium, and blood. The clustering-based methods consist in aggregating the similar data within the same classes. This clustering may be operated by K-means [25] or by fuzzy C-means, and the latter allows partial belonging to classes [26]. After grouping into distinct regions, the cavity is extracted by the computation of the distance to a circle [25].

5.2.3 Statistical shape model-based approaches

The active shape model (ASM) is a statistical model whose parameters are optimized so that they adjust to image graphical objects [27]. This framework is quite similar to the famous active contours, originally introduced by Kass in the formalism of snakes [28], except that they integrate an a priori information about the shape searched inside the image. This knowledge is formalized with the point distribution model (PDM) constructed from learned shapes. This kind of method assumes that points of a shape can be detected within different contexts. These shapes are centered, oriented, and scaled thanks to an algorithm of generalized Procrust analysis. Then the principal variation modes are obtained by principal component analysis of the covariance matrix of normalized points. Each shape can thus be expressed as a linear combination of principal objects. The associated eigenvalues represent the variability of objects and fix the limits of the space of admissible shapes by bounding the coefficients by considering a normal distribution. This active appearance model (AAM) is a generalization of the ASM, which models the distribution of the intensity of points, besides the one of their positions, on the same principle of linear decomposition.

To apply these methodologies on cardiac images, several modifications have been proposed. First, the precision of the algorithm can be improved by the use of independent component analysis (ICA) instead of the PCA [29]. O'Brien et al. [30] present a ASM extended to the multi-contour segmentation of anatomical structures. The 3D segmentation is conducted by the propagation of a 2D ASM. This model considers the endocardium and the epicardium as a single structure, and the authors have an a priori constraint to force the epicardium to stay outside the endocardium. As the endocardial wall is detected with a higher reliability, its energy is minimized first. Thanks to the fact that the endocardium and the epicardium are approximately concentric, a histogram of contour frequency is generated for each value of the epicardium's gradient. For the 3D case, a first segmentation is computed on the basal slice and then a statistical estimation permits to approximate the shape at the next slice. Wijnhout et al. [31] propose an automatic segmentation algorithm using statistical models of 2D AAM and 3D ASM. The final contour of epicardium is obtained by a FCM, which establishes a clustering between three classes: blood/fat, air, and myocardium.

5.3   A polygonal model-based approach

5.3.1   Parametric active polygonal model

The first stage of the myocardium segmentation we propose in this section consists in adjusting, at a coarse scale, a simple shape model to the contour of the endocardium. In order to cover the variability of shapes that the region defined by the endocardium contour can present in MRI images, it is necessary to have a model flexible enough to make a good approximation in each situation. The optimization of such a simple model will give a first idea of the shape of the endocardium that can later be adjusted more precisely to the contour in the image.

We define a parametric polygonal model as a symmetric shape defined by only 12 points. To ensure the properties of regularity and symmetry of the shape, those 12 points are built based on two points defining the symmetry axis of the shape and a reduced set of five generative parameters accounting for the basic characteristics of elongation, skewness, and local roundness of the shape, in the spirit of what had been done for vegetal objects [6]. Such a model, with a very small set of degrees of freedom, can easily reproduce a variety of shapes one can encounter in the myocardium images.

The idea is then to optimize the position of the two control points and the values of the five shape parameters defining the model by an iterative process to make it fit the content of the image. Much like the common approach regarding deformable models, this optimization is seen as an energy minimization problem, with an energy decomposed in an internal energy term and an external, or image attachment, energy term. It is this last term that will guide the evolution of the polygonal model toward the desired region, and it is designed to find a region of consistent intensity within the image.

5.3.2   Intensity dissimilarity map

The external energy term that links the polygonal shape to the content of the image relies on an interpretation of the intensity in the image. As the model is an approximation of the shape, the contour information (gradient or Laplacian) could not be used as such, and we chose to rely only on the intensity level. To fill the energy term, we need a measure over the image that will be minimal for the pixels belonging to the object of interest, and maximal outside of it.

Therefore, we define an intensity dissimilarity measure estimating for each pixel how well it fits with the intensity distribution of the object to segment. In the case of the myocardium, the region inside the endocardium generally presents a rather homogeneous intensity. This is, however, not distinctive enough to detect it in the image, and we use a small supervision to help locate it with a circle drawn by the user inside the right ventricle.

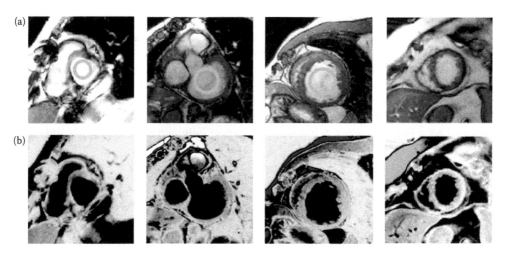

Figure 5.5 Intensity dissimilarity maps for the left ventricle (b) obtained for different myocardium MRI images with manual circle drawings (a).

This initial region is used to estimate a Gaussian distribution of the intensity values of the left ventricle. The parameters $(\bar{I}_{LV}, \sigma_{LV})$ of this Gaussian are used to compute, for each pixel $(x; y)$ in the image, the dissimilarity of its intensity $I(x, y)$ to the estimated intensity distribution:

$$d_{LV}(x, y) = \left(\frac{1}{\sigma_{LV}^2} \left(I(x, y) - \bar{I}_{LV} \right)^2 \right)^{\frac{1}{2}} \tag{5.2}$$

The representation of this dissimilarity $d_{LV}(x, y)$ once normalized over the whole image produces an intensity dissimilarity map such as those displayed in Figure 5.5, where the objects consistent with the intensity model appear in dark and intensity-distant pixels in lighter color.

5.3.3 *Model optimization and guided active contour segmentation*

The problem of optimizing the parametric polygonal model consists in determining the optimal values of the model's parameters that will generate a region Π^* containing as many similar pixels as possible while leaving out dissimilar pixels. To ensure this outcome, we define the image attachment energy, using a maximal acceptable dissimilarity $d_{\max}$ that acts as an implicit threshold:

$$E_{ext}(\Pi) = \sum_{(x;y) \in \Pi} \left(d_{LV}(x, y) - d_{\max} \right) \tag{5.3}$$

The parameter $d_{\max}$ can also be seen as the intensity of a balloon force that pushes the region Π to grow. In addition, an internal energy term is added, by measuring the distance of the values of the construction parameters to reference values, therefore ensuring that the polygonal shapes remain plausible for the object to segment.

Starting from an initial position derived from the manual supervision, the values of the parameters are iteratively optimized by an energy gradient descent approach, where the

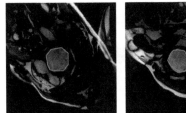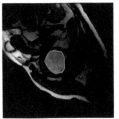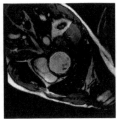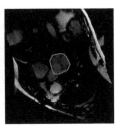

Figure 5.6 Optimized polygonal models on endocardium contours over different myocardium images.

deformation leading to the greatest decrease of energy is selected at each step. The reduced number of parameters involved in the model's construction makes the search space limited. Still, to avoid that the model gets stuck in local minima of energy, we perform a heuristic close to simulated annealing, where nonoptimal deformations might be selected, with a decreasing probability. This optimization process performs a quick estimation of the shape of the endocardium as depicted in Figure 5.6.

To obtain the exact contour of the endocardium, this optimal polygonal model will actually fulfill the role of both initial guess and shape constraint. We perform this segmentation using active contours under the binary level-set framework [32] based on the same energy, to which we add a guiding energy term to constrain the contour to remain close to the polygon. Since the contour is now precise enough, we also add another image attachment term taking into account the gradient information, and a smoothness term to limit the noisiness of the contour.

These so-called guided active contours (GAC) attach to high values of the gradient while avoiding intensity-dissimilar pixels, and are limited in their evolution by the shape prior defined by the optimal polygon. This provides a great robustness to the method, that has been highlighted in the context of leaf segmentation. The result of such segmentation can be seen in Figure 5.8.

5.3.4   From endocardium to epicardium

The computation of the epicardium contour is an easier problem when the endocardium is known, and we chose to use the previous segmentation as a base to perform a segmentation of the myocardium and retrieve its external contour. The major problem comes from the fact that the intensity distribution of the myocardium is different from the one estimated for the LV. To have an appropriate image energy term for the myocardium, we use a dilated region outside the endocardium contour as an initial region on which we estimate a Gaussian model of intensity $(\bar{I}_{My}, \sigma_{My})$ to compute a dissimilarity map $d_{My}(x, y)$ as shown in Figure 5.7.

The segmentation of the epicardium contour is then performed using the same guided active contour method, with a polygonal shape constraint that will be slightly extended compared to the endocardium case. After evolution, this results in a second region, which in the external contour corresponds to the epicardium. Figure 5.8 presents results of this twofold segmentation of both contours of the myocardium on various MR images.

This polygonal model-based approach provides a robust way to segment complex shapes, as the constraints contained in the construction of the model ensure that it will adjust to the best-fitting object in the image without possibility of overflow. Using this

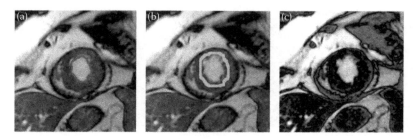

Figure 5.7 Construction of the dissimilarity map for the myocardium region: segmented endocardium contour (a), dilated contour as an initial region for the myocardium (b), and intensity dissimilarity map (c).

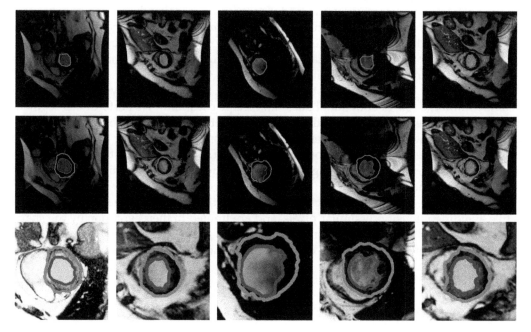

Figure 5.8 Results of polygonal model optimization and endocardium and epicardium segmentation using guided active contours on several MR images.

shape as a guide for an active contour segmentation limits the risk of wrong segmentation in the areas of the image where signal is noisy, while leaving it free to adjust to object boundaries when they are well-defined. This is a robust compromise that guarantees a high-precision segmentation of homogeneous objects.

5.4   A B-spline model-based approach

5.4.1   The dual B-spline model

The B-spline snake, originally introduced by Brigger et al. [33], is a compact representation that deals with the problems raised by the Kass's model [28] and by B-snake [34]: a long convergence due to a high number of parameters, a difficult determination of the correct constraints of elasticity and rigidity, and a description of the curve by a list of disconnected points. As described further, the B-spline snake model is defined by the nodal points of a B-spline curve, which are a simple way to manipulate and to update it. It has been demonstrated that the parametrization of the B-spline is an optimal solution for the regularization of the snake, because the constraint of minimal curve is implicitly related to the parametrization [33]. We base our work on the model of B-spline $\Gamma(s)$, parametrized by the curvilinear abscissa s defined as:

$$\Gamma = \sum_{i=0}^{N-1} \mathbf{Q}_i B_i^3(s), s \in [s_0, s_{N-1}], \tag{5.4}$$

where $\mathbf{Q}_i$ are the control points, $B_i^3(s)$ are the basis functions of B-splines. These control points (not belonging to Γ) can be obtained thanks to the nodal points of the curve by a filtering expressed in Brigger et al. [33], based on this relation:

$$\Gamma(i) = \mathbf{P}_i = \frac{1}{6}(\mathbf{Q}_{i-1} + 4\mathbf{Q}_i + \mathbf{Q}_{i+1}), \tag{5.5}$$

This property is interesting as it permits to any user to control B-splines by only manipulating the nodal points $\mathbf{P}_i$, instead of the control points $\mathbf{Q}_i$.

The model proposed in Bianchi et al. [5] groups the representation of all parts of the LV (epicardium, endocardium, and myocardium) by using two coupled B-spline contours Γ_{endo} and Γ_{epi}. These two curves are parametrized from a median curve Γ_{mid} and a half-thickness term b, inspired from the work [35]:

$$\Gamma_{endo}(s) = \Gamma_{mid}(s) - b(s)\mathbf{N},$$

$$\Gamma_{epi}(s) = \Gamma_{mid}(s) + b(s)\mathbf{N}, \tag{5.6}$$

where $\mathbf{N}$ is the normal vector of Γ_{mid}. This model, named dual B-spline snake (DBS), is also illustrated in Figure 5.9. In this framework, the median curve is constructed by combining

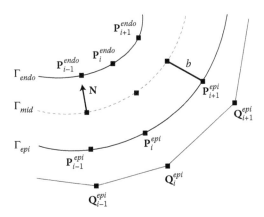

Figure 5.9 The dual B-spline snake model and notations. $\mathbf{P}_i^{epi}$, $\mathbf{P}_i^{endo}$ are the nodal points of the endocardial and epicardial curves, while $\mathbf{Q}_i^{epi}$ are the control points of Γ_{epi}.

two heterogeneous energies and an elastic force:

$$E = \alpha E_1(\Gamma_{endo}) + \beta E_2(\Gamma_{epi}) + \eta E_3(\Gamma_{endo}, \Gamma_{epi}), \tag{5.7}$$

where α, β, and η are scalar weights, $E_1(\Gamma_{endo})$ is a region energy from Chan and Vese [36] dedicated to endocardium, and $E_2(\Gamma_{epi})$ a boundary energy based on the gradient vector flow (GVF) [37] for epicardium. As the contrast of epicardium may be very low due to the lack of gradient information, an elastic force $E_3(\Gamma_{endo}, \Gamma_{epi})$ is applied between the two contours Γ_{endo} and Γ_{epi}. Moreover, the nodal points are forced to move along the limits of the cardiac segmentation defined by the AHA [2] (see also Figure 5.2). The combination of the elastic force together with the constraints implied by the B-spline curves and the movement of nodal points ensure the conservation of the geometry of the final segmentation w.r.t. the myocadium's shape.

5.4.2 Distance map by path propagation

To detect correctly the endocardium, the Chan and Vese term we have mentioned previously needs that the segmented object may be composed of an homogeneous region. To enhance the homogeneity of the myocardium and the one of the cavity, we have adapted the minimum barrier distance (MBD) transform [38,39] to our context. For a path $\pi\colon [0,1] \to \mathbb{R}$, the barrier along π is $\tau_A(\pi) = \max_t f_A(\pi(t)) - \min_t f_A(\pi(t))$, that is, the difference between the maximal and minimal values along this path. In this case, the MBD between two points p and q is defined as:

$$\rho_A(p,q) = \inf_{\pi \in \Pi_{p,q}} \tau_A(\pi). \tag{5.8}$$

Intuitively, $\rho_A(p,q)$ is given by the path between p and q with the minimal barrier. The points of Γ_{epi} and Γ_{endo} are used as seeds for a wave front propagation algorithm adapted from Kårsnäs et al. [38]. Since we have employed a GVF energy for the epicardium case, we need to have a clear gradient information within the processed images. However, the contrast between the myocardium and the surrounding organs may be insufficiently low, as we have shown in Figure 5.4 (see also Figure 5.10 for the application of MBD for endocardium enhancement). To tackle this problem, we conduct a second enhancement of the myocardium, consisting in calculating two MBD transforms based on a geodesic distance. The first one represents the distance between points belonging to the myocardium to the

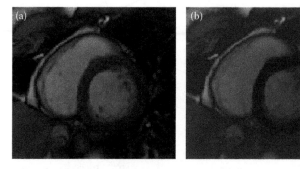

Figure 5.10 Impact of MBD transform on a cardiac MRI slice for endocardium enhancement. (a) Original image. (b) Enhanced image.

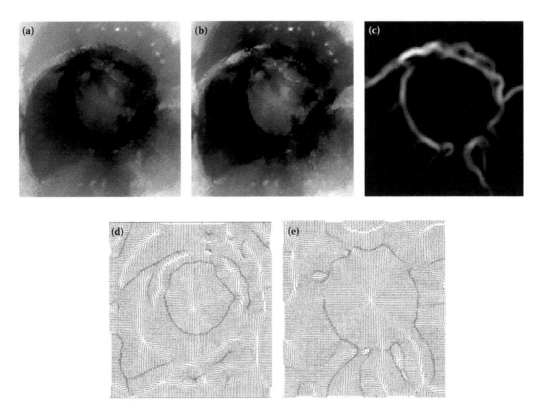

Figure 5.11 Impact of MBD transform with geodesic distance on the GVF calculation. (a) Distance map D_1: myocardium versus background. (b) Distance map D_2: background versus myocardium. (c) Difference between D_1 and D_2. (d) Original GVF. (e) GVF obtained with the difference between D_1 and D_2.

background, while the second one is associated to the reciprocal distance (between points of the background to the myocardium). Then, we compute the absolute difference between both of the two distance maps obtained by these processes; this final map serves as input to the GVF algorithm, and enhances the orientation of the output gradient vectors for a correct extraction of the epicardium. Figure 5.11 groups a collection of images presenting this complete process.

5.4.3   Minimization by gradient descent

The minimization of the global energy of our model (Equation 5.7) implies that we develop the derivatives of the three energies E_1, E_2, and E_3 w.r.t. the nodal points $\mathbf{P}_i$ and the half-thicknesses b_i. As an example, these respective derivatives for the energy E_1 are:

$$
\begin{aligned}
\frac{\partial E_1}{\partial \mathbf{P}_i} &= \left(\frac{\partial E_1}{\partial \Gamma_{mid}} \right)^T \frac{\partial \Gamma_{mid}}{\partial \mathbf{P}_i} \\
&= \frac{\partial E_1}{\partial \Gamma_{mid}} \cdot \frac{\partial \Gamma_{mid}}{\partial \mathbf{P}_i}
\end{aligned}
$$

$$= \left[\left(\frac{\partial E_1}{\partial \Gamma_{endo}} \right)^T \frac{\partial \Gamma_{endo}}{\partial \Gamma_{mid}} \right] \cdot \frac{\partial \Gamma_{mid}}{\partial \mathbf{P}_i}$$

$$= \left[\left(\frac{\partial E_1}{\partial \Gamma_{endo}} \right)^T \left(\mathbf{I}_2 - b \frac{\partial \mathbf{N}_{mid}}{\partial \Gamma_{mid}} \right) \right] \cdot \frac{\partial \Gamma_{mid}}{\partial \mathbf{P}_i}$$

$$= \frac{\partial E_1}{\partial \Gamma_{endo}} \cdot \left[\frac{\partial \Gamma_{mid}}{\partial \mathbf{P}_i} - b \left(\frac{\partial \mathbf{N}_{mid}}{\partial \Gamma_{mid}} \right)^T \frac{\partial \Gamma_{mid}}{\partial \mathbf{P}_i} \right]$$

$$\approx - \frac{\partial E_1}{\partial \Gamma_{endo}} \cdot \frac{\partial \Gamma_{mid}}{\partial \mathbf{P}_i}, \tag{5.9}$$

where we assume that the derivative of the normal vector of the curve Γ_{mid} w.r.t. their nodal points is negligible, and

$$\frac{\partial E_1}{\partial b_i} = \left(\frac{\partial E_1}{\partial \Gamma_{endo}} \right)^T \frac{\partial \Gamma_{endo}}{\partial b_i}$$

$$= - \frac{\partial E_1}{\partial \Gamma_{endo}} \cdot \mathbf{N}_{mid}. \tag{5.10}$$

The combination of those partial derivatives then permits to develop the complete derivative of E w.r.t. the nodal points and to the half thickness terms. To minimize this global energy E, we have utilized the gradient descent with variable steps. This algorithm first calculates the forces applied on nodal points of the median curve, the new position of the points, and the partial derivatives for the update of the half-thickness terms. The endocardial and epicardial curves are updated with the new values of the position of the median curve and the half-thicknesses thanks to Equation 5.6.

Figure 5.12 groups the outputs of this segmentation, composed of the two myocardium contours on several MRI slices.

We also present in Figure 5.13 the use of our algorithm in an interactive application where the user may move nodal points so that the computed curves are corrected. Once the dual B-spline snake has converged on a local minimum of the energy E, any movement of a

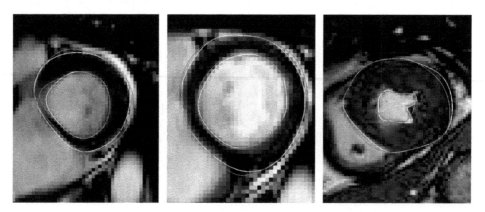

Figure 5.12 Myocardial wall segmentation issues with dual B-spline snake (red curves) compared to expert delineation (white curves).

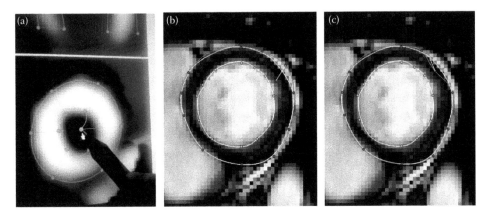

Figure 5.13 (a) Moving a point for the interaction correction of the curves thanks to an interactive screen and a pen. (b) The image-based force is aligned with the interaction and guides toward the global minima of the energy. (c) This force opposes the user who gets away from the minimum.

point implies the calculation in real time of feedback forces acting against the user: they are minimal at the expected place of a global minimum. The action of the user can extract the model from a local minimum thanks to a sufficient opposition to these antagonist image-based forces.

5.5   Experimental evaluations

In this section, we propose to present a quantitative and visual experimental evaluation of the two approaches developed in this chapter: GAC (g from Section 5.3) and DBS (from Section 5.4).

In clinical practice, the endocardial and epicardial contours are employed to quantify the cardiac function. In the specific case of the LV, the clinicians (radiologists, nuclear physicians, etc.) are mainly interested in two clinical indexes: the ventricular mass (VM) and the volume of the cavity (VC). The latter is necessary to compute the ejection fraction (EF), which is the percentage of blood ejected within the cavity. The EF depends only on the endocardium's geometry, whereas the VM is deduced from both myocardium walls. The calculation of these clinical indexes is based on the telediastolic and telesystolic times, which are bound the cardiac cycle.

The evaluation conducted within the challenge provided in Radau et al. [7] concern the epicardial and endocardial contours at both cardiac times. All the images of this challenge are acquired during an apnea of 10–15 seconds, and have a temporal resolution of 20 images per cardiac cycle. Their spatial resolution is 256×256 pixels, with a space of 8 mm between slices, and the voxels' size is $1.37 \times 1.37 \times 8$ mm^3. The dataset of Radau et al. [7] is decomposed in four groups of patients presenting various left ventricle pathologies (cardiac insufficiency with and without ischemia, etc.). Besides the calculation of the VM and the EF mentioned earlier, this challenge also extracts the values of the Dice coefficient (denoted by DI in the rest of the chapter) and the mean orthogonal distance (MOD). For a contour delineated by an expert (i.e., reference) A_m, and a contour computed automatically A_a, the Dice coefficient is defined as:

$$A_{am} = \frac{2 * |A_a \cup A_m|}{|A_a| + |A_m|}. \tag{5.11}$$

The MOD is defined as the mean of the distance between points of A_a and their closest associated points (following the curve's normals) in A_m. The Dice coefficient is a statistical evaluation of the similarity between the two segmentation, while the MOD reveals the closeness of the geometries of the contours.

In Figure 5.14, we present a visual comparison between the contours obtained by the two approaches and the expert delineation. The association between the contours (manual vs. automatic) leads to the computation of the MOD. It should be noted that the original MR images are part of the challenge group of patients suffering from cardiac insufficiency with ischemia, the so-called HF-I.

Table 5.1 presents the values of the MOD and DI measures for three patients of the dataset proposed in Radau et al. [7], meaning that the algorithms have been applied on three MRI sequences of 20 images with a spatial resolution of 256 × 256 pixels. The EF values for the same patients are shown in Table 5.2.

5.6   Discussion and conclusions

In this chapter, we have presented two segmentation algorithms devoted to extract the myocardium within cardiac MRI sequences. The result of this process is of high interest for medical practice, since it permits to automatically deduce the values of important clinical indexes as ejection fraction or the left ventricle mass. The common point of these two approaches is to use prior models of the myocardium to guide the segmentation toward an iterative optimization process. The models implied (polygonal coarse model [6] vs. B-spline model with sectorization [5]) bring robustness within this operation, and prevents the segmentation to exceed the myocardium's geometry in an excessive manner. We have also presented the possibility to interact with the output of DBS, by moving the nodal points of the endocardial and epicardial curves. This property could be studied for the first polygonal model GAC, where each point of the polygon may be manipulated by the user to correct the segmentation.

This matter of interaction in segmentation could be improved by the use of advanced devices, as force-feedback arms or tangible user interfaces for example. The simple use case we have illustrated with an interactive screens shows that there may be more applications of image processing methodologies with these devices.

Another common point of the two approaches is the use of distance transforms to enhance the input MR slices. In each case, the proposed operation is directly related to the structure of the concerned a priori model. This enhancement is a very important step in the treatment of MR images, since they are subject to acquisition noise and kinetic blurring. An alternative could be to use noise reduction filtering. The algorithm we have designed in Vacavant et al. [40] is an interesting option to improve the segmentation's quality.

The experiments we have illustrated in this chapter represent the global behavior of the algorithm with the whole dataset provided by Radau et al. [7]. In these cases, the Dice coefficient is always greater than 90%, which shows consistency in the segmentation obtained by these approaches. The original hypothesis of using a guiding model helps in preventing to alter the ratio of image points correctly classified (myocardium or background). The MOD measure demonstrates that the DBS is an efficient method to extract the epicardium, while the GAC approach shows a good stability to segment the endocardium (even if the MOD are generally greater than the ones of DBS). It should be noted that the GAC algorithm was originally designed for vegetal objects, and the adaptation of the associated tree leaf model to the myocardium shows interesting results that encourage us to keep on improving this methodology. As a general point of view, the precision and the robustness

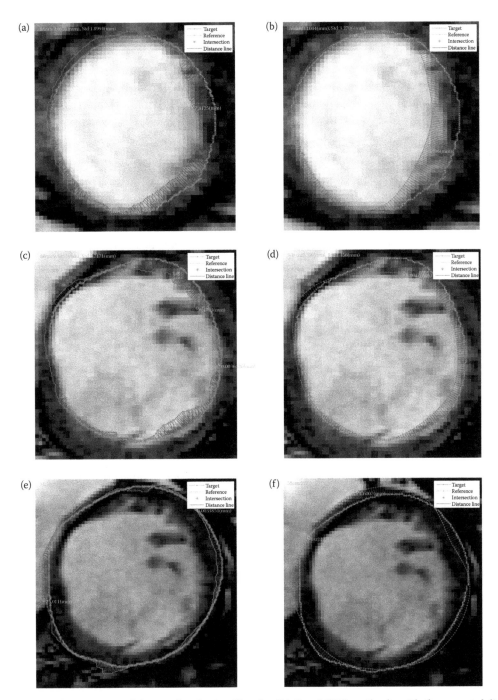

Figure 5.14 Comparison of the results obtained by the GAC and DBS methods with the expert delineation. For each image selected from the challenge [7], the red line represents the contour computed by the concerned algorithm (A_a); the green curve is the expert contour (A_m); the purple points are the closest points of A_m to A_a, linked by a blue line. The mean of these blue segments leads to the calculation of the MOD. (a) GAC, endocardium, patient SC-HF-I-10, frame 188. (b) DBS, endocardium, patient SC-HF-I-10, frame 188. (c) GAC, endocardium, patient SC-HF-I-11, frame 20. (d) DBS, endocardium, patient SC-HF-I-11, frame 20. (e) GAC, epicardium, patient SC-HF-I-11, frame 20. (f) DBS, epicardium, patient SC-HF-I-11, frame 20.

Table 5.1 Evaluation of the segmentations obtained by the two approaches, DBS and GAC, for some patients represented in the MICCAI challenge

	GAC				DBS			
Patient	MOD endo (mm)	MOD epi (mm)	DI endo	DI epi	MOD endo (mm)	MOD epi (mm)	DI endo	DI epi
SC-HF-I-09	3.50	4.25	0.90	0.91	3.69	2.25	0.88	0.95
SC-HF-I-10	3.14	3.60	0.90	0.92	2.67	2.01	0.91	0.95
SC-HF-I-11	2.48	3.55	0.91	0.90	2.16	1.73	0.91	0.94

Source: From P. Radau et al., "Evaluation framework for algorithms segmenting short axis cardiac MRI," *MIDAS Journal*, 2009.

Note: In this table, the MOD (in mm) and DI measures are expressed for endocardial and epicardial contours.

Table 5.2 Evaluation of the segmentations obtained by the two approaches, DBS and GAC, for some patients represented in the MICCAI challenge

	GAC	DBS	Manual
Patient	EF (%)	EF (%)	EF (%)
SC-HF-I-09	0.73	6.42	9.71
SC-HF-I-10	12.32	16.10	16.75
SC-HF-I-11	13.73	14.48	13.74

Source: From P. Radau et al., Evaluation framework for algorithms segmenting short axis cardiac MRI, *MIDAS Journal*, 2009.

Note: In this table, the EF (in %) is expressed in each patient, compared with the expert value (manual).

of our approaches are sufficient to bound the left ventricle's displacement field, deducing then the myocardial strain.

Even if the shape of the segmentation may be evaluated as of good quality by DI or MOD, the clinical indexes that we compute thanks to our segmentations of myocardium are not coherent with the clinicians' expertise. We have presented this phenomenon by depicting the EF values deduced from our segmentation. This fact is first due to the calculation of these factors along a whole cardiac MRI sequence, implying that the slight errors we suffer on each images are accumulated and alter the EF measurement significantly. Moreover, it should be noted that the delineation of the endocardium by a clinician always include the heart's pillars, which is generally not the case in our algorithms. The future model we will design should integrate more information from clinical expertise, as learned practices for example. These new features will allow us to determine more precisely the geometry of the myocardium, w.r.t. the final clinical needs, and to deduce (possibly by extending in 3D) the values of clinical indexes and the components of the strain.

References

1. Wikipedia, Ventricle (heart)—Wikdipedia, the free encyclopedia, 2014. Online. Available: http://en.wikipedia.org/wiki/Ventricle.
2. W. C. Members, R. C. Hendel, M. J. Budoff, J. F. Cardella, C. E. Chambers, J. M. Dent, D. M. Fitzgerald et al., ACC/AHA/ACR/ASE/ASNC/HRS/NASCI/RSNA/SAIP/SCAI/

SCCT/SCMR/SIR 2008 key data elements and definitions for cardiac imaging: A report of the American College of Cardiology/American Heart Association Task Force on Clinical Data Standards (Writing Committee to Develop Clinical Data Standards for Cardiac Imaging), *Circulation*, vol. 119, no. 1, pp. 154–186, 2009.

3. L. Ernande, Détection précoce des anomalies de la fonction myocardique au cours du diabète de type 2: Apport de léchocardiographie en mode speckle tracking imaging et de l'imagerie par résonance magnétique, Ph.D. dissertation, Université de Lyon, 2011.

4. C. Petitjean, N. Rougon, and P. Cluzel, Assessment of myocardial function: a review of quantification methods and results using tagged MRI, *Journal of Cardiovascular Magnetic Resonance*, vol. 7, no. 2, pp. 501–516, 2005.

5. K. Bianchi, A. Vacavant, R. Strand, P. Terv, and L. Sarry, Dual B-spline snake for interactive myocardial segmentation. in *MIUA*, 2013, pp. 131–136.

6. G. Cerutti, L. Tougne, A. Vacavant, and D. Coquin, A parametric active polygon for leaf segmentation and shape estimation, in *ISVC*, 2011, pp. 202–213.

7. P. Radau, Y. Lu, K. Connelly, G. Paul, A. Dick, and G. Wright, Evaluation framework for algorithms segmenting short axis cardiac MRI, *MIDAS Journal*, 2009.

8. C. Petitjean and J. Dacher, A review of segmentation methods in short axis cardiac MR images, medical image analysis, in *IEEE WACV*, vol. 15, 2011, pp. 169–184.

9. V. Tavakoli and A. Amini, A survey of shaped-based registration and segmentation techniques for cardiac images, *Computer Vision and Image Understanding*, vol. 117, no. 9, pp. 966–989, 2013.

10. A. Goshtasby and D. Turner, Segmentation of cardiac cine MR images for extraction of right and left ventricular chambers, *IEEE Transactions on Medical Imaging*, vol. 14, no. 1, pp. 56–64, 1995.

11. J. Weng, A. Singh, and M. Chiu, Learning-based ventricle detection from cardiac MR and CT images, *IEEE Transactions on Medical Imaging*, vol. 16, no. 4, pp. 378–391, 1997.

12. E. Nachtomy, R. Cooperstein, V. M., E. Bosak, Z. Vered, and S. Akselrod, Automatic assessment of cardiac function from short-axis MRI: procedure and clinical evaluation, *Magnetic Resonance Imaging*, vol. 16, pp. 365–376, 1998.

13. A. Gupta, L. von Kurowski, A. Singh, D. Geiger, C. Liang, M. Chiu, L. Adler, M. Haacke, and D. Wilson, Cardiac MR image segmentation using deformable models, in *IEEE CCC*, 1993, pp. 747–750.

14. D. Geiger, A. Gupta, L. Costa, and J. Vlontzos, Dynamic programming for detecting, tracking and matching deformable contours, *IEEE Transactions on Pattern Analysis and Machine Intelligence*, vol. 19, no. 6, pp. 294–302, 1995.

15. A. Lalande, L. Legrand, P. M. Walker, F. Guy, Y. Cottin, S. Roy, and F. Brunotte, Automatic detection of left ventricular contours from cardiac cine magnetic resonance imaging using fuzzy logic, *Investigative Radiology*, no. 3, pp. 211–217, 1999.

16. Y. Lu, P. Radau, K. Connelly, A. Dick, and G. Wright, Segmentation of left ventricle in cardiac cine MRI: An automatic image-driven method, *MIDAS Journal, Cardiac MR Left Ventricle Segmentation Challenge, MICCAI*, 2009.

17. S. Huang, J. Liu, L. C. Lee, S. K. Venkatesh, L. L. S. Teo, C. Au, W. L. Nowinski, Segmentation of the left ventricle from cine mr images using a comprehensive approach, *MIDAS Journal, Cardiac MR Left Ventricle Segmentation Challenge, MICCAI*, 2009.

18. J. K. Udupa and S. Samarasekera, Fuzzy connectedness and object definition: Theory, algorithms, and applications in image segmentation, *Graphical Models*, vol. 58, no. 3, pp. 246–261, 1996.

19. Y. Boykov and V. Kolmogorov, An experimental comparison of min-cut/max-flow algorithms for energy minimization in vision, *IEEE Transactions on Pattern Analalysis and Machine Intelligence*, vol. 26, no. 9, pp. 1124–1137, 2004.

20. G. Kedenburg, C. A. Cocosco, U. Köthe, W. J. Niessen, E. Vonken, and M. A. Viergever, Automatic cardiac MRI myocardium segmentation using graph-cut, 2006.

21. D. Mahapatra, Cardiac image segmentation from cine cardiac MRI using graph cuts and shape priors, *Journal of Digital Imaging*, vol. 26, no. 4, pp. 721–730, 2013.

22. L. Marak, J. Cousty, L. Najman, and H. Talbot, 4D morphological segmentation and the MIC-CAI LV-segmentation grand challenge, *MIDAS Journal, Cardiac MR Left Ventricle Segmentation Challenge, MICCAI*, 2009.

23. J. Cousty, G. Bertrand, L. Najman, and M. Couprie, Watershed cuts: Minimum spanning forests and the drop of water principle, *IEEE Transactions on Pattern Analysis and Machine Intelligence*, vol. 31, no. 8, pp. 1362–1374, 2009.

24. M. Jolly, Fully automatic left ventricle segmentation in cardiac cine MR images using registration and minimum surfaces, *MIDAS Journal, Cardiac MR Left Ventricle Segmentation Challenge, MICCAI*, 2009.

25. M. Lynch, O. Ghita, and P. Whelan, Automatic segmentation of the left ventricle cavity and myocardium in MRI data, *Computer Biology and Medicine*, vol. 36, no. 4, pp. 389–407, 2006.

26. A. Boudraa, Automated detection of the left ventricular region in magnetic resonance images by fuzzy C-means model, vol. 13, no. 4, pp. 347–355, 1997.

27. T. Cootes, C. Taylor, D. Cooper, and J. Graham, Active shape models—their training and application, *Computer Vision and Image Understanding*, vol. 61, no. 1, pp. 38–59, 1995.

28. M. Kass, A. Witkin, and D. Terzopoulos, Snakes: Active contour models, *International Journal of Computer Visison*, vol. 1, no. 4, pp. 321–331, 1988.

29. M. Üzümcü, R. van der Geest, C. Swingen, J. Reiber, and B. Lelieveldt, Time continuous tracking and segmentation of cardiovascular magnetic resonance images using multidimensional dynamic programming, *Investigative Radiology*, vol. 41, no. 1, pp. 52–62, 2006.

30. S. O'Brien, O. Ghita, and P. Whelan, Segmenting the left ventricle in 3D using a coupled ASM and a learned non-rigid spatial model, *MIDAS Journal, Cardiac MR Left Ventricle Segmentation Challenge, MICCAI*, 2009.

31. J. Wijnhout, D. Hendriksen, H. Van Assen, and R. Van der Geest, LV challenge LKEB contribution: Fully automated myocardial contour detection, *MIDAS Journal, Cardiac MR Left Ventricle Segmentation Challenge, MICCAI*, 2009.

32. Y. Shi and W. C. Karl, A real-time algorithm for the approximation of level set-based curve evolution, *IEEE Transactions on Image Processing*, vol. 17, no. 5, pp. 645–656, 2008.

33. P. Brigger, J. Hoeg, and M. Unser, B-spline snakes: a flexible tool for parametric contour detection, *IEEE Transactions on Image Processing*, vol. 9, no. 9, pp. 1484–1496, 2000.

34. S. Menet, P. Saint-Marc, and G. Medioni, B-snakes: Implementation and application to stereo, in *DARPA Image Understanding Workshop*, 1990, pp. 720–726.

35. I. Ghorbel, F. Rossant, I. Bloch, and M. Paques, Modeling a parallelism constraint in active contours. application to the segmentation of eye vessels and retinal layers, in *IEEE ICIP*, 2011, pp. 445–448.

36. T. Chan and L. Vese, Active contours without edges, *IEEE Transactions on Image Processing*, vol. 10, no. 2, pp. 266–277, 2001.

37. C. Xu and J. L. Prince, Snakes, shapes, and gradient vector flow, *IEEE Transactions on Image Processing*, vol. 7, no. 3, pp. 359–369, 1998.

38. A. Kårsnäs, R. Strand, and P. K. Saha, The vectorial minimum barrier distance, in *IEEE ICPR*, 2012, pp. 792–795.

39. R. Strand, K. C. Ciesielski, F. Malmberg, and P. K. Saha, The minimum barrier distance, *Computer Vision and Image Understanding*, vol. 117, no. 4, pp. 429–437, 2013.

40. A. Vacavant, A. Albouy-Kissi, P. Y. Menguy, and J. Solomon, Fast smoothed shock filtering, in *IEEE ICPR*.

chapter six

Incorporating shape variability in implicit template deformation for image segmentation

Raphael Prevost, Remi Cuingnet, Benoit Mory, Laurent D. Cohen, and Roberto Ardon

Contents

Abstract

In this chapter, we propose a method to learn and use prior knowledge on shape variability in the implicit template deformation framework. This shape prior is learned via an original and dedicated process in which both an optimal template and principal modes of variations are estimated from a collection of shapes. This learning strategy does not require one-to-one correspondences between shape sample points and is not biased by a prealignment of the training shapes. We then generalize the implicit template deformation formulation to automatically select the most plausible deformation as a shape prior. This novel framework maintains the two main properties of implicit template deformation: topology preservation and computational efficiency. Our approach can be applied to any organ with a possibly complex shape but fixed topology. We validate our method on myocardium segmentation from cardiac magnetic resonance short-axis images and demonstrate segmentation improvement over standard template deformation.

6.1   Introduction

Implicit template deformation is a model-based segmentation framework involves deforming an initial template to segment an image. When one applies it to a particular clinical problem, the first step is to choose an adequate template. Indeed as we are working with diffeomorphisms, the template must have the same topology as the organ that we want to segment. But it also needs to be "close" to the target object, since the magnitude of the deformation is penalized. While it is always possible to build a synthetic template (e.g., a hyperquadric or superquadric for a ventricle [1,2], or an ellipsoid for the kidney in Cuingnet et al. [3]), one feels that this choice is probably suboptimal in other applications. The purpose of this chapter is to answer the following questions: how can we use a database to design an optimal (in some sense) template? Can we learn the shape variability from this database so that we can take it into account within the deformation penalization?

In this chapter, we present two variational approaches for training and segmentation, respectively. Both phases rely on the implicit template deformation framework [4–7]. While this framework has been successfully applied in several contexts [3,8], its prior knowledge is limited to a single given shape. To introduce shape variability in the same framework, its segmentation functional is used as a measure of dissimilarity between shapes during a training step. This step estimates both the mean shape and a set of principal deformations through joint segmentation of all training shapes (Figure 6.1). The segmentation step then extends implicit template deformation framework by incorporating these computed statistics in the regularization term. It ensures preservation of the template topology and automatically selects the most plausible deformation as a shape prior, with very limited additional complexity.

This chapter is organized as follows: Section 6.2 introduces the problem and lists some of the related work available in the literature. Section 6.3 introduces the main notations and recalls the implicit template deformation framework. In Section 6.4, we describe an original learning process that is tailored to the implicit template deformation framework. The learned statistics will be used in a generalized formulation of the segmentation algorithm introduced in Section 6.5. Validation proving the benefits of our approach is provided in Section 6.6 in the application of myocardium segmentation in 2D MR images. Finally, discussion on potential improvements and conclusion conclude the chapter in Section 6.7 and 6.8.

A short version of this chapter was presented at the MICCAI 2013 conference [9].

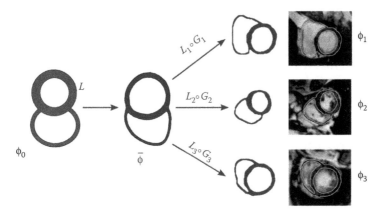

Figure 6.1 Given an initial synthetic shape ϕ_0, a set of shapes $\{\phi_n\}_n$ is simultaneously segmented via implicit template deformation while an intermediate mean shape $\bar{\phi} = \phi_0 \circ L$ is estimated. The topology of ϕ_0 is preserved during the process.

6.2 Implicit template deformation

6.2.1 Motivation

Model-based methods are particularly effective and popular in medical image segmentation. Among them, implicit template deformation has recently been used in various applications [3,4,7,8,10] for its interesting properties (computational efficiency, topology preservation, compatibility with user interactions). This variational method consists in seeking a segmenting implicit function as a deformed implicit template. This template, acting as a shape prior, is therefore of paramount importance. However, in previous works, the initial template was either set as a synthetic model (e.g., an ellipsoid for a kidney [3,7,8]) or as a segmented organ from a single arbitrary image [4]. Despite the consensus that learning shape priors is a powerful approach to improving robustness [11,12], this has never been proposed in the context of segmentation by implicit template deformation. As public databases are developed and become available, it is important to think about how we can exploit them to validate but also improve our algorithms.

Here we aim at (i) learning statistics from a database of shapes (i.e., the most likely shape and the main variations around it) on organs that present a possibly complex shape but a consistent topology, (ii) proposing a method to exploit such learned information within the segmentation framework of implicit template deformation. Naturally, our approaches have to maintain the interesting characteristics of implicit template deformation, namely the computational efficiency and the topology preservation. These two properties are usually incompatible notwithstanding their ability to guarantee both by generalizing the formulation of the implicit template deformation. A combination of learned shapes will be used not to directly segment the images but rather within the regularization term. Thus they will act as a shape prior that is automatically updated during the segmentation.

6.2.2 Previous work and our shape learning approach

The shape learning literature is considerably large, so we include only the well-known or closely related techniques in this section.

In the early and popular active shape model [13], objects are represented by an explicit parameterization of their boundary vertices. Statistics (mean shape and variations) are computed on these vertices coordinates, thus a suitable one-to-one vertices correspondence is needed across the database. This correspondence can be complicated to obtain: either tedious when relying on manually labeled points or lacking robustness when automatically obtained [14]. Due to boundary self-intersections, shape topology may also be lost.

Implicit methods [15–18] represent objects through the signed distance functions to their boundary to estimate statistics. Although the correspondence of vertices is no longer needed during the learning step, this representation is still inadequate for topology preservation. Rousson and Paragios [16] built a probabilistic model in order to estimate a mean implicit function ϕ_m (and an associated variance at each pixel) from a dataset of signed distance functions. Unlike most previous works, they constrained ϕ_m to be a true distance function, that is, $\|\nabla \phi_m\| = 1$, and not just any implicit function. Although more satisfying, this approach requires complex optimization schemes and the constraint is only enforced during the learning (and not the subsequent segmentations). Furthermore, it is still inadequate for topology preservation.

Finally, closely related with this paper, a third class of methods uses statistics on diffeomorphisms of implicit shape representations [19,20] or on currents [21]. While they present elegant and appealing theoretical properties and do preserve shape topology, they are also much more computationally expensive. Most of their applications therefore lie in offline shape analysis and they were not used for segmentation purposes (apart from atlas-based segmentation methods [22], which are not compatible with real-time or user interactions).

Here, we propose an approach that is closely related to this third class of methods, since implicit template deformation consists in seeking a space transformation. We thus introduce a dedicated learning approach by using the template deformation energy as a pre-metric in the shapes space. This idea was inspired by the seminal paper of Joshi et al., in which they construct an unbiased mean template by minimizing a sum of distances to a database [23]. As they were motivated by registration applications, they worked directly on images. When applied to shapes, this approach yields a cosegmentation process (sharing some ideas with Yezzi and Soatto [24] to a certain extent), within which an optimal shape is estimated (see Figure 6.1). However, we go further than both the papers by also learning (and subsequently exploiting) the variability of the shape around this mean. This means we also capture further information by building a space of main deformations around this template. Finally, we introduce a generalization of the template deformation formulation by using the computed statistics in the regularization term. The proposed framework is generic and can be applied to any organ with a possibly complex and variable shape but a fixed topology. We demonstrate its efficiency and interest by addressing the problem of myocardium segmentation in 2D cine-MR images.

6.3   Segmentation by implicit template deformation

Implicit template deformation [4,7] is a variational framework for image segmentation. The segmentation is defined through the zero level set of an implicit function $\phi : \Omega \to \mathbb{R}$, and ϕ is positive (resp. negative) inside (resp. outside) the segmentation. In this framework, the set of admissible segmentations $\mathbb{S}$ is defined via an implicit template $\phi_0 : \Omega \to \mathbb{R}$ as the set of all implicit functions with the same topology as ϕ_0, that is, $\mathbb{S} = \{\phi : \Omega \to \mathbb{R} \text{ s.t. } \phi = \phi_0 \circ \psi, \psi \text{ is diffeomorphic}\}$. The unknown is thus the transformation $\psi : \Omega \to \Omega$, which is sought as a minimum of a region competition energy:

$$\min_{\psi} \left\{ \int_{\Omega} H(\phi_0 \circ \psi)\, r_{\text{int}} + \int_{\Omega} (1 - H(\phi_0 \circ \psi))\, r_{\text{ext}} + \lambda\, \mathcal{R}(\psi) \right\}, \tag{6.1}$$

where H denotes the Heaviside function ($H(a) = 1$ if $a > 0$, 0 otherwise) while r_{int} and r_{ext} are image-based functions such as $r_{\text{int}}(\mathbf{x})$ is lower (resp. higher) than $r_{\text{ext}}(\mathbf{x})$ if voxel $\mathbf{x}$ seems to belong to the target object (resp. background). $\mathcal{R}(\psi)$ is a constraint term on ψ that prevents the segmentation $\phi = \phi_0 \circ \psi$ to deviate too much from the initial template ϕ_0; it is weighted by a parameter λ. In Mory et al. [7], ψ is decomposed into (i) a global transformation $\mathcal{G} \in \mathbb{G}$ (e.g., a similarity) accounting for the pose of the template in the image, and (ii) a diffeomorphism $\mathcal{L} \in \mathbb{D}(\Omega)$ that yields local deformation and does change the shape of the template. This decomposition allows to define the regularization as a function of the deformation only $\mathcal{R}(\psi) = \mathcal{R}(\mathcal{L}) = \frac{1}{2}\|\mathcal{L} - Id\|_2^2$. The problem finally reads

$$\min_{\mathcal{L},\mathcal{G}} \left\{ \int_{\Omega} H(\phi_0 \circ \mathcal{L} \circ \mathcal{G})\, r_{\text{int}} + \int_{\Omega} (1 - H(\phi_0 \circ \mathcal{L} \circ \mathcal{G}))\, r_{\text{ext}} + \frac{\lambda}{2}\|\mathcal{L} - Id\|_2^2 \right\}. \tag{6.2}$$

In such a setting, ϕ_0 not only fixes the topology of the segmentation but also acts as a shape prior, which makes its choice of paramount importance. Moreover, the term $\mathcal{R}$ could be improved by taking into account shape variability of the considered organ. In the following sections, we develop a framework to tackle both problems by estimating statistics on a collection of shapes.

6.4 A learning process dedicated to template deformation

Given a training set of variables $(X_n)_{n=1...N} \subset \mathbb{S}^N$, one can define its mean (more precisely its Fréchet-mean or Karcher-mean [25]) as the solution of the following problem:

$$\bar{X} = \underset{X \in \mathbb{S}}{\operatorname{argmin}} \frac{1}{N} \sum_{n=1}^{N} d^2(X, X_n) \tag{6.3}$$

This definition therefore depends both on the space $\mathbb{S}$ that is used to represent shapes and the distance d that defines their similarity. We will use these two degrees of freedom to build a mean shape that is tailored for the implicit template deformation.

6.4.1 A dedicated estimation of a mean model

The first choice concerns the space of shapes $\mathbb{S}$. Shapes can be represented by different types of objects (i.e., vertices [13], implicit functions [17], deformations [23], currents [21], etc.). Our goal here is to estimate a model for the implicit template deformation framework, so we will choose an implicit representation. However, we would like to specify and fix the topology of the considered shapes. This information will be given by an initial implicit template ϕ_0, on which the space of admissible shapes will depend:

$$\mathbb{S}_{\phi_0} = \{\phi : \Omega \to \mathbb{R} \text{ such that } \phi = \phi_0 \circ L \text{ with } L \in \mathbb{D}(\Omega)\} \tag{6.4}$$

which can be thought of as the orbit of ϕ_0 in the set of shapes. Note that such a space is stable under any diffeomorphism. Its dependency on ϕ_0 is rather low (except the topology) as it is identical to any $\mathbb{S}_\phi$ such that $\phi \in \mathbb{S}_{\phi_0}$. For the sake of simplicity, in the following, we will omit the index and denote this space $\mathbb{S}$.

In order to estimate statistics in $\mathbb{S}$, we then define a metric-like function in this space, which should be related to our segmentation framework. To do so, we point out that any shape $\phi_1 \in \mathbb{S}$ can be warped to another shape $\phi_2 \in \mathbb{S}$ via implicit template deformation. Indeed, we can segment an image representing ϕ_2 using ϕ_1 as template. With the notations of Equation 6.2, we simply have to set $\phi_0 := \phi_1$, $r_{\text{int}}^{\phi_2} := \max(-\phi_2, 0)$ and $r_{\text{ext}}^{\phi_2} := \max(\phi_2, 0)$. The definition of $r_{\text{int}}^{\phi_2}$ and $r_{\text{ext}}^{\phi_2}$ is not unique and we could have selected other functions that represent the interior and the exterior of ϕ_2. The rationale behind this particular choice is that the difference $r_{\text{int}}^{\phi_2} - r_{\text{ext}}^{\phi_2}$ is then equal to $-\phi_2$. This leads to a tailored definition of shape dissimilarity d^2.

Definition 6.1

The shape dissimilarity from shape ϕ_1 to shape ϕ_2 is defined as

$$d^2(\phi_1, \phi_2) = \min_{\substack{L \in \mathbb{D}(\Omega) \\ G \in \mathbb{G}}} \int_\Omega H(\phi_1 \circ L \circ G) \, \max(-\phi_2, 0)$$

$$+ \int_\Omega (1 - H(\phi_1 \circ L \circ G)) \, \max(\phi_2, 0)$$

$$+ \frac{\lambda}{2} \|L - Id\|_U^2, \tag{6.5}$$

or equivalently

$$d^2(\phi_1, \phi_2) = C(\phi_2) + \min_{\substack{L \in \mathbb{D}(\Omega) \\ G \in \mathbb{G}}} - \int_\Omega H(\phi_1 \circ L \circ G) \, \phi_2 + \frac{\lambda}{2} \|L - Id\|_U^2, \tag{6.6}$$

where $C(\phi_2)$ is a constant that only depends on ϕ_2.

In this definition, the U-norm represents the natural norm in the Gaussian reproducing kernel Hilbert space (see Aronszajn [26] for more details), which can usually also be the L^2 norm.

Remark 6.1

The shape constraint parameter λ should be chosen carefully, since a too high value will prevent ϕ_1 to be exactly matched to ϕ_2 and the learning will be biased. In practice, however, it is not difficult to find a suitable value.

This shape dissimilarity measure is not a distance but a pre-metric, as it is not symmetric and does not verify triangular inequality. The lack of symmetry is directly inherited from the segmentation process itself as the template ϕ_0 has a very particular role. Triangular inequality does not either appear as an important property for our application. Cremers et al. discussed these properties in Cremers and Soatto [27] and point out that defining a true distance between implicit shapes is still an open problem. But anyway, this function does measure a closeness between two shapes and we can still use it to define our dedicated notion of mean shape.

Definition 6.2

An implicit function $\bar{\phi}$ is a mean of the set $\{\phi_n\}_{n=1..N}$ (in the sense of implicit template deformation) if it is a local minimum of the shape dissimilarity to all the elements of this set, that is,

$$\bar{\phi} = \underset{\phi \in \mathbb{S}}{\operatorname{argmin}} \frac{1}{N} \sum_{n=1}^{N} d^2(\phi, \phi_n). \tag{6.7}$$

It is important to note that we seek the mean shape $\bar{\phi}$ as an element of $\mathbb{S}$. Indeed, in our application, the mean shape has to preserve the topology of the training shapes. This means that there exists $L \in \mathbb{D}(\Omega)$ such that $\bar{\phi} = \phi_0 \circ L$. The mean shape expression can thus be reformulated as

$$\bar{\phi} = \phi_0 \circ \left\{ \underset{L \in \mathbb{D}(\Omega)}{\operatorname{argmin}} \frac{1}{N} \sum_{n=1}^{N} d^2(\phi_0 \circ L, \phi_n) \right\}. \tag{6.8}$$

Expanding the segmentation costs and neglecting constant terms in Equation 6.8 yields the following optimization problem to solve:

$$\underset{\substack{L \in \mathbb{D}(\Omega) \\ (L_n)_n \in \mathbb{D}(\Omega)^N \\ (G_n)_n \in \mathbb{G}^N}}{\min} E_{\text{learn}} = -\sum_{n=1}^{N} \int_{\Omega} H(\phi_0 \circ L \circ L_n \circ G_n) \, \phi_n + \sum_{n=1}^{N} \frac{\lambda}{2} \|L_n - \mathbf{Id}\|_U^2. \tag{6.9}$$

This can be interpreted as segmenting simultaneously all training shapes $(\phi_n)_n$ starting from ϕ_0 while estimating an optimal common intermediate shape $\phi_0 \circ L$ (see Figure 6.1). In Equation 6.9, the energy E_{learn} is minimized with respect to three kinds of variables:

- The global transformations $(G_n)_n$, called the poses, which register all shapes to ϕ_0 with translation, rotation, and scaling (as they are part of the optimization process, they do not bias the learning, as a fixed prealignment [16,17] would do).
- The *common deformation L*, which includes the common parts of the deformations from ϕ_0 to all the training shapes
- The local deformations $(L_n)_n$, called the *residual deformations*, are the residual components of the deformations from $\phi_0 \circ L$ to ϕ_n. Unlike L, their magnitude is penalized so that any deformation that is common to all the training set will be preferably included in L.

The optimal common deformation L^* can be used to define the optimal shape (in the sense of the segmentation algorithm) as $\bar{\phi} = \phi_0 \circ L^*$. This shape globally minimizes the magnitude of residual deformations to each shape of the dataset. Note that the magnitude of L is not penalized so the choice of ϕ_0 defines the topology of $\bar{\phi}$ but does not affect it further (apart from the smoothness enforced to L). In our experiments, running a second time the learning process with $\phi_0 := \bar{\phi}$ did not alter the results.

Remark 6.2

We assumed that the set of training shapes $\{\phi_n\}_n$ was a subset of $\mathbb{S}_{\phi_0}$. It is a very natural hypothesis and ϕ_0 should be chosen accordingly. However, those training shapes will probably come from manual annotations of images and, as such, prone to errors. As a consequence, it may occur that some training shapes do not have the correct topology. This does not question the soundness of our learning because, in such cases, we will implicitly learn the "closest shapes" with the topology of ϕ_0.

Details on the resolution of Equation 6.9 are provided in the next section.

6.4.2 Numerical optimization

Problem 6.9 presents some mathematical similarities with the co-segmentation method Prevost et al. [28,29]. It is therefore minimized similarly, with a gradient descent simultaneously on each of the unknowns. The gradient directions with respect to $\mathbf{p}_{n,i}$ (the i-th parameter of G_n), the common deformation L, and the residual deformations L_n are given by the following equations[*]:

$$\nabla_{\mathbf{p}_{n,i}} E_{\text{learn}} = \int_{\Omega_0} \delta(\phi_0 \circ L \circ L_n)\, \phi_n \circ G_n^{-1} \left| J_{G_n}^{-1} \right|$$

$$\left\langle \nabla \phi_0 \circ L \circ L_n,\, DL \circ L_n \,.\, DL_n \circ \frac{\partial G_n}{\partial \mathbf{p}_{n,i}} \circ G_n^{-1} \right\rangle \qquad (6.10)$$

$$\nabla_L E_{\text{learn}} = K_\sigma * \left[\sum_{n=1}^{N} \delta(\phi_0 \circ L)\, \phi_n \circ G_n^{-1} \circ L_n^{-1} \,.\, \left| J_{L_n \circ G_n}^{-1} \right| \,.\, DL \,.\, \nabla \phi_0 \circ L \right]$$

$$\nabla_{L_n} E_{\text{learn}} = K_\sigma * \left[\delta(\phi_0 \circ L \circ L_n)\, \phi_n \circ G_n^{-1} \,.\, \left| J_{G_n}^{-1} \right| \,.\, DL_n \,.\, \nabla \phi_0 \circ L \circ L_n \right] + \lambda(L_n - \mathbf{Id})$$

The first gradient—with respect to the poses—is used in a standard gradient procedure, while the two others, with respect to the common and residual deformations, are exploited in a topology-preserving optimization scheme since the space is not stable under linear combinations. The appropriate way is to combine diffeomorphisms via composition since $(\mathbb{D}(\Omega), \circ)$ is a group. Following Saddi et al. [4], we therefore update any diffeomorphism $\mathcal{L}$ in the following way:

$$\mathcal{L}^{(n+1)} \leftarrow (Id - \Delta t\, \nabla_{\mathcal{L}} E) \circ \mathcal{L}^{(n)}. \qquad (6.11)$$

The regularity is enforced by a Gaussian filtering of the gradient as in Mory et al. [7].

All these integrands actually have a very small support (the zero level set of an implicit function), which makes the computations fast. Moreover, the three kinds of gradients have a lot of terms in common.

Remark 6.3

Some terms depends on inverses of diffeomorphisms L_n^{-1}. These deformations are built iteratively and simultaneously to the direct transformations L_n.

---

[*] They are obtained with standard calculus of variation, but we omit the tedious details here.

Remark 6.4

Although the computations needed for the training process are relatively fast, there is a high memory requirement (especially in 3D) since a high number of implicit functions and deformation fields have to be stored simultaneously. A possible solution would be to use a stochastic gradient descent [30], that is, at each iteration only consider a randomly chosen subset of the training set.

6.4.3   Building a space of deformation priors

As seen in the previous section, minimization of Equation 6.9 yields a mean shape. However, the optimal residual deformations $(L_n^*)_n$ are also available and can be used to capture further information on the variability of the training shapes.

We build a space of principal deformations $\mathbb{L}$ to constrain future segmentation of new images. Similar to Rueckert et al. [31], a principal component analysis (PCA) [32] is applied to the residual deformations to find a suitable parameterization of such a space. The goal of this analysis is to find a reduced number of orthogonal vectors that maximize the explained variance of the residual deformations. This is accomplished by first computing the mean residual deformation

$$\bar{\ell} = \frac{1}{N} \sum_{n=1}^{N} L_n^* \tag{6.12}$$

and then performing a singular value decomposition (SVD) of the sample covariance matrix

$$S = \frac{1}{N-1} \sum_{n=1}^{N} (L_n^* - \bar{\ell})(L_n^* - \bar{\ell})^T. \tag{6.13}$$

Any deformation ℓ in agreement with the variability of the training data can then be approximated by a linear combination of the offset $\bar{\ell}$ and $(\ell_k)_{k=1..M}$ the first M singular vectors of S. It is parametrized by the vectors of its weights $w \in \mathbb{R}^M$:

$$\ell \approx \ell[w] = \bar{\ell} + \sum_{k=1}^{M} w_k \, \ell_k. \tag{6.14}$$

We denote $\mathbb{L}$ the set of such transformations. M can be empirically chosen using the distribution of the modes' eigenvalues. To each singular vector ℓ_k corresponds a singular value λ_k that represents the amount of variance of the residual deformations, which are explained with this mode of variation.

Remark 6.5

Note that even if the PCA is applied to the residual deformations, $\bar{\ell}$ is non-null (though with a very small magnitude) because it denotes a mean with respect to a different metric than L^*.

The space of diffeomorphisms is not stable under linear combinations. There is, therefore, no guarantee that an element of $\mathbb{L}$ is actually a diffeomorphism. Nevertheless, as shown in the next section, it is possible to use this space indirectly in a topology-preserving segmentation framework.

6.5   Generalized implicit template deformation

The previously estimated statistical information can be used to robustify and improve future segmentations. In order to incorporate such information in the segmentation process, we propose a generalization of the implicit template deformation framework.

6.5.1   An improved formulation for segmentation

A first improvement is achieved by replacing the original template ϕ_0 by the mean template $\bar{\phi} = \phi_0 \circ L^*$. Second, the estimation of the deformation can also be enhanced by using the space of principal deformations $\mathbb{L}$. In most previous works [13,15,17], the learned variable is expressed as a linear combination of modes. When dealing with deformations, this does not guarantee topological preservation. Therefore, we rather use such linear combinations indirectly. More specifically, we modify the regularization term so that the diffeomorphism L is constrained with respect to the set $\mathbb{L}$ instead of the identity (see Figure 6.2). Thus, only deformations that cannot be explained through the learned space $\mathbb{L}$ are penalized. The new segmentation energy therefore reads

$$E_{\text{seg}}(L, G, w) = \int_{\Omega} H(\bar{\phi} \circ L \circ G)\, r_{\text{int}} + (1 - H(\bar{\phi} \circ L \circ G))\, r_{\text{ext}} + \frac{\lambda}{2}\|L - \ell[w]\|^2_{\mathcal{U}}. \qquad (6.15)$$

This represents a generalization of the standard template deformation formulation. The novel regularization term can be interpreted as a shape prior that depends on the image. Thus, even if the target organ has a high variability around the mean, we can learn it in order to automatically select the most plausible shape that is implicitly used to constrain the segmentation.

A related approach was proposed in Rousson et al. [33] with implicit functions. In this paper, the authors defined the regularization term as a distance between the segmenting implicit function and a linear combination of implicit modes previously learned. However, our method presents a major advantage over theirs. Indeed, as explained above in Section 6.4.2, using Equation 6.11 we are able to let the deformation L evolve while preserving its diffeomorphic properties (and therefore maintaining the topology of the template ϕ_0). Conversely, it is not possible to easily enforce such a constraint into the evolution of an implicit function.

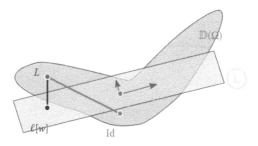

Figure 6.2 Comparison of the penalization of the deformation L with the standard regularization term toward the identity (red) and the novel term toward the space $\mathbb{L}$ (blue) that is centered in $\bar{\ell}$ and spanned by the modes $(\ell_k)_k$. The new prior $\ell[w]$ is the projection of L onto the set $\mathbb{L}$. Note that all transformations of $\mathbb{L}$ are not diffeomorphisms but L is constrained to be one.

6.5.2 Numerical optimization

Minimization of Equation 6.15 can be performed with a two-step alternate scheme:

Update of the segmentation: With $\ell[w]$ fixed, the energy is minimized through a gradient descent-like scheme on L and G (see Mory et al. [7,34]).

Update of the shape prior: With L and G fixed, the update of $\ell[w]$ can be seen as a projection of L onto $\mathbb{L}$. Indeed, the energy comes down to a simple quadratic function, whose minimizers are obtained by solving a simple linear system, as stated by the following proposition.

Proposition 6.1

The minimum of $E_{\text{seg}}(L, G, \cdot)$ is reached at $w^* \in \mathbb{R}^M$ such that

$$Aw^* = b_L \tag{6.16}$$

where A is a $M \times M$ matrix whose entries are $(A_{ij}) = <\ell_i, \ell_j>_U$ while $b_L \in \mathbb{R}^M$ is defined by $(b_{L,i}) = <L - \bar{\ell}, \ell_i>_U$.

Proof. With L and G fixed, the minimization problem comes down to

$$\underset{w \in \mathbb{R}^M}{\operatorname{argmin}} E_{\text{seg}}(L, G, w) = \underset{w \in \mathbb{R}^M}{\operatorname{argmin}} \left\| L - \bar{\ell} - \sum_{k=1}^{M} w_k \ell_k \right\|_U^2 . \tag{6.17}$$

Setting to zero its derivative with respect to the weight of the mode k_0 yields

$$0 = \frac{d}{dw_{k_0}} \left\langle L - \bar{\ell} - \sum_{k=1}^{M} w_k \ell_k, \ L - \bar{\ell} - \sum_{k=1}^{M} w_k \ell_k \right\rangle_U (w^*), \tag{6.18}$$

$$0 = \left\langle L - \bar{\ell} - \sum_{k=1}^{M} w_k^* \ell_k, \ \ell_{k_0} \right\rangle_U, \tag{6.19}$$

$$\sum_{k=1}^{M} w_k^* \langle \ell_k, \ \ell_{k_0} \rangle_U = \langle L - \bar{\ell}, \ \ell_{k_0} \rangle_U. \tag{6.20}$$

Each k_0 yields a linear equation in w, hence the result.

Note that the matrix A has a quite small size, so this system is very easy to solve. Actually, we can even precompute the inverse of A since it only involves learned variables.

However, we may simplify this solution further by making some hypotheses. Recall that by construction via the PCA, the $(\ell_k)_k$ are L^2-orthogonal. If we assume that they are also nearly U-orthogonal, then the matrix M is diagonal and the solutions are given by

$$\forall k \in \{1, ..., M\}, \ w_k^* = \frac{\langle L - \bar{\ell}, \ell_k \rangle_U}{\langle \ell_k, \ell_k \rangle_U} . \tag{6.21}$$

The values of w_k^* are subsequently clipped in the interval $[-3\sqrt{\lambda_k}; 3\sqrt{\lambda_k}]$, as these bounds represent the lengths of the semiaxes of the ellipsoid estimated by the PCA. Any deformation obtained with weights beyond this interval are not in agreement with the training set and thus should not be considered as possible priors. Other possibilities of computing these weights will be mentioned in Section 6.7.

To summarize, the first step is similar to the standard implicit template deformation formulation, and the second one is straightforward. Therefore, the computational efficiency of the method is maintained while topology preservation is still guaranteed.

6.6 Application: Myocardium segmentation in 2D MR images

We validated our method in the context of myocardium analysis and segmentation in cardiac short-axis 2D cine-MR images. Quantitative assessment on the heart muscle is critical for diagnosis or therapy planning. This task is particularly challenging for model-based approaches because of the complex topology of the target object, that is, a band around left and right ventricles.

6.6.1 Material

Our dataset is composed of 245 magnetic resonance (MR) images coming from 61 different patients (for each case, several slices in the z-direction are available). The acquisitions have been synchronized so that each heart is in the same cardiac phase. The typical images size was 256×256 with resolution 1.56×1.56 mm. In every image, a myocardium segmentation has been manually performed by a radiologist. Based on the geometric information, we set for our method the scale of the deformation field σ to 10 mm. The initial synthetic template ϕ_0 used is shown in Figure 6.1. Global transformations are sought in the set $\mathbb{G}$ of similarities (accouting for translation, rotation, and isotropic scaling). The dataset was randomly split into a training set including 120 images from 30 patients and a testing set composed of the remaining 125 images coming from 31 patients.

6.6.2 Experiments on the learned information

6.6.2.1 Synthetic experiments

First, we conducted controlled experiments to assess quantitatively the estimation of the mean model. Random myocardium shapes were generated by applying random deformation fields to an original myocardium. We aim at recovering this original shape by estimating a mean model from subsets of these synthetically generated shapes. The efficiency of a learning process is evaluated by computing the Dice coefficient between the ground truth and the estimated mean shape. To avoid randomness bias, the experiments have been performed 100 times and the results were averaged.

We reported in Figure 6.3 a comparison of three fully automatic methods using this metric: the implicit shape model proposed in Tsai et al. [17], the active shape framework [13] with point correspondences estimated by ICP [14], and the proposed method. For any number of used shapes, our method provided statistically significantly better estimates of the original shape than the two others. These results can be better understood with Figure 6.4 showing the spatial localization of the errors. Indeed, the implicit method fails to recover the entire muscle around the right ventricle: working directly on signed distance function is not adapted to thin structures. This area also causes high errors for the explicit

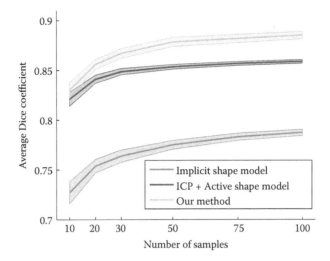

Figure 6.3 Dice coefficients (averaged over the 100 experiments) between the estimated mean model and the original model as a function of the number of samples using the implicit shape model [17], ICP [14] + active shape model [13], and the proposed method. Bands around the curves delineate the 95% confidence interval.

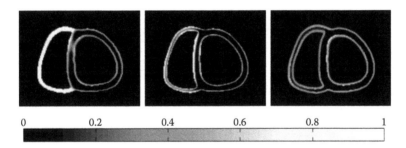

Figure 6.4 Repartition of errors on the estimated model using the implicit shape model [17] (left), ICP [14] + active shape model [13] (middle), and the proposed method (right). Color indicates the pixelwise empirical probability of bad classification (inside vs. outside the shape).

method, which retrieves but underestimates this part of the band. Conversely, errors for our method are lower and more evenly distributed.

6.6.2.2   Mean model and principal modes

We now provide a qualitative comparison between the different approaches on learned information from clinical data. The initial dataset was randomly split into a training set including 120 images from 30 patients and a testing set composed of 125 images coming from the remaining 31 patients.

The mean shape and first two modes of variation are shown in Figure 6.5 for each method. As expected from the results of the previous section, the implicit method fails at recovering the true topology of the mean shape, but also with the first modes of variations. The explicit method performs better and provides a reasonable mean model. However, the modes of variation are not satisfying because very irregular and difficult to interpret.

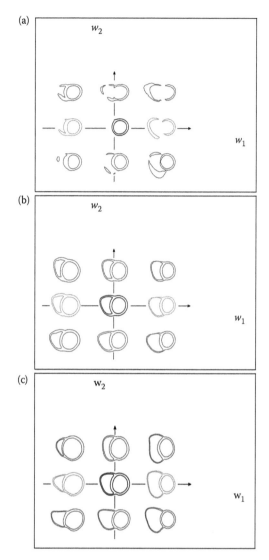

Figure 6.5 Mean model and first two modes of the variation of the myocardium, learned on the training dataset using the implicit shape model [17] (a), ICP [14] + active shape model [13] (b), and the proposed method (c). For our approach, the visualized shapes are the zero level sets of $\bar{\phi} \circ (\bar{\ell} + w_1 \ell_1 + w_2 \ell_2)$.

On the other hand, the results obtained with our method show a much better preservation of the topology and seem more realistic. Moving along the first principal components changes the relative size of the ventricles. This corresponds to the variability observed when moving on the axial direction of a given heart. This variation was expected because the training set include several slices of each heart. The second principal component controls the global anisotropic scaling of the hearts, which seems to rather represent an intersubject variability. Such variations were not taken into account by the global poses because their scaling were isotropic.

6.6.3 Validation of the improved segmentation

We finally evaluate how learned information improves segmentation via implicit template deformation of unseen images. Myocardiums have been segmented in test images using (i) the synthetic model ϕ_0 as template, (ii) the estimated mean model $\bar{\phi}$ as template, and (iii) the new deformation model-based regularization term in addition to the mean model $\bar{\phi}$ (with five modes).

The image-based classification functions r_{int} and r_{ext} were set to

$$r_{\text{int}}(\mathbf{x}) = -\log(p_{\text{int}}(\mathbf{x})) \quad \text{and} \quad r_{\text{ext}}(\mathbf{x}) = -\log(p_{\text{ext}}(\mathbf{x})). \tag{6.22}$$

where p_{int} and p_{ext} are of intensity probability distributions inside and outside the myocardium (estimated from the training datasets). For the intensities to be comparable, all the images were normalized beforehand.

The performance of each algorithm is quantified using Dice coefficients between the segmentation and the expert ground truth. The results on the whole testing set are summarized in Figure 6.6. Changing the template from ϕ_0 to the learned $\bar{\phi}$ makes the algorithm more robust as the minimum Dice coefficient greatly increases from 0.46 to 0.69. Modifying the regularization term by taking into account the deformation model further raises it 0.86. The proposed method globally enhances the algorithm on most images of the test database as the median goes from 0.85 for the baseline method to 0.92 with our modifications. These improvements are statistically significant with a p-value of $< 10^{-4}$ for a Wilcoxon signed-rank test [35].

Figure 6.7 shows segmentation results in three different cases, for the classical regularization term with two values of the shape constraint parameter $\lambda \in \{1, 2\}$ and the new model-based regularization term. In all settings, the template was the mean model $\bar{\phi}$. Consider Case #1 (first row). Since the image term is reliable, a satisfying result is obtained with

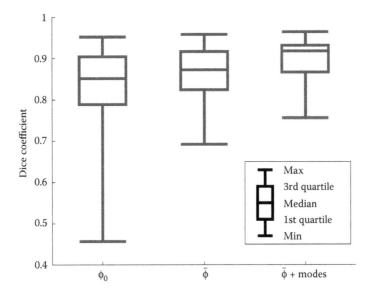

Figure 6.6 Boxplot of the Dice coefficients for myocardium segmentation in MR images via implicit template deformation with synthetic model ϕ_0 (left), mean model $\bar{\phi}$ (middle), mean model $\bar{\phi}$, and deformation modes (right).

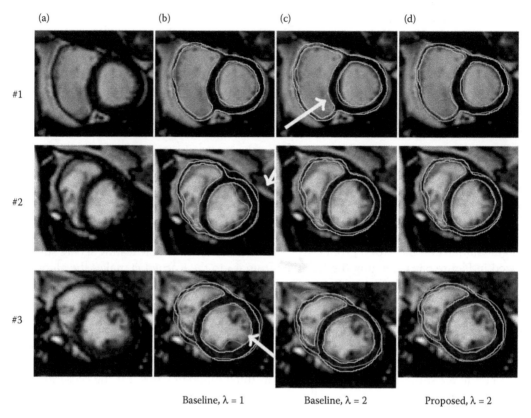

Figure 6.7 Segmentation results (red) of different cases versus ground truths (green). Main failures are highlighted by yellow arrows. (a) Original images. (b,c) Standard method with small ($\lambda = 1$) and high ($\lambda = 2$) shape constraint. (d) Proposed method.

a small shape constraint. However, the myocardium deviates significantly from the mean shape: using a too strong constraint ($\lambda = 2$) prevents the algorithm to converge toward the right solution. Conversely in Case #2, the image information is much more ambiguous. This provokes some leaks (e.g., in papillary muscles of the left ventricle) with $\lambda = 1$, which shows there is no fixed value that allows a good segmentation in the first two cases. Yet, by introducing the new regularization (fourth column), likely deformations are not penalized. This widens the capture range while still maintaining a high constraint on the shape and therefore avoiding unrealistic leaks. Finally, Case #3 illustrates that our method may also improve the result even if no λ was originally successful.

6.7   Discussion

Here, we discuss some limitations of the current work and propose several ideas for future work.

- *From 2D to 3D:* Although we first proved the potential of our approach on a 2D application, it should be noted that the whole method can be directly extended to 3D shapes, thanks to the implicit representation of shapes. Another advantage of our approach is that it does not require point-to-point correspondences between shapes, which can be particularly challenging for obtaining 3D shapes. We are thus currently investigating 3D applications, such as learning the shape variability of the liver.

- *Penalizing the weights of the modes:* In this chapter, we proposed to replace the regularization term on the deformation L from

$$\|L - Id\|^2 \qquad \text{to} \qquad \min_w \|L - \ell[w]\|^2 \text{ with } \ell[w] \in \mathbb{L} \qquad (6.23)$$

which basically consists in removing the penalization on all deformations in the affine space $\mathbb{L}$. The rationale was that $\mathbb{L}$ is composed of deformations in agreement with the database. However, the weights w should be not too large: with a Gaussian assumption, the training shapes are supposed to have their weight w_k in $[-3\sqrt{\lambda_k}; 3\sqrt{\lambda_k}]$. Our solution was to clip each weight into this interval, but there is a more elegant approach. We could decompose the original term $\|L - Id\|_U^2$ into

$$\min_{w \in \mathbb{R}^M} \|L - \ell[w]\|^2 + \|\ell[w] - \bar{\ell}\|^2 + \|\bar{\ell} - Id\|^2 \qquad (6.24)$$

where the first term is the same as in Equation 6.23. The third term is constant and can therefore be discarded in the minimization. Finally, the second term penalizes the distance between $\ell[w]$ and $\bar{\ell}$ that are both deformations in $\mathbb{L}$. Instead of using the standard L^2- or U-norms, we can exploit the assumption of Gaussian distribution around $\bar{\ell}$ and define a Mahalanobis distance in $\mathbb{L}$ as follows:

$$\|\ell[w] - \bar{\ell}\|^2 = \nu \sum_{k=1}^{M} \frac{w_k^2}{\lambda_k^2} \qquad (6.25)$$

where ν is a normalization factor. This simply means that modes with high variance are less penalized. Minimization remains easy as Equation 6.21 becomes

$$\forall k \in \{1, ..., M\}, \ w_k^* = \frac{\langle L - \bar{\ell}, \ell_k \rangle_U}{\langle \ell_k, \ell_k \rangle_U + \nu \frac{1}{\lambda_k}} \qquad (6.26)$$

The weights of the modes are slightly shifted down, according to the variance of the corresponding mode.

- *Choice of the dimension reductions method:* In order to build the space $\mathbb{L}$, we used as a dimension reduction approach, the principal component analysis (PCA), since it is a standard and easy-to-implement method. However, we might try other methods such as independent component analysis (ICA) [36] which, unlike PCA, does not aim at capturing the largest variance with orthogonal vectors but with decorrelated ones.

To understand the potential benefits of ICA over PCA, consider the following simple "thought experiment": in all the training shapes, only two disjoint zones Ω_A and Ω_B differ from the mean model. These zones are the same in each shape but they vary independently from each other. PCA will capture all the changes in a single mode, while ICA needs two modes (one for each region). Now, let's imagine the segmentation of a corrupted image in which there is no information in Ω_A. With both methods, the weights of the shape prior will solely be determined by the information available in Ω_B. However, since the two regions are in the same PCA mode, the shape prior will also change in Ω_A if we use the PCA approach. This is clearly not desirable since the two variations were independent: there is no reason for Ω_A to influence Ω_B. The correct behavior (i.e., the prior in Ω_A should be only the mean model unless there exists some statistical correlation with other regions) is obtained with the ICA modes.

- *Learning on logarithms:* We mentioned earlier, that diffeomorphisms are not stable under linear combinations. This was the reason why we did not use the modes of the PCA directly in the segmentation step. However, we may question the learning step itself: is it really sensible to perform a PCA in a space that is not linear? The answer is probably negative from a purely theoretical point of view.

   One possible solution would be to perform the PCA on the logarithms of the residual deformations $(L_i^*)_i$, since the logarithm of a diffeomorphism is a vector field that does lie in a linear space [19]. Preliminary experiments that we are currently conducting, however, suggest that both learning and segmentation results do not significantly change when working on logarithms, whereas the efficiency of the algorithm is lost.

6.8   Conclusion

In this chapter, we have presented an approach to include organ shape variability in the implicit template deformation framework. By computing a mean over a database of shapes defined with a dedicated distance, we constructed a shape template that is tailored to our algorithm. We even used further statistics by estimating (and then exploiting for the segmentation of unseen images) the main modes of variations of the deformations. The remarkable properties of this approach are its computational efficiency and the topology preservation of the initial model. A variational approach was proposed to extract statistical information (mean and principal variations) from a collection of shapes. This training method is automatic, does not require landmarks correspondance, and relies upon a definition of shape dissimilarity that is directly derived from the implicit template deformation functional. We also proposed a generalization of the original segmentation algorithm in which the shape prior is automatically adapted to the current image during the deformation process while still maintaining both the computational efficiency and the topology preservation of the method (segmentation takes around one second on a standard computer). Quantitative results demonstrated the improvement over implicit template deformation for a 2D application. Our approach is very generic and can be used to segment any object with a complex shape but a fixed topology that shall be preserved. Furthermore, extension in 3D or to multiple objects (e.g., brain structures) is straightforward thanks to the implicit representation of shapes. Despite its paramount importance, the image-based term was not investigated as we focused on incorporating shape information on top of any pixelwise classifier.

All in all, this approach is very promising and was proven to be both effective and efficient on the addressed clinical application. It also paves the way for numerous further investigations: for instance in Prevost et al. [37], we go beyond and learn not only the shape variability but also the local appearance of the organ of interest.

References

1. I. Cohen and L. D. Cohen, A hybrid hyperquadric model for 2-D and 3-D data fitting, *Computer Vision and Image Understanding*, vol. 63(3), pp. 527–541, 1996.

2. E. Bardinet, L. D. Cohen, and N. Ayache, A parametric deformable model to fit unstructured 3D data. *Computer Vision and Image Understanding*, vol. 71(1), pp. 39–54, 1998.

3. R. Cuingnet, R. Prevost, D. Lesage, L. D. Cohen, B. Mory, and R. Ardon, Automatic detection and segmentation of kidneys in 3D CT images using random forests, in *MICCAI*, vol. 7512 of *LNCS*, pp. 66–74, Springer, 2012.

4. K. Saddi, C. Chefd'hotel, M. Rousson, and F. Cheriet, Region-based segmentation via non-rigid template matching, *Proceedings of IEEE International Conference on Computer Vision (ICCV'07)*, pp. 1–7, 2007.

5. Xiaolei Huang, Zhiguo Li, and Dimitris Metaxas, Learning coupled prior shape and appearance models for segmentation, in *Medical Image Computing and Computer-Assisted Intervention—MICCAI 2004*, pp. 60–69, Springer, 2004.

6. X. L. Huang and D. N. Metaxas, Metamorphs: Deformable shape and appearance models, *IEEE Transactions on PAMI*, vol. 30(8), pp. 1444–1459, 2008.

7. B. Mory, O. Somphone, R. Prevost, and R. Ardon, Real-time 3D image segmentation by user-constrained template deformation, in *MICCAI*, vol. 7510 of *LNCS*. Berlin: Springer, 2012, pp. 561–568.

8. R. Prevost, B. Mory, J.-M. Correas, L. D. Cohen, and R. Ardon, Kidney detection and real-time segmentation in 3D contrast-enhanced ultrasound images, in *Proceedings of IEEE ISBI 2012*, pp. 1559–1562, 2012.

9. R. Prevost, R. Cuingnet, B. Mory, L. D. Cohen, and R. Ardon, Incorporating shape variability in image segmentation by implicit template deformation, in *MICCAI*, vol. 8151 of *LNCS*. Berlin: Springer, 2013, pp. 82–89.

10. O. Somphone, B. Mory, S. Makram-Ebeid, and L. D. Cohen, Prior-based piecewise-smooth segmentation by template competitive deformation using partitions of unity, in *ECCV*, October 2008.

11. D. Cremers, M. Rousson, and R. Deriche, A review of statistical approaches to level set segmentation: integrating color, texture, motion and shape, *International Journal of Computer Vision*, vol. 72(2), pp. 195–215, 2007.

12. T. Heimann and H.-P. Meinzer, Statistical shape models for 3D medical image segmentation: A review, *Medical Image Analysis*, vol. 13(4), p. 543, 2009.

13. T. F. Cootes, C. J. Taylor, D. H. Cooper, and J. Graham, Active shape models—Their training and application, *Computer Vision and Image Understanding*, vol. 61(1), pp. 38–59, 1995.

14. P. J. Besl and N. D. McKay, A method for registration of 3D shapes, *IEEE Transactions on Pattern Analysis and Machine Intelligence*, vol. 14(2), pp. 239–256, 1992.

15. M. E. Leventon, W. E. L. Grimson, and O. Faugeras, Statistical shape influence in geodesic active contours, in *Proceedings of CVPR 2000*, pp. 316–323, 2000.

16. M. Rousson and N. Paragios, Shape priors for level set representations, *Proceedings of ECCV 2002*, pp. 416–418, 2002.

17. A. Tsai, A. Yezzi Jr, W. Wells, C. Tempany, D. Tucker, A. Fan, W. E. Grimson, and A. Willsky, A shape-based approach to the segmentation of medical imagery using level sets, *Medical Imaging, IEEE Transactions on*, vol. 22(2), pp. 137–154, 2003.

18. D. Cremers, T. Kohlberger, and C. Schnorr, Shape statistics in kernel space for variational image segmentation, *Pattern Recognition*, vol. 36(9), pp. 1929–1943, 2003.

19. V. Arsigny, O. Commowick, X. Pennec, and N. Ayache, A log-Euclidean framework for statistics on diffeomorphisms, in *Medical Image Computing and Computer-Assisted Intervention—MICCAI 2006*. Berlin: Springer, 2006, pp. 924–931.

20. M. Vaillant, M. I. Miller, L. Younes, and A. Trouve,' Statistics on diffeomorphisms via tangent space representations, *NeuroImage*, vol. 23(1), p. 161, 2004.

21. S. Durrleman, Statistical models of currents for measuring the variability of anatomical curves, surfaces and their evolution, These de sciences (PhD thesis), Universite' de Nice-Sophia Antipolis (March 2010), 2010.

22. A. R. Khan, L. Wang, and M. F. Beg, Freesurfer-initiated fully-automated subcortical brain segmentation in MRI using large deformation diffeomorphic metric mapping, *NeuroImage*, vol. 41(3), pp. 735–746, 2008.

23. S. Joshi et al., Unbiased diffeomorphic atlas construction for computational anatomy, *NeuroImage*, vol. 23(1), p. 151, 2004.

24. A. J Yezzi and S. Soatto, Deformotion: Deforming motion, shape average and the joint registration and approximation of structures in images, *International Journal of Computer Vision*, vol. 53(2), p. 153–167, 2003.

25. H. Karcher, Riemannian center of mass and mollifier smoothing, *Communications of Pure and Applied Mathematics*, vol. 30(5), pp. 509–541, 1977.

26. N. Aronszajn, Theory of reproducing kernels, *Transactions of the American Mathematical Society*, vol. 68(3), pp. 337–404, 1950.

27. D. Cremers and S. Soatto, A pseudo-distance for shape priors in level set segmentation, *in 2nd IEEE Workshop on Variational, Geometric and Level Set Methods in Computer Vision*, pp. 169–176, 2003.

28. R. Prevost, R. Cuingnet, B. Mory, J.-M. Correas, L. D Cohen, and R. Ardon, Joint co-segmentation and registration of 3D ultrasound images, in *Information Processing in Medical Imaging*. Berlin: Springer, 2013, pp. 268–279.

29. R. Prevost, B. Romain, R. Cuingnet, B. Mory, L. Rouet, O. Lucidarme, L. D. Cohen, and R. Ardon, Registration of free-breathing 3D+t abdominal perfusion CT images via co-segmentation, in *MICCAI*, vol. 8150 of *LNCS*. Berlin: Springer, 2013, pp. 99–107.

30. L. Bottou, Online learning and stochastic approximations, *Online Learning in Neural Networks*, vol. 17, no. 9, 1998.

31. D. Rueckert, A. Frangi, and J. Schnabel, Automatic construction of 3D statistical deformation models using non-rigid registration, *Proceedings of MICCAI 2001*, pp. 77–84, 2001.

32. I. T Jolliffe, *Principal Component Analysis*, vol. 487. New York: Springer-Verlag, 1986.

33. M. Rousson, N. Paragios, and R. Deriche, Implicit active shape models for 3D segmentation in MR imaging, in *Medical Image Computing and Computer-Assisted Intervention—MICCAI 2004*. Berlin: Springer, 2004, pp. 209–216.

34. B. Mory, O. Somphone, R. Prevost, and R. Ardon, Template deformation with user constraints for live 3D interactive surface extraction, in *MICCAI Workshop MeshMed*, 2011.

35. F. Wilcoxon, Individual comparisons by ranking methods, *Bio-metrics Bulletin*, vol. 1, no. 6, pp. 80–83, 1945.

36. P. Comon, Independent component analysis, a new concept? *Signal Processing*, vol. 36, no. 3, pp. 287–314, 1994.

37. R. Prevost, R. Cuingnet, B. Mory, L. D. Cohen, and R. Ardon, Tagged template deformation, in *Medical Image Computing and Computer-Assisted Intervention MICCAI 2014*, vol. 8673 of *Lecture Notes in Computer Science*, P. Golland, N. Hata, C. Barillot, J. Hornegger, and R. Howe, Eds. Berlin: Springer International Publishing, 2014, pp. 674–681.

chapter seven

Exudate detection in fundus images using active contour methods and region-wise classification

Balazs Harangi and Andras Hajdu

Contents

Abstract

Diabetic retinopathy is one of the most common causes of blindness in the world. Exudates are among the early signs of this disease, so the proper detection of these lesions is a very important task to prevent the worsening of health status. In this chapter, we propose an automated approach for exudate detection which is based on the combination of active contours obtained for the image after different preprocessing algorithms. First, we identify possible regions containing exudates using grayscale morphology. Then, we minimize the Chan–Vese energy function to achieve nearly accomplished boundary on the differently preprocessed images. Considering an appropriate combination of the extracted contours we derive the final candidate region. To exclude false candidates having sufficiently strong borders to pass the active contour method we use a region-wise classifier. Hence, we extract many shape features for each candidate and let a boosted Naïve–Bayes classifier to eliminate the false candidates. To test our approach, we consider publicly available color retinal image sets, where we measure the accuracy of the segmentation of exudate regions and the recognition rate of the presence of exudates at image level.

7.1   Introduction

In this chapter, we introduce a method for the automatic detection of exudates in digital fundus images using an active contour-based approach. The method can be divided into three main stages: candidate extraction, precise contour segmentation and the labeling of candidates as true or false exudates. For candidate detection, a grayscale morphology-based method is applied to identify possible regions containing these bright lesions. The result of candidate detection is used for initializing active contour methods. In this way, the usually manual or semiautomatic active contour-based segmentation can be made fully automatic. To increase the accuracy of segmentation, we extract additional possible contours by taking advantage of the diverse behavior of different preprocessing methods. After selecting an appropriate combination of the extracted contours, a region-wise classifier is applied to remove the false exudate candidates. For this task, we consider several region-based features, and extract an appropriate feature subset to train a Naïve–Bayes classifier optimized further by an adaptive boosting technique. Regarding experimental studies, the method is tested on publicly available databases both to measure the accuracy of the segmentation of exudate regions and to recognize their presence at the image level.

In the corresponding literature, a large number of exudate detection algorithms have been proposed. In general, we can divide these approaches into two main groups. The first group contains algorithms based on grayscale morphology [1–3], while the second one consists of methods considering pixel/region-wise classification [4–8]. Furthermore, we can find some special approaches [9–11] falling out of these groups. Walter et al. [1] proposed a method using morphological closing to eliminate blood vessels, and then the local standard deviation is calculated and thresholded to find the candidate regions. Finally, morphological reconstruction is applied to find the contours of the exudates. Sopharak et al. [2] introduced a technique based on optimally adjusted morphological operations. Since the optic disk is also a bright patch, it is eliminated and Otsu's algorithm is used for thresholding to locate regions with high intensities. Welfer et al. [3] applied morphological operations and H-maxima transform after contrast enhancement on the channel L in the color space CIE 1976 L*u*v*. Sopharak et al. [4] proposed a method using fuzzy c-means clustering in order to determine whether a pixel belongs to an exudate or not. Then, morphological operations are applied to refine the segmentation result. Sopharak et al. [5] designed an algorithm for exudate detection, which applies pixel-based classification. Namely, a Naïve–Bayes classifier sorts each pixel-based on five extracted features. The method proposed by Sánchez et al. [6] also considers pixel-based classification, but the training database is defined for each analyzed image separately. That is, the algorithm first detects small isolated exudates and uses those pixels as a positive training set. Then, the rest of the image pixels are classified based on their corresponding properties. Niemeijer et al. [7] proposed a multilevel classification approach for segmentation of pixels which belongs to bright lesions with high probability. These pixels are grouped into clusters and the clusters are labeled as exudates, cotton wool spots, or drusens. Jaafar et al. [9] proposed exudate detection based on a split-and-merge technique. This algorithm splits the images into disjoint regions first, and merges them based on local variance afterwards. Finally, a histogram-based adaptive thresholding is applied to each merged region. Ali et al. [10] proposed an atlas-based method to detect exudates. Harangi et al. [11] published an active contour-based method for exudate detection using only the green intensity channel of the image.

In the rest of this chapter, the combination of these mainstream approaches (morphology and classification) within a single framework is introduced. The aim is to take advantage of several image enhancement methods for recognizing the precise boundaries of candidates extracted by a morphology-based candidate extractor. The motivation behind this objective is that the features extracted from the precisely segmented regions are more appropriate to differentiate the true exudates from the false ones. For precise boundary detection, we consider several different preprocessing algorithms to extract contour candidates by an active contour method for each preprocessed image. The final exudate contour is found by a combination of these contour candidates. Finally, a region-wise classifier is applied to decide whether the candidates should be considered as exudates or not. In Section 7.2, the clinical background and the publicly available datasets are introduced. In Section 7.3, we describe the algorithm [1] applied for rough candidate extraction, list the involved image preprocessing methods and present the methodology which is based on active contour segmentation. Section 4 is dedicated to comparative experimental results regarding some other state-of-the-art exudate detection methods. Finally, some discussions and conclusions are given in Section 7.5.

7.2 Clinical background

More than 360 million people suffered from diabetes in 2012 worldwide. The number of the diagnosed cases has grown rapidly in the last few years and this tendency is estimated to continue [12]. Long-term diabetes also affects the eyes, resulting in a disease called diabetic retinopathy (DR). See Figure 7.1a for a healthy retinal (fundus) image with the main anatomical parts, and also an abnormal case in Figure 7.1b, which contains several DR-related lesions.

If DR remains undiagnosed or is treated inappropriately, it can lead to loss of vision. Moreover, DR is the most common cause of blindness in the world. However, there exist suitable ways of treatment to slow down this damage of the eye. Thus, an automatic screening system for DR would have great importance mainly in developing countries, where nearly 40% of the cases remain undiagnosed. Such a system is useful if it is able to detect the first signs of the disease. Such signs of DR are microaneurysms and exudates. Exudates arise when fluid exudes from tissue due to its injured capillaries. Since the fluid contains protein, cellular debris and white blood cells, exudates appear as yellowish, bright patches

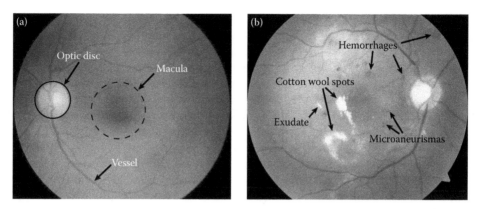

Figure 7.1 Retinal (fundus) images. (a) Healthy case and main anatomical parts, (b) abnormal case with lesions corresponding to diabetic retinopathy.

on the retinal background. That is, considering intensity differences, exudates can be distinguished more efficiently from the background than microaneurysms from blood vessel segments. On the other hand, the fluid can flow without restrain, so the exudates have various sizes and irregular shapes as it can be seen in Figure 7.2, which makes the automatic detection of exudates rather challenging.

In the corresponding literature, we can find some publicly available datasets that contain both healthy and abnormal images showing the signs of DR. These datasets are supplied with manual annotations of ophthalmologists and this data can be used for

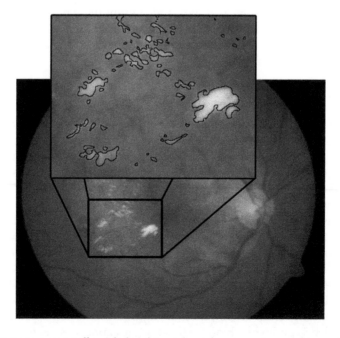

Figure 7.2 Exudates appear as yellowish, bright patches of various sizes and irregular shapes.

the evaluation of the automatic detection and segmentation methods regarding anatomical parts and lesions. Currently, the two commonly used datasets for exudate detection are DIARETDB1 (Standard Diabetic Retinopathy Database) [13] and HEI-MED (Hamilton Eye Institute Macular Edema Dataset) [14]. The dataset DIARETDB1 contains 89 fundus images with a 50° field of view (FOV) and resolution of 1500 × 1152 pixels. Fifty-three images contain exudates based on the labeling of four clinical experts. Each expert marked manually the most representative points of the exudates in these images, and the coordinates of these points are stored in text files. Based on these manually marked anchor points, a local ophthalmologist segmented manually the exudates further in these images. Thus, we have gained 53 binary masks containing the precise exudate boundaries. For feature selection and the training of the region-wise classifier (more details will be given in Section 3.4), the dataset DIARETDB1 is divided into a training and a test part by taking the distribution of normal and abnormal images also into account as proposed by Kauppi et al. [13]. The training set consists of 24 images containing exudates and four images with no such lesions. The dataset HEI-MED consists of 169 images of resolution 2196 × 1958 pixels with a 45° FOV, among which 54 images are classified manually by an ophthalmologist as containing exudates. The binary images containing the manually segmented exudates for HEI-MED images are not available, so we use this image set for evaluation at image-level only. For both image sets, the images have been captured from patients belonging to heterogeneous ethnic groups so the datasets do not correspond to any typical population (see Kauppi et al. [13] and Giancardo et al. [14]). Consequently, the retinal pigmentations of these images are quite diverse as it can be observed in Figure 7.3, as well.

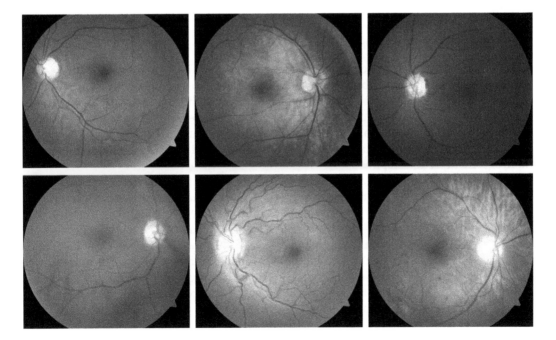

Figure 7.3 Sample retina fundus images from DIARETDB1 and HEI-MED datasets.

7.3   Methodology

In this section, we introduce an automatic exudate detector, which combines the advantage of several image preprocessing methods and applies a novel exudate detection approach using an active contour method (ACM). The candidate extractor technique [1] is based on grayscale morphology and has high sensitivity, since it basically marks every bright region as an exudate. To keep up this high sensitivity, but also to increase the specificity, we aim to reduce the number of false-positive regions. For this purpose, we exclude the nonexudate regions by region-wise classification and to enhance the accuracy of this classification we detect the precise boundaries of the exudates, since the features used for region-wise classification are based on the contour, shape and composing pixels of the region.

The method starts with rescaling the images to normalize the resolution to common height of 1500 pixels. Next, a rough candidate extractor is applied to retrieve the possible exudate regions. Because of the high similarity in appearance between the exudates and the optic disk, we exclude the optic disk (OD) region from the candidate ones. For the localization of the OD, we apply an ensemble-based method [15]. The main motivation of this approach is to compensate for the weaknesses of the different OD detectors by fusing their results. In this way, the performance of the individual OD detectors can be outperformed. The combined result is considered to be the final OD region. After OD removal, the boundaries of the remaining exudate candidates are used to initialize an ACM. To determine the precise boundaries, the ACM method is applied separately on nine different enhanced varieties of the input image having different intensities and contrast. Then, the nine extracted boundaries are combined. Finally, some features are extracted from each candidate, and a properly adjusted Naïve–Bayes classifier labels each candidate as an exudate or nonexudate. The schematic workflow of the proposed approach is also given in Figure 7.4.

7.3.1   Candidate extraction

A morphology-based technique for exudate detection given by Walter et al. [1] can extract candidate regions quite reliably. However, this method works improperly on the retinal images of young patients, where shiny regions spread along the temporal arcade (main vessels). Moreover, the boundaries of the detected exudates are less natural due to the applied structural elements and the method detects several false-positives, as well. For these reasons, we use the results obtained by Walter et al. [1] only as an initial mask for a more precise detection step.

Walter et al. [1] consider high local contrast and intensity in the green channel of the fundus image as the most important properties of exudates. Since there is also a high contrast between the vessels and the background, the method eliminates the vascular system by a simple grayscale morphological closing. On the vessel-free image, the local variation is calculated at each pixel inside a window and the regions with low local variations are excluded. The OD is also eliminated from the image, because it is similar to exudates regarding brightness and contrast. The remaining bright regions are excluded from the original image and the holes are filled in by morphological reconstruction. The result looks like a healthy image without bright lesions, so when it is subtracted from the original one, the difference image contains the bright exudate candidates only. Finally, thresholding is performed on the remaining candidates to eliminate false exudate pixels (partial results of the candidate extraction can be seen in Figure 7.5). This algorithm has three parameters: The size of the window ($W = 11$), the contrast threshold ($\alpha_1 = 3$)

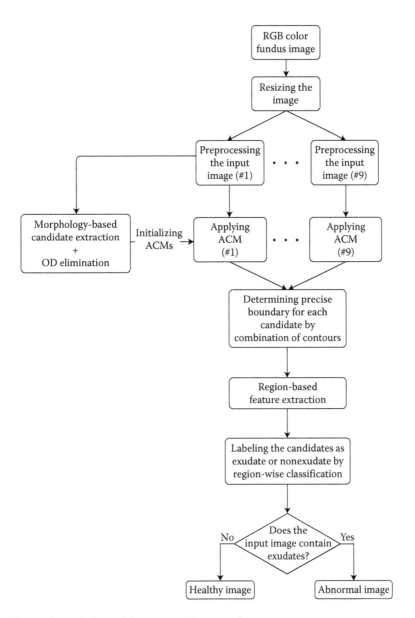

Figure 7.4 Schematic workflow of the proposed approach.

and the brightness threshold ($\alpha_1 = 8$), which are set as proposed by Walter et al. [1]. The boundaries of these extracted regions will be used as initial positions for the active contour segmentation method.

7.3.2 Image preprocessing methods

Several papers dealing with digital fundus image processing propose the green channel G for image analysis, since it provides the highest contrast between the anatomical parts, lesions and the retinal background. According to this recommendation, we simply extract

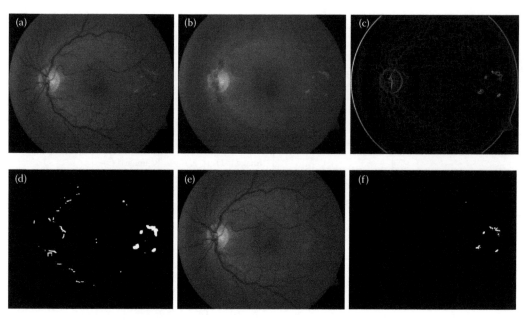

Figure 7.5 (a) Green channel of the input image, (b) vessel free image after morphological closing, (c) the local variation at each pixel, (d) extracting bright regions by adjusted thresholding, (e) result of morphological reconstruction, and (f) result of candidate extraction.

the G from the RGB fundus image. Moreover, we consider the channel I from the color space HSI, where I is defined as the average of the R, G, and B channel. In this way, we can keep some relevant information also from the red and blue channels. Besides using the intensity images G and I, we apply seven more preprocessing methods proposed in the literature of retinal image analyses focusing mainly on exudate detection [1,3,5,6,9]. The corresponding preprocessing algorithms highlight several typical features of exudates to increase the accuracy of the detection and our aim is to exploit the advantage of all of them. For this reason, an ACM (see Section 3.3) minimizes the energy function regarding the result of each preprocessing algorithm. The reason for selecting these specific seven methods [6,16–21] also lies in the fact that they provide larger image contrast compared to others [22–27] and thus have proved to be efficient in combining with an ACM. Also note that the selected preprocessing algorithms provide different intensity values inside and outside the contour of the lesions which is necessary to apply an ACM. Thus, the preprocessing methods which provide nearly zero values at both inside and outside the expected contour, cannot be applied here. We will now a short description for the nine applied preprocessing methods and include Figure 7.6 to show their results.

7.3.2.1   *Chromaticity normalization*

Chromaticity normalization [16] can normalize the green intensity channel according to the portion of the green among the colors as:

$$I_{CN} = \frac{G}{R + G + B},$$ (7.1)

where I_{CN} is the resulting intensity channel, and R, G, and B are the original intensity channels of the image in the color space RGB, respectively. This method is usually applied,

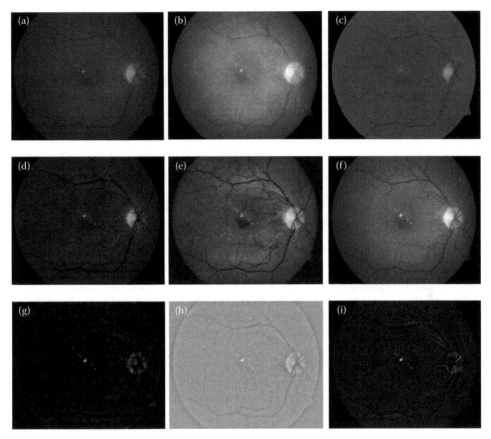

Figure 7.6 Nine different enhanced variants of the input image. (a) G, (b) I, (c) I_{CN}, (d) I_{CE}, (e) I_{CL}, (f) I_{GN}, (g) I_{IC}, (h) I_{IE}, (i) I_{WT}.

when the scene is captured by a camcorder and the illumination of the object is not uniform in a video. In our case, it is suited to reduce the bright reflection of retinal images of young patients.

7.3.2.2 Contrast enhancement

A robust contrast enhancement method has been proposed by Sanchez et al. [6]. To follow the instructions of the authors to enhance the image for further analysis, we convert the RGB image to the color space YIQ and replace the channel Y by the weighted sum of the channels $Y, I,$ and Q as:

$$Y_{mod} = 1.5 * Y + (-1) * I + (-1) * Q \tag{7.2}$$

After this modification, we convert $Y_{mod}IQ$ back to RGB. In the resulting image I_{CE}, the bright regions become brighter, while the dark ones darker.

7.3.2.3 Contrast-limited adaptive histogram equalization

Contrast-limited adaptive histogram equalization (CLAHE) [17] improves the contrast of the image locally. The sufficiently high contrast of the fundus image is very important, since besides high intensity, the contrast is another useful feature in exudate detection.

After applying CLAHE, the exudates can be better distinguished from the background on the resulting image I_{CL}.

7.3.2.4 Gray-world normalization

Gray-world normalization [18] divides each color channel by its respective average intensity, so it is suitable to suppress shining along temporal arcades. As the green channel contains the largest amount of information about the lesions and anatomical parts, we consider only the gray world normalization of the green channel as:

$$I_{GN} = \frac{G}{\bar{G}}, \tag{7.3}$$

where G is the original green intensity channel of the input image, I_{GN} is the resulting intensity channel, and $\bar{G}$ is the average intensity of the green channel respectively.

7.3.2.5 Illumination correction

The illumination is usually nonuniform in retinal images due to the variation of the retinal tissues and the spherical shape of the eye. To suppress nonuniform illumination, we apply illumination correction [19]. To perform this image enhancement technique, a spatially large (90 × 90) pixels median filter is applied to the input image. To get the corrected image I_{IC}, the blurred image is subtracted from the original one.

7.3.2.6 Illumination equalization

Besides illumination correction, we also simulate uniform illumination by using illumination equalization [20]. The adjusted intensity values are derived for each pixel as:

$$I_{IE}(x,y) = G(x,y) + m - \bar{G}_w(x,y), \tag{7.4}$$

where $G(x,y)$ is the original green intensity value at the position (x,y), m is the desired average intensity (in our case $m = 128$), and $\bar{G}_w(x,y)$ is the mean intensity value within a local (45 × 45) pixels neighborhood of the pixel (x,y) respectively.

7.3.2.7 White top-hat transformation

White top-hat transformation [21] is a morphological operator designed for extracting bright regions from the image. Since the opening operator realizes an erosion followed by a dilation, the darker regions will suppress the brighter ones on the opened image. When this relatively dark image is subtracted from the original one, the intensity peaks are enhanced and the exudates can be distinguished better from the background on the resulting image I_{WT}.

7.3.3 Precise boundary detection for each candidate

To detect the precise exudate boundaries, we propose the application of an active contour method, which minimizes the energy function regarding the nine variants $G, I, I_{CN}, I_{CE}, I_{CL}, I_{GN}, I_{IC}, I_{IE}, I_{WT}$ of the input image after which we combine the nine extracted contours. Our aim is to determine the most precise boundary for each exudate candidate to improve the accuracy of the region-wise classification. Toward this aim, we examine three different active contour methods and select the most efficient one for exudate contour detection. First, we apply a gradient vector flow field-based active contour model (known as snake) [28] and then we determine the boundary of the exudates by a Markov random field and a graph-cut algorithm [29]. Finally, the Chan–Vese energy function is minimized by an optimized level set method [30]. The proper details are given below.

7.3.3.1   Gradient vector flow and snake model

A traditional snake is a curve $X(s) = [x(s), y(s)]$, $s \in [0, 1]$, that moves through the spatial domain of an image to minimize the energy function:

$$E = \int_0^1 \frac{1}{2} \left(\alpha \, |X'(s)|^2 + \beta \, |X''(s)|^2 \right) + E_{ext}(X(s)) ds, \qquad (7.5)$$

where α and β are weighting parameters that control the tension and rigidity of the snake. $X'(s)$ and $X''(s)$ denote the first and second derivate of $X(s)$ with respect to s. The external energy function E_{ext} is derived from the image so that it takes its smaller values at the features of interest, for example boundaries.

A snake that minimizes Equation 7.5 must satisfy the following Eulerian equation:

$$\alpha X''(s) - \beta X''''(s) - \nabla E_{ext} = 0, \qquad (7.6)$$

where $\alpha X''(s) - \beta X''''(s)$ can be considered as an internal force E_{int} which discourages stretching and blending while the external potential force $-\nabla E_{ext}$ pulls the snake towards the desired image contour.

To find a solution for Equation 7.6, the snake is made dynamic by treating X as also a function of time t. Then, the partial derivate of X with respect to t can be set as the left hand side of (6) as follows:

$$X_t(s, t) = \alpha X''(s, t) - \beta X''''(s, t) - \nabla E_{ext}. \qquad (7.7)$$

A solution to Equation 7.7 can be found by discretizing the equation and solving the discrete system iteratively.

Xu and Prince defined a new non-irrotational external force field, which is called the gradient vector flow (GVF) field in Xu and Prince [28]. First, they define a gradient field ∇f based on the edge map of the image having the property that it is larger near the image edges. ∇f consists of vectors pointing toward the edges, but it has a narrow capture range, in general. Furthermore, in homogeneous regions, the field is zero, and therefore no information about nearby or distant edges are available. Finally, GVF is defined to be the vector field $v(x, y) = (u(x, y), v(x, y))$ that minimizes the following energy function:

$$\varepsilon = \int \int \mu(u_x^2 + u_y^2 + v_x^2 + v_y^2) + |\nabla f|^2 \, |v - \nabla f|^2 \, dxdy, \qquad (7.8)$$

where μ is a regularization parameter. This parameter should be set according to the amount of noise on the image. After computing $v(x, y)$, the external potential force $-\nabla E_{ext}$ in the dynamic snake Equation 7.7 can be replaced by $v(x, y)$. Using a force balance condition and the GVF potential force field in (7), a GVF snake can be defined. The GVF field points toward the object boundary in its close surrounding, and varies smoothly over homogeneous image regions.

The weaknesses of the GVF snake lie in the hard selection of the parameters and its sensitivity for its initialization. Moreover, it is not an appropriate tool for exudate boundary detection, since the energy function prefers high image gradients and smooth curvature of the contour. However, high contrast may be present close to the vessels in fundus images and the curvature of the contour of the exudates varies irregularly. These drawbacks of the GVF snake for this task can also be checked in Figure 7.7.

7.3.3.2 *Markovian segmentation model*

Markov random field (MRF) provides a robust tool to find exact boundaries of objects by minimizing a specific energy function. To find the global minimum for the usual energy function is an *NP*-hard problem, however, certain energy functions can be minimized in polynomial time by graph cuts. Lesko et al. [29] proposed a segmentation algorithm, which requires user interaction to mark an initial set of foreground/background pixels. Then, segmentation is performed via graph cut in real time.

As a well-known approach, segmentation can be considered as a labeling problem, where labels $\omega_s \in \{0,1\}$, $s \in S$ are assigned to the pixels $S = \{s_1, \ldots, s_N\} \subset \mathbb{Z}^2$ based on some observed features $\mathcal{F} = \{f_s\}$ of them. Based on the Bayesian theorem, the posterior probability can be factorized as $P(\omega|\mathcal{F}) \propto P(\mathcal{F}|\omega)P(\omega)$, where the optimal segmentation $\hat{\omega}$ is obtained as the maximum a posteriori (MAP) estimate. Based on the Hammersley–Clifford theorem [31], $\hat{\omega}$ can be found by specifying MRF with clique potentials and minimizing Gibbs energy. The main contribution of Lesko et al. [29] is to construct the Gibbs energy function in a way that it can be minimized via standard max-flow/min-cut. Namely, the full gradient information is exploited as magnitude and direction next to the gray-level

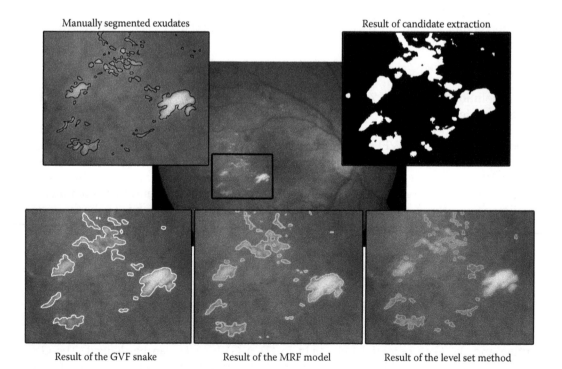

Figure 7.7 Precise exudate contour detection.

intensity and only the pairwise interactions (doubleton cliques) are considered. In this way, the constructed Gibbs energy can be represented by a graph and an exact MAP solution can be determined by computing the minimum *s-t-cut* on the graph [32] in polynomial time.

For the precise segmentation of the candidates, we apply this optimized MRF model with a modification to make the method automatic. So to eliminate user interaction, we define the initial foreground and background pixels as the result of candidate extraction. Based on our experiments, the MRF model initialized automatically provides near precise boundaries of candidates. The result of the MRF model can be seen in Figure 7.7.

7.3.3.3   Level set method and Chan–Vese energy function

A level set framework considers the 2D contour C as an embedded part of a 3D surface and C is represented as the zero level set, where the 3D surface is intersected by the image plane. This approach allows the contour to vary iteratively from pixel to pixel by modifying the 3D surface and the image is divided into separate regions so that the defined energy function is minimized. There are two main drawbacks of level set methods. Namely, the handling of the 3D surface makes them rather slow, and the definition of the initial contour is also difficult.

To reduce the computational time, Whitaker proposed the sparse field method (SFM) [30]. Here, the 3D surface is represented by lists of points $L_0, L_{-1}, L_{+1}, L_{-2}, L_{+2}, \ldots$ according to the distance of the points from the intersection image plane, where L_0 contains the pixels of the zero level set, and L_{-1}/L_{+1} contains the inner and outer adjacent pixels, respectively. The changes of the 3D surface are followed by moving the pixels from and to the appropriate lists. To initialize the zero level set, we use the boundary points of the extracted candidates found by the candidate extractor. In this way, the level set method can determine the zero level set for the next iteration automatically by minimizing the following Chan–Vese energy function:

$$E_{Chan-Vese} = F_1(C) + F_2(C). \tag{7.9}$$

The energy function (7.9) is suitable for exudate boundary detection (see also Figure 7.7), since it depends only on the difference of the pixel intensities $p_{x,y}$ and the respective average intensities inside (c_1) and outside (c_2) the contour C as formulated in the following way:

$$F_1(C) = \sum_{(x,y)\in \ inside(C)} \left| p_{x,y} - c_1 \right|^2, \tag{7.10}$$

$$F_2(C) = \sum_{(x,y)\in \ outside(C)} \left| p_{x,y} - c_2 \right|^2. \tag{7.11}$$

The energy function (7.9) takes its minimum, when both the inside and outside regions are the most homogeneous regarding pixel intensities.

7.3.3.4   Combination of the extracted contours

As we had described in Section 7.3.2, besides the intensity channels G and I we consider seven different image preprocessing methods to improve the contrast and the information content of the input image regarding exudates. After extracting $G, I, I_{CN}, I_{CE}, I_{CL}, I_{GN}, I_{IC}, I_{IE}$, and I_{WT} from the input fundus image, the previously discussed ACMs minimize their energy function on each of these variants of the input image. With the energy function, an

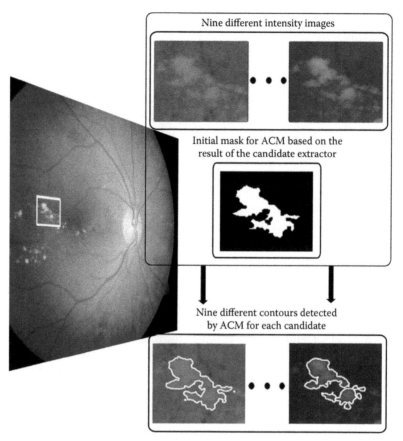

Figure 7.8 Different contours $(B_1, \ldots, B_9)$ for the nine preprocessed input images for an exudate candidate.

ACM is applied separately on the nine disparate enhanced images to produce nine different contours $B_1, \ldots, B_9$ for each exudate candidate as shown in Figure 7.8. These regions, bounded by the contours $B_1, \ldots, B_9$, are denoted by $R_1, \ldots, R_9$ respectively.

The next step is to extract a precise boundary for the candidate based on these nine contours or regions. Precise boundary detection has been found to be essential to provide appropriate features for a region-wise classification of true or false candidates. To let the different preprocessors take an effect on the final contour or region of a specific candidate, we fuse the corresponding extracted information in terms of combining the regions $R_i (i = 1, \ldots, 9)$ in the following way. First, we create the union of the regions as $\mathcal{R} = \cup_{i=1}^{9} R_i$, and to each pixel $p \in \mathcal{R}$ we assign a score as:

$$Score(p) = \left| \{ i : p \in R_i, i = 1, \ldots, 9 \} \right|, \qquad (7.12)$$

where $|.|$ represents the set cardinality, that is, the number of detected regions R_i ($i = 1, \ldots, 9$) containing p. If p falls out of all the regions R_i it gets score 0, whereas it falls inside all of them, it gets score 9. This assignment leads to nine new regions $R'_1, \ldots, R'_9$ as:

$$R'_i = \left\{ p \in \mathcal{R} : Score(p) \geq i \right\}, \quad i = 1, \ldots, 9 \qquad (7.13)$$

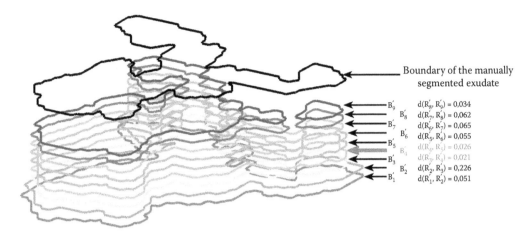

Boundary of the manually segmented exudate

B_9' $d(R_8', R_9') = 0,034$
B_8' $d(R_7', R_8') = 0,062$
B_7' $d(R_6', R_7') = 0,065$
B_6' $d(R_5', R_6') = 0,055$
B_5' $d(R_4', R_5') = 0,026$
B_3' $d(R_3', R_4') = 0,021$
B_2' $d(R_2', R_3') = 0,226$
B_1' $d(R_1', R_2') = 0,051$

Figure 7.9 The boundaries B_i' of the combined regions $R_i'(i = 1, \ldots, 9)$ and the boundary of a manually segmented exudate. The red arrow shows the selected region, which has the smallest total distance from its neighbors.

with R_i' consisting of pixels having score greater than or equal to i. Note that, we have $R_1' \supseteq R_2' \supseteq \ldots \supseteq R_9'$, with $R_1' = \mathcal{R}$. In this way, we merge the nine extracted regions $R_i(i = 1, \ldots, 9)$ and determine nine new regions $R_i'(i = 1, \ldots, 9)$ with their respective boundaries $B_i'(i = 1, \ldots, 9)$. Besides fusing the regions $R_i(i = 1, \ldots, 9)$, we have found that the final region should represent a stable state as well. That is, we select that $R_1', \ldots, R_9'$ as the final region, which is the most similar to its neighbors R_{i-1}' and R_{i+1}' regarding the fusion. As extreme, less meaningful cases, $R_1' = \cup_{i=1}^9 R_i'$ and $R_9' = \cap_{i=1}^9 R_i'$ are excluded from this analysis. For a precise formulation of this process, we measure the similarities between two adjacent regions by computing their symmetric difference as:

$$d(R_i', R_{i+1}') = \frac{\left|\left(R_i' \cup R_{i+1}'\right) \setminus \left(R_i' \cap R_{i+1}'\right)\right|}{|R_i'|}, \quad i = 1, \ldots, 8, \tag{7.14}$$

where $\setminus$ denotes the set difference operator. The denominator $|R_i'|$ in Equation 7.14 is applied for scale-invariance. According to our experimental results, that R_F' with $F \in \{2, \ldots, 8\}$ should be selected as the final exudate region for which:

$$d\left(R_{F-1}', R_F'\right) + d\left(R_F', R_{F+1}'\right) = \min_{i=2,\ldots,8} \left(d\left(R_{i-1}', R_i'\right) + d\left(R_i', R_{i+1}'\right)\right). \tag{7.15}$$

This procedure is performed for each candidate separately to have the set of the candidates with precisely detected contours. Naturally, some candidates are not true exudates, but we determine the best fitted boundary for each candidate individually to improve the accuracy of the region-wise classification. An example for this procedure is also shown in Figure 7.9, where the measured similarities are also included.

7.3.4 Region-wise classification

As we have mentioned in Section 7.3.1, the method used for candidate extraction has high sensitivity, since it finds almost all exudates in the input image. At the same time,

Table 7.1 Region-wise descriptors to classify exudate candidates

	Region-based features	Boundary-based features
Based[a] on the intensity images $G, I, I_{CN}, I_{GN},$ $I_{CL}, I_{CE}, I_{IC}, I_{IE}, I_{WT}$ (9×10 features)	Mean Standard deviation Minimum value Maximum value Range (difference of minimum and maximum value)	Mean Standard deviation Minimum value Maximum value Range (difference of minimum and maximum value)
Based on the magnitude of gradient image of the green channel (10 features)	Mean Standard deviation Minimum value Maximum value Range (difference of minimum and maximum value)	Mean Standard deviation Minimum value Range (difference of minimum and maximum value) Range (difference of minimum and maximum value)
Morphological (shape) descriptors (6 features)	Compactness Area Number of holes Elongatedness Eccentricity	Perimeter

[a] The intensity based descriptors extracted separately for the images $G, I, I_{CN}, I_{CE}, I_{CL}, I_{GN}, I_{IC}, I_{IE}, I_{WT}$.

it marks each bright region (mainly the ones are close to vessels on retinal images of youngsters) as an exudate that leads to many false-positive hits. If we consider all these candidates as the result of detection of exudates, the specificity of the automatic screening system drops. To exclude the false-positive candidates besides keeping up high sensitivity, we propose a region-wise classification step, which labels each candidate region as exudate or nonexudate. This step can be considered as a postprocessing step, where each candidate region with precisely detected boundary is classified by an optimally adjusted Naïve–Bayes classifier based on region-based features.

For this region-wise classification, we extract descriptors from each exudate candidate found by the candidate extractor method [1]. These descriptors are based on the respective intensity values of pixels composing the properly detected candidate and are calculated from the morphological behavior (shape) of the precisely detected region and its boundary. In this way, for candidate classification initially we consider 106 region-wise descriptors listed in Table 7.1.

In Table 7.1, we have provided all the descriptors extracted from the candidate regions of a training dataset regardless of their classification performance, so it contains such descriptors that are less efficient for this task. To select the meaningful features for classification, we have evaluated their corresponding performance by two-sample t-tests. We have tested some commonly used classifiers (Naïve–Bayes, k-nearest neighbors) with several feature selection methods like PCA, relative entropy, minimum attainable classification error, ROC analysis, Wilcoxon test, etc. based on class separability criteria. We have found that the Naïve–Bayes classifier and the two-sample t-test are the most efficient for our case. Namely, the Naïve–Bayes classifier reached the highest *Accuracy* value (84.37%) when it used features selected by two-sample t-test for labeling. For the sake of completeness, we list the highest *Accuracy* values of Naïve–Bayes, when it used features selected by other methods. The following feature selection methods are included (with highest *Accuracy* is also indicated): PCA (80.38%), minimum attainable classification error (Bhattacharyya) (80.44%), relative entropy (80.51%), ROC analysis (81.09%), and Wilcoxon test (81.61%). Now we give the proper description of feature selection based on the two-sample *t*-test.

To rank the descriptors based on their performance obtained by the two-sample *t*-test, we used 28 training images from the dataset DIARETDB1. These images were considered as input to the candidate extractor method. Then, we generated the nine different preprocessed images, finally determined the precise boundary for each candidate by the proposed boundary detection algorithm. The output binary images contained exudate candidates (1239 regions) with precise boundary and we labeled manually the candidates as true exudates (955 true-positive) or not (284 false-positive), according to the manually segmented binary images described in Section 3.7.2. Based on this labeling, the *t*-test can be performed for each descriptor given in Table 7.1 according to the following formula:

$$t_j = \frac{(\mu_{j_F} - \mu_{j_T})\sqrt{\frac{nm(n+m-2)}{n+m}}}{\sqrt{(n-1)\sigma_{j_F}^2 + (m-1)\sigma_{j_T}^2}}, \tag{7.16}$$

where t_j denotes the performance of the *j*-th descriptor, n the number of the true exudate regions (955), and m the number of the false ones (284) considering the whole set of the candidates for the training set. μ_{j_F} (resp. μ_{j_T}) denotes the mean, while σ_{j_T} (resp. σ_{j_F}) denotes the standard deviation of the *j*-th descriptor of all true (resp. false) exudates respectively.

To find the meaningful descriptors, we ranked them based on their performance values t_j, and tried to find the k descriptors, which provided highest accuracy. For this aim, we divided the set of 1239 manually labeled regions extracted from 28 training images into training and test parts. Then, a Naïve–Bayes classifier was trained on the first k ($k = 1, \ldots, 106$) region-wise features extracted from the training regions. Next, we observed the performance of the classifier on the test regions using these k features. We found that the Naïve–Bayes classifier reached the highest *Accuracy* value (derived from the number of true-positive, true-negative, false-positive, and false-negative cases), when the first $k = 29$

Table 7.2 Selected region-wise descriptors to classify exudate candidates

	Region-based features	Boundary-based features
Based[a] on the intensity images G, I_{CL}, I_{CE} (3 × 6 features)	Standard deviation Maximum value Range (difference of minimum and maximum value)	Standard deviation Maximum value Range (difference of minimum and maximum value)
Based on the magnitude of gradient image of the green channel (5 features)	Mean Maximum value Mean Minimum value Maximum value	
Morphological (shape) descriptors (6 features)	Compactness Area Number of holes Elongatedness Eccentricity	Perimeter

[a] The intensity based descriptors extracted separately for the images G, I_{CL}, I_{CE}.

descriptors (see them in Table 7.2) were selected from the ranked list as features (see Figure 7.10a). For this evaluation, we separated the regions into a training and test set by *K*-fold cross validation (*K* = 10) and evaluated the performance of the classifier for a given feature set at 10 times. For the sake of completeness, the accuracies of different combination of classifiers (Naïve–Bayes, *k*-nearest neighbors) and feature selection methods regarding the numbers of features are enclosed in Figure 7.10a,b. These empirical results also serve

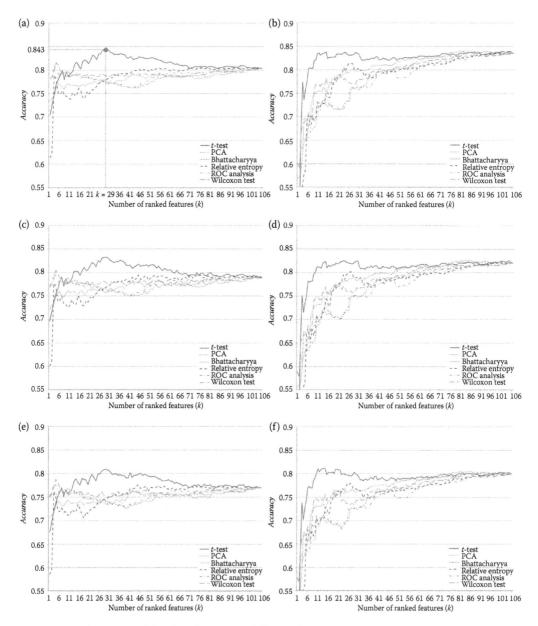

Figure 7.10 Peformance of the classifiers using different feature selection methods. Naïve–Bayes classifier with (a) level set method, (c) MRF, and (e) GVF snake. *k*-Nearest neighbors classifier with (b) level set method, (d) MRF, and (f) GVF snake.

as further proof for our former claim that the applied Chan–Vese energy function minimized by level set method is the most appropriate tool for the detection of the irregularly
variable contours of the exudates. As it can be observed in Figure 7.10c–f, the accuracies of
classifiers decrease if the exudate candidates are extracted by the MRF or the GVF snake.

The simple Naïve–Bayes classifier reaches relatively high accuracy regarding the
correct labeling of the exudate candidates using the selected 29 features. As for implementation, the built-in MATLAB® R2010b class of Naïve–Bayes [33] is used. To increase further
the performance of the Naïve–Bayes classifier, we apply the adaptive boosting (AdaBoost)
technique [34]. To realize the idea that the performance of ensemble learning is usually
better than single learning, to set up an ensemble of classifiers, the training dataset is separated into two disjoint sets T_1 and T_2. The first classifier learns on T_1 and classifies the
elements of T_2. In the next turn, the new classifier is trained on mainly the previously mis-
classified elements to teach it for the instances that are hard to classify, and so on. Finally,
these classifiers make a decision about a label of a new instance by weighted majority voting, where the weights come from the individual accuracies of the classifier. In this way, an
ensemble of several Naïve–Bayes classifiers can achieve 10% higher accuracy in labeling
the candidates as exudates or nonexudates in our framework.

7.4   Results

We have evaluated our proposed exudate detection method on the test part of the dataset
DIARETDB1 and on the whole dataset HEI-MED. The accuracy of the proposed method
has been evaluated at both image and lesion-level as described next.

7.4.1   Classification results at image level

The test part of DIARETDB1 includes 29 (from 61) and that of HEI-MED 54 (from 169)
images that contain exudates according to the publicly available annotation of clinical
experts. Based on this knowledge, we measured the performance of the proposed method
first at the image level. Namely, we considered the classification result for an image as
a true positive (resp. true negative) if the input image contained (resp. did not contain)
exudates according to both our proposed method and the ground truth. We had a false-
positive, when the proposed method recognized bright regions of the input image as
exudates, though based on the ground truth no exudates were labeled manually. We had a
false-negative in the reversed case. Based on the true/false-positive/negative cases, we calculated *Sensitivity* (also known as true-positive rate), *Specificity* (also known as *true-negative
rate*, which equals to 1-*false-positive rate*), and *Accuracy* as follows:

Accuracy

$$= \frac{\text{\# of true positives} + \text{\# of true negatives}}{\text{\# of true positives} + \text{\# of false negatives} + \text{\# of false positives} + \text{\# of true negatives}},$$
(7.17)

to measure the performance at the image level.

Based on these measures, we were able to compare the proposed exudate detector
with some other state-of-the-art exudate detector algorithms quantitatively. As we can see

Table 7.3 Comparative results for image-level classification for the proposed method on the dataset DIARETDB1

	Sensitivity	Specificity	Accuracy
Exudate detection by level set method	0.92	0.68	**0.82**
Sopharak et al. [2]	0.73	0.87	**0.79**
Sánchez et al. [6]	0.66	0.92	**0.77**
Exudate detection by MRF	0.90	0.54	**0.75**
Walter et al. [1]	1.00	0.32	**0.72**
Exudate detection by GVF snake	0.81	0.54	**0.70**
Welfer et al. [3]	0.79	0.55	**0.69**
Sopharak et al. [4]	1.00	0.14	**0.64**
Sopharak et al. [5]	1.00	0.02	**0.59**
Jaafar et al. [9]	1.00	0.06	**0.61**

in Tables 7.3 and 7.4, in these tests, the proposed algorithm outperformed the algorithms [1–6,9] involved in our comparative study with respect to the *Accuracy* value. Note that, *Accuracy* can also be derived from *Sensitivity* and *Specificity*, so *Accuracy* is high if and only if both *Sensitivity* and *Specificity* are large. Moreover, it can be observed that the application of all the nine preprocessing methods simultaneously and the detection of the precise boundary of the candidates lead to a meaningful improvement in region-wise classification, as well.

For the sake of completeness, we also enclose the receiver operating characteristics (ROC) results of the proposed method in Figure 7.11 to demonstrate its robustness at image level on the datasets DIARETDB1 and HEI-MED. To create the ROC curve, we applied different threshold levels for the weighted majority voting result of the boosted Naïve–Bayes classifiers to accept exudate candidates as true ones. As in Sopharak et al. [2,4,5], Welfer et al. [3], and Jaafar et al. [9], the authors did not define an adjustable parameter, a complete ROC analysis cannot be done for them. Instead, we indicate only their single available (*Sensitivity*, 1-*Specificity*) figures in Figure 7.11. However, a full comparative ROC analysis with Walter et al. [1] and Sánchez et al. [6] and the proposed method without

Table 7.4 Comparative results for image-level classification for the proposed method on the dataset HEI-MED

	Sensitivity	Specificity	Accuracy
Exudate detection by level set method	0.87	0.86	**0.86**
Sopharak et al. [2]	0.65	0.90	**0.82**
Sánchez et al. [6]	0.62	0.90	**0.81**
Exudate detection by MRF	0.83	0.79	**0.80**
Welfer et al. [3]	0.70	0.84	**0.79**
Exudate detection by GVF snake	0.74	0.77	**0.76**
Sopharak et al. [4]	0.91	0.68	**0.75**
Walter et al. [1]	0.93	0.65	**0.74**
Sopharak et al. [5]	0.93	0.60	**0.70**
Jaafar et al. [9]	0.88	0.65	**0.72**

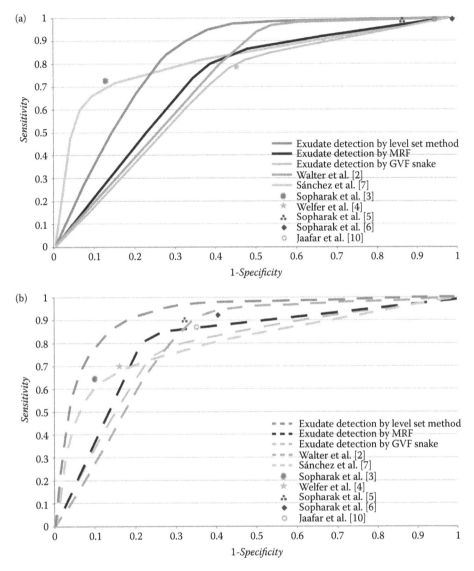

Figure 7.11 Comparative analysis for receiver operating characteristics (ROC) on the datasets: (a) DIARETDB1, (b) HEI-MED.

precise boundary detection is included in the figure. The competitiveness of the proposed method can be observed regarding ROC analysis, as well.

7.4.2 Precise segmentation of exudates

We also show the accuracy of our proposed method regarding the precise detection of the exudates. For this evaluation, we used such 53 binary images as ground truth, which were created manually by a local eye specialist based on the rough labeling of four experts defining the ground truth for DIARETDB1.

For the comparison of a ground truth binary image R_m with a segmentation result R_s of a detector, Walter et al. [1] proposed the following true-positive, false-negative, and false-positive measures:

$$\text{true positive} = |R_m \cap R_s| \tag{7.18}$$

$$\text{false negative} = |R_m \setminus (R_m \cap (R_s \otimes B))| \tag{7.19}$$

$$\text{false positive} = |R_s \setminus ((R_m \otimes B) \cap R_s)| \tag{7.20}$$

where $\otimes B$ is a morphological dilation executed with a 3×3 pixels structuring element B. Based on these definitions, we considered *Sensitivity* and *Positive Predicted Value* (*PPV*) to calculate the *F-Score* for performance measurement at lesion-level as:

$$PPV = \frac{true\ positive}{true\ positive + false\ positive} \tag{7.21}$$

$$F\text{-}Score = \frac{2 * \text{Sensitivity} * \text{PPV}}{\text{Sensitivity} + \text{PPV}} \tag{7.22}$$

As a comparative study, in Table 7.5, we have enclosed the performance of the algorithms [1–5]. It can be seen that the level set method-based exudate detection outperformed the other contour detection algorithms and all the other detectors at lesion-level considering the *F-Score*. Note that, *F-Score* is the most important performance measure in our case, since it is high if and only if both *Sensitivity* and *PPV* are large (see also Equation 7.20). The algorithms given in Sánchez et al. [6] and Jaafar et al. [9] are not involved in this lesion-level comparison, since they were not optimized for precise exudate boundary detection. The low accuracy figures for some algorithms may come from the fact that they were tested on smaller databases with images having low resolution.

For the sake of completeness, Figure 7.12 demonstrates the differences between the results of the proposed algorithm and the state-of-the-art methods involved in our comparative study. Figure 7.12 includes the final outputs of Walter et al. [1], Sopharak et al. [2,4,5], Welfer et al. [3], Sánchez et al. [6], and Jaafar et al. [9] and the proposed method for a sample image containing both hard and soft exudates.

Table 7.5 Comparative results at the lesion level on the dataset DIRAETDB1

	Sensitivity	PPV	F-Score
Exudate detection by level set method	0.86	0.84	**0.85**
Exudate detection by MRF	0.73	0.69	**0.71**
Exudate detection by GVF snake	0.69	0.67	**0.68**
Walter et al. [1]	0.76	0.59	**0.67**
Sopharak et al. [2]	0.40	0.91	**0.56**
Welfer et al. [3]	0.19	0.92	**0.31**
Sopharak et al. [4]	0.49	0.09	**0.16**
Sopharak et al. [5]	0.82	0.06	**0.11**

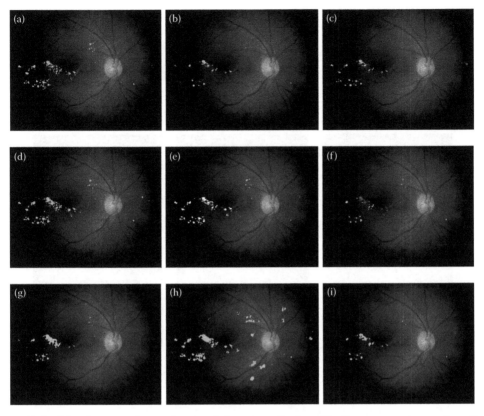

Figure 7.12   Visual comparison of state-of-the-art methods with the proposed one. Results of (a) proposed method, (b) [2], (c) [6], (d) [1], (e) manual segmentation, (f) [3], (g) [4], (h) [5], and (i) [9].

In Figure 7.13, we show some detection results obtained by the proposed algorithm for images having different intensity appearance. See Figures 7.14 through 7.16 for a visual comparison between the result of the proposed level set-based precise contour detection with region-wise classification and the final output of Walter et al. [1], Sopharak et al. [2,4,5], Welfer et al. [3], Sánchez et al. [6], and Jaafar et al. [9] on these images with different intensity behavior. As can be observed in these sample images, our approach basically detects all the exudates that consist of bright pixels and have irregular, sharp border. In Figure 7.17, we also demonstrate the performance of the proposed algorithm for the detection of other, more expanded bright lesions like drusens and cotton wool spots. Since the candidate extraction step locates all the bright regions, we can initialize the proposed precise boundary segmentation method with them. It makes the region-wise classifier identify these lesions as exudates if they share sufficiently many from the considered features. As it can be seen in Figure 7.17, the algorithm works well till the point, when the sharp edges of the lesion start to disappear and the features of the detected regions become more different from those of the exudates (e.g., number of holes, edge properties). This consideration suggests that with a different feature set, our framework might be tuned also for the detection of other bright lesions besides exudates. However, we have not performed quantitative analysis for drusens and cotton wool spots, since the corresponding manual annotations are hardly available publicly at the moment.

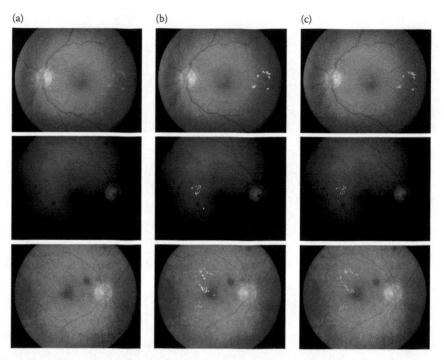

Figure 7.13 Detection results of the proposed method. (a) Original images with different intensity behavior, (b) corresponding ground truth images, and (c) results of detection.

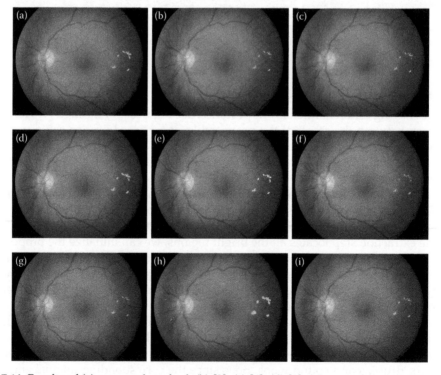

Figure 7.14 Results of (a) proposed method, (b) [2], (c) [6], (d) [1], (e) manual segmentation, (f) [3], (g) [4], (h) [5], and (i) [9] for the input image shown in Figure 7.13a (top).

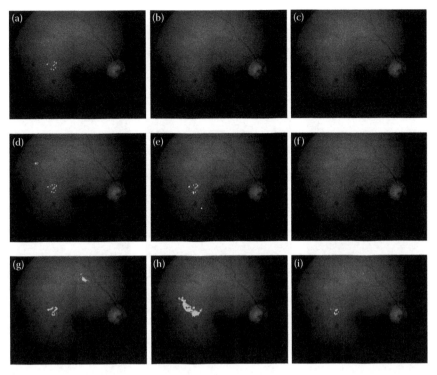

Figure 7.15 Results of (a) proposed method, (b) [2], (c) [6], (d) [1], (e) manual segmentation, (f) [3], (g) [4], (h) [5], and (i) [9] for the input image shown in Figure 7.13a (middle).

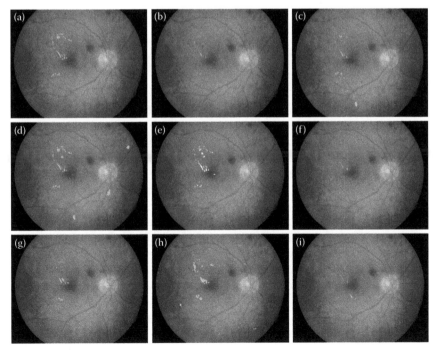

Figure 7.16 Results of (a) proposed method, (b) [2], (c) [6], (d) [1], (e) manual segmentation, (f) [3], (g) [4], (h) [5], and (i) [9] for the input image shown in Figure 7.13a (bottom).

(a)   (b)   (c)

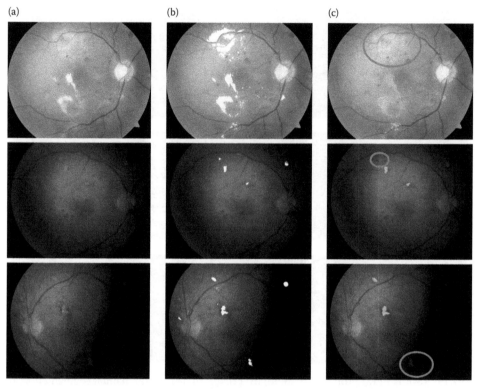

Figure 7.17 Detection results of the proposed method also for drusens and cotton wool spots. (a) Original images, (b) result of candidate extraction, (c) result of detection (red ellipses mark the false negative regions).

7.5   Discussion and conclusion

In this chapter, we have presented an exudate segmentation approach, which is based on the combination of grayscale morphology, active contour method, and region-wise classification. The result of a grayscale morphology–based exudate detection method is considered as the initial mask for the level set method. We apply sparse field algorithm as a level set method to minimize the Chan–Vese energy function. Nine different image enhancement results are involved for minimizing the energy function, and from the extracted nine regions, we select the most appropriate one. The proposed exudate segmentation method finds the contours more precisely and reduces the number of false-positive pixels and improves the reliability of the region-based features. The candidates are labeled as exudate or nonexudate through a region-wise classification step. For this task, we extract carefully selected descriptors for each candidate. For feature selection, we used a two-sample *t*-test, while for classification the Naïve–Bayes classifier is optimized by AdaBoost.

Considering the image-level accuracy, our proposed method achieved *Accuracy* values of 86% and 80% on the publicly available datasets DIARETDB1 and HEI-MED, respectively. With these results, the proposed technique gained higher accuracy in comparison to several other state-of-the-art approaches.

(a)   (b)

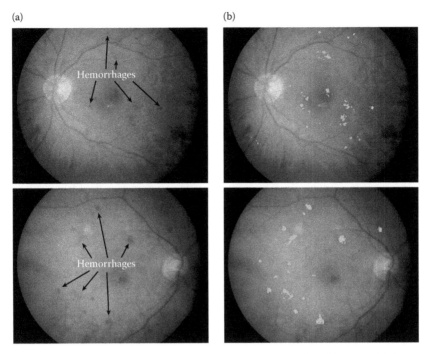

Figure 7.18 Results of the proposed approach in the segmentation of dark lesions. (a) Original images and (b) outputs of the modified proposed method.

Note that the proposed combined framework is dedicated to the detection of bright lesions caused by diabetic retinopathy, especially for exudates. That is, the selected pre-processing methods enhance the contrast between the bright lesions and their dark background. The candidate extractor method finds the regions that might contain these bright lesions, while the consequent region-wise classifier is trained to select the bright patches with irregular contours as exudates. Naturally, if we change the components of the approach appropriately, it could be applied also for the segmentation of expanded dark lesions like hemorrhages with some examples shown in Figure 7.18. That is, a future attempt can be to find the necessary modifications to specialize our approach also for the detection of dark retinal lesions.

According to Abramoff et al. [35], such screening algorithms cannot be recommended for clinical practice. However, our proposed methodology with its high *Accuracy* at image-level can be a solid component of a complex system to make the decision about the further clinical investigation of the patient. Precise boundary detection has an implicitly important influence on clinical practice to increase image-level accuracy.

The presented method was implemented in MATLAB, and we used a single core 2.4 GHz CPU with 2GB memory for testing. The precise boundary for each candidate is extracted using sequential computations. Moreover, the applied candidate extractor algorithm provides a large number of candidates. These are the reasons for the currently relatively high computational time 31 seconds per image by using the proposed level set methods (17 seconds per image by using the MRF and 51 seconds per image by using the GVF snake), which could be drastically decreased, for example, with parallel implementation. For the sake of completeness, we enclose the computational times of the reimplemented algorithms, which are involved in our comparative studies: Sopharak et al. [2], 6.63 seconds; Sánchez et al. [6], 27 seconds; Welfer et al. [3], 9.75 seconds; Sopharak et al. [4], 86 seconds; Walter et al. [1], 6.42 seconds; Sopharak et al. [5], 17 seconds; and Jaafar et al. [9], 12 seconds. These times do not include the optic disk detection step.

Acknowledgment

This work was partly supported by the project DRSCREEN: Developing a Computer-Based Image Processing System for Diabetic Retinopathy Screening of the National Office for Research and Technology of Hungary (Contract no.: OM-00194/2008, OM-00195/2008, OM-00196/2008); and the TÁMOP-4.2.2.C-11/1/KONV-2012-0001 Project and the European Union and the State of Hungary, cofinanced by the European Social Fund in the framework of TÁMOP-4.2.4.A/ 2-11/1-2012-0001 National Excellence Program.

References

1. T. Walter, J. C. Klein, P. Massin, and A. Erginay, A contribution of image processing to the diagnosis of diabetic retinopathy—detection of exudates in color fundus images of the human retina, *IEEE Transactions on Medical Imaging*, vol. 21, no. 10, pp. 1236–1243, 2002.
2. A. Sopharak, B. Uyyanonvara, S. Barman, and T. H. Williamson, Automatic detection of diabetic retinopathy exudates from non-dilated retinal images using mathematical morphology methods, *Computerized Medical Imaging and Graphics*, vol. 32, no. 8, pp. 720–727, 2008.
3. D. Welfer, J. Scharcanski, and D. R. Marinho, A coarse-to-fine strategy for automatically detecting exudates in color eye fundus images, *Computerized Medical Imaging and Graphics*, vol. 34, no. 3, pp. 228–235, 2010.
4. A. Sopharak, B. Uyyanonvara, and S. Barman, Automatic exudate detection from nondilated diabetic retinopathy retinal images using fuzzy c-means clustering, *Sensors*, vol. 9, no. 3, pp. 2148–2161, 2009.
5. A. Sopharak, M. N. Dailey, B. Uyyanonvara, S. Barman, T. Williamson, K. T. Nwe, and Y. A. Moe, Machine learning approach to automatic exudate detection in retinal images from diabetic patients, *Journal of Modern Optics*, vol. 57, no. 2, pp. 124–135, 2010.
6. I. Sánchez, R. Hornero, M. I. López, M. Aboy, J. Poza, and D. Abásolo, A novel automatic image processing algorithm for detection of hard exudates based on retinal image analysis, *Medical Engineering & Physics*, vol. 30, no. 3, pp. 350–357, 2008.
7. M. Niemeijer, B. van Ginneken, S. R. Russell, M. S. Suttorp-Schulten, and M. D. Abramoff Automated detection and differentiation of drusen, exudates, and cotton-wool spots in digital color fundus photographs for diabetic retinopathy diagnosis, *Investigative Ophthalmology & Visual Science*, vol. 48, no. 5, pp. 2260–2267, 2007.
8. M. García, C. I. Sánchez, M. I. López, D. Abásolo, and R. Hornero, Neural network based detection of hard exudates in retinal images, *Computer Methods and Programs in Biomedicine*, vol. 93, no. 1, pp. 9–19, 2009.
9. H. F. Jaafar, A. K. Nandi, and W. Al-Nuaimy, Detection of exudates in retinal images using a pure splitting technique, in *Conference of the Engineering in Medicine and Biology Society (EMBC 2010)*, pp. 6745–6748, 2010.
10. S. Ali, D. Sidibé, K. M. Adal, L. Giancardo, E. Chaum, T. P. Karnowski, and F. Mériaudeau, Statistical atlas based exudate segmentation, *Computerized Medical Imaging and Graphics*, vol. 37, no. 5, pp. 358–368, 2013.
11. B. Harangi, I. Lazar, and A. Hajdu, Automatic exudate detection using active contour model and regionwise classification, *Conference of the Engineering in Medicine and Biology Society (EMBC 2012)*, pp. 5951–5954, 2012.
12. J. E. Shaw, R. A. Sicree, and P. Z. Zimmet, Global estimates of the prevalence of diabetes for 2010 and 2030, *Diabetes Research and Clinical Practice*, vol. 87, no. 1, pp. 4–14, 2010.

13. T. Kauppi, V. Kalesnykiene, J. K. Kmrinen, L. Lensu, I. Sorri, A. Raninen, R. Voutilainen, H. Uusitalo, H. Klviinen, and J. Pietil, DIARETDB1 diabetic retinopathy database and evaluation protocol, *Conference on Medical Image Understanding and Analysis (MIUA 2007)*, pp. 61–65, 2007.

14. L. Giancardo, F. Meriaudeau, T.P. Karnowski, Y. Li, S. Garg, Jr K. W. Tobin, and E. Chaum, Exudate-based diabetic macular edema detection in fundus images using publicly available datasets, *Medical Image Analysis*, vol. 16, no. 1, pp. 216–226, 2012.

15. R. J. Qureshi, L. Kovacs, B. Harangi, B. Nagy, T. Peto, and A. Hajdu, Combining algorithms for automatic detection of optic disc and macula in fundus images, *Computer Vision and Image Understanding*, vol. 116, no. 1, pp. 138–145, 2012.

16. J. B. Martinkauppa and M. Piettikäinen, Facial skin color modeling, *Handbook of Face Recognition*. Berlin: Springer, 2005, pp. 113–135.

17. K. Zuiderveld, Contrast limited adaptive histogram equalization, *Graphics Gems IV*. New York: Academic Press Professional, 1994, pp. 474–485.

18. K. A. Goatman, A. D. Whitwam, A. Manivannan, J. A. Olson, and P. F. Sharp, Colour normalisation of retinal images, *Conference on Medical Image Understanding and Analysis (MIUA 2003)*, pp. 49–52, 2003.

19. A. Frame, P. Undrill, M. Cree, J. Olson, K. McHardy, P. Sharp, and J. Forrester, A comparison of computer based classification methods applied to the detection of microaneurysms in ophthalmic fluorescein angiograms, *Computers in Biology and Medicine*, vol. 28, pp. 225–238, 1998.

20. A. Hoover and M. Goldbaum, Locating the optic nerve in a retinal image using the fuzzy convergence of the blood vessels, *Transaction on Medical Imaging*, vol. 22, no. 8, pp. 951–958, 2003.

21. F. Meyer, Contrast feature extraction, in *Symposium on Quantitative Analysis of Microstructures in Material Science. Biology and Medicine*, pp. 374–380, 1977.

22. A. A. A. Youssif, A. Z. Ghalwash, and A. S. Ghoneim, Comparative study of contrast enhancement and illumination equalization methods for retinal vasculature segmentation, *Cairo International Biomedical Engineering Conference (CIBEC 2006)*, pp. 21–24, 2006.

23. A. A. A. Youssif, A. Z. Ghalwash, and A. S. Ghoneim, A comparative evaluation of preprocessing methods for automatic detection of retinal anatomy, in *International Conference on Informatics and Systems (INFOS 2007)*, pp. 24–26, 2007.

24. M. Sonka, V. Hlavac, and R. Boyle, *Image Processing, Analysis, and Machine Vision*, 2nd ed. Pacific Grove, CA: Thomson-Engineering, 1998.

25. M. Foracchia, E. Grisan, and A. Ruggeri, Luminosity and contrast normalization in retinal images, *Medical Image Analysis*, vol. 9, no. 3, pp. 179–190, 2005.

26. H. Peregrina-Barreto, A. M. Herrera-Navarro, L. A. Morales-Hernández, and I. R. Terol-Villalobos, Morphological rational operator for contrast enhancement, *Journal of the Optical Society of America A*, vol. 28, no. 3, pp. 455–464, 2011.

27. S. Ravishankar, A. Jain, and A. Mittal, Automated feature extraction for early detection of diabetic retinopathy in fundus images, *Computer Vision and Pattern Recognition (CVPR 2009)*, pp. 210–217, 2009.

28. C. Xu and J.L. Prince, Gradient vector flow: A new external force for snakes, *Computer Vision and Pattern Recognition (CVPR 1997)*, pp. 66–71, 1997.

29. M. Lesko, Z. Kato, A. Nagy, I. Gombos, Zs. Török, L. Vígh Jr., and L. Vígh, Live cell segmentation in fluorescence microscopy via graph cut, *International Conference on Pattern Recognition (ICPR 2010)*, pp. 1485–1488, 2010.

30. R. T. Whitaker, A level-set approach to 3D reconstruction from range data, *International Journal of Computer Vision*, vol. 29, no. 3, pp. 203–231, 1998.

31. S. Geman and D. Geman, Stochastic relaxation, Gibbs distributions, and the Bayesian restoration of images, *IEEE Transactions on Pattern Analysis and Machine Intelligence*, vol. 6, no. 6, pp. 721–741, 1984.

32. V. Kolmogorov and R. Zabih, What energy functions can be minimized via graph cuts? *IEEE Transactions on Pattern Analysis and Machine Intelligence*, vol. 26, no. 2, pp. 147–159, 2004.

33. G. H. John and P. Langley. Estimating continuous distributions in Bayesian classifiers, *Uncertainty in Artificial Intelligence (UAI 1995)*, pp. 338–345, 1995.

34. R. Polikar, Ensemble based system in decision making, *IEEE Circuits and Systems Magazine*, vol. 6, no. 3, pp. 21–45, 2006.

35. M. D. Abramoff, M. Niemeijer, M. S. Suttorp-Schulten, M. A. Viergever, S. R. Russell, and B. van Ginneken, Evaluation of a system for automatic detection of diabetic retinopathy from color fundus photographs in a large population of patients with diabetes, *Diabetes Care*, vol. 31, no. 2, pp. 193–198, 2008.

chapter eight

Preprocessing local features and fuzzy logic-based image segmentation

Umer Javed, Muhammad Mohsin Riaz, Abdul Ghafoor, and Tanveer Ahmed Cheema

Contents

Abstract

In this chapter, preprocessing, local features, and fuzzy active contours based image segmentation technique is presented. Image preprocessing techniques are used to mitigate the effects of different artifacts (noise, contrast degradation, and low resolution). Local features are then computed and are assigned weights using fuzzy logic to enhance the segmentation boundaries. Modified active contour based image segmentation technique is developed, which provides better accuracy in terms of visual and quantitative analysis.

8.1 Introduction

The medical image acquisition devices have improved tremendously to give images of high quality and resolution. However, the recorded images often represent a degraded version of the original scene (as the conditions under which images are obtained are not ideal). The image acquisition introduces degradations (like noise, blur, and poor contrast) and therefore, to represent the object adequately, image processing (preprocessing, feature extraction, and segmentation) is required.

Image preprocessing is a fundamental step in computer-aided diagnosis. It is used to improve the spatial resolution, reduce the noise effect, remove blur, and enhance the contrast distribution in an image. Some order statistic functions, such as the mean and median filters, leading to a simple generalization of the box filter, can be used for this purpose [1]. Some techniques based on image derivatives (such as adaptive smoothing [2–4] and anisotropic diffusion [5]) have been successfully used for preprocessing.

Feature extraction (captures visual contents of the image) represents the image in its reduced form. Object(s) can be represented by using a range of feature space (such as color, geometric, topological, statistical, and texture features [1]) because in some applications, only a few features do not capture sufficient information.

Segmentation is another important part of computer-aided diagnosis system. It is used to separate different components or objects like bones, soft tissues, and tumor in the images. Accurate segmentation greatly affects the overall performance. Segmentation requires a careful assessment of the various image features. Generally, the medical images are segmented by experienced radiologists, as the tumor and soft tissues have overlapping boundaries. However, the manual segmentation is time-consuming, subjective, and prone to human error. To overcome these issues, image analysis techniques are frequently used. Besides other components, the accurate segmentation of tumor is essential for clinical analysis, determining the efficacy of radiation therapy and effective diagnosis. Several algorithms have been proposed to achieve accurate image segmentation [6–19].

In this work, a brief review of image preprocessing techniques and feature extraction is given. Two fuzzy-weighted active contour based segmentation schemes are proposed (a brief version appears in Javed et al. [18]). These schemes utilize the texture information present in the images. A weighting factor based on texture information is introduced in the active contour model for fast convergence. Mamdani inference engine (MIE) and Takagi Sugeno (TS) inference engine are used to compute the optimal weights. Various simulations are performed to verify the proposed schemes.

8.2   Image preprocessing

Since the performance of segmentation algorithms are directly dependent on the quality of input images, preprocessing becomes an essential step.

8.2.1   Filtering or edge preserving smoothing

Image filtering is performed to enhance the desired information while minimizing the unwanted artifacts.

8.2.1.1   Domain transform filtering

Edge-preserving smoothing filters are of vital importance in several applications [4]. In Gastal and Oliveira [20], a transform-based edge-preserving technique defines the isometry between curves on the image and line. Recently, several techniques have been proposed to improve edge-aware smoothing [4,21,22]. However, these solutions natively only handle gray scale [8,15], are not sufficiently fast for real-time performance [4] and are restricted to a certain scale [21].

In Gastal and Oliveira [20], three variations of 1D edge preserving filters are presented namely, normalized convolution (NC), interpolated convolution (IC), and recursive filtering (RF). These approaches consume less computation time, less memory, and computation cost, thus making them applicable for color images at arbitrary scales in real time. In Knutsson and Westin [23], the nonuniform signal is filtered by assuming it as a uniform signal with missing samples. The optimal results are extracted by using NC method. The NC performs basic convolution operations on data of signal type. In Gastal and Oliveira [20], a moving average approach is used for performing NC with a box filter. This box filter estimates the population mean and have a constant radius. The IC method [24] is also used for interpolating the irregularly sampled data. It works as a linear diffusion process on the given signal. The RF method [20] uses a recursive edge-preserving filter for discrete samples. These domain transform and edge-preserving filters (NC, IC, and RF) are easy to implement and suitable for real-time image and video processing [20].

8.2.1.2 L0 gradient minimization

For image smoothing and noise removal, bilateral filter is frequently used and is proven simple and effective [2]. This filter is effective for smoothing small intensity variations while preserving the strong edges. However, it provides limited performance at arbitrary scales [4]. In Farbman et al. [4], a weighted least square optimization based alternative edge-preserving smoothing operator is used for progressive coarseness of images for multiscale detail extraction. This scheme reduces the ringing effect while reducing image blur in presence of noise. Anisotropic diffusion [5] also mitigates the noise and preserves image details [2].

In Xu et al. [2], edge-preserving image smoothing is performed using a sparse gradient counting scheme. L0 norm based method is used for determining the number of intensity changes that occur among pixel neighborhood. This method effectively removes unimportant details and reduces blur and noise.

8.2.2 Contrast enhancement techniques

Contrast enhancement (plays a vital role in image processing system) techniques are used for increasing the dynamic range of an image. If the contrast of an image is concentrated in a specified range, then information cannot be viewed properly. Histogram equalization is commonly used for contrast enhancement [25–28]. Histogram equalization can be applied on an image either globally or locally. Global histogram equalization obtains the transformation function based on cumulative distribution function of the whole image. It tends to spread the intensity distribution uniformly. On the contrary, the local histogram equalization technique divides the image into subimages and performs the histogram equalization on each subimage independently [28].

8.2.2.1 Nonparametric modified histogram equalization

Histogram equalization leads to overenhancement of the image and the image appears unnatural [25]. A nonparametric modified histogram equalization (NMHE) based contrast enhancement technique is proposed in Poddar et al. [26] for improving the quality of an image. The spikes from the input image histogram are removed as a preliminary step, by using method given in Arici et al. [27]. The modified histogram is further used for computing un-equalization measure, which indicates the nonuniform distribution of histogram and is utilized for computing the nonparametric modified histogram. This scheme is simple and efficient.

8.2.2.2   *Contrast enhancement using image decomposition*

In Pei et al. [3], an image decomposition based visual enhancement method decomposes the image into base and detail layers using L0 gradient-based method. A median-preserving gamma correction is applied to compensate the scaled down base layer. The detail layer is enhanced by visual profile and saliency maps. The image decomposition is based on constrained L0 gradient (CG) minimization. The L0 norm of gradient represents the number of gradients and forces the minimization to produce an approximated version of the original image. A median-preserving gamma correction method is used for adjusting the dynamic range of the processed image. Furthermore, the detail layer of a given image is enhanced by human perception based nonlinear boosting method. This method takes into consideration the smallest difference observable by humans. Saliency maps are generated by calculating the image curvature.

8.2.3   *Image resolution enhancement*

Several medical imaging modalities (computed tomography, magnetic resonance imaging (MRI), and positron emission tomography, etc.) provide complementary information. Some of them provide anatomical information whereas others provide functional information. The resolution of such imaging systems is based on operational conditions, imaging sensors, and physical constraints [29]. In order to analyze the medical images in a better way, high resolution is desirable. Super-resolution techniques are developed for addressing this issue [29,30]. In Dong et al. [30], a learning-based deblurring and super-resolution technique uses a set of autoregressive model (ARM) based learning method. The image nonlocal self-similarity and sparsity measure are used as regularization parameters.

8.3   *Feature extraction*

8.3.1   *Local entropy and variance*

Local entropy, as a regional descriptor, is concerned with the intensity variations in an image. The local energy $L_E(u, v)$ is

$$L_E(u, v) = -\frac{1}{u_1 \times v_1} \sum_{i_s} p(i_s) \log_2 p(i_s) \tag{8.1}$$

where $p(i_s)$ represents the intensity histogram, $i_s \in [0, 1]$ are intensities in $u_1 \times v_1$ matrix of an image centered at (u, v) pixel. High-intensity variation leads to a higher local entropy and vice versa. The total energy functional is then integrated into a variational level set formulation.

Let $L_V(u, v)$ be the local variance,

$$L_V(u, v) = \frac{1}{(2u_1 + 1)(2v_1 + 1)} \sum_{k=u-u_1}^{k=u+u_1} \sum_{l=v-v_1}^{l=v+v_1} \left(I(k, l) - \bar{I}(u, v) \right)^2 \tag{8.2}$$

where $\bar{I}(u, v)$ denotes the mean value of $u_1 \times v_1$ window situated at (u, v) pixel.

8.3.2   Fractal transform and lacunarity

Texture analysis relates to the study of intensity variation in an image. In Al-Kadi and Watson [31], fractal dimension and lacunarity features are used for the purpose of texture analysis. Images are transformed to fractal features by using the differential box counting algorithm (DBC) [31,32]. This algorithm assesses image at different scales and then analyze texture. DBC approach provides promising and accurate results for computing fractals and is commonly used when dealing with large data values [31,32].

In natural images, the similarity between shapes (seen at different scales) is generally approximate and is considered to be random. In biological structures, the fractal dimension of a structure is self-similar for a finite scaling range [31]. The structure of natural fractal may become smooth or rough for examining it below and above the finite range, respectively. The fractal dimension of visually different structures may turn out to be similar. In order to address this issue, lacunarity of the fractal dimension is computed. It quantizes the nature of gaps in texture images. Higher values of lacunarity in a fractal area indicate higher inhomogeneity and vice versa [31,33].

8.4   Image segmentation

Active contours are being extensively used for image segmentation [8,11,12,15]. The theories of surface evolution and geometric flows are combined with classic energy minimization problem to solve the image segmentation problem. The surface evolution problem is frequently solved by using level set method [8,10,15]. Active contours are categorized into edge-based [11,12] and region-based [8,13,15] methods. The edge-based methods use edge information and are in general sensitive to the initial conditions. These methods often fail to work for images with weak object boundaries [16]. Region-based methods use region descriptors (based on statistical information) for identifying region of interests and do not rely on the image gradients and therefore they are less sensitive to initial conditions. Conventional region-based methods assume piecewise homogeneous intensities [8,15]. The performance of these methods become limited for medical images (because of inhomogeneities in intensities).

In He et al. [17], the existing region scalable fitting (RSF) energy [16] is replaced with local entropy based weighted energy. A major limitation of this model is use of single regional descriptor (which is sometimes not sufficient). Different region descriptors behave differently depending on the input conditions. Moreover, if different region descriptors are combined in an intelligent manner, the segmentation results can be improved. In Li et al. [16] and He et al. [17], a Gaussian kernel function $K(u', v')$ is used for selecting the local region size and is defined as

$$K(u', v') = \left(\frac{1}{2\pi\rho^2}\right) \exp\left(\frac{-||u' - v'||^2}{2\rho^2}\right) \tag{8.3}$$

Weighted average values $f_1(u, v)$ and $f_2(u, v)$ are used for estimating the local image intensities in Ω_1 and Ω_2 are [16]

$$f_1(u, v) = \frac{K(u, v) * [H_{\phi(u,v)}I(u, v)]}{K(u, v) * H_{\phi(u,v)}}$$

$$f_2(u, v) = \frac{K(u, v) * [(1 - H_{\phi(u,v)})I(u, v)]}{K(u, v) * (1 - H_{\phi(u,v)})} \tag{8.4}$$

where $H_{\phi(u,v)}$ denotes the Heaviside function, $*$ denotes the convolution operator, $\{m, n, u, v\} \in \Omega$, and $u' = m - u, v' = n - v$, ρ represent the standard deviation. The smooth approximation of $H_{\phi(u,v)}$ and its derivative $\delta_{\phi(u,v)}$ are

$$H_{\phi(u,v)} = \frac{1}{2}\left[1 + \frac{2}{\pi}\tan^{-1}\left(\frac{\phi(u,v)}{\epsilon}\right)\right]$$

$$\delta_{\phi(u,v)} = H'_{\phi(u,v)} = \frac{\epsilon}{\pi(\epsilon^2 + \phi^2(u,v))} \tag{8.5}$$

where ϵ is a constant value and ϕ represents the level set function. The weighted local intensity fitting energy is given as

$$\frac{\partial \phi(m,n)}{\partial t} = \delta_{\phi(mn)}\left[\eta div\left(\frac{\nabla \phi(m,n)}{|\nabla \phi(m,n)|}\right) - \lambda_1 \int_{\Omega} K(u',v')W_{EV}(u,v)|I(m,n) - f_1(u,v)|^2 du\, dv\right.$$

$$\left. + \lambda_2 \int_{\Omega} K(u',v')W_{EV}(u,v)|I(m,n) - f_2(u,v)|^2 du\, dv\right]$$

$$+ \ddot{\mu}_2\left(\nabla \phi(m,n) - div\left(\frac{\nabla \phi(m,n)}{|\nabla \phi(m,n)|}\right)\right) \tag{8.6}$$

where W_{EV} are the weights computed using fuzzy system.

Note that, for $W_{EV}(u,v) = 1$ and $W_{EV}(u,v) = L_E(u,v)$ the gradient flow in Equation 8.6 transforms to the gradient flow given in Li et al. [16] and He et al. [17], respectively.

The weights not only improve the segmentation accuracy but also result in a faster convergence. Two fuzzy weight assessment methods namely, MIE and TS inference methods, for active contour segmentation are proposed. These methods combine the characteristics of dissimilar local features [19]. Fuzzy inference engine (FIE) is utilized to assign high weights to pixels having small local entropy and local variance, and low weights to pixels having large local entropy and local variance values.

8.4.1   Mamdani inference based weight computation

The fuzzy rule base has been based upon observation that pixels with less local entropy and local variance should be assigned higher weights and vice versa. This higher weight causes contour to approach the desired region faster than the existing technique. The fuzzy IF–THEN rules for propose scheme are

$Ru^{(1)}$: IF $L_E(u,v)$ is A^1 and $L_V(u,v)$ is B^1 THEN $W_{EV}(u,v)$ is C^1
$Ru^{(2)}$: IF $L_E(u,v)$ is A^1 and $L_V(u,v)$ is B^2 THEN $W_{EV}(u,v)$ is C^2
$Ru^{(3)}$: IF $L_E(u,v)$ is A^2 and $L_V(u,v)$ is B^1 THEN $W_{EV}(u,v)$ is C^2
$Ru^{(4)}$: IF $L_E(u,v)$ is A^1 and $L_V(u,v)$ is B^3 THEN $W_{EV}(u,v)$ is C^3
$Ru^{(5)}$: IF $L_E(u,v)$ is A^2 and $L_V(u,v)$ is B^2 THEN $W_{EV}(u,v)$ is C^3
$Ru^{(6)}$: IF $L_E(u,v)$ is A^3 and $L_V(u,v)$ is B^1 THEN $W_{EV}(u,v)$ is C^4
$Ru^{(7)}$: IF $L_E(u,v)$ is A^2 and $L_V(u,v)$ is B^3 THEN $W_{EV}(u,v)$ is C^4
$Ru^{(8)}$: IF $L_E(u,v)$ is A^3 and $L_V(u,v)$ is B^2 THEN $W_{EV}(u,v)$ is C^4
$Ru^{(9)}$: IF $L_E(u,v)$ is A^3 and $L_V(u,v)$ is B^3 THEN $W_{EV}(u,v)$ is C^5

where A^1, A^2, and A^3 are high, medium, and low membership functions (MF) for L_E and B^1, B^2, and B^3 are high, medium, and low MF for L_V. $\mathcal{C}^c$ for $c \in 1, 2, \ldots, 5$ are five output MFs, with $\mathcal{C}^1$ and $\mathcal{C}^5$ corresponds to lowest and highest values, respectively.

The inputs are fuzzified using Gaussian MF, passed through inference engine using the above rule base and defuzzified using center average defuzzifier to obtain W_{EV}^{MIE}.

$$W_{EV}^{MIE}(u,v) = \frac{\sum\limits_{c=1}^{5} \bar{y}^{(c)} \varpi^{(c)}}{\sum\limits_{c=1}^{5} \varpi^{(c)}} \tag{8.7}$$

where $\varpi^{(c)}$ is height of $\mu_{\mathcal{C}'}(y)$ in output MF.

8.4.2 TS inference based weighting

In contrast to the MIE [34], the TS inference offers the freedom to adjust output MF using optimization techniques [35]. The TS rule base for computing weights is

IF $L_E(u,v)$ is $A^{(i_1)}$ AND $L_V(u,v)$ is $B^{(i_2)}$ THEN

$$z^{(i_1+i_2-1)}(u,v) = \left(\frac{1}{1 + e^{-\eta_1 \ L_E(u,v)} + e^{-\eta_2 L_V(u,v)}} \right)^{i_1+i_2-1} \tag{8.8}$$

where η_1 and η_2 are constants and control the contribution of $L_E(u,v)$ and $L_V(u,v)$, respectively. Note that large $i_1 + i_2$ reduces the output of fuzzy weights (which is desirable). The computed weights W_{EV}^{TS} are

$$W_{EV}^{TS}(u,v) = \frac{\sum\limits_{i_1=1}^{3} \sum\limits_{i_2=1}^{3} z^{(i_1+i_2-1)} t\{\mu_{A^{i_1}}(L_E), \mu_{B^{i_2}}(L_V)\}}{\sum\limits_{i_1=1}^{3} \sum\limits_{i_2=1}^{3} t\{\mu_{A^{i_1}}(L_E), \mu_{B^{i_2}}(L_V)\}} \tag{8.9}$$

8.5 Results and discussion

The existing and proposed techniques are simulated on a Dell Inspiron, Intel Core i3 CPU, 2.1 GHz Processor, 4 GB RAM using MATLAB 7.13. Above 130 real MRI images belonging to different classes, that is, normal, astrocytoma, meningioma, sarcoma, glioma, and so forth, are used. The T1- and T2-weighted brain MRI images of 256×256 spatial resolution are obtained from the Harvard Medical School [36] and National Center for Biotechnology Information [37]. The parameters that are used during the experiments are initialized as $\eta = 0.001 \times (255)^2$ [16], $\lambda_1 = 1$ and $\lambda_2 = 1$, $\mu = 1$, $\kappa = 2$, and $\rho = 3$. The kernel window size, $u_1 \times v_1$, is selected as 3×3 unless otherwise specified. A small kernel size is preferable for images having high-intensity inhomogeneities.

In Figure 8.1, the results of local filters applied on low-grade glioma and high-grade astrocytoma images are shown. Figure 8.1a,k shows original MRI images whereas noisy

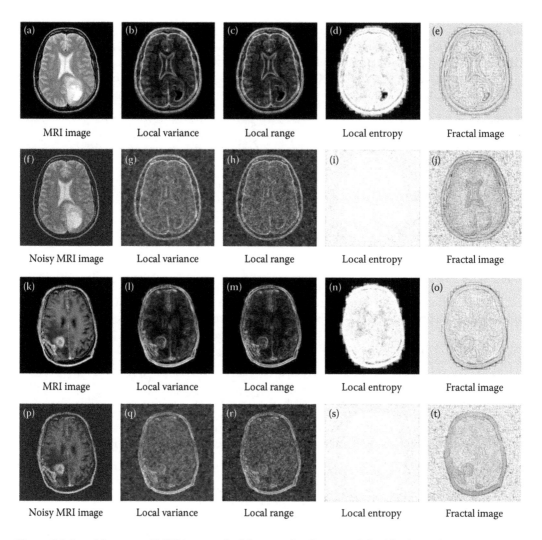

Figure 8.1 Local features of MRI images: (a–j) low-grade glioma and (k–t) high-grade astrocytoma.

MRI images are given in Figure 8.1f,p. The local features are computed for both noisy and noiseless images. It is observed that the local features fail to provide significant information in the presence of noise. Therefore, in the preprocessing step, filtering is required in order to mitigate the effect of noise.

The results, after applying domain transformation and L0 filters on noisy low-grade glioma image (Figure 8.1f), is given in Figure 8.2. Figure 8.2a,f,k,p shows the outputs of filters and Figure 8.2b–e,g–j,l–o,q–t shows the corresponding local features. Note that, although domain transform filters have sufficiently suppressed the noise effects, however, the results of L0 filter are significantly improved.

Similarly, the effects of applying domain transformation and L0 filters on noisy high-grade astrocytoma image (Figure 8.1p) are presented in Figure 8.3.

In Figure 8.4, the results after applying contrast enhancement techniques on low-grade glioma image (Figure 8.1a) is given. Figure 8.4a shows the result after processing the MRI image through NMHE [26] filter and Figure 8.4b–e shows local features. Figure 8.4f

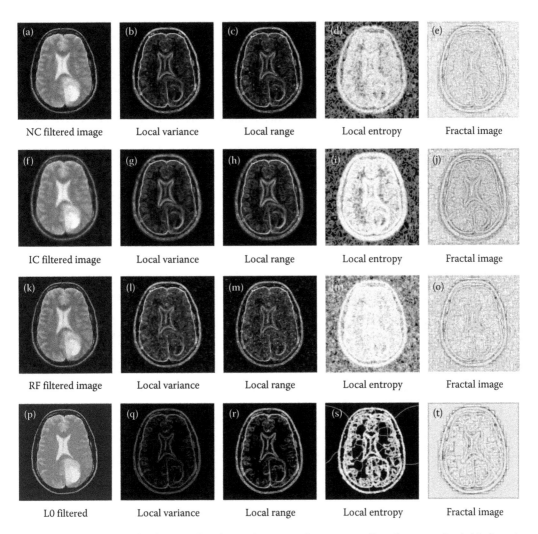

Figure 8.2 Denoising the low-grade glioma image and corresponding features: (a, f, k) domain transformation filters [20], (p) L0 filter [2], and (b–e, g–j, l–o, q–t) local features.

shows the result after processing the MRI image through CG [3] filter and Figure 8.4g–j shows corresponding local features. Similarly, the results of contrast enhancement techniques on high-grade astrocytoma images are given in Figure 8.5. It is observed that contrast-enhanced images results in improved local feature values.

The improvement in spatial resolution can be achieved by applying ARM [30] on MRI images. Figure 8.6 shows the results of enhancing the spatial resolution three times of given MRI images. Figure 8.6a,c shows low-grade glioma and high-grade astrocytoma images, respectively. Figure 8.6b,d is the transformed image with improved spatial resolution.

The segmentation results of three different examples are presented now. These three examples provide unique scenario in terms of intensity variations, which greatly affect the robustness and accuracy of different segmentation techniques. Figure 8.7a shows a low-grade glioma image. The results of local entropy and variance are shown in Figure 8.7b,c,

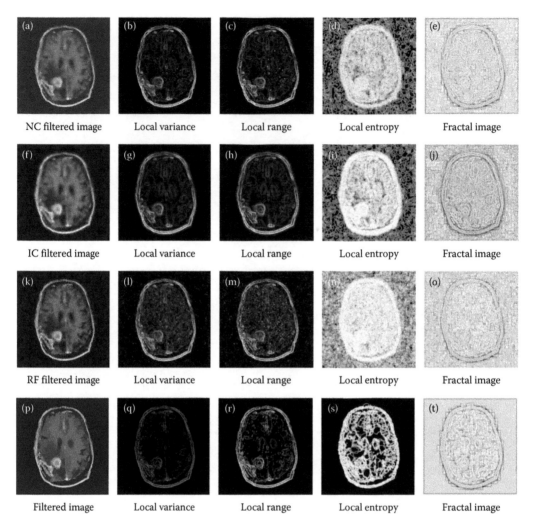

NC filtered image   Local variance   Local range   Local entropy   Fractal image

IC filtered image   Local variance   Local range   Local entropy   Fractal image

RF filtered image   Local variance   Local range   Local entropy   Fractal image

Filtered image   Local variance   Local range   Local entropy   Fractal image

Figure 8.3 Denoising a high-grade astrocytoma image and corresponding features: (a, f, k) domain transformation filters [20], (p) L0 filter [2], and (b–e, g–j, l–o, q–t) local features.

respectively. Note that the input image has inhomogeneous intensity due to which the segmentation of all the objects becomes difficult. The segmentation result of the existing RSF technique, after 35 iterations is given in Figure 8.7d. The MIE and TS based proposed techniques have effectively segmented the objects present inside an image in 30 iterations (shown in Figure 8.7e and Figure 8.8f, respectively). For this example, the parameters are set as $\eta = 0.001 \times (255)^2$ [16], $\lambda_1 = 1$ and $\lambda_2 = 1$. This reveals the ability of the proposed method to handle weak boundaries, complex background, and intensity inhomogeneities.

In Figure 8.8a, shows a grade IV astrocytoma image. The outputs of local entropy and variance are shown in Figure 8.8b,c, respectively. Figure 8.8d, shows the segmentation result of the RSF method, after 30 iterations. The proposed MIE and TS based techniques (shown in Figure 8.8e,f) have successfully segmented the objects present inside an image in

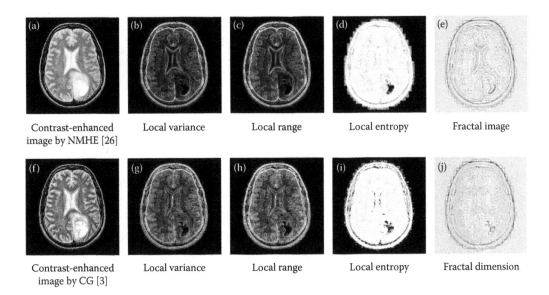

Figure 8.4 Contrast enhancement and features for low-grade glioma: (b–e, g–j) local features.

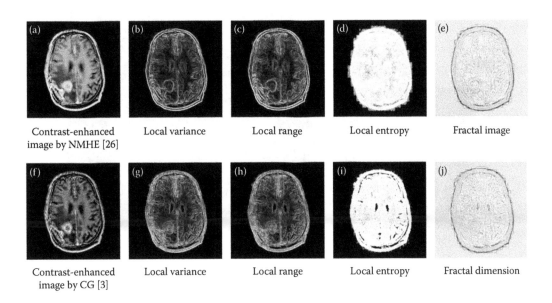

Figure 8.5 Contrast enhancement and features for low-grade glioma: (b–e, g–j) local features.

25 and 20 iterations, respectively. The MIE-based segmentation technique has successfully segmented the regions lying in MR image as compared to RSF and TS based schemes.

For quantitative analysis, the results of proposed and existing RSF models are shown by using probability rand index (PRI) and global consistency error (GCE) [14]. Figure 8.9 presents the PRI and GCE graphs for 46 different images. In Figure 8.9a, results are plotted

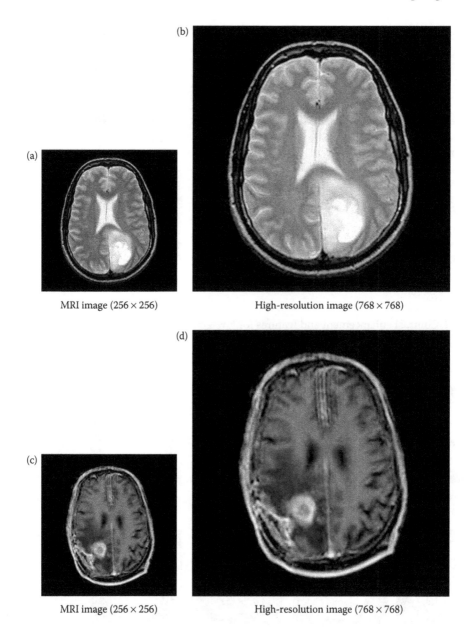

(a) MRI image (256 × 256)   **(b)** High-resolution image (768 × 768)

(c) MRI image (256 × 256)   **(d)** High-resolution image (768 × 768)

Figure 8.6 Enhancing spatial resolution of MRI images.

for 50 iterations, since proposed technique, (in general), successfully segmented the ROI within these iterations. Figure 8.9b,c uses MRI images for computing PRI and GCE, respectively. It can be seen that PRI lies around 0.8 and 0.9 for majority of the images using the proposed technique, whereas, for the existing RSF model the PRI lies between 0.6 and 0.7. Similarly, the GCE values lies between 0.1 and 0.2 for most of the images using proposed technique whereas for existing RSF model the GCE lies between 0.3 and 0.4.

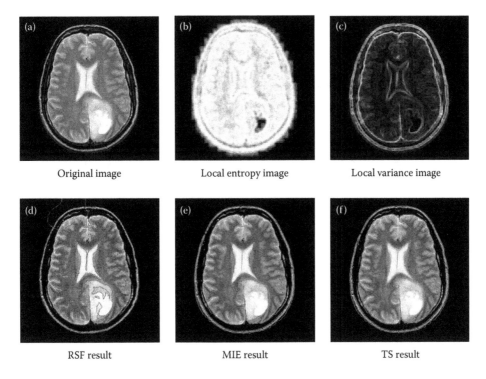

Figure 8.7 Segmentation results for low-grade glioma image.

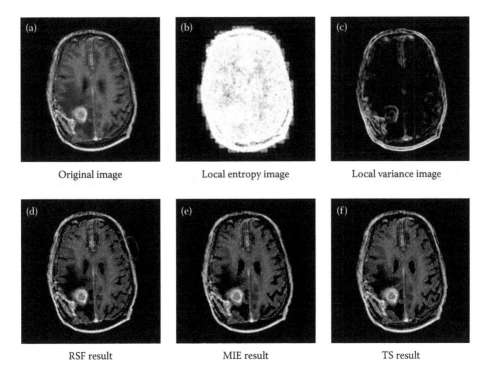

Figure 8.8 Segmentation results for grade IV astrocytoma image.

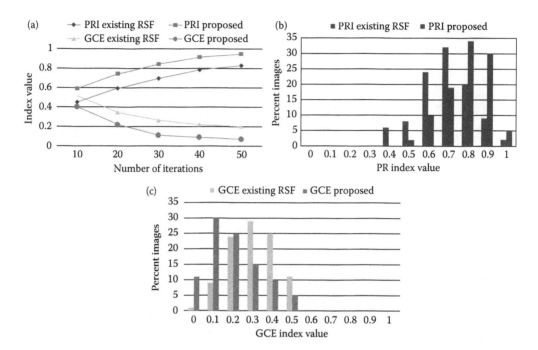

Figure 8.9 PRI and GCE graphs for existing RSF model and proposed technique: (a) PRI and GCE values, (b) PRI distribution of percent images, and (c) GCE distribution of percent images.

8.6   Conclusion

In this chapter, a brief review of image preprocessing techniques and feature extraction is presented. Fuzzy-weighted active contour based image segmentation is proposed, which utilizes texture information present for fast convergence. Simulation results on various images prove the significance of the proposed schemes.

References

1. R. C. Gonzales and R. E. Woods, *Digital Image Processing*, 2nd ed. Englewood Cliffs, NJ: Prentice Hall, 2002.
2. L. Xu, C. Lu, Y. Xu, and J. Jia, Image smoothing via L0 gradient minimization, *ACM Transaction on Graphics*, vol. 30, no. 6, pp. 1–11, 2011.
3. S. C. Pei, C. T. Shen, and T. Y. Lee, Visual enhancement using contrained L0 gradient image decomposition for low backlight displays, *IEEE Signal Processing Letters*, vol. 19, no. 12, pp. 813–816, 2012.
4. Z. Farbman, R. Fattal, D. Lischinski, and R. Szeliski, Edge-preserving decompositions for multi-scale tone and detail manipulation, *ACM Transactions on Graphics*, vol. 27, no. 3, pp. 1–10, 2008.
5. M. J. Black, G. Sapiro, D. H. Marimont, and D. Heeger, Robust anisotropic diffusion, *IEEE Transactions on Image Processing*, vol. 7, no. 3, pp. 421–432, 1998.
6. P. Truc, T. Kim, S. Lee, and Y. Lee, Homogeneity and density distance-driven active contours for medical image segmentation, *Computers in Biology and Medicine*, vol. 41, pp. 292–301, 2011.
7. C. Li, R. Huang, Z. Ding, J. Gatenby, and D. Metaxas, A level set method for image segmentation in the presence of intensity inhomogeneities with application to MRI, *IEEE Transactions on Image Processing*, vol. 20, no. 7, pp. 2007–2016, 2011.

8. T. Chan and L. Vese, Active contours without edges, *IEEE Transactions on Image Processing*, vol. 10, no. 2, pp. 266–277, 2001.

9. D. Mumford and J. Shah, Optimal approximations by piecewise smooth functions and associated variational problems, *Communications on Pure and Applied Mathematics*, vol. 42, no. 9, pp. 577–685, 1989.

10. N. Paragios and R. Deriche, Geodesic active regions and level set methods for supervised texture segmentation, *International Journal on Computer Vision*, vol. 46, no. 3, pp. 223–247, 2002.

11. V. Caselles, R. Kimmel, and G. Sapiro, Geodesic active contours, *International Journal on Computer Vision*, vol. 22, no. 1, pp. 61–79, 1997.

12. N. K. Paragios, Geodesic active regions and level set methods: Contributions and applications in artificial vision, PhD thesis, University of Nice Sophia Antipolis, 2000.

13. R. Ronfard, Region-based strategies for active contour models, *International Journal of Computer Vision*, vol. 13, no. 2, pp. 229–251, 1994.

14. R. Unnikrishnan, C. Pantofaru, and M. Hebert, A measure for objective evaluation of image segmentation algorithms, in *Computer Vision and Pattern Recognition Workshops*, San Diego, USA, pp. 34–34, 2005.

15. L. Vese and T. Chan, A multiphase level set framework for image segmentation using the Mumford and Shah model, *International Journal on Computer Vision*, vol. 50, no. 3, pp. 271–293, 2002.

16. C. Li, C. Kao, J. C. Gore, and Z. Ding, Minimization of region-scalable fitting energy for image segmentation, *IEEE Transactions on Image Processing*, vol. 17, no. 10, pp. 1940–1949, 2008.

17. C. He, Y. Wang, and Q. Chen, Active contours driven by weighted region-scalable fitting energy based on local entropy, *Signal Processing Journal*, vol. 92, pp. 587–600, 2012.

18. U. Javed, M. M. Riaz, A. Ghafoor, and T. A. Cheema, Fuzzy logic and local features based medical image segmentation, in *International Conference on Image Processing*, Melbourne, Australia, pp. 1148–1152, 2013.

19. C. Darolti, A. Mertins, C. Bodensteiner, and U. Hofmann, Local region descriptors for active contours evolution, *IEEE Transactions on Image Processing*, vol. 17, no. 12, pp. 2275–2288, 2008.

20. E. S. L. Gastal and M. M. Oliveira, Domain transformation for edge aware image and video processing, *ACM Transactions on Graphics*, vol. 30, no. 4, pp. 1–12 , 2011.

21. R. Fattal, Edge-avoiding wavelets and their applications, *ACM Transaction on Graphics*, vol. 28, no. 3, pp. 22.1–22.9, 2009.

22. J. Chen, S. Paris, and F. Durand, Real-time edge aware image processing with the bilateral grid, *ACM Transaction on Graphics*, vol. 26, no. 3, pp. 103.1–103.9, 2007.

23. H. Knutsson and C. F Westin, Normalized and differential convolution: Methods for interpolation and filtering of incomplete and uncertain data, *Computer Vision and Pattern Recognition*, pp. 515–523, 1993.

24. R. Piroddi and M. Petrou, Analysis of irregularly sampled data: A review, *Advances in Imaging and Electron Physics*, vol. 132, pp. 109–165, 2004.

25. S.-D. Chen and A. R. Ramli, Preserving brightness in histogram equalization based contrast enhancement techniques, *Digital Signal Processing*, vol. 14, no. 5, pp. 413–428, 2014.

26. S. Poddar, S. Tewary, D. Sharma, V. Karar, A. Ghosh, and S. K. Pal, Non-parametric modified histogram equalisation for contrast enhancement, *IET Image Processing*, vol. 7, no. 7, pp. 641–652, 2013.

27. T. Arici, S. Dikbas, Y. Altunbasak, A histogram modification framework and its application for image contrast enhancement, *IEEE Transactions on Image Processing*, vol. 18, no. 9, pp. 1921–1935, 2009.

28. S. M. Pizer, E. P. Amburn, J. D. Austin, R. Cromartie, A. Geselowitz, T. Greer, B. T. H. Romeny, and J. B. Zimmerman, Adaptive histogram equalization and its variations, *Computer Vision, Graphics, and Image Processing*, vol. 49, no. 3, pp. 355–368, 1987.

29. H. Greenspan, Super-Resolution in Medical Imaging, *The Computer Journal*, vol. 52, no. 1, pp. 43–63, 2009.

30. W. Dong, L. Zhang, G. Shi, and X. Wu, Image deblurring and super-resolution by adaptive sparse domain selection and adaptive regularization, *IEEE Transaction on Image Processing*, vol. 20, no. 7, pp. 1838–1857, 2011.

31. O. S. Al-Kadi and D. Watson, Texture analysis of aggressive and nonaggressive lung tumor CE CT Images, *IEEE Transaction on Biomedical Engineering*, vol. 55, no. 7, pp. 1822–1830, 2008.

32. K. M. Iftekharuddin, W. Jia, and R. Marsh, Fractal analysis of tumor in brain MR images, *Machine Vision and Applications*, vol. 13, pp. 352–362, 2003.

33. K. I. Kilic and R. H. Abiyev, Exploiting the synergy between fractal dimension and lacunarity for improved texture recognition, *Signal Processing*, vol. 91, no. 10, pp. 2332–2344, 2011.

34. R. Yager and D. Filev, *Essentials of Fuzzy Modeling and Control*. New York: Wiley, 1994.

35. T. Takagi and M. Sugeno, Fuzzy identification of systems and its applications to modeling and control, *IEEE Transactions on Systems, Man and Cybernetics*, vol. 15, no. 1, pp. 116–132, 1985.

36. Harvard Medical Atlas Database, http://www.med.harvard.edu/AANLIB/home.html. Accessed January 15, 2015.

37. National Center for Biotechnology Information, http://www.ncbi.nlm.nih.gov/. Accessed January 10, 2015.

chapter nine

Model-based curvilinear network extraction toward quantitative microscopy

Ting Xu, Chao Zhou, and Xiaolei Huang

Contents

Abstract

Curvilinear networks in cells and tissues are routinely imaged by fluorescence microscopy and sometimes optical coherence microscopy
(OCM). Gaining insight into the structural and mechanical properties
of these curvilinear networks and understanding the mechanisms
of their formation require image analysis methods for automated
quantification of massive image datasets. The diversity of these
networks as well as low image quality make reliable extraction challenging. This chapter presents a recent body of work that provides
a complete framework for extracting the geometry and topology of
multidimensional curvilinear networks in microscopy images. The
proposed multiple Stretching Open Active Contours (SOACs) are
automatically initialized and evolve along the network centerlines
synergically: they can merge with others, stop upon collision, and
reconfigure with others to allow smooth continuation across network
junctions. The approach is generally applicable to 2D/3D images of
curvilinear networks with varying signal-to-noise ratio (SNR). Qualitative and quantitative evaluation using simulated and experimental
images demonstrate its effectiveness and potential.

9.1 Introduction

9.1.1 Biological network extraction

Network structures made of filamentous biopolymers or vessels are ubiquitous among biological systems. These curvilinear networks are essential for the lives of cells and tissues.
For instance, actin filaments form dynamic meshworks that organize in structures such
as stress fibers, actin cables, and contractile rings that are of fundamental importance for
the cell [1]. The structure and connectivity of collagen and fibrin networks are crucial to
their mechanical properties in the tissue [2–4]. Angiogenesis, the formation of new blood
vessels from the existing ones, plays an essential role in many physiological conditions
such as wound healing, embryonic development, and granulation formation. Dysregula-
tion of angiogenesis contributes to numerous diseases such as cancer, ischemic disease,
and infectious and immune disorders [5–7].

Biophysicists and cell biologists routinely use static and time-lapse confocal microscopy to image intracellular networks of actin filaments [8,9] and microtubules [10,11] as
well as extracellular polymers such as fibrin [3,12], both in vitro and in live cells or model
organisms. Biological engineers use confocal microscopy and optical coherence microscopy
(OCM) to study angiogenesis, a highly organized morphogenetic process including vessel initiation, formation, branching, maturation, and remodeling [5]. Understanding the
fundamental morphogenetic processes of how cells organize to form new vessels and
determining the function of various angiogenic factors that regulate angiogenesis is
essential for developing novel therapeutic strategies.

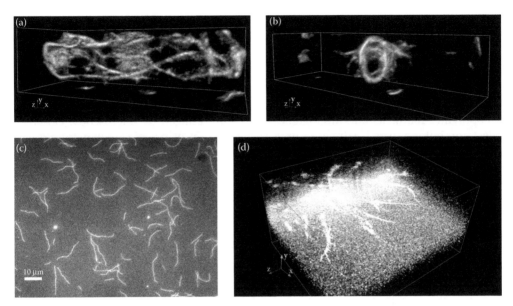

Figure 9.1 Examples of curvilinear networks in 2D and 3D. (a,b) 3D meshworks of actin cables labeled by GFP-CHD in a fission yeast cell (radius is 1.73 μm) [17]. Images were acquired at different times during the cell's life cycle. The cells were treated with CK-666 [20] that disassembled actin patches and allowed clearer images of actin cable structures. (c) Intersecting actin filaments in one frame of a 2D TIRFM time-lapse sequence [15]. (d) An OCM image of vascular network of sprouting vessels rendered by maximum intensity projection [18].

The appearance of curvilinear networks in cells and tissues can be diverse. Figure 9.1a,b shows 3D networks of actin cables imaged by spinning disk confocal microscopy. Actin cables promote polarized cell growth by directing the transport of vesicles towards the growing cell tip. They are highly dynamic, changing their distribution inside the cell within minutes. During mitosis, actin reorganizes and forms a dynamic meshwork in the cell center (Figure 9.1b). This meshwork condenses into a contractile ring whose constriction drives the separation of the cell into two daughters [13,14]. Figure 9.1c shows fluorescently labeled actin filaments imaged by total internal reflection fluorescence microscopy (TIRFM) in a study of actin polymerization in vitro [15]. In this experiment, the filaments grew parallel to a glass slide by polymerization and intersected with each other as they elongated. Figure 9.1d shows a 3D image of angiogenic sprouting vessels acquired on the microengineered blood vessel device [7] and imaged by an ultrahigh-resolution OCM system [16].

To gain insight into the structural, dynamic, and mechanical properties of these biological networks and to understand the mechanisms of their formation, image analysis methods are required to obtain quantitative information from images of these networks. For the purpose of analysis, manual inspection of microscopy images is still often used, which is time-consuming, error-prone, and subjective. To achieve automated quantification of massive datasets, computerized image analysis methods are needed not only to facilitate objective and reproducible analysis but also help quantify and model mesoscale phenomena in cells and tissues, which give insights into their biological functions.

This chapter presents a review of several recently developed image analysis methods [16–19], which are aimed at extracting the centerline geometry of all the filaments or vessels and their connectivity (network topology), for the quantitative study of spatial and physical properties of these networks.

9.1.2 Literature review

This section reviews literature on segmenting curvilinear structures with an emphasis on biopolymer filaments and angiogenic vasculature imaged by microscopy. One of the earliest computer-assisted extraction and reconstruction of protein fiber networks, with human inputs playing a major role, was developed by Baradet et al. [21] who analyzed fibrin networks. Since then, semiautomatic and fully automatic identification of biopolymer networks has become an active research topic.

9.1.2.1 Morphological thinning

One popular category of methods uses morphological skeletonization on binarized images. Wu et al. [22] and Stein et al. [4] reconstructed collagen fiber networks by tracing maximal ridges in the Euclidean distance maps of binarized images. Mickel et al. [23] extracted the skeleton of collagen fiber networks by distance-ordered homotopic thinning using the Chamfer distance map. Herberich et al. [24,25] extracted networks of microtubules and intermediate filaments by binarizing and thinning the image filtered by vessel enhancement filters based on Hessian analysis [26,27]. To remove artifacts caused by binarization, Beil et al. [28] and Lück et al. [29] further pruned the obtained skeletons, eliminating outliers such as open branches or loops. Binarization and skeletonization has also been used to segment and quantify angiogenic vasculature [30,31].

9.1.2.2 Template matching

A more robust way of extracting curvilinear networks is to use template matching [32–35], where prior knowledge about the target is incorporated into a database of 2D or 3D templates. These template-based detection methods are more selective and impose stronger constraints than simple intensity thresholding used in binarization. Another form of template matching is to use Hough/Radon transform to extract linear structures. Sandberg and Brega [36] and Winkler et al. [37] adopted localized Radon transform to extract thin line network of microtubules and actin filaments. In Rusu et al. [38], actin filaments in cryo-ET datasets were segmented by a stochastic template-based search, which combines a genetic algorithm and a bidirectional expansion strategy. However, the method does not resolve the possible template overlap when tracing converging branches and the network junctions are left undetected.

9.1.2.3 Active contour models

Fluorescent microscopy images of polymer fiber networks usually suffer from low signal-to-noise ratio (SNR). Active contour-based methods increase the robustness of segmentation by incorporating prior information about the object shape. Unlike the previous image processing or template matching based methods, open curve parametric active contours (Snakes) [39] explicitly model the linear topology of filaments or vessels, and have been successfully applied to extract centerlines of actin filaments [40–43], microtubules [44–48], and axons [49]. These methods focus on segmenting an individual line structure instead of extracting both geometry and topology of the entire network. Saban and Manjunath [45] used 2D open Snakes to track microtubules but their method does not handle intersection of microtubules. In their method, the extent of elongating or shrinking the Snakes relies on thresholded outputs of a line detector, which may cause over- or under-segmentation in case of large intensity variations in foreground and background regions.

Different from parametric active contours, implicit active contours [50,51] have been used for segmenting the contours of curvilinear structures such as bronchi [52], blood vessels [53], white matter tracts [54], and road networks [55]. While implicit active contours can naturally handle topology changes in the contours, they are more computationally expensive compared to parametric models and are difficult to evolve open curves in the level set framework. One attempt on centerline extraction using implicit active contours is due to Basu et al. [56], who evolved 2D open curves implicitly by deriving the medial axis from the zero level set. It is not clear how this formulation can be extended to higher dimensions. Moreover, as topology change is handled implicitly, additional steps are needed to detect junctions and retrieve topological information.

To more robustly handle corrupted data and anomalies, minimal path approaches [57,58] have also been used to extract the centerlines of curvilinear networks, as these methods can find the global optimal path between two points. These methods are usually interactive, requiring the user to specify the extremities of a line structure before extracting its centerline. For instance, the method from Hadjidemetriou et al. [57] requires manual input of one starting point for each microtubule in 2D. It would be cumbersome to make such methods adapt to 3D segmentation tasks, however, since it would be difficult for the user to specify ending points of filaments in a 3D network, especially when the network is dense. A method that specifies initial seed points automatically was proposed by Sargin et al. [58], but the seed points must not be on a filament gap or intersection.

Other explicit models such as generalized cylinder [59] and super-Gaussian functions [60] are also used to trace and quantify the geometry of curvilinear networks, but the topological information of the network, such as junction locations, is not retrieved.

9.1.3   Outline

The remainder of this chapter is organized as follows. Section 9.2 introduces the multiple Stretching Open Active Contours (SOACs) for 2D/3D network extraction. Section 9.3 demonstrates the power of the multiple SOACs method on various kinds of curvilinear networks arising from cells, tissues, and angiogenesis by experimental results and quantitative evaluation. Discussion and conclusion are presented in Sections 9.4 and 9.5.

9.2   Method

9.2.1   Overview of multiple SOAC methods

The overall strategy is to extract curvilinear networks using a large number of Stretching Open Active Contours (SOACs) [40]. A SOAC is an open curve variant of parametric active contours (snakes) [39] evolving on the centerline of a curvilinear structure by stretching itself until it reaches the extremities of the structure. Unlike previous methods that focus on extracting an individual line structure, the proposed method [17–19] extracts the geometry and topology of the entire network by evolving and configuring a set of SOACs.

Multiple SOACs are first initialized automatically at image intensity ridges and then evolve along the centerlines of line structures. Because of their large quantities, these initial SOACs can extract the entire network but may be redundant. The proposed mechanisms can eliminate any duplicate extraction by allowing SOACs to merge, stop at junctions, and transform into closed curve forms. After all SOACs are converged, network junctions are detected by clustering nearby meeting points (referred to as "T-junctions") of different SOACs. A physical network topology is enforced by maintaining the smoothness of SOACs across detected network junctions by dissecting and reconnecting them at each junction.

The output of the above framework includes multiple SOACs, each representing an extracted filament or vessel in the curvilinear network. The distributions of orientation and curvature of line structures can be computed from the densely sampled points of SOACs. The branch intensities can be estimated by the image intensity along the curve. Furthermore, information on network topology, including locations of all network junctions and the connectivity among branches, can also be retrieved.

9.2.2   Stretching open active contours

A SOAC is an open parametric curve $r(s)$ in $\mathbb{R}^n$ with stretching forces applied at its two tips, where $s \in [0, L]$ is the arc-length parameter and L is its total length. A contour energy functional $\mathcal{E}(r) = \mathcal{E}_{int}(r) + \mathcal{E}_{ext}(r)$ is defined for it, where $\mathcal{E}_{int}(r)$ and $\mathcal{E}_{ext}(r)$ are the internal and external energy functional, respectively. Minimizing $\mathcal{E}_{int}(r)$ maintains the continuity and smoothness of the curve; minimizing $\mathcal{E}_{ext}(r)$ elongates and pushes the curve towards salient image features such as edges or intensity ridges. $\mathcal{E}_{int}(r)$ is defined as

$$\mathcal{E}_{int}(r) = \int_0^L \alpha(s) \left| r'(s) \right|^2 + \beta(s) \left| r''(s) \right|^2 ds, \qquad (9.1)$$

where $\alpha(s)$ and $\beta(s)$ are weights for curve tension and rigidity at length s, respectively. The external energy functional $\mathcal{E}_{ext}(r)$ is a weighted combination of an image potential energy function $E_{img}(x)$ and a stretching energy function $E_{str}(r)$,[*]

$$\mathcal{E}_{ext}(r) = \int_0^L k_{img} E_{img}(r(s)) + k_{str} E_{str}(r(s)) \, ds, \qquad (9.2)$$

where k_{img} and k_{str} are respective weights. The image potential energy function $E_{img}(x)$ is the Gaussian-smoothed input image $E_{img}(x) = I(x) * G_\sigma(x)$, where $I(x)$ is the input image and $G_\sigma(x)$ is the Gaussian kernel with standard deviation σ. Thus the image force exerted on the SOAC is the gradient field, which points toward the intensity ridges.

$$\nabla E_{img}(x) = \nabla (I * G_\sigma)(x) = (I * \nabla G_\sigma)(x). \qquad (9.3)$$

The tangential stretching force $F(r(s))$ exerted at tips ($s = 0, L$) elongates the SOAC:

$$F(r(s)) = \begin{cases} -F(r(s)) \frac{r'(s)}{|r'(s)|}, & s = 0, \\ F(r(s)) \frac{r'(s)}{|r'(s)|}, & s = L, \\ 0, & 0 < s < L \end{cases} \qquad (9.4)$$

where $F(r(s))$ is the magnitude of the stretching force. It is made adaptive to local image appearance to address the problem of over- or underextraction in the presence of intensity

---

[*] Strictly speaking, the tangential stretching force cannot be derived as the gradient of potential energy function like $E_{str}(r)$ [61]. It is used loosely here for the formulation of energy functional minimization.

variations (Section 9.2.3). Combining the image and stretching forces, the overall external force field exerted on $r(s)$ is

$$\nabla \mathcal{E}_{ext}(r(s)) = k_{img} \cdot (I * \nabla G_\sigma)(r(s)) + k_{str} \cdot F(r(s)) \tag{9.5}$$

Overall, minimizing the contour energy $\mathcal{E}(r)$ makes SOACs grow along the intensity ridges until the internal and external forces balance out and reach an equilibrium. Solving this optimization problem numerically requires discretized SOACs. A SOAC can be represented as a linearly ordered sequence of l points: $r = \{(x_{i,0}, x_{i,1})\}$ for 2D and $r = \{(x_{i,0}, x_{i,1}, x_{i,2})\}$ for 3D, $i = 0, \ldots, l-1$, with a uniform spacing $\delta = L/l$. Let $X_k = (x_{0,k}, \ldots, x_{i,k}, \ldots, x_{l-1,k})^T$, $k = 0, 1$ for 2D and $k = 0, 1, 2$ for 3D, be the vector containing all the kth-dimension coordinates of SOAC points, X_k^t at iteration t can be computed iteratively after deriving the Euler–Lagrange equation [39],

$$X_k^t = (A + \gamma I)^{-1}(\gamma X_k^{t-1} - \partial \mathcal{E}_{ext}(X_0^{t-1}, X_1^{t-1})/\partial x_k), \quad \text{(2D)} \tag{9.6}$$

$$X_k^t = (A + \gamma I)^{-1}(\gamma X_k^{t-1} - \partial \mathcal{E}_{ext}(X_0^{t-1}, X_1^{t-1}, X_2^{t-1})/\partial x_k), \quad \text{(3D)} \tag{9.7}$$

where A is the pentadiagonal banded matrix containing the internal continuity and smoothness constraints defined by Equation 9.1. The openness of SOACs requires $\alpha(0) = \alpha(L) = \beta(0) = \beta(L) = 0$ to introduce position and tangent discontinuity at two tips. I is the identity matrix, and γ is the viscosity coefficient that controls the step size for the dynamic evolution of the curve [39]. The larger γ is, the smaller the step size will be. All SOACs are resampled to maintain the point spacing δ after each iteration. A SOAC is considered to be converged if every point changes its position for less than 0.05 voxels after 100 iterations.

9.2.3 Adaptive tangential stretching force

To address over and undersegmentation caused by variations in foreground and background intensity, the magnitude of stretching force, $F(r(s))$ in Equation 9.4, needs to be adaptive. It is defined to be the normalized local image contrast around the tip:

$$F(r(s)) = \frac{I(r(s)) - I_{lb}(r(s))}{I(r(s))} = 1 - \frac{I_{lb}(r(s))}{I(r(s))}, \qquad s = 0, L \tag{9.8}$$

where $I(r(s)|_{s=0,L})$ is the image intensity at a SOAC tip and $I_{lb}(r(s)|_{s=0,L})$ is the local background intensity around it.

An effective way to estimate $I_{lb}(r(s)|_{s=0,L})$ is to sample local intensities around a tip on a set of perpendicular concentric circles of radii between R_{near} and R_{far} and then compute their average, as shown in Figure 9.2 for the 3D case. Sample points are located on a plane that passes through the tip and has its normal as the tip tangent.

The above local contrast estimation makes the SOAC's stretching force adaptable to the local appearance of the line structure: the higher the contrast, the more SOAC will stretch itself. This can avoid undersegmentation in dim backgrounds or oversegmentation in bright backgrounds, as in previous methods that rely on a global intensity contrast [19,40,43].

To account for the anisotropic resolution of confocal microscopy along the z direction, the z coordinates of the local samples are scaled by a fixed value (usually around 3). As a result, the local sampling region can be a concentric circle or an ellipse depending on the orientation of the tangent at a SOAC's tip (Figure 9.3).

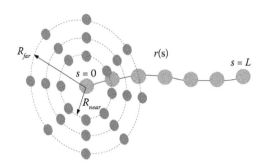

Figure 9.2 Estimation of local background around a SOAC's tip [17]. Red points are local background samples, all located on the plane perpendicular to the tangent at the SOAC tip ($r(0)$ here) and delimited by radii R_{near} and R_{far}. The angle step size is $\pi/4$.

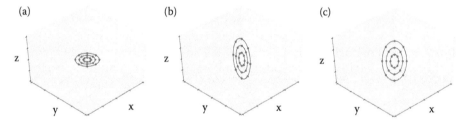

Figure 9.3 Local background sampling regions for different tips with different tangent orientations. (a) Sampling regions are circular when the tip tangent aligns with the z-axis. (b,c) Sampling regions are elliptical in all other cases. (b) Tip tangent is $(1,0,0)^T$. (c) Tip tangent is $(1,1,1)^T$.

9.2.4   *Automatic initialization of multiple SOACs*

Since a large number of SOACs are employed to extract the network, manual initialization is not an option, especially in 3D. SOACs are automatically initialized on intensity "ridge points," obtained by scanning the Gaussian smoothed image gradient. Vessel enhancement filters such as Hessian analysis [26] and optimally oriented flux [62] assume the cross-section of a 3D curvilinear structure is circular. Detecting ridge points based on these filter outputs may lead to many false-negatives because of the shape irregularity of the cross-section of many biopolymer filaments imaged by confocal microscopy.

9.2.4.1   *Ridge point detection*

Without loss of generality, the foreground intensity is assumed to be higher than background intensity. The ridge point detection algorithm is based on this observation: In 2D, a point on the centerline of a line structure is a local intensity maximum along at least one axis direction; in 3D, the centerline point is local intensity maxima along at least two axis directions. Thus, a ridge point x can be detected by searching for the plus-to-minus sign change in the spatial derivatives of image $\widetilde{I}(x)$, obtained after convolving input image $I(x)$ with a Gaussian kernel of standard deviation σ [63]. Let $\partial_k \widetilde{I}(x) = \frac{\partial(G_\sigma(x)*I(x))}{\partial x_k}$ denote the

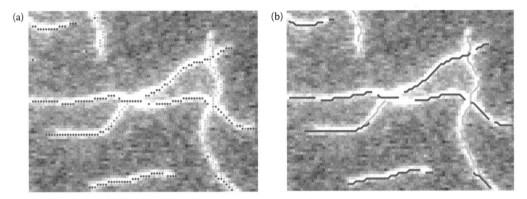

Figure 9.4 Ridge points and initialized SOACs in a 2D TIRFM image (Figure 9.1c) [19]. (a) Ridge points detected along x (green), y (blue), and both (red) directions. (b) SOACs along x (blue) and y (green) are initialized from ridge points in y and x directions, respectively.

image derivative along the kth axis direction. x is a ridge point in that direction if

$$\exists m > 0 : \begin{cases} \partial_k \tilde{I}(\ldots, x_k - \lfloor m/2 \rfloor, \ldots) > \tau \\ \partial_k \tilde{I}(\ldots, x_k + \lceil m/2 \rceil, \ldots) < -\tau \\ |\partial_k \tilde{I}(\ldots, x_k + l, \ldots)| < \tau, \forall l \in (-\lfloor m/2 \rfloor, \lceil m/2 \rceil) \end{cases} \qquad (9.9)$$

where ridge threshold $\tau > 0$ is the minimum change of intensity to trigger the detection of a ridge point. Here m, l are integers and $m > 0$. Along the kth axis direction, this defines the middle point on a ridge of m pixels wide: the first two conditions requires that the intensity slope must change from positive to negative (to ensure a ridge not a valley) and that the intensity difference be significant enough; the third condition states there should be no slope greater or equal to τ in between, requiring the intensity across the ridge (or plateau) is relatively uniform. Figure 9.4a and the second row of Figure 9.5 show detected ridge points in a 2D TIRFM image and a 3D confocal microscopy image, respectively.

9.2.4.2 Selecting and linking ridge points into initial SOACs

Ridge points, detected along various axis directions, are then linked up into initial SOACs. Since the orientation of line structures is unknown, SOACs are initialized along axis directions. To link ridge points into a SOAC along a particular axis direction, a subset of them are used. In 2D, SOACs along x are linked by ridge points detected along y, and *vice versa* (Figure 9.4b). In 3D, a SOAC along x is linked by ridge points in both of the other two axis directions, namely, y and z. Similarly, a SOAC along y is linked by ridge points in both x and z, and a SOAC along z is linked by ridge points in both x and y. The third row of Figure 9.5 shows selected ridge points for initializing SOACs along different axis directions in 3D.

Selected ridge points for a particular axis direction are then linked in the ascending coordinate in that axis. To start tracing an initial SOAC along an axis direction k, we first find an unused selected ridge point $x = (\ldots, x_k, \ldots)$ that has the smallest kth coordinate. Then we repeatedly add a new point that has the kth coordinate incremented by 1, $x' = (\ldots, x_k + 1, \ldots)$, and is 8-connected (2D) or 26-connected (3D) to x, until no such unused selected point can be found. Figure 9.4b and the fourth row of Figure 9.5 demonstrate the result of tracing initial SOACs along all axis directions.

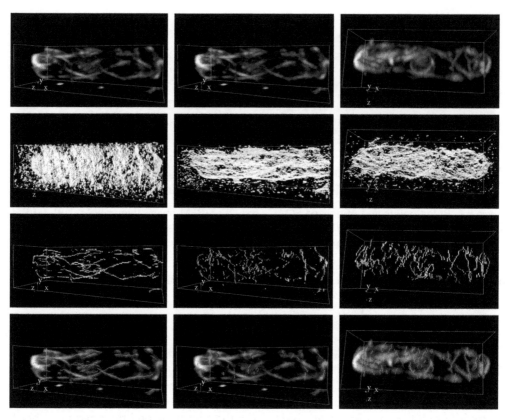

Figure 9.5 3D SOAC initialization on the image in Figure 9.1a [17]. Image intensity is normalized to [0, 1] followed by Gaussian smoothing with $\sigma = 1.0$. First row: Input image with the first two share the same view while the third one is different. Second row: Detected ridge points ($\tau = 0.003$). Third row: Selected ridge points for initialization along each axis direction. Fourth row: Initialized SOACs using corresponding selected ridge points. Columns from left to right correspond to initialization along x-, y-, and z-axis directions, respectively. All images are rendered by Maximum Intensity Projection.

After the points on a SOAC are determined, we resample the SOAC with uniform spacing δ. The initial SOACs may be redundant but they will be regulated to generate a concise and clear representation of the network structure after their subsequent evolution.

9.2.5   *Sequential evolution of multiple SOACs*

Initialized SOACs will evolve until convergence, one after another, in a sequential manner. A set of evolution regulation mechanisms keep a SOAC free of overlap with others and itself.

A brute-force strategy to detect overlap involves calculating the Euclidean distance from each point of an evolving SOAC to all converged SOACs: if its distance to a converged SOAC is small enough, an overlap is detected. If this is done after each iteration, it would be too expensive and would dramatically slow down the evolution process. If, otherwise, overlap is checked after all the SOACs have converged, then a lot of computation time would be wasted when SOACs extend onto structures that have already been extracted.

To detect overlaps efficiently, a balanced strategy is adopted. SOAC overlaps can be categorized into two types: tip overlap and body overlap. The former is an overlapping portion that starts from the SOAC's tip, and is usually introduced by SOAC elongation. The second type of overlap is the one that does not include any SOAC tips, and is usually caused by multiple SOACs' body drifting across weak boundaries toward the same bright intensity ridge. For the sake of efficiency, tip overlaps are detected and eliminated after each SOAC's iteration in order to timely avoid aforementioned duplicate extraction. Meanwhile, as each tip can overlap with at most one converged SOAC, most of the time only two tips need to be checked. Body overlaps are more expensive to detect since every point on a SOAC will need to be checked; therefore checks for this type of overlap are only done once after a newly converged SOAC is obtained.

To facilitate a detailed discussion on detecting both types of overlap, let $r_{ev}(s), s \in [0, L_{ev}]$ denote the current evolving SOAC, where L_{ev} is its total length. r_{ev} is checked against each one of converged SOACs, denoted by $r_j(s), s \in [0, L_j]$, for overlap.

9.2.5.1 Checks for tip overlap and self-intersection

After each iteration of evolution of r_{ev}, following Equation 9.6, the Euclidean distances from the two tips of r_{ev} to r_j are computed; if the distances are greater than a threshold d_e, no overlap between r_{ev} and r_j is detected, otherwise, the first point of r_{ev} (starting from a tip) with a distance to r_j greater than the threshold d_e is identified (P in Figure 9.6).

It is possible that the other tip of r_{ev} is reached before P is found; this means that all points of r_{ev} overlap with r_j, thus r_{ev} is deleted. If P is found before reaching the other tip (as the case in Figure 9.6), the overlapping part on r_{ev}, starting from the overlapping tip to the first nonoverlapping point P, is deleted. The closest point on r_j to P, denoted by Q, is assigned as the new tip for r_{ev}, forming a "T-junction" at Q.

Once a T-junction is formed, the stretching force at that tip is set to zero, and the tip is pinned down from stretching further. The connectivity at this T-junction is also recorded for subsequent network reconfiguration. It is possible that the network junction is actually a cross junction where two line structures intersect. Although not allowing the evolving SOAC to stretch across the junction, it is expected that if the line structure continues across the junction, the remaining part will be extracted by another SOAC that is initialized on that part of the branch. The topology will be fixed in the subsequent network reconfiguration stage.

To detect loopy structures in a network (Figure 9.1b) and avoid infinite elongation of SOACs on them, self-intersection is checked after each iteration. Specifically, a SOAC

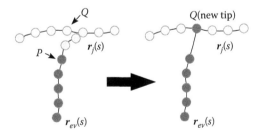

Figure 9.6 Tip overlap check after each SOAC iteration [17]. (Left) The tip overlap (yellow) of an evolving SOAC r_{ev} with a converged SOAC r_j. P is the first nonoverlap point on r_{ev}. Q is the point of r_j that is the closest to P. (Right) Deletion of the overlapping part, and making Q the new tip for r_{ev}, which will be resampled (not shown). Q is recorded as a "T-junction."

self-intersects if there are two SOAC points on the curve that are sufficiently apart along the curve length but are spatially very close, that is, $\|r_{ev}(s_1) - r_{ev}(s_2)\| < d_e$ and $|s_1 - s_2| > \kappa$ where κ is a threshold typically set to be one-tenth of the curve length L_{ev}. If so, r_{ev} is divided into three sub-SOACs, which correspond to the parts of $r_{ev}(s)$ with $s \in [0, s_1]$, $s \in [s_1, s_2], s \in [s_2, L_{ev}]$, respectively. The second sub-SOAC will reevolve as a closed curve, followed by other two sub-SOACs.

9.2.5.2 Checks for body overlap
After convergence of the current SOAC r_{ev}, body overlap with any other converged SOACs is checked. This is the second type of overlap, which features an overlapping part that does not include any tip of r_{ev}, and so would not have been detected during the SOAC's evolution. If an overlap is detected in the middle of r_{ev}'s body (i.e., no tips included), r_{ev} is dissected into several sub-SOACs; any sub-SOAC that overlaps with another SOAC will be discarded, and any remaining nonoverlapping sub-SOACs will be treated as new independent SOACs and will evolve again on their own and allowed to form new T-junctions. As discussed above, this postconvergence body overlap check is necessary in that the body of a SOAC may drift away from the original intensity ridge that initialized the SOAC. This happens when the SOAC was initialized on some faint line structures with weak edges but drifted toward other brighter ones nearby during its evolution.

9.2.6 Reconfiguration of network topology
The result of sequential evolution is a network of SOACs connected with one another at "T-junctions" (vertices of order 3) or else have an unconnected end corresponding to a dangling line structure tip, as illustrated in Figure 9.7b. The T-junctions would capture actin cytoskeletal networks that consist of branches off of mother filaments, such as those formed by the Arp2/3 complex [1]. Actin networks may also contain crosses (vertices of order 4) when two filaments are linked by a cross-linker [64,65]. Actin bundles may also form star shapes (vertices of order 5 and higher) [66]. While vertices of order higher than 3 are not addressed during evolution, the extracted filaments are subsequently reconfigured by joining nearby T-junctions into a network junction. Meanwhile, the main filament and branches are reassigned based on the "smoothness constraint": junctions in cytoskeletal filament networks typically involve straight fibers crossing one another or side branches forming off straight filaments.

This reconfiguration process corrects the topology of converged SOAC network. The network of converged SOACs may not be topologically correct for three reasons. First, the sequential evolution is designed to form T- or corner-junctions only, without any cross junctions or even higher-order junctions. Second, because SOACs evolve one after another, those SOACs that evolve first have a better chance to extend along multiple branches. When they elongate across intersections of branches, artificial corners may occur. For example, suppose there is a "T"-shape network composed of a horizontal line structure and a vertical branch. If the first SOAC to evolve is initialized on the lower branch of "T," it may continue to grow onto one of the horizontal branches and exhibit an nonphysical corner around the junction. Lastly, artificial "sharp turns" can also be introduced by the influence of strong external force field such as a very bright nearby branch.

To retrieve a topologically correct network, converged SOACs are cut at each T-junction into "SOAC segments" using the recorded connectivity information (Figure 9.7c). SOAC segments of length less than a threshold d_g are discarded. Next an undirected graph $G = (V, E)$ is constructed, where V is the set of end points of SOAC segments. For any two

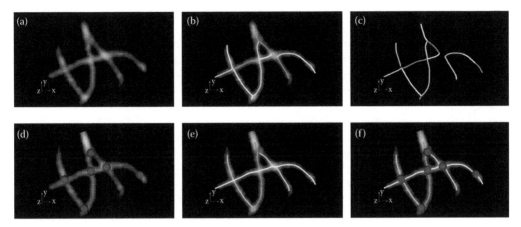

Figure 9.7 Network reconfiguration on a 3D simulated image rendered by maximum intensity projection [17]. (a) One part of the 3D image. (b) Converged SOACs. Different colors indicate different SOACs. (c) Dissect converged SOACs into segments (shown in different colors) at each T-junction. (d) Cluster nearby T-junctions into a single higher-degree junction (blue spheres). Note the rightmost junction is not a false-positive as there is a branch perpendicular to this image plane (not shown). (e) New SOACs formed by reconfiguration and linking of grouped segments. (f) Reconfigured SOACs and detected junctions.

vertices, $u, v \in V$, an edge $(u, v) \in E$ if $\|u - v\|_2 < d_g$. Then connected components analysis is performed on G to detect clusters of vertices, where each cluster represents a network junction (Figure 9.7d).

The smoothness between a pair of end points is defined as the angle between the tangential vectors of SOAC segments at the two end points. For each network junction, the smoothest pair of end points is greedily linked up across the junction, until all pairs are linked or the angle between current smoothest pair is less than a threshold θ. All the SOAC segments that are linked up become one longer SOAC (Figure 9.7e). The linked SOACs then evolve with their tip fixed to remove kinks that resulted from cutting and linking. Finally the detected network junctions are pruned by deleting the one that has only one SOAC crossing it. Figure 9.7f shows an example of the reconfigured SOACs and detected network junctions.

9.3   Validation and applications

The Multiple SOACs method is validated using various kinds of simulated and experimental images, including 2D TIRFM Images of actin filaments, 3D spinning disk confocal microscopy images of actin cable meshwork in fission yeast, and 3D optical coherence microscopy (OCM) images of angiogenic sprouting vessels. The method is implemented in C++, with support functions from the Insight Toolkit (ITK),[*] Visualization Toolkit (VTK)[†] and Qt.[‡] The experiments were carried out on a PC workstation with Intel Xeon 3.00 GHz and 4Gb memory. Please see the project website http://www.cse.lehigh.edu/~idealab/soax/ for the source code and build instructions.

[*] www.itk.org. ITK is used for routine image processing.
[†] www.vtk.org. VTK is used for 3D visualization and user interaction.
[‡] www.qt-project.org. Qt is used for building the user interface.

9.3.1   Tests on simulated images

The goal of testing on simulated images is to quantitatively evaluate the accuracy and robustness of the proposed method. Two types of images are synthetically generated: one is to mimic confocal microscopy images of fission yeast actin meshworks labeled by GFP-CHD, and the other is to mimic OCM images of networks of angiogenic sprouting vessels.

9.3.1.1   Generation of simulated images of actin meshwork

Thirteen confocal microscopy images with their corresponding manual segmentation results are collected, nines of which are images of actin cable meshworks and the rest contain actin contractile ring structures. The manual segmentation was obtained by a semiautomatic tool [43]. The manual segmentation results also serve as ground truth when evaluating results on real experimental images. These results, like SOACs, are represented as open curves consisting of sequences of points.

From the manual segmentation results, 14 images with different levels of Gaussian noise are generated for each real experimental image, making a test bed of $13 \times 14 = 182$ images (see Figure 9.9 for four sample images). Let the real experimental image and the simulated image denoted by $I_r(x)$ and $I_s(x)$, respectively. $I_s(x)$ is computed as

$$I_s(x) = (W(x) \cdot I_r(x) - \mu_b) * G_{psf}(x) + N(x) \tag{9.10}$$

where $\mu_b \approx 230$ is the estimated mean background intensity of the experimental images. $G_{psf}(x)$ is an anisotropic point spread function of the imaging system, simulated by a Gaussian kernel with $\sigma_{psf} = (1.5, 1.5, 4.32)^T$; $N(x)$ is the additive Gaussian noise with μ_b and $\sigma_b = 2, 4, 6, \ldots, 26, 28$. $W(x)$ is a window function

$$W(x) = \begin{cases} 1, & \text{if } x \in R_{gt} \\ 0, & \text{otherwise} \end{cases} \tag{9.11}$$

with R_{gt} being the point set of ground truth curves.

The SNR of simulated images is defined as

$$\text{SNR} = \frac{E(I_s(x)|_{|x-R_{gt}|<2\sigma_{psf}} - \mu_b)}{\sigma_b} \tag{9.12}$$

where the foreground voxels are those within $2\sigma_{psf}$ to the ground truth centerlines.

9.3.1.2   Generation of simulated images of angiogenic sprouting vessels

Similar to the generation of simulated images of actin meshwork, extraction results on real OCM images are used as the skeleton of simulated vessels, which are then diffused by an isotropic Gaussian kernel $G_{psf}(x)$ with $\sigma_{psf} = (3.0, 3.0, 3.0)^T$. The intensity is then rescaled back to $[0, 255]$. Finally, the resultant image is corrupted by a multiplicative speckle noise. The 8-bit simulated image $I_s(x)$ is computed as

$$I_s(x) = ((aW(x) \cdot I_r(x) + b) * G_{psf}(x)) \cdot Y \tag{9.13}$$

where $W(x)$ and $I_r(x)$ are defined as before. The scale and shift factor a and b are used for scaling up the intensity and generating a constant background. $Y \sim \Gamma(\frac{1}{\sigma_\Gamma^2}, \sigma_\Gamma^2)$ is a random variable of Gamma distribution. Setting $a = 10, b = \{0, 1, \ldots, 9\}, \sigma_\Gamma = 0.5, 1$ gives 20 simulated images of different degradation quantified by the peak signal-to-noise ratio (PSNR) between I_s and the clean image.

9.3.1.3   Tests for extraction accuracy

The extraction accuracy is measured by the mean and maximum disparity between the resultant SOAC point sets R_c and ground truth point sets R_{gt}. The mean distance measure d_V, referred as "vertex error," is the average distance between points of the result and their closest points on the ground truth:

$$d_V(R_c, R_{gt}) = \frac{1}{2|R_c|} \sum_{x_c \in R_c} \min_{x_{gt} \in R_{gt}} \|x_c - x_{gt}\| + \frac{1}{2|R_{gt}|} \sum_{x_{gt} \in R_{gt}} \min_{x_c \in R_c} \|x_{gt} - x_c\| \qquad (9.14)$$

similar to the "error per face" in Narayanaswamy et al. [67]. The max distance measure d_H is the Hausdorff distance between R_c and R_{gt},

$$d_H(R_c, R_{gt}) = \max\{\max_{x_c \in R_c} \min_{x_{gt} \in R_{gt}} \|x_c - x_{gt}\|, \max_{x_{gt} \in R_{gt}} \min_{x_c \in R_c} \|x_{gt} - x_c\|\} \qquad (9.15)$$

where x_c and x_{gt} are SOAC point in the set of R_c and R_{gt}, respectively.

The mean and standard deviation of d_V and d_H against image SNR are plotted in Figure 9.8. The method performs well even on very noisy images; the vertex error is around one voxel when the SNR is greater than 4. The Hausdorff distances between the result and ground truth are around 10 voxels when the SNR is greater than 5. The increase in false-positives and false-negatives becomes an issue when SNR is less than 4. The estimated SNR values for real experimental images in the experiments range from 4.85 to 6.52, with a mean of 5.72. Some sample extraction results are shown in Figure 9.9, obtained using the same parameter settings (Table 9.1).

For simulated images of angiogenic sprouting vessels, the d_V-PSNR and d_H-PSNR curves for these 20 images are plotted in Figure 9.10, which shows the extraction error (in terms of vertex error and Hausdorff distances) is very low on images with PSNR greater than 25 dB. An example result for one of the simulated images is shown in Figure 9.11.

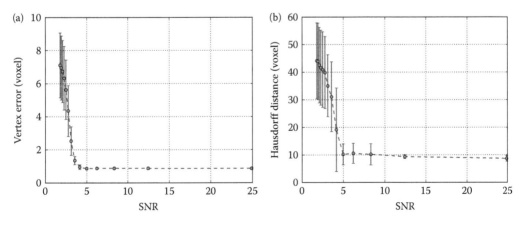

Figure 9.8 Statistics of vertex error (a) and Hausdorff distance (b) versus image signal-to-noise ratio (SNR) for experiments on 182 simulated images [17].

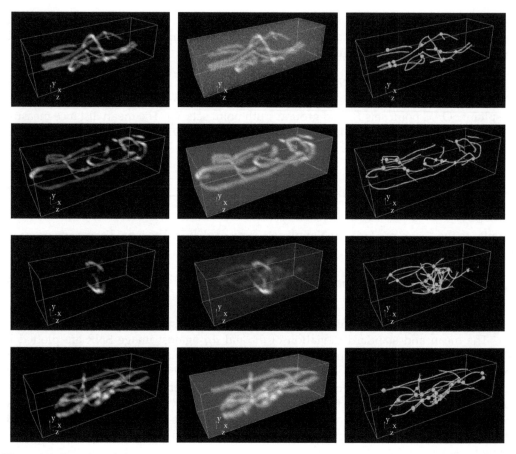

Figure 9.9 Samples of clean image, noisy image, and resultant SOACs extracted from noisy image overlaid with ground truth SOACs [17]. Left column: Clean images. Middle column: Noisy images (Gaussian noise $\sigma_b = 12$). Right column: Resultant SOACs (translucent purple) overlaid with ground truth (light yellow), linked by network junctions (green spheres). Images are rendered by maximum intensity projection.

Table 9.1 Parameters for SOAC initialization and evolution used in experiments on simulated images

γ	α	β	k_{img}	k_{str}	σ	τ	d_e	θ	R_{near}	R_{far}	d_g
2	0.01	0.1	1	0.5	1	0.005	2.0	$2\pi/3$	3	6	4

Note: The intensities of all images are scaled to be in the range $[0, 1]$.

Comparing the three results in Figure 9.12 shows that the number of false-positives drastically decreases as PSNR increases.

9.3.1.4 *Tests for rotational sensitivity*

To test how sensitive Multiple SOACs method is to image rotation, the set of 182 simulated images of actin meshworks are rotated by 45 degrees around z-axis. Results on rotated images are compared against the rotated SOACs extracted from the un-rotated images.

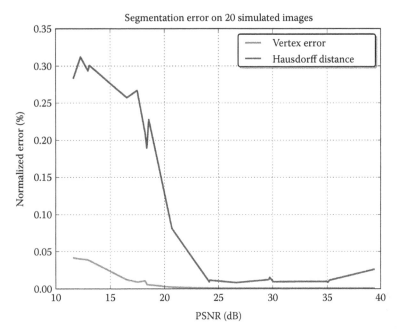

Figure 9.10 d_V-PSNR and d_H-PSNR curve [18]. The error is in a fraction of the length of the diagonal of the image volume.

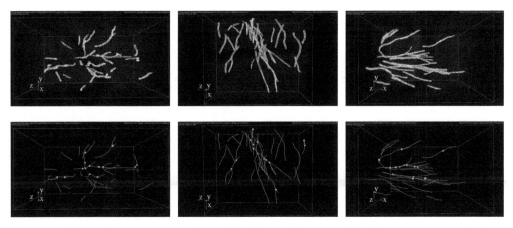

Figure 9.11 Three orthogonal views of a simulated image (upper row) and its extraction result shown in same view (lower row). SOACs (magenta) are shown with the detected junction points (green) [18].

As shown in Figure 9.13, the disparity measured by vertex error between results on rotated simulated images and rotated results on original simulated images is about 0.5 voxels when the SNR is greater than 5, and Hausdorff distance is below 10 voxels. Rotational sensitivity increases when the SNR is less than 5. When the SNR drops even further, both measurements first drastically increase and then decrease. The decrease is because both results have a large number of false positive points that are close by, when the SNR gets very low.

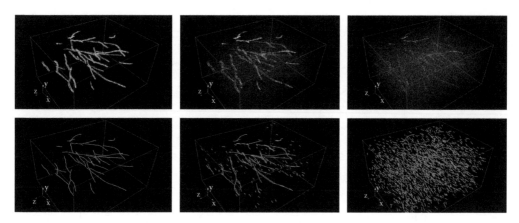

Figure 9.12 Comparison of results on images with different PSNR values [18]. First column: PSNR = 26.6 dB (image same as in Figure 9.11). Second column: PSNR = 16.5 dB. Third column: PSNR = 12.3 dB. Note the different number of false-positives introduced.

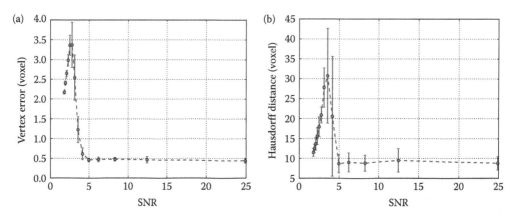

Figure 9.13 Disparities between results on rotated simulated images and rotated results on original simulated images versus SNR [17]. (a) Vertex error. (b) Hausdorff distance.

9.3.2   *Tests on 2D TIRMF images of actin filaments*

TIRFM image sequences from Fujiwara et al. [15] is used for 2D validation. In the experiment, polymerization of muscle Mg-ADP-actin is monitored in the presence of inorganic phosphate (Pi) and actin monomers. The pixel size is 0.17 μm. The last frame of a sequence is used because of more filaments and intersections are present than in previous frames. Its nonuniform illumination makes a global magnitude of stretching force inappropriate.

Approximately, 55 filaments are selected from the frame for evaluation. For each filament, a SOAC generated by Smith et al. [43] and subsequently modified by a human expert serves as the ground truth. The body distance d_b between resultant SOAC r_c and the corresponding ground truth curve r_{gt} is defined as

$$d_b(r_c, r_{gt}) = \max_{x_c \in r_c} \min_{x_{gt} \in r_{gt}} \|x_c - x_{gt}\|_2 \tag{9.16}$$

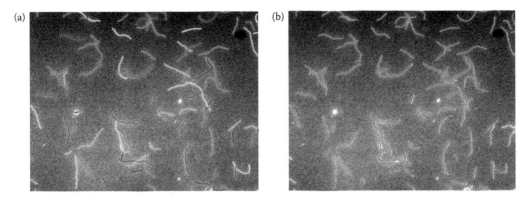

Figure 9.14 Extraction of actin filaments on a 2D TIRFM image (Figure 9.1c) [19]. (a) Resultant SOACs. (b) Ground truth curves.

Table 9.2 Body and tip extraction error statistics of 55 filaments (unit: pixel)

	Mean	Maximum	Standard deviation
Body	2.7312	8.3775	2.0266
Tip1	2.3645	11.2704	2.2668
Tip2	2.1377	8.3775	1.7210

where x_c and x_{gt} are SOAC points of r_c and r_{gt}, respectively. The Euclidean distances between tips of resultant SOACs and ground truth are also computed. Figure 9.14a shows the extraction results, compared with the ground truth (Figure 9.14b). Table 9.2 shows the extraction error statistics.

9.3.3 Tests on spinning disk confocal microscopy images

To evaluate the performance on real images, the proposed method is tested on experimental images of fission yeast cells expressing fluorescent protein GFP-CHD that attaches to the sides of actin filaments.[*] These cell images acquired by spinning disk confocal microscopy show actin cables in nondividing cells (Figure 9.1a), actin contractile rings and medial actin cables in dividing cells (Figure 9.1b). The voxel spacing is 0.0694 μm in the x and y directions and 0.2 μm in the z direction. The images were first interpolated using the sinc function with Lanczos window to make the voxel spacing equal to 0.0694 μm in all directions.

Figure 9.15 shows results on extracting 3D networks of actin cables. The parameter settings are shown in Table 9.3. Since it is still an open question how to get reliable ground truth for these types of real experimental images, qualitative evaluation is performed first by visually inspecting the results against the image and counting the number of false-negatives and false-positives, for four different experimental images (left column of Figure 9.15). If a filament in an image is not extracted by any SOAC, then it counts as a false-negative; if a SOAC does not appear to extract any filament, then it counts as a

---

[*] The images were provided by I-Ju Lee and Jian-Qiu Wu at the Ohio State University.

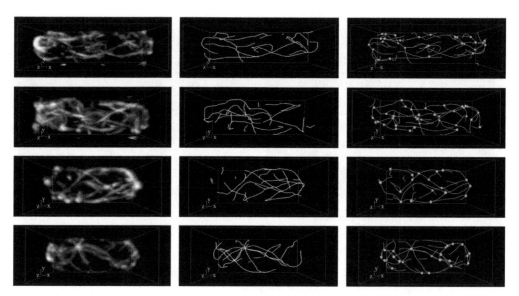

Figure 9.15 Results on confocal microscopy images of actin cables in yeast cells [17]. Left column: Four experimental images rendered by maximum intensity projection along z direction. Middle column: Manual segmentation with the semiautomatic tool in Smith et al. [43]. Right column: Resultant SOACs with junctions (green spheres).

Table 9.3 Parameters for SOAC initialization and evolution used in experiments on confocal microscopy images

γ	α	β	k_{img}	k_{str}	σ	τ	d_e	θ	R_{near}	R_{far}	d_e
2	0.01	0.4	1	0.7	0.5	0.01	1.0	$2\pi/3$	3	6	4

Note: The intensities of all images are scaled to be in the range $[0, 1]$.

Table 9.4 Number of false-negatives (FN) and false-positives (FP) counted by inspecting the results (right column in Figure 9.15) against the image (left column in Figure 9.15). The total number of resultant SOACs for each image is shown in the fourth column (# SOACs). The percentage of (FP + FN) is shown in the last column

Image no.	FP	FN	# SOACs	%(FP + FN)
1	6	4	41	24.4
2	4	2	34	17.6
3	2	4	22	27.3
4	1	2	26	11.5

false-positive. The number and the percentage of false-positives and false-negatives against the total number of SOACs are shown in Table 9.4.

For quantitative evaluation on the extraction accuracy, the resultant SOACs are compared against manual extraction using vertex error and Hausdorff distance. Manual extractions were obtained by asking an expert to use the semiautomatic tool [43] to manually delineate actin cables that he can identify. Despite the effort, the manual segmentation is often incomplete, missing some cables that are near cell boundary or have faint intensity.

Table 9.5 Vertex error and Hausdorff distance between
automated results and manual segmentation results on four
different experimental images

Image no.	Vertex error	Hausdorff distance
1	2.607	29.240
2	2.193	18.170
3	2.019	18.147
4	2.501	19.053

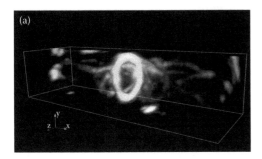 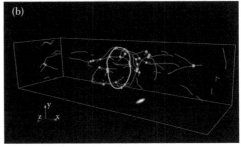

Figure 9.16 Result on confocal microscopy images of dividing fission yeast cells that assemble a contractile actin ring [17]. (a) Image rendered by maximum intensity projection. (b) Extraction result. The closed-form SOAC capturing the ring is highlighted.

In comparison, the proposed method can extract some cables that are present in the image but are missed by a human. For quantitative comparison, all SOACs that have corresponding manually extracted curves are selected. The vertex error and Hausdorff distance between the resultant SOACs and the manual curve counterparts are calculated in Table 9.5.

Figure 9.16 shows the result on an image of dividing yeast cells that assemble a contractile actin ring. Owing to the mechanism for self-intersection detection (Section 9.2.5.1), a closed-form SOAC (highlighted in Figure 9.16b) is formed to capture the ring structure in the center of the cell. In other scenarios, a closed-form SOAC could also form through reconfiguration, where relinked SOAC segments form a loop.

The method is also tested on a 3D network of actin filaments cross-linked by α-actinin (Figure 9.17a). Visual comparison between the results (Figure 9.17b) and the images show that the proposed method extracts the geometry and topology of these curvilinear networks accurately in the presence of foreground and background intensity variations.

In terms of efficiency, the Multiple SOACs method is much more efficient than the single-SOAC, semiautomatic tool in Smith et al. [43]. Using the single-SOAC method, it typically took 20–30 minutes for a human to segment the cytoskeletal network from a 3D image like the ones shown in Figure 9.15. By the proposed method, the time is reduced by more than 10-fold, since the program completes a segmentation in 2 minutes. Furthermore, the method also outputs information about the topology of the extracted network.

9.3.4   Tests on 3D optical coherence microscopy images

In addition to fluorescence microscopy images, the proposed method is also tested on images acquired using ultrahigh-resolution optical coherence microscopy (OCM) to study

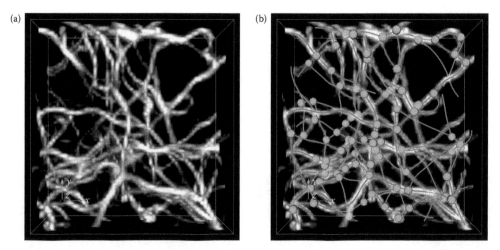

Figure 9.17 (a) A 3D network of actin filaments cross-linked by α-actinin [65]. (b) Extraction result overlaid with the original image [17].

angiogenesis in microengineered devices [16]. The success of in vitro vascular models that closely mimic in vivo conditions point towards the potential of using this platform to investigate fundamental questions pertaining to angiogenesis and its role in disease progression.

Optical coherence tomography (OCT) is a noninvasive optical imaging modality that can provide 3D, high-resolution images of biological tissues without staining and processing [68,69]. Optical coherence microscopy (OCM), which is an extension of OCT, combines the advantages of OCT and confocal microscopy using high numerical aperture objectives to provide cellular-resolution images [70]. Compared with confocal microscopy, OCM provides greater imaging depth, higher acquisition speed, and free of fluorescent labeling or external contrast agents. OCT has been used for obtaining images of natural physiological blood vessels [71] and engineered biological tissues [72–75]. However, few studies have utilized OCM to evaluate microstructural organization and development in engineered tissues [72,76].

In this study, an ultrahigh-resolution OCM (UHR-OCM) system is used to evaluate angiogenic sprouting in a microengineered device. The in vitro organotypic model of angiogenic sprouting was developed by putting type-I collagen into a polydimethylsilaxone (PMDS) mold/gasket shown in Figure 9.18 [7]. Two needles were originally placed into the collagen matrix, and extracted during the polymerization of the collagen to create two cylinder channels. Endothelial cells were injected into one channel and adhere to form an endothelium. The other channel was filled with angiogenic factors to establish a gradient across the collagen matrix, which induced angiogenesis from the endothelium. The device was placed on a rocker to provide flow across the channels. Throughout the experiment, the device was placed in an incubator at 37°C, 5% CO_2, and 85%–90% humidity at the University of Pennsylvania. Media and angiogenic factors in both channels were replenished daily [7]. After about 4 days, the device was fixed with 3.7% formaldehyde and subsequently submerged in phosphate-buffered saline (PBS) before it was transported and imaged at Lehigh University with the UHR-OCM system.

The system was developed using a supercontinuum light source, which enabled 1.5 μm axial resolution in tissue. A 175-degree conical lens [77,78] was used in combination with a

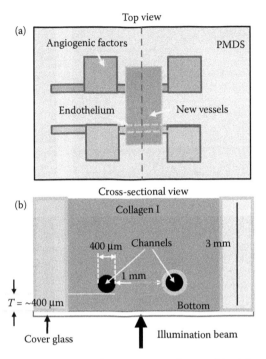

Figure 9.18 Diagrams of the top view (a) and cross-sectional view (b) of the microengineered device [16]. The orange region shows the type-I collagen matrix. Sprouting vessels shown as green lines start from the channel lined with endothelial cells (green) toward the channel filled with angiogenic factors (blue). The two channels are marked as black circles in (b).

10× objective to provide an extended depth-of-field of 200 μm and a traverse resolution of 2.3 μm. Data acquisition was performed at 20,000 A-scans/s with over 100 dB sensitivity. 3D OCM images were acquired on the artificial blood vessel device [7] with voxel size 1.0 × 1.0 × 1.0 μm.

The goal is to accurately delineate the morphology of the vascular network and identify vessel junction points. Figure 9.19 shows one result of applying the method. The output includes multiple SOACs, each representing an individual vessel in the vascular network. The length of each SOAC is used to estimate the length of the vessel.

9.3.5   Parameter selection

Parameter tuning is often needed when different types of experimental images need to be analyzed. The most critical two parameters are τ (Equation 9.9) and k_{str} (Equation 9.2). τ influences the quantity of initialized SOACs and is chosen empirically. In a rescaled image with intensity values in [0,1], depending on the contrast between background and foreground, the appropriate value of τ can range from 10^{-4} to 0.1. If τ is large, fewer image points will be considered as a ridge point, thus fewer SOACs will be initialized. Given a new type of experimental image, one can adjust this parameter in a semiautomatic fashion. k_{str} acts as a global parameter that controls the final magnitude of stretching force. One can use a larger k_{str} if the image is undersegmented and a smaller value if SOACs are overelongated.

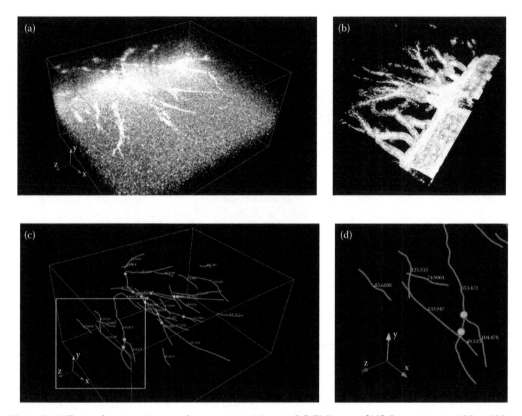

Figure 9.19 Example extraction results on an experimental OCM image [18]. Image size is 480 × 300 × 600. (a) An OCM image of vascular network of sprouting vessels rendered by maximum intensity projection. (b) Volume rendering of sprouting vessels using the extraction results in (c). (c) Resultant SOACs and junction points (green spheres). (d) A zoomed-in view of a portion of the extracted network, the area enclosed by the white square in (b). Estimated vessel lengths (Unit: μm) are displayed as text labels.

As discussed in Section 9.2.3, the radius range $[R_{near}, R_{far})$ specifies the range where local background intensities are sampled. They are empirically chosen based on the size and density of line structures which depend on the type of image and the point spread function (PSF) of the imaging process. Specifically, the actin cables in the experimental images have radii ≤ 3 voxels, so $R_{near} = 3$ to set apart the foreground and background region. R_{far} is influenced by the density of the curvilinear structures in the image. Nearby foreground voxels should not be included for background intensity estimation, so a small value is preferred for R_{far} when the curvilinear network is dense. Keeping R_{far} not too large makes the intensity estimation local. For the type of actin cable images used, $R_{far} = 6$ voxels, since the distance between filaments are usually greater than this value when they are not crossing each other. When they do cross, a small magnitude of stretching force is usually generated because areas near the junction are mostly occupied by foreground filaments. This makes the SOAC stop elongating at junctions but this works fine as the sequential evolution stage discourages a SOAC to go across junctions in the first place. Similarly for the OCM images of blood vessels, R_{near} and R_{far} are set according to the vessel scale and density.

The viscosity coefficient γ, controlling the step size, is set to 2 for the rescaled image where the intensity ranges from 0 to 1, in all the experiments. γ is inversely proportional to the step size: the larger γ is, the smaller step size will be. For typical images that have sufficiently high SNR to allow visual recognition of curvilinear structures, it is found that any $\gamma \geq 2$ can converge without any stability issue if the model is resampled after each iteration. Although larger step size can give quicker convergence, it could cause oscillation around the solution.

9.4   Discussion

Compared to other methods that use open parametric active contours for tracing filamentous structures such as microtubules in cellular electron tomography [48] and neurons in confocal microscopy images [49], the novel aspects in the proposed work include an n-dimensional automatic initialization scheme, a principled way to exert adaptive stretching forces at a SOAC's tips, regularization mechanisms to resolve SOAC collision and overlap issues, and also the greedy algorithm for reconfiguration of a SOAC network, which regroups SOAC segments at detected network junctions according to physical constraints. Thus, the proposed method is applicable to extraction of general curvilinear network structures with complex topology whereas previous methods were often tested on filamentous structures that are mostly parallel to each other or form simple tree-like topology (e.g., microtubules and neurons).

The computational efficiency of the method depends on the quantity of initialized SOACs. On a PC workstation with 3.00 GHz CPU and 4Gb RAM, the program completes the extraction of a 3D cytoskeletal network from a simulated image of size $200 \times 60 \times 60$ voxels in 20 seconds; it takes longer (usually less than 90 seconds) to segment a real confocal microscopy image of similar size, since more SOACs are initialized on noisy experimental images. The run time will decrease significantly with a parallel computing implementation.

Several mechanisms in the proposed method help reduce extraction time. First, detection of collision and redundancy prevents a SOAC from elongating to a region already covered by other SOACs. Second, differentiating two types of overlap keeps the overhead of regulation low: most of the time only tips are checked after each iteration while the more expensive body overlap check is performed only after convergence. Third, evolution order can have an impact on efficiency. The initial SOACs are sorted based on their length and let longer ones evolve first to reduce the total evolution time.

To achieve best result using the proposed method, parameter tuning is often needed for different types of experimental images. Manual testing in search of appropriate set of parameters is often needed for each *type* of images. However, the set of parameters can be fixed for a certain type of experimental images that share the same image characteristics. One only needs to tune parameters for one example of a new type of images, and then can utilize these same parameters for batch segmentation of all such images without any human intervention.

9.5   Conclusion

In this chapter, we reviewed an image segmentation method based on multiple Stretching Open Active Contours for the extraction of centerlines of curvilinear networks in 2D/3D confocal microscopy images and 3D OCM images. Complex issues that arise in 3D are addressed and mechanisms are proposed to make the approach robust to heavy image noise, nonuniform foreground and background intensity, and anisotropic sampling as are typical in many 3D experimental images. Validation on simulated images shows the robustness of the method; experiments on real experimental images show the potential of the method in extracting the geometry and topology of curvilinear networks accurately and efficiently. The method is also generally applicable to other types of curvilinear networks with varying image SNR.

References

1. T. D. Pollard and J. A. Cooper, Actin, a central player in cell shape and movement, *Science*, vol. 326, no. 5957, pp. 1208–1212, 2009.
2. C. Storm, J. J. Pastore, F. C. MacKintosh, T. C. Lubensky, and P. A. Janmey, Nonlinear elasticity in biological gels, *Nature*, vol. 435, no. 7039, pp. 191–194, 2005.
3. I. K. Piechocka, R. G. Bacabac, M. Potters, F. C. MacKintosh, and G. H. Koenderink, Structural hierarchy governs fibrin gel mechanics, *Biophysical Journal*, vol. 98, no. 10, pp. 2281–2289, 2010.
4. A. M. Stein, D. A. Vader, L. M. Jawerth, D. A. Weitz, and L. M. Sander, An algorithm for extracting the network geometry of three-dimensional collagen gels, *Journal of Microscopy*, vol. 232, no. 3, pp. 463–475, 2008.
5. P. Carmeliet, Angiogenesis in health and disease, *Nature Medicine*, vol. 9, no. 6, pp. 653–660, 2003.
6. J. Folkman, Angiogenesis in cancer, vascular, rheumatoid and other disease, *Nature Medicine*, vol. 1, no. 1, pp. 27–30, 1995.
7. D.-H. T. Nguyen, S. C. Stapleton, M. T. Yang, S. S. Cha, C. K. Choi, P. A. Galie, and C. S. Chen, Biomimetic model to reconstitute angiogenic sprouting morphogenesis in vitro, *Proceedings of the National Academy of Sciences*, vol. 110, no. 17, pp. 6712–6717, 2013.
8. S. Köhler, V. Schaller, and A. R. Bausch, Structure formation in active networks, *Nature Materials*, vol. 10, no. 6, pp. 462–468, 2011.
9. A.-C. Reymann, R. Boujemaa-Paterski, J.-L. Martiel, C. Guèrin, W. Cao, H. F. Chin, M. Enrique, M. Thèry, and L. Blanchoin, Actin network architecture can determine myosin motor activity, *Science*, vol. 336, no. 6086, pp. 1310–1314, 2012.
10. T. Sanchez, D. T. Chen, S. J. DeCamp, M. Heymann, and Z. Dogic, Spontaneous motion in hierarchically assembled active matter, *Nature*, vol. 491, no. 7424, pp. 431–434, 2012.
11. M. Bailey, L. Conway, M. W. Gramlich, T. L. Hawkins, and J. L. Ross, Modern methods to interrogate microtubule dynamics, *Integrative Biology*, vol. 5, no. 11, pp. 1324–1333, 2013.
12. E. Kim, O. V. Kim, K. R. Machlus, X. Liu, T. Kupaev, J. Lioi, A. S. Wolberg, D. Z. Chen, E. D. Rosen, Z. Xu, and M. Alber, Correlation between fibrin network structure and mechanical properties: An experimental and computational analysis, *Soft Matter*, vol. 7, no. 10, pp. 4983–4992, 2011.
13. D. Vavylonis, J.-Q. Wu, S. Hao, B. O'Shaughnessy, and T. D. Pollard, Assembly mechanism of the contractile ring for cytokinesis by fission yeast, *Science*, vol. 319, no. 5859, pp. 97–100, 2008.
14. T. D. Pollard and J.-Q. Wu, Understanding cytokinesis: Lessons from fission yeast, *Nature Reviews Molecular Cell Biology*, vol. 11, no. 2, pp. 149–155, 2010.
15. I. Fujiwara, D. Vavylonis, and T. D. Pollard, Polymerization kinetics of adp-and adp-pi-actin determined by fluorescence microscopy, *Proceedings of the National Academy of Sciences*, vol. 104, no. 21, pp. 8827–8832, 2007.
16. F. Li, T. Xu, D.-H. T. Nguyen, X. Huang, C. S. Chen, and C. Zhou, Label-free evaluation of angiogenic sprouting in microengineered devices using ultrahigh-resolution optical coherence microscopy, *Journal of Biomedical Optics*, vol. 19, no. 1, pp. 016 006–016 006, 2014.
17. T. Xu, D. Vavylonis, and X. Huang, 3D actin network centerline extraction with multiple active contours, *Medical Image Analysis*, vol. 18, no. 2, pp. 272–284, 2014.

18. T. Xu, F. Li, D.-H. T. Nguyen, C. S. Chen, C. Zhou, and X. Huang, Delineating 3D angiogenic sprouting in OCT images via multiple active contours, in *Augmented Reality Environments for Medical Imaging and Computer-Assisted Interventions*. Berlin: Springer, 2013, pp. 231–240.
19. T. Xu, H. Li, T. Shen, N. Ojkic, D. Vavylonis, and X. Huang, Extraction and analysis of actin networks based on open active contour models, in *Biomedical Imaging: From Nano to Macro, 2011 IEEE International Symposium on*. IEEE, 2011, pp. 1334–1340.
20. B. J. Nolen, N. Tomasevic, A. Russell, D. W. Pierce, Z. Jia, C. D. McCormick, J. Hartman, R. Sakowicz, and T. D. Pollard, Characterization of two classes of small molecule inhibitors of arp2/3 complex, *Nature*, vol. 460, no. 7258, pp. 1031–1034, 2009.
21. T. C. Baradet, J. C. Haselgrove, and J. W. Weisel, Three-dimensional reconstruction of fibrin clot networks from stereoscopic intermediate voltage electron microscope images and analysis of branching, *Biophysical Journal*, vol. 68, no. 4, pp. 1551–1560, 1995.
22. J. Wu, B. Rajwa, D. L. Filmer, C. M. Hoffmann, B. Yuan, C. Chiang, J. Sturgis, and J. P. Robinson, Automated quantification and reconstruction of collagen matrix from 3D confocal datasets, *Journal of Microscopy*, vol. 210, no. 2, pp. 158–165, 2003.
23. W. Mickel, S. Münster, L. M. Jawerth, D. A. Vader, D. A. Weitz, A. P. Sheppard, K. Mecke, B. Fabry, and G. E. Schröder-Turk, Robust pore size analysis of filamentous networks from three-dimensional confocal microscopy, *Biophysical Journal*, vol. 95, no. 12, pp. 6072–6080, 2008.
24. G. Herberich, A. Ivanescu, I. Gamper, A. Sechi, and T. Aach, Analysis of length and orientation of microtubules in wide-field fluorescence microscopy, in *Pattern Recognition*. Berlin: Springer, 2010, pp. 182–191.
25. G. Herberich, R. Windoffer, R. Leube, and T. Aach, 3D segmentation of keratin intermediate filaments in confocal laser scanning microscopy, in *Engineering in Medicine and Biology Society, EMBC, 2011 Annual International Conference of the IEEE*. IEEE, 2011, pp. 7751–7754.
26. A. F. Frangi, W. J. Niessen, K. L. Vincken, and M. A. Viergever, Multiscale vessel enhancement filtering, in *Medical Image Computing and Computer-Assisted Intervention–MICCAI'98*. Berlin: Springer, 1998, pp. 130–137.
27. Y. Sato, S. Nakajima, N. Shiraga, H. Atsumi, S. Yoshida, T. Koller, G. Gerig, and R. Kikinis, Three-dimensional multi-scale line filter for segmentation and visualization of curvilinear structures in medical images, *Medical Image Analysis*, vol. 2, no. 2, pp. 143–168, 1998.
28. M. Beil, H. Braxmeier, F. Fleischer, V. Schmidt, and P. Walther, Quantitative analysis of keratin filament networks in scanning electron microscopy images of cancer cells, *Journal of Microscopy*, vol. 220, no. 2, pp. 84–95, 2005.
29. S. Lück, M. Sailer, V. Schmidt, and P. Walther, Three-dimensional analysis of intermediate filament networks using SEM tomography, *Journal of Microscopy*, vol. 239, no. 1, pp. 1–16, 2010.
30. S. Blacher, L. Devy, M. F. Burbridge, G. Roland, G. Tucker, A. Noël, and J.-M. Foidart, Improved quantification of angiogenesis in the rat aortic ring assay, *Angiogenesis*, vol. 4, no. 2, pp. 133–142, 2001.
31. A. Niemisto, V. Dunmire, O. Yli-Harja, W. Zhang, and I. Shmulevich, Robust quantification of in vitro angiogenesis through image analysis, *Medical Imaging, IEEE Transactions on*, vol. 24, no. 4, pp. 549–553, 2005.
32. D. Mayerich and J. Keyser, Hardware accelerated segmentation of complex volumetric filament networks, *Visualization and Computer Graphics, IEEE Transactions on*, vol. 15, no. 4, pp. 670–681, 2009.
33. A. Rigort, D. Günther, R. Hegerl, D. Baum, B. Weber, S. Prohaska, O. Medalia, W. Baumeister, and H.-C. Hege, Automated segmentation of electron tomograms for a quantitative description of actin filament networks, *Journal of Structural Biology*, vol. 177, no. 1, pp. 135–144, 2012.
34. B. Weber, G. Greenan, S. Prohaska, D. Baum, H.-C. Hege, T. Müller-Reichert, A. A. Hyman, and J.-M. Verbavatz, Automated tracing of microtubules in electron tomograms of plastic embedded samples of *Caenorhabditis elegans* embryos, *Journal of Structural Biology*, vol. 178, no. 2, pp. 129–138, 2012.
35. P. Krauss, C. Metzner, J. Lange, N. Lang, and B. Fabry, Parameter-free binarization and skeletonization of fiber networks from confocal image stacks, *PloS One*, vol. 7, no. 5, p. e36575, 2012.

36. K. Sandberg and M. Brega, Segmentation of thin structures in electron micrographs using orientation fields, *Journal of Structural Biology*, vol. 157, no. 2, pp. 403–415, 2007.

37. C. Winkler, M. Vinzenz, J. V. Small, and C. Schmeiser, Actin filament tracking in electron tomograms of negatively stained lamellipodia using the localized radon transform, *Journal of Structural Biology*, vol. 178, no. 1, pp. 19–28, 2012.

38. M. Rusu, Z. Starosolski, M. Wahle, A. Rigort, and W. Wriggers, Automated tracing of filaments in 3D electron tomography reconstructions using Sculptor and Situs, *Journal of Structural Biology*, vol. 178, no. 2, pp. 121–128, 2012.

39. M. Kass, A. Witkin, and D. Terzopoulos, Snakes: Active contour models, *International Journal of Computer Vision*, vol. 1, no. 4, pp. 321–331, 1988.

40. H. Li, T. Shen, M. B. Smith, I. Fujiwara, D. Vavylonis, and X. Huang, Automated actin filament segmentation, tracking and tip elongation measurements based on open active contour models, in *Biomedical Imaging: From Nano to Macro, 2009. ISBI'09. IEEE International Symposium on*. IEEE, 2009, pp. 1302–1305.

41. H. Li, T. Shen, D. Vavylonis, and X. Huang, Actin filament tracking based on particle filters and stretching open active contour models, in *Medical Image Computing and Computer-Assisted Intervention–MICCAI 2009*. Berlin: Springer, 2009, pp. 673–681.

42. H. Li, T. Shen, D. Vavylonis, and X. Huang, Actin filament segmentation using spatiotemporal active-surface and active-contour models, in *Medical Image Computing and Computer-Assisted Intervention–MICCAI 2010*. Berlin: Springer, 2010, pp. 86–94.

43. M. B. Smith, H. Li, T. Shen, X. Huang, E. Yusuf, and D. Vavylonis, Segmentation and tracking of cytoskeletal filaments using open active contours, *Cytoskeleton*, vol. 67, no. 11, pp. 693–705, 2010.

44. K. Y. Kong, A. I. Marcus, J. Y. Hong, P. Giannakakou, and M. D. Wang, Computer assisted analysis of microtubule dynamics in living cells, in *Engineering in Medicine and Biology Society, 2005. IEEE-EMBS 2005. 27th Annual International Conference of the*. IEEE, 2005, pp. 3982–3985.

45. M. A. El-Saban and B. S. Manjunath, Tracking curvilinear structures using active contours and application to microtubule videos, University of California, Santa Barbara, Tech. Rep., 2005.

46. M. A. El-Saban, A. Altinok, A. Peck, C. Kenney, S. Feinstein, L. Wilson, K. Rose, and B. S. Manjunath, Automated tracking and modeling of microtubule dynamics, in *Biomedical Imaging: Nano to Macro, 2006. 3rd IEEE International Symposium on*. IEEE, 2006, pp. 1032–1035.

47. A. Altinok, M. A. El-Saban, A. J. Peck, L. Wilson, S. C. Feinstein, B. S. Manjunath, and K. Rose, Activity analysis in microtubule videos by mixture of hidden Markov models, in *Computer Vision and Pattern Recognition, 2006 IEEE Computer Society Conference on*, vol. 2. IEEE, 2006, pp. 1662–1669.

48. D. Nurgaliev, T. Gatanov, and D. J. Needleman, Automated identification of microtubules in cellular electron tomography, *Methods in Cell Biology*, vol. 97, pp. 475–495, 2010.

49. Y. Wang, A. Narayanaswamy, C.-L. Tsai, and B. Roysam, A broadly applicable 3-D neuron tracing method based on open-curve snake, *Neuroinformatics*, vol. 9, no. 2–3, pp. 193–217, 2011.

50. R. Malladi, J. A. Sethian, and B. C. Vemuri, Shape modeling with front propagation: A level set approach, *Pattern Analysis and Machine Intelligence, IEEE Transactions on*, vol. 17, no. 2, pp. 158–175, 1995.

51. V. Caselles, R. Kimmel, and G. Sapiro, Geodesic active contours, *International Journal of Computer Vision*, vol. 22, no. 1, pp. 61–79, 1997.

52. L. M. Lorigo, O. D. Faugeras, W. E. L. Grimson, R. Keriven, R. Kikinis, A. Nabavi, and C.-F. Westin, Curves: Curve evolution for vessel segmentation, *Medical Image Analysis*, vol. 5, no. 3, pp. 195–206, 2001.

53. A. Vasilevskiy and K. Siddiqi, Flux maximizing geometric flows, *Pattern Analysis and Machine Intelligence, IEEE Transactions on*, vol. 24, no. 12, pp. 1565–1578, 2002.

54. J. Melonakos, E. Pichon, S. Angenent, and A. Tannenbaum, Finsler active contours, *Pattern Analysis and Machine Intelligence, IEEE Transactions on*, vol. 30, no. 3, pp. 412–423, 2008.

55. M. Rochery, I. H. Jermyn, and J. Zerubia, Higher order active contours, *International Journal of Computer Vision*, vol. 69, no. 1, pp. 27–42, 2006.

56. S. Basu, D. P. Mukherjee, and S. T. Acton, Implicit evolution of open ended curves, in *Image Processing, 2007. ICIP 2007. IEEE International Conference on*, vol. 1. IEEE, 2007, pp. I-261–I-264.

57. S. Hadjidemetriou, D. Toomre, and J. S. Duncan, Segmentation and 3D reconstruction of microtubules in total internal reflection fluorescence microscopy (TIRFM), in *Medical Image Computing and Computer-Assisted Intervention–MICCAI 2005*. Berlin: Springer, 2005, pp. 761–769.

58. M. E. Sargin, A. Altinok, K. Rose, and B. Manjunath, Tracing curvilinear structures in live cell images, in *Image Processing, 2007. ICIP 2007. IEEE International Conference on*, vol. 6. IEEE, 2007, pp. VI-285–VI-288.

59. M.-A. Abdul-Karim, K. Al-Kofahi, E. B. Brown, R. K. Jain, and B. Roysam, Automated tracing and change analysis of angiogenic vasculature from in vivo multiphoton confocal image time series, *Microvascular Research*, vol. 66, no. 2, pp. 113–125, 2003.

60. J. A. Tyrrell, V. Mahadevan, R. T. Tong, E. B. Brown, R. K. Jain, and B. Roysam, A 2-D/3-D model-based method to quantify the complexity of microvasculature imaged by in vivo multiphoton microscopy, *Microvascular Research*, vol. 70, no. 3, pp. 165–178, 2005.

61. C. Xu and J. L. Prince, Snakes, shapes, and gradient vector flow, *Image Processing, IEEE Transactions on*, vol. 7, no. 3, pp. 359–369, 1998.

62. M. W. Law and A. C. Chung, Three dimensional curvilinear structure detection using optimally oriented flux, in *Computer Vision–ECCV 2008*. Berlin: Springer, 2008, pp. 368–382.

63. S. Chang, C. A. Kulikowski, S. M. Dunn, and S. Levy, Biomedical image skeletonization: A novel method applied to fibrin network structures, *Studies in Health Technology and Informatics*, no. 2, pp. 901–905, 2001.

64. O. Pelletier, E. Pokidysheva, L. S. Hirst, N. Bouxsein, Y. Li, and C. R. Safinya, Structure of actin cross-linked with α-actinin: A network of bundles, *Physical Review Letters*, vol. 91, no. 14, p. 148102, 2003.

65. T. T. Falzone, M. Lenz, D. R. Kovar, and M. L. Gardel, Assembly kinetics determine the architecture of α-actinin crosslinked f-actin networks, *Nature Communications*, vol. 3, p. 861, 2012.

66. D. Vignjevic, D. Yarar, M. D. Welch, J. Peloquin, T. Svitkina, and G. G. Borisy, Formation of filopodia-like bundles in vitro from a dendritic network, *The Journal of Cell Biology*, vol. 160, no. 6, pp. 951–962, 2003.

67. A. Narayanaswamy, S. Dwarakapuram, C. S. Bjornsson, B. M. Cutler, W. Shain, and B. Roysam, Robust adaptive 3-D segmentation of vessel laminae from fluorescence confocal microscope images and parallel GPU implementation, *Medical Imaging, IEEE Transactions on*, vol. 29, no. 3, pp. 583–597, 2010.

68. D. Huang, E. A. Swanson, C. P. Lin, J. S. Schuman, W. G. Stinson, W. Chang, M. R. Hee, T. Flotte, K. Gregory, C. A. Puliafito, et al., Optical coherence tomography, *Science*, vol. 254, no. 5035, pp. 1178–1181, 1991.

69. J. A. Izatt, E. A. Swanson, J. G. Fujimoto, M. R. Hee, and G. M. Owen, Optical coherence microscopy in scattering media, *Optics Letters*, vol. 19, no. 8, pp. 590–592, 1994.

70. W. Drexler, U. Morgner, F. X. Kärtner, C. Pitris, S. A. Boppart, X. D. Li, E. P. Ippen, and J. G. Fujimoto, In vivo ultrahigh-resolution optical coherence tomography, *Optics Letters*, vol. 24, no. 17, pp. 1221–1223, 1999.

71. S. Makita, Y. Hong, M. Yamanari, T. Yatagai, and Y. Yasuno, Optical coherence angiography, *Optics Express*, vol. 14, no. 17, pp. 7821–7840, 2006.

72. Y. Yang, A. Dubois, X.-p. Qin, J. Li, A. El Haj, and R. K. Wang, Investigation of optical coherence tomography as an imaging modality in tissue engineering, *Physics in Medicine and Biology*, vol. 51, no. 7, p. 1649, 2006.

73. P. O. Bagnaninchi, Y. Yang, N. Zghoul, N. Maffulli, R. K. Wang, and A. J. E. Haj, Chitosan microchannel scaffolds for tendon tissue engineering characterized using optical coherence tomography, *Tissue Engineering*, vol. 13, no. 2, pp. 323–331, 2007.

74. H.-J. Ko, W. Tan, R. Stack, and S. A. Boppart, Optical coherence elastography of engineered and developing tissue, *Tissue Engineering*, vol. 12, no. 1, pp. 63–73, 2006.

75. X. Liang, B. W. Graf, and S. A. Boppart, Imaging engineered tissues using structural and functional optical coherence tomography, *Journal of Biophotonics*, vol. 2, no. 11, pp. 643–655, 2009.

76. Y. Zhao, B. W. Graf, E. J. Chaney, Z. Mahmassani, E. Antoniadou, R. DeVolder, H. Kong, M. D. Boppart, and S. A. Boppart, Integrated multimodal optical microscopy for structural and functional imaging of engineered and natural skin, *Journal of Biophotonics*, vol. 5, no. 5–6, pp. 437–448, 2012.

77. R. A. Leitgeb, M. Villiger, A. H. Bachmann, L. Steinmann, and T. Lasser, Extended focus depth for Fourier domain optical coherence microscopy, *Optics Letters*, vol. 31, no. 16, pp. 2450–2452, 2006.

78. T. Bolmont, A. Bouwens, C. Pache, M. Dimitrov, C. Berclaz, M. Villiger, B. M. Wegenast-Braun, T. Lasser, and P. C. Fraering, Label-free imaging of cerebral β-amyloidosis with extended-focus optical coherence microscopy, *The Journal of Neuroscience*, vol. 32, no. 42, pp. 14 548–14 556, 2012.

chapter ten

Level set-based cell segmentation using convex energy functionals

Jan-Philip Bergeest and Karl Rohr

Contents

Abstract

Accurate and efficient segmentation of cells in fluorescence microscopy images, in particular, from high-throughput experiments, is of central importance for the quantification of protein expression and the understanding of cell function. We present an approach for segmenting cell nuclei, which is based on level set active contours and convex minimization. Our approach employs different convex energy functionals and uses an efficient numeric scheme for minimization. Compared to previous work using non-convex energy functionals, our approach determines the global solution. Thus, the approach does not suffer from local minima and the segmentation result does not depend on the initialization. We consider two different well-known non-convex energy functionals for level set-based segmentation and introduce convex formulations of these functionals. The performance of our approach has been evaluated using fluorescence microscopy images from different experiments comprising different cell types. We have also performed a quantitative comparison with previous segmentation approaches.

10.1   Introduction

One of the most important tasks in analyzing and quantifying fluorescence microscopy images is cell nucleus segmentation. In particular, the enormous amount of image data generated by high-throughput experiments makes semiautomatic and manual analysis infeasible. Thus, automatic methods are needed, which efficiently cope with different cell types and image artifacts such as intensity inhomogeneities.

In previous work on the segmentation of cell nuclei in fluorescence microscopy images various approaches have been proposed. Often, thresholding approaches are applied, which, however, suffer from intensity inhomogeneities within nuclei and over a whole image. To separate clustered nuclei, watershed-based techniques are frequently used. In Wählby et al. [1], a watershed algorithm for cell segmentation was proposed followed by cluster splitting based on concavity regions. Lin et al. [2] introduced an approach that uses an improved distance transform by combining the intensity gradient and a geometric distance followed by statistical model-based merging. Cheng and Rajapakse [3] as well as Jung and Kim [4] proposed marker-controlled watershed approaches for cluster splitting, where the optimal number of markers is determined based on the H-minima transform.

A main class of cell segmentation approaches is based on deformable models, which allow incorporation of a priori knowledge and can capture a wide spectrum of different shapes. One can distinguish between parametric models [5] and implicit models [6]. *Parametric models* are based on an explicit representation of objects [7–9]. Zimmer and Olivo-Marin [7] introduced a region-based parametric energy functional, which includes a coupling term for multiple contours and a penalty term to prevent merging. An extension of this approach was described by Wang et al. [8], which includes texture-adaptive weights for the external energy of the active contour model to cope with internal pseudo-edges and low-contrast cell boundaries. In Butenuth and Heipke [9], a combination of a parametric active contour model with a graph-based approach was introduced. However, parametric models have the disadvantage that they depend on the parametrization, an extension from 2D to 3D is difficult, and these models have problems with topological changes.

Implicit models using level sets have gained increased interest for cell segmentation since topological changes can be handled naturally [10–25]. Ortiz de Solórzano et al. [10] developed a two-step level set approach for segmenting cells, which employs a gradient-based energy functional. Dufour et al. [11] introduced an energy functional that integrates multiple active contours and combines gradient-based and region-based terms. To reduce the high computational cost of representing each cell with one level set, Nath et al. [12] introduced an approach that can cope with an arbitrary number of cells by using only four level sets (analogously to the four color theorem). In Chang et al. [13], regions corresponding to single cells are determined by Voronoi tessellation and then a region-based energy functional is employed within each of these regions. Palaniappan et al. [14] developed a level set approach based on a Bayesian energy functional, which uses the flux tensor for initialization. Maška et al. [16] first separate foreground and background of cell images using a gradient-based level set approach and second perform cluster splitting using topology preserving level sets. Mosaliganti et al. [17] proposed an energy functional based on an appearance model of cells. Padfield et al. [18] introduced a level set approach for cell tracking, which considers tracking as a spatio temporal volume segmentation problem and which includes size and shape constraints in the energy functional. In Dzyubachyk et al. [20], a level set approach based on a Bayesian energy functional and a non-PDE-based minimization scheme is described. A combination of level set approaches and graph partitioning approaches within in a variational framework was proposed in Ersoy et al. [19], Xu et al. [21], and Maška et al. [23]. In Ersoy et al. [19], a multi phase graph partitioning active contour approach using regional density functions was introduced. Xu et al. [21] described a two-step level set approach for cell segmentation in histopathological images, where first, a geodesic active contour model is initialized by a hierarchical normalized cuts scheme and second, a level set functional is used. In Maška et al. [23], an approach for segmentation and tracking of cells was proposed, which uses graph-cuts for the minimization of a region-based energy functional integrating a topological prior. Whereas in graph-cut based approaches discrete optimization is employed, with level set-based approaches continuous optimization of the energy functionals is used. Approaches using multiple coupled level sets, where one level set corresponds to one cell nucleus were introduced in Dufour et al. [11], Nath et al. [12], Yan et al. [15], Mosaliganti et al. [17], Ersoy et al. [19], Qi et al. [22], Yang and Padfield [24], and Lu et al. [25]. A two-step segmentation approach was proposed in Qi et al. [22], which first determines initial seed points for the level sets by iterative voting and then couples the level sets with a repulsion force. In Yang and Padfield [24], a fast non-PDE-based minimization for coupled level sets was presented where the initialization was performed using wavelet-based segmentation. In Lu et al. [25], a multistep approach for the segmentation of cell clumps was described. First, cell clumps are detected, then nuclei within the cell clumps are detected, and finally a level set optimization using a shape prior for single cells is employed. A disadvantage of previous level set approaches is that the underlying energy functionals lead to non-convex minimization problems. Hence, the optimization function has local minima and the global solution is generally not found (using local optimization methods which are typically applied). In addition, the segmentation result depends on the initialization.

In this chapter, we describe an approach for cell nucleus segmentation in fluorescence microscopy images, which is based on active contours and level sets. Compared to previous work, our approach is based on energy functionals that lead to convex minimization problems for which global solutions are determined. We consider two functionals and take advantage of the combination of the Bayesian functional in Rousson and Deriche [26], which was used for cell segmentation in Dzyubachyk et al. [20], and the region-scalable fitting energy functional in Li et al. [27]. A convex formulation for the region-based functional of Chan and Vese [28] was derived in Chan et al. [29] and Goldstein et al. [30] and we employ this formulation for two different energy functionals. We consider the Bayesian functional in Rousson and Deriche [26] and the region-scalable fitting energy functional in Li et al. [27] to cope with intensity inhomogeneities and clustered cell nuclei. We reformulate these two functionals leading to convex optimization problems. For the two convex functionals, we use an efficient minimization scheme using the split Bregman method. Based on the convex functionals, we developed a two-step approach for cell nucleus segmentation, which combines the convex Bayesian functional and the convex region-scalable fitting energy functional. An advantage of the two-step approach is that it can cope with both global and local intensity inhomogeneities. We have successfully applied our two-step approach to 2D fluorescence microscopy images from four different experiments comprising different cell types, and we have compared the results with previous approaches.

This chapter is organized as follows. In the following Section 10.2, we describe a general non-convex formulation of level set-based energy functionals and we state the corresponding convex formulation. In Section 10.3, we present the two non-convex energy functionals, which we employ in our approach for cell segmentation. In Section 10.4, we use the general formulation from Section 10.2 to reformulate the non-convex energy functionals to convex functionals. In Section 10.5, we describe our two-step cell segmentation approach, which combines the two convex functionals. Finally, we show experimental results in Section 10.6 and give a discussion in Section 10.7.

10.2   Non-convex and convex energy functionals

In this section, we describe a general non-convex formulation of energy functionals commonly used for cell segmentation. Then, we reformulate the energy functional using level sets and we derive the corresponding convex formulation.

A commonly used class of non-convex energy functionals can be stated as

$$
E(\Theta, \partial\Omega) = \lambda \left(\kappa_0 \int_{\Omega_0} g_0(\mathbf{x}, \Theta)d\mathbf{x} + \kappa_1 \int_{\Omega_1} g_1(\mathbf{x}, \Theta)d\mathbf{x} \right) + |\partial\Omega|, \tag{10.1}
$$

where $\partial\Omega$ denotes the boundaries between the background region Ω_0 and the foreground region Ω_1, $\mathbf{x}$ is the pixel position (x, y), $|\partial\Omega|$ corresponds to the length of $\partial\Omega$, and $\kappa_0, \kappa_1, \lambda$ are weighting factors [28,31]. The integrands $g_0(\mathbf{x}, \Theta)$ and $g_1(\mathbf{x}, \Theta)$ with parameter vector Θ are chosen to model properties of the background and foreground region (e.g., intensity distribution) of fluorescence microscopy images.

Using a level set representation for the energy functional E in Equation 10.1 by embedding the contour $\partial\Omega$ in a level set function ϕ with

$$
\partial\Omega = \{\mathbf{x} : \phi(\mathbf{x}) = 0\} \tag{10.2}
$$

leads to the functional

$$
E(\Theta, \phi) = \lambda \left(\kappa_0 \int_{\Omega} g_0(\mathbf{x}, \Theta)(1 - H(\phi(\mathbf{x})))d\mathbf{x} + \kappa_1 \int_{\Omega} g_1(\mathbf{x}, \Theta)H(\phi(\mathbf{x}))d\mathbf{x} \right) + \int_{\Omega} |\nabla H(\phi(\mathbf{x}))|, \tag{10.3}
$$

with $H(x)$ being the Heaviside function

$$
H(x) = \begin{cases} 0, & x < 0 \\ 1, & x \geq 0 \end{cases} \tag{10.4}
$$

Note, that the integration in Equation 10.3 is performed over the whole image region Ω (in comparison to Equation 10.1). Since the level set function ϕ assumes negative values in the background region and positive values in the foreground region, the respective region is obtained using $1 - H(\phi(\mathbf{x}))$ and $H(\phi(\mathbf{x}))$. Using the Euler–Lagrange equation for Equation 10.3 leads to the gradient flow for the level set function ϕ

$$
\frac{\partial\phi(\mathbf{x})}{\partial t} = -\lambda \left(-\kappa_0 g_0(\mathbf{x}, \Theta) + \kappa_1 g_1(\mathbf{x}, \Theta) - \nabla \cdot \frac{\nabla\phi}{|\nabla\phi|} \right) H'(\phi(\mathbf{x})), \tag{10.5}
$$

where $H'(x)$ is the derivative of the Heaviside function.

In Chan et al. [29], it was shown that certain non-convex minimization problems can be reformulated as convex problems. Following Chan et al. [29], the Heaviside function in Equation 10.5 is omitted since Equation 10.5 and the following gradient descent equation have the same steady-state solution

$$
\frac{\partial\phi(\mathbf{x})}{\partial t} = -\lambda r + \nabla \cdot \frac{\nabla\phi}{|\nabla\phi|}, \tag{10.6}
$$

where

$$r = \kappa_1 g_1(\mathbf{x}, \Theta) - \kappa_0 g_0(\mathbf{x}, \Theta) \tag{10.7}$$

Then, the corresponding energy functional can be stated as

$$E(\Theta, \phi) = \lambda \langle \phi, r \rangle + |\nabla \phi|_1, \tag{10.8}$$

where $\langle \cdot, \cdot \rangle$ denotes the inner product and $| \cdot |_1$ is the $L1$-norm. This energy is homogenous of degree 1 in ϕ (which means that if ϕ is multiplied by a factor then the energy scales by the same factor), and thus does not have a minimizer in general. However, a global minimum can be guaranteed by restricting ϕ to lie in a finite interval, for example, $[0, 1]$, and by solving the following convex problem for the normalized ϕ_n:

$$\min_{0 \leq \phi_n \leq 1} E^c(\Theta, \phi_n) = \lambda \langle \phi_n, r \rangle + |\nabla \phi_n|_1 \tag{10.9}$$

Based on the solution $\phi_n(\mathbf{x})$, the segmentation result Ω is determined by comparing the level set function with a threshold $\alpha \in {]0, 1[}$:

$$\Omega = \{\mathbf{x} : \phi_n(\mathbf{x}) > \alpha\} \tag{10.10}$$

10.3   Non-convex energy functionals for cell segmentation

Our segmentation approach for cell nuclei in fluorescence microscopy images is based on two energy functionals. The first functional is the energy functional in Li et al. [27] and is called region-scalable fitting energy functional:

$$E_1(\Theta, \partial\Omega) = \lambda \left(\sum_{i=0}^{1} \kappa_i \int_{\Omega_i} \int_{\Omega_i} K_\sigma(\mathbf{x} - \mathbf{y}) |I(\mathbf{y}) - f_i(\mathbf{x})|^2 d\mathbf{y} d\mathbf{x} \right) + Per(\Omega_1), \tag{10.11}$$

with $\Theta = (f_0(\mathbf{x}), f_1(\mathbf{x}))$, where $f_0(\mathbf{x})$ and $f_1(\mathbf{x})$ approximate the image intensities locally in a region centered at the position $\mathbf{x}$ in the background region Ω_0 and the foreground region Ω_1, respectively. $\partial\Omega$ denotes the boundaries between the regions Ω_i, $I(\mathbf{x})$ is the image intensity at position $\mathbf{x}$, $Per(\Omega_1)$ is the perimeter of Ω_1, and $\kappa_0, \kappa_1, \lambda$ are weighting factors. K is chosen to be a Gaussian kernel

$$K_\sigma(\mathbf{u}) = \frac{1}{\sqrt{2\pi}\sigma} e^{-\frac{|\mathbf{u}|^2}{2\sigma^2}}$$

with scale parameter $\sigma > 0$. The scale parameter σ is used to control the size of the region in which the image intensities are approximated (local mean value). The center of the region is at the position $\mathbf{x}$. The intensity information is exploited locally due to the strong decrease of $K_\sigma(\mathbf{x} - \mathbf{y})$ to zero as the distance between $\mathbf{y}$ and $\mathbf{x}$ increases. An advantage of E_1 is that for each position a locally varying mean value is computed.

The second functional employed in our approach was proposed in Rousson and Deriche [26] and was derived based on a Bayesian approach:

$$E_2(\Theta, \partial\Omega) = \lambda \left(\sum_{i=0}^{1} \int_{\Omega_i} -\log P(I(\mathbf{x})|\Omega_i) d\mathbf{x} \right) + Per(\Omega_1), \tag{10.12}$$

with $\Theta = (\mu_0, \mu_1, \sigma_0, \sigma_1)$, where μ_i and σ_i are the mean intensities and standard deviations of the regions Ω_i. $P(I(\mathbf{x})|\Omega_i)$ is the conditional probability that pixel $\mathbf{x}$ with intensity $I(\mathbf{x})$ belongs to region Ω_i. Here, we assume a Gaussian distribution

$$P(I(\mathbf{x})|\Omega_i) = \frac{1}{\sqrt{2\pi}\sigma_i}e^{-(I(\mathbf{x})-\mu_i)^2/2\sigma_i^2}.$$

for the background region Ω_0 and the foreground region Ω_1, respectively. Note that this is different to E_1 where, for each image position, a different mean value is taken into account. Note also that the weights κ_i are not needed, but are implicitly included via the standard deviations σ_i, which are estimated from the image data.

Using a level set representation for E_1 and E_2 and applying the Euler–Lagrange equation leads to the gradient flow for the level set function ϕ

$$\frac{\partial \phi(\mathbf{x})}{\partial t} = \left(-\lambda r_j + \nabla \cdot \frac{\nabla \phi}{|\nabla \phi|}\right) H'(\phi(\mathbf{x})), \tag{10.13}$$

The term r_j corresponds to the external image forces of the two energies $E_j, j = 1, 2$, and is defined as

$$r_1 = \kappa_1 \int K_\sigma(\mathbf{y} - \mathbf{x}) |I(\mathbf{x}) - f_1(\mathbf{y})|^2 d\mathbf{y} -$$

$$\kappa_0 \int K_\sigma(\mathbf{y} - \mathbf{x}) |I(\mathbf{x}) - f_0(\mathbf{y})|^2 d\mathbf{y} \tag{10.14}$$

$$r_2 = \log P(I(\mathbf{x})|\Omega_1) - \log P(I(\mathbf{x})|\Omega_0) \tag{10.15}$$

The parameter vector Θ can be computed directly from the image data:

$$\mu_0 = \frac{\int I(\mathbf{x})(1 - H(\phi(\mathbf{x})))d\mathbf{x}}{\int (1 - H(\phi(\mathbf{x})))d\mathbf{x}} \qquad \mu_1 = \frac{\int I(\mathbf{x})H(\phi(\mathbf{x}))d\mathbf{x}}{\int H(\phi(\mathbf{x}))d\mathbf{x}}$$

$$\sigma_0^2 = \frac{\int (I(\mathbf{x}) - \mu_0)^2(1 - H(\phi(\mathbf{x})))d\mathbf{x}}{\int (1 - H(\phi(\mathbf{x})))d\mathbf{x}} \qquad \sigma_1^2 = \frac{\int (I(\mathbf{x}) - \mu_1)^2 H(\phi(\mathbf{x}))d\mathbf{x}}{\int H(\phi(\mathbf{x}))d\mathbf{x}}$$

$$f_0(\mathbf{x}) = \frac{K_\sigma(\mathbf{x}) * [(1 - H(\phi(\mathbf{x})))I(\mathbf{x})]}{K_\sigma(\mathbf{x}) * (1 - H(\phi(\mathbf{x})))} \qquad f_1(\mathbf{x}) = \frac{K_\sigma(\mathbf{x}) * [H(\phi(\mathbf{x}))I(\mathbf{x})]}{K_\sigma(\mathbf{x}) * H(\phi(\mathbf{x}))},$$

where $*$ denotes the convolution.

10.4   Convex energy functionals for cell segmentation

In this section, we use the general formulation in Section 10.2 to reformulate the non-convex energy functionals in Section 10.3 to convex functionals. The integrands $g_0(\mathbf{x}, \Theta)$ and $g_1(\mathbf{x}, \Theta)$ of the general energy functional E in Equation 10.3 are chosen to model properties of the background and foreground region of fluorescence microscopy images. For the non-convex region-scalable fitting energy E_1 in Equation 10.11 the corresponding model is based on locally varying mean intensity values:

$$g_{i,1}(\mathbf{x}, \Theta) = \int_\Omega K_\sigma(\mathbf{x} - \mathbf{y})|I(\mathbf{y}) - f_i(\mathbf{x})|^2 M_i(\phi(\mathbf{y}))d\mathbf{y}, \quad i = 1, 2 \tag{10.16}$$

For the non-convex Bayesian energy E_2 in Equation 10.12 the corresponding model is based on a Gaussian distribution of the intensity values:

$$g_{i,2}(\mathbf{x}, \Theta) = -\log P(I(\mathbf{x})|\Omega_i)M_i(\phi(\mathbf{x})), \quad i = 1, 2 \tag{10.17}$$

where the functions $M_0 = 1 - H(\phi)$ and $M_1 = H(\phi)$ are used to select the background and foreground region, respectively. This leads to the level set formulation of the energies E_1 and E_2 in Equations 10.11 and 10.12

$$E_j(\Theta, \phi) = \lambda \left(\sum_{i=0}^{1} \kappa_i \int_{\Omega} g_{i,j}(\mathbf{x}, \Theta)M_i(\phi(\mathbf{x}))d\mathbf{x} \right) + \int_{\Omega} |\nabla H(\phi(\mathbf{x}))| \tag{10.18}$$

Note that the weights κ_i for the Bayesian energy E_2 are not needed and can be set to 1. The corresponding gradient descent formulation is obtained by using the Euler–Lagrange equation

$$\frac{\partial \phi(\mathbf{x})}{\partial t} = \left(-\lambda r_j + \nabla \cdot \frac{\nabla \phi}{|\nabla \phi|} \right) H'(\phi(\mathbf{x})) \tag{10.19}$$

Following the derivation in Section 10.2 the corresponding convex formulation is

$$\min_{0 \leq \phi_n \leq 1} E_j^c(\Theta, \phi_n) = \lambda \langle \phi_n, r_j \rangle + |\nabla \phi_n|_1 \tag{10.20}$$

To solve the minimization problem (Equation 10.20), we use the split Bregman method. This method is a general technique for efficiently solving L1-regularized problems and for iteratively finding extrema of convex functionals [30]. The method consists of variable splitting and Bregman iteration. Variable splitting is achieved by introducing the auxiliary vector $\mathbf{d}$ (with dimension according to the image domain) and by using a quadratic penalty term to enforce the constraint $\mathbf{d} = \nabla \phi_n$. For (Equation 10.20) this leads to

$$(\phi_n^*, \mathbf{d}^*) = \arg \min_{0 \leq \phi_n \leq 1, \mathbf{d}} \left(\lambda \langle \phi_n, r_j \rangle + |\mathbf{d}|_1 + \frac{\nu}{2}|\mathbf{d} - \nabla \phi_n|_2^2 \right), \tag{10.21}$$

where ϕ_n^* and $\mathbf{d}^*$ denote the iteratively computed solution, and ν is a weighting factor. In Equation 10.21, $\nabla \phi_n$ is no longer associated with the L1-norm, however, the constraint $\mathbf{d} = \nabla \phi_n$ is only weakly enforced. To enforce the constraint exactly, the Bregman iteration technique is applied. With this technique, a vector $\mathbf{b}$ is included in the penalty function and an alternating minimization is carried out:

$$(\phi_n^k, \mathbf{d}^k) = \arg \min_{0 \leq \phi_n \leq 1, \mathbf{d}} \left(\lambda \langle \phi_n, r_j \rangle + |\mathbf{d}|_1 + \frac{\nu}{2}|\mathbf{d} - \nabla \phi_n - \mathbf{b}^{k-1}|_2^2 \right), \tag{10.22}$$

$$\mathbf{b}^k = \mathbf{b}^{k-1} + \nabla \phi_n^k - \mathbf{d}^k, \tag{10.23}$$

where ϕ_n^k and $\mathbf{d}^k$ represent the solution at iteration k. The problem in Equations 10.22 and 10.23 is first solved w.r.t. ϕ_n, while $\mathbf{d}$ and $\mathbf{b}$ are fixed and second w.r.t. $\mathbf{d}$. In our case, we use a fast iterative Gauss–Seidel solver for the first minimization. The second minimization is obtained explicitly using the vector-valued shrinkage operator:

$$\mathbf{d}^k = \max\{|\mathbf{b}^{k-1} + \nabla \phi_n^k|_2 - \nu, 0\} \frac{\mathbf{b}^{k-1} + \nabla \phi_n^k}{|\mathbf{b}^{k-1} + \nabla \phi_n^k|_2} \tag{10.24}$$

10.5   Two-step cell segmentation approach based on convex energy functionals

We have developed a two-step approach for cell nuclei segmentation which combines the two convex energy functionals E_1^c and E_2^c in Equation 10.20 (see Figure 10.1). In the first step, we perform a segmentation of the whole image using the convex region-scalable fitting functional E_1^c. In the second step, we minimize the convex Bayesian functional E_2^c independently for all regions-of-interest that were segmented using E_1^c (we used a somewhat enlarged bounding box obtained by dilation). Note that doing this we use multiple level sets for the segmentation of an image. This is similar to multiple level set approaches [11,12,15,19,17,22,24,25]. However, in our case, we do not need a coupling term to prevent level sets from merging because we perform the minimization within previously segmented regions.

Since the functional E_1^c in the first step takes into account locally varying mean intensities, we can deal with varying background intensities and with clustered cell nuclei. The second step is used because the first step cannot cope well with inhomogeneities at the border of cell nuclei (see Figure 10.2b and note the nonsmooth contours of the segmented regions that do not well agree with the borders of the cell nuclei). At the same time, the sensitivity of E_1^c to inhomogeneities within cell nuclei allows effective handling of clustered cells. Using E_1^c, even small intensity differences in a small region between two neighboring cell nuclei or overlapping cell nuclei make cell splitting feasible (see Figures 10.2 and 10.3).

10.6   Experimental results

We have applied our approach to 2D fluorescence microscopy images of cell nuclei from four different experiments comprising four different cell types. We used two datasets from Coelho et al. [32] for which ground truth is available. The first dataset consists of 48 images with a size of 1349 × 1030 pixels, which include in total 1831 U20S Hoechst stained cell nuclei (see Figure 10.4a). The second dataset contains 49 images with a size of 1344 × 1024 pixels comprising in total 2178 NIH3T3 Hoechst stained nuclei (Figure 10.4b). Note that several images in the second dataset are heavily affected by intensity inhomogeneities and visible artifacts. Therefore, automatic analysis of the second set is more challenging compared to the images in the first set. Furthermore, we have applied our approach to a dataset of 7 2D fluorescence microscopy images of mouse neuroblastoma cells from Yu et al. [33]. Each image has a size of 1392 × 1040 pixels and the dataset includes in total

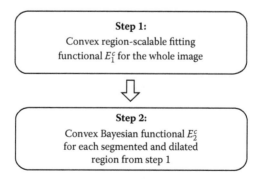

Figure 10.1 Diagram of the two-step segmentation approach.

(a)   (b)   (c)

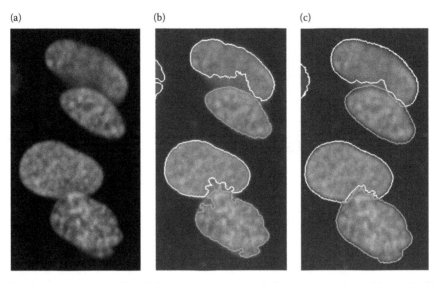

Figure 10.2 Segmentation results of the two-step approach (contour overlay with original images): (a) Original image, (b) two-step approach after the first step, and (c) after the second step. For better visibility, in (b) and (c) the contours of adjacent cells have been displayed with different gray values.

389 N1E115 DAPI stained cell nuclei (Figure 10.4c). The ground truth for these images was obtained by manually outlining the cell nuclei borders. In addition, we have applied our approach to the dataset of Drosophila cells used in Jones et al. [34] for which ground truth is available. The dataset consists of 16 images with a size between 400×400 and 512×512 pixels and includes approximately 1280 cell nuclei (Figure 10.4d). In total, we used 120 real microscopy images, which include 5678 cells.

To evaluate the performance of our approach, we determined region-based and contour-based measures. As region-based measure, we used the Dice coefficient and as contour-based measures we employed the normalized sum of distances (NSD [32]) and the Hausdorff distance. The Dice coefficient is defined as

$$Dice(R, S) = \frac{2|R \cap S|}{|R| + |S|},$$

(10.25)

(a)   (b)   (c)

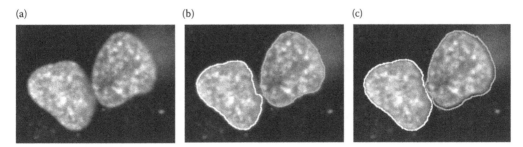

Figure 10.3 Segmentation results of the two-step approach (contour overlay with original images): (a) Original image, (b) two-step approach after the first step, and (c) after the second step.

(a)   (b)

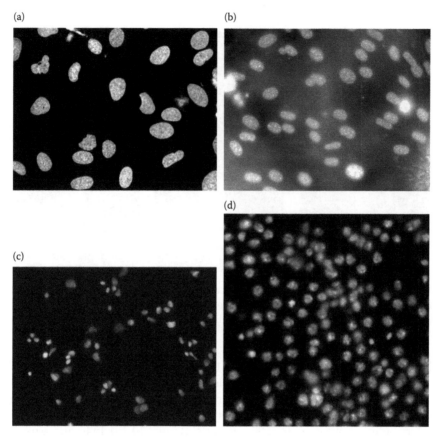

(d)

(c)

Figure 10.4 Original images of the four different datasets. (a) U20S cells, (b) NIH3T3 cells, (c) N1E115 cells, (d) Drosophila cells.

where R is the binary reference image, and S is the binary segmented image. The NSD is defined as

$$\text{NSD}(R, S) = \frac{\sum_{i \in R \cup S \setminus R \cap S} D(i)}{\sum_{i \in R \cup S} D(i)}, \qquad (10.26)$$

where $D(i)$ is the minimal Euclidean distance of pixel i to the contour of the reference object. The Hausdorff distance is defined as

$$h(R, S) = \max_{i \in S_c}\{D(i)\}, \qquad (10.27)$$

with S_c being the contour of the segmented object. We also used two detection measures, namely the number of false-positives (FP) and the number of false-negatives (FN). FP corresponds to spuriously segmented nuclei and FN corresponds to nuclei that have not been segmented. In all our experiments, we used for our two-step segmentation approach in the first step the parameter values $\nu = 0.5$ and $\lambda = 100$, and in the second step, $\nu = 10$ and $\lambda = 1000$. The values for λ and ν were chosen empirically based on a subset of the data and yielded the best results. The scale parameter σ was chosen empirically based on the observed average size of cell nuclei. For the U20S, NIH3T3, and N1E115 datasets we used $\sigma = 16$ and for the Drosophila dataset, we chose $\sigma = 3$. Note, that for the Drosophila dataset, the resolution of the images is much smaller compared to the other three datasets. Therefore, the cells are much smaller in the images and a smaller value for the scale parameter is better suited. For the U20S and NIH3T3 datasets, we used a dilation of the segmented regions by $d = 28$ (second step of our approach), and for the N1E115 and Drosophila datasets we used $d = 5$. To initialize the minimization scheme, we used the image intensities normalized with respect to the maximum intensity.

Table 10.1 shows the results of our two-step segmentation approach for the different performance measures averaged over all images in the U20S and NIH3T3 datasets. Table 10.2 shows the results averaged over all images in the N1E115 and Drosophila datasets. As a comparison, we also give the results for Otsu thresholding [35] as well as for the watershed algorithm [36] and the merging algorithm [2] applied to the mean thresholded image. The latter approach uses an improved watershed algorithm followed by statistical model-based region merging to cope with oversegmentation and yielded the best results in the evaluation study of Coelho et al. [32]. Also, we included the result of the non-convex functional E_2 in Equation 10.12 from Rousson and Deriche [26], which was used in Dzyubachyk et al. [20]. We also provided the result of the non-convex functional E_1 in Equation 10.11 from Li et al. [27]. In addition, we show the results for the convex functional E_1^c and the convex functional E_2^c. Moreover, we included the result of manual segmentation (for a subset of five images for each dataset) by a different observer than the one who provided the ground truth (second row, "Manual").

From Table 10.1, it can be seen that the two-step approach yields the best results for the Dice coefficient, the NSD, and the Hausdorff distance for both datasets, and that the results are comparable to the results by the different observer ("Manual"). In particular, for the more challenging NIH3T3 images, we obtain significantly better results than previous approaches. Furthermore, it can be seen that the two-step approach yields better results than the convex Bayesian functional E_2^c (which is the second step of the two-step approach). Also, the two-step approach yields better results than the convex region-scalable fitting functional E_1^c (which is the first step of the two-step approach). Thus, the multiple step scheme is advantageous. In addition, it can be seen that the convex Bayesian functional E_2^c yields better results than the non-convex Bayesian functional E_2. Also, the convex region-scalable fitting functional E_1^c yields better results than the corresponding non-convex functional E_1. For the FP value the results of the two-step approach are equally good or comparable to the best results of the other approaches. Compared to the merging algorithm, the two-step approach allows better splitting of clustered cell nuclei, copes better with spurious objects (see Figure 10.5c,e), and yields more accurate results for the cell nuclei shapes (see Figure 10.5d,f).

The results in Table 10.2 for the N1E115 and Drosophila datasets are similar to those in Table 10.1. It can be seen that for both datasets our two-step approach yields the best results for the Dice coefficient, the NSD, the Hausdorff distance, and that the results are comparable to those by the different observer ("Manual"). Note that for this dataset Otsu thresholding and watershed yield good results for the Dice coefficient and the NSD, however, Otsu thresholding has a relatively high FP value and watershed has a relatively high FN value. The non-convex Bayesian functional E_2 and the convex Bayesian functional E_2^c yield not so good results because the contrast between cells within large clusters often is too low and therefore the cells are merged in the segmentation. Compared to E_2 and E_2^c, the non-convex and convex region-scalable fitting functionals E_1 and E_1^c yield better results. Regarding the FP value, the two-step approach yields results comparable to the best result for the N1E115 dataset and intermediate results for the Drosophila dataset. For the FN value, the two-step approach yields the best results.

Table 10.1 Quantitative results for U20S and NIH3T3 datasets using different segmentation approaches

Approach	U20S cells (48 images)					NIH3T3 cells (49 images)				
	Dice	NSD	Hausdorff	FP	FN	Dice	NSD	Hausdorff	FP	FN
Manual	0.93	0.04	9.8	0.6	2.2	0.87	0.07	12.1	0.0	3.2
Otsu	0.87	0.12	34.8	**0.3**	5.5	0.64	0.35	36.7	1.7	26.4
Watershed	0.69	0.36	34.3	1.9	3.0	0.62	0.37	19.1	11.6	5.5
Merging algorithm	0.92	0.08	13.3	1.0	3.3	0.70	0.28	19.0	7.0	5.8
Non-convex E_1 in Equation 10.11	0.84	0.14	20.6	2.4	4.9	0.78	0.18	15.6	4.8	4.7
Convex E_1^c in Equation 10.20	0.89	0.09	16.7	1.0	3.5	0.78	0.19	15.4	5.3	**4.7**
Non-convex E_2 in Equation 10.12	0.88	0.15	25.2	1.5	**2.8**	0.76	0.24	21.9	3.5	5.2
Convex E_2^c in Equation 10.20	0.93	0.11	18.1	1.4	3.2	0.84	0.23	21.0	3.3	8.6
Two-step approach	**0.94**	**0.05**	**12.8**	0.5	3.8	**0.85**	**0.12**	**14.2**	2.8	6.1

Table 10.2 Quantitative results for N1E115 and Drosophila datasets using different segmentation approaches

Approach	N1E115 cells (7 images)					Drosophila cells (16 images)				
	Dice	NSD	Hausdorff	FP	FN	Dice	NSD	Hausdorff	FP	FN
Manual	0.92	0.06	4.9	0.0	1.8	0.80	0.24	4.4	1.2	0.4
Otsu	0.82	0.17	10.0	4.7	8.1	0.82	0.20	5.5	9.3	4.0
Watershed	0.49	0.71	24.2	**0.0**	7.7	0.80	0.23	4.7	0.9	10.5
Merging algorithm	0.72	0.34	13.6	0.14	4.1	0.67	0.43	9.7	**0.0**	18.1
Non-convex E_1 in Equation 10.11	0.88	0.10	8.4	0.6	3.7	0.79	0.23	5.2	7.6	8.9
Convex E_1^c in Equation 10.20	0.88	0.10	8.3	0.3	3.4	0.82	0.19	4.7	3.3	3.4
Non-convex E_2 in Equation 10.12	0.71	0.37	21.0	1.9	4.0	0.43	0.77	24.1	1.4	33.7
Convex E_2^c in Equation 10.20	0.73	0.33	18.5	1.1	3.4	0.51	0.66	20.0	2.3	29.6
Two-step approach	**0.90**	**0.10**	**6.7**	0.4	**3.0**	0.82	**0.19**	**4.0**	2.9	**3.4**

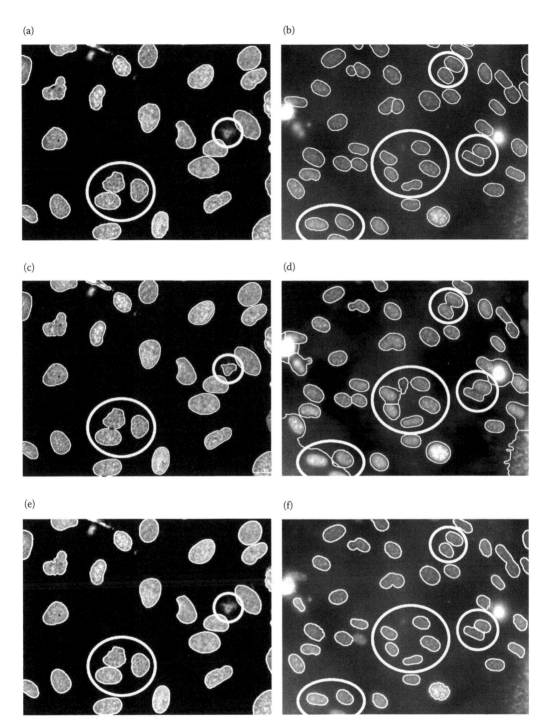

Figure 10.5 Segmentation results of different approaches (contour overlays with original images). First column: U20S cells, second column: NIH3T3 cells; first row: ground truth, second row: merging algorithm of Lin et al. [2], third row: two-step approach.

In our approach, the minimization of the convex Bayesian functional E_2^c in Equation 10.20 for a whole image with a size of 1349×1030 pixels converges after about five iterations and the computation time is approximately 15 seconds per image (using an Intel Xeon CPU X5550, 2.67GHz, with 48 GB RAM, and Linux 64 bit). In comparison, using a standard level set scheme for the non-convex Bayesian functional E_2 in Equation 10.12 with gradient descent optimization needs about 400 iterations and the computation time is about 9 minutes. For the convex region-scalable fitting functional E_1^c, our approach converges after about 10 iterations (ca. 100 seconds) while the optimization for the non-convex functional E_1 in Equation 10.11 needs about 1000 iterations (ca. 35 minutes). Thus, our approach is significantly faster. As convergence criterion we used the average Euclidean distance between the contours of segmented objects in two successive iterations.

10.7 Discussion

We have described a level set approach based on convex energy functionals for cell nuclei segmentation in fluorescence microscopy images. Since convex functionals are used, the global solution is obtained compared to non-convex functionals, which suffer from local minima. Our approach employs two different convex energy functionals, the convex region-scalable fitting energy functional and the convex Bayesian functional, and consists of two main steps. In the first step, the region-scalable fitting energy functional is used, which can cope with spatially local mean intensity values in comparison to the Bayesian functional, which is based on global mean intensity values. In the second step, the Bayesian functional is used, which allows us to deal with inhomogeneities at the border of cell nuclei. By combining the two convex functionals, we can cope with both global intensity inhomogeneities and local intensity inhomogeneities. Another advantage of our two-step approach is that small intensity differences between neighboring cell nuclei or even between overlapping cell nuclei make cluster splitting feasible. To minimize the convex energy functionals, we use the split Bregman method, which is an efficient method for $L1$-regularized problems and which significantly reduces the computation time compared to standard level set approaches. Thus, our approach is suitable for high-throughput applications and very large datasets. We have demonstrated the applicability of our approach using fluorescence microscopy image datasets from four different experiments comprising four different cell types. From the experiments, it turned out that the two-step approach can cope with images of different cell types. We also found that the two-step approach yields superior results compared to previous approaches. Recently, we extended our approach for application to 3D image data [37].

Acknowledgments

Support of the BMBF projects FANCI and ImmunoQuant (e:Bio) and the EU project SysPatho (FP7) is gratefully acknowledged. We thank Luis Pedro Coelho (CMU) for help with his software.

References

1. C. Wåhlby, J. Lindblad, M. Vondrus, E. Bengtsson, and L. Björkesten, Algorithms for cytoplasm segmentation of fluorescence labelled cells, *Analytical Cellular Pathology*, vol. 24, no. 2, pp. 101–111, 2002.

2. G. Lin, U. Adiga, K. Olson, J. F. Guzowski, C. A. Barnes, and B. Roysam, A hybrid 3D watershed algorithm incorporating gradient cues and object models for automatic segmentation of nuclei in confocal image stacks, *Cytometry A*, vol. 56, no. 1, pp. 23–36, 2003.

3. J. Cheng and J. C. Rajapakse, Segmentation of clustered nuclei with shape markers and marking function, *IEEE Transactions on Biomedical Engineering*, vol. 56, no. 3, pp. 741–748, 2009.

4. C. Jung and C. Kim, Segmenting clustered nuclei using H-minima transform-based marker extraction and contour parameterization, *IEEE Transactions on Biomedical Engineering*, vol. 57, no. 10, pp. 2600–2604, 2010.

5. M. Kass, A. Witkin, and D. Terzopoulos, Snakes: Active contour models, *International Journal of Computer Vision*, vol. 1, no. 4, pp. 321–331, 1988.

6. S. Osher and J. A. Sethian, Fronts propagating with curvature-dependent speed: algorithms based on Hamilton-Jacobi formulations, *Journal of Computational Physics*, vol. 79, no. 1, pp. 12–49, 1988.

7. C. Zimmer and J. C. Olivo-Marin, Coupled parametric active contours, *IEEE Transactions on Pattern Analysis and Machine Intelligence*, vol. 27, no. 11, pp. 1838–1842, 2005.

8. X. Wang, W. He, D. Metaxas, R. Mathew, and E. White, Cell segmentation and tracking using texture-adaptive snakes, in *Proc. IEEE International Symposium on Biomedical Imaging (ISBI 2007)*, IEEE. Washington DC, April 2007, pp. 101–104.

9. M. Butenuth and C. Heipke, Network snakes: Graph-based object delineation with active contour models, *Machine Vision and Applications*, vol. 23, no. 1, pp. 1–19, 2011.

10. C. Ortiz de Solórzano, R. Malladi, S. Lelievre, and S. J. Lockett, Segmentation of nuclei and cells using membrane related protein markers, *Journal of Microscopy*, vol. 201, no. 3, pp. 404–415, 2001.

11. A. Dufour, V. Shinin, S. Tajbakhsh, N. Guillen-Aghion, J.-C. Olivo- Marin, and C. Zimmer, Segmenting and tracking fluorescent cells in dynamic 3-D microscopy with coupled active surfaces, *IEEE Transactions on Image Processing*, vol. 14, no. 9, pp. 1396–1410, 2005.

12. S. K. Nath, K. Palaniappan, and F. Bunyak, Cell segmentation using coupled level sets and graph-vertex coloring, in *Proceedings of the International Conference on Medical Image Computing and Computer-Assisted Intervention (MICCAI 2006), Part I*, Vol. 4190, Lecture Notes in Computer Science, R. Larsen, M. Nielsen, and J. Sporring, Eds. Heidelberg: Springer, 2006, pp. 101–108.

13. H. Chang, Q. Yang, and B. Parvin, Segmentation of heterogeneous blob objects through voting and level set formulation, *Pattern Recognition Letters*, vol. 28, no. 13, pp. 1781–1787, 2007.

14. K. Palaniappan, I. Ersoy, and S. Nath, Moving object segmentation using the flux tensor for biological video microscopy, *Advances in Multimedia Information Processing (PCM 2007)*, pp. 483–493, 2007.

15. P. Yan, X. Zhou, M. Shah, and S. T. C. Wong, Automatic segmentation of high-throughput RNAi fluorescent cellular images, *IEEE Transactions on Information Technnology in Biomedicine*, vol. 12, no. 1, pp. 109–117, 2008.

16. M. Maška, O. Daněk, C. Ortiz de Solórzano, A. Muñoz-Barrutia, M. Kozubek, and I. García, A two-phase segmentation of cell nuclei using fast level set-like algorithms, *16th Scandinavian Conference on Image Analysis*, pp. 390–399, 2009.

17. K. Mosaliganti, A. Gelas, A. Gouaillard, R. Noche, N. Obholzer, and S. Megason, Detection of spatially correlated objects in 3D images using appearance models and coupled active contours, *Proceedings of the International Conference on Medical Image Computing and Computer-Assisted Intervention (MICCAI 2009), Part II*, Vol. 5762, Lecture Notes in Computer Science G.-Z. Yang, D. J. Hawkes, D. Rueckert, J. Alison Noble, and C. J. Taylor, Eds. Heidelberg: Springer, 2009, pp. 641–648.

18. D. Padfield, J. Rittscher, N. Thomas, and B. Roysam, Spatio-temporal cell cycle phase analysis using level sets and fast marching methods, *Medical Image Analysis*, vol. 13, no.1, pp. 143–155, 2009.

19. I. Ersoy, F. Bunyak, V. Chagin, M. Cardoso, and K. Palaniappan, Segmentation and classification of cell cycle phases in fluorescence imaging, *Proceedings of the International Conference on Medical Image Computing and Computer-Assisted Intervention (MICCAI 2009), Part II*, Vol. 5762, Lecture

Notes in Computer Science, G.-Z. Yang, D. J. Hawkes, D. Rueckert, J. Alison Noble, and C. J. Taylor. Heidelberg: Springer, 2009, pp. 617–624.

20. O. Dzyubachyk, W. A. van Cappellen, J. Essers, W. J. Niessen, and E. H. W. Meijering, Advanced level set-based cell tracking in time-lapse fluorescence microscopy, *IEEE Transactions on Medical Imaging*, vol. 29, no. 3, pp. 852–867, 2010.

21. J. Xu, A. Janowczyk, S. Chandran, and A. Madabhushi, A high-throughput active contour scheme for segmentation of histopathological imagery, *Medical Image Analysis*, vol. 15, no. 6, pp. 851–862, 2011.

22. X. Qi, F. Xing, D.J. Foran, and L. Yang, Robust segmentation of overlapping cells in histopathology specimens using parallel seed detection and repulsive level set, *IEEE Transactions on Biomedical Engineering*, vol. 59, no. 3, pp. 754–765, 2012.

23. M. Maška, O. Daněk, S. Garasa, A. Rouzaut, A. Muñoz-Barrutia, and C. Ortiz de Solórzano, Segmentation and shape tracking of whole fluorescent cells based on the Chan–Vese model, *IEEE Transactions on Medical Imaging*, vol. 32, no. 6, pp. 995–1006, 2013.

24. X. Yang and D. Padfield, Wavelet-initialized 3D level-set cell segmentation with local background support, in *Proc. IEEE International Symposium on Biomedical Imaging (ISBI 2014)*. IEEE. Beijing, China, April 2014, pp. 814–817.

25. Z. Lu, G. Carneiro, and A.P. Bradley, An improved joint optimization of multiple level set functions for the segmentation of overlapping cervical cells, *IEEE Transactions on Image Processing*, vol. 24, no. 4, pp. 1261–1272, 2015.

26. M. Rousson and R. Deriche, A variational framework for active and adaptative segmentation of vector valued images, in: *Proceedings of the Workshop on Motion and Video Computing*, IEEE Computer Society, 2002, pp. 56–62.

27. C. Li, C.Y. Kao, J.C. Gore, and Z. Ding, Minimization of region-scalable fitting energy for image segmentation, *IEEE Transactions on Image Processing*, vol. 17, no. 10, pp. 1940–1949, 2008.

28. T. F. Chan and L. A. Vese, Active contours without edges, *IEEE Transactions on Image Processing*, vol. 10, no. 2, pp. 266–277, 2001.

29. T. F. Chan, S. Esedoglu, and M. Nikolova, Algorithms for finding global minimizers of image segmentation and denoising models, *SIAM Journal on Applied Mathematics*, vol. 66, pp. 1632–1648, 2006.

30. T. Goldstein, X. Bresson, and S. Osher. Geometric applications of the split Bregman method: Segmentation and surface reconstruction, *Journal of Scientific Computing*, vol. 45, no. 1, pp. 272–293, 2010.

31. D. Mumford and J. Shah, Optimal approximations by piecewise smooth functions and associated variational problems, *Communications on Pure and Applied Mathematics*, vol. 42, no. 5, pp. 577–685, 1989.

32. L. P. Coelho, A. Shariff, and R. F. Murphy, Nuclear segmentation in microscope cell images: a hand-segmented dataset and comparison of algorithms, in *Proceedings of the IEEE International Symposium on Biomedical Imaging (ISBI 2009)*, Boston, MA, June 2009, pp. 518–521.

33. W. Yu, H. K. Lee, S. Hariharan, W. Bu, and S. Ahmed, Evolving generalized Voronoi diagrams for accurate cellular image segmentation, *Cytometry A*, vol. 77, no. 4, pp. 379–386, 2010.

34. T. Jones, A. Carpenter, and P. Golland, Voronoi-based segmentation of cells on image manifolds, in *Proceedings of the First International Workshop on Computer Vision for Biomedical Image Applications*. Berlin: Springer, 2005, pp. 535–543.

35. N. Otsu. A threshold selection method from gray-level histograms, *IEEE Trans actions on Systems and Managing Cybernetics*, vol. 9, no. 1, pp. 62–66, 1979.

36. L. Vincent and P. Soille, Watersheds in digital spaces: An efficient algorithm based on immersion simulations, *IEEE Transactions on Pattern Analysis and Machine Intelligence*, vol. 13, no. 6, pp. 583–598, 1991.

37. J.-P. Bergeest and K. Rohr, Segmentation of cell nuclei in 3D microscopy images based on level set deformable models and convex minimization, in *Proceedings of the IEEE International Symposium on Biomedical Imaging (ISBI 2014)*, Beijing, China, April 2014, pp. 637–640.

chapter eleven

Histogram-based level set methods for medical image segmentation

Wei Yu and Jifeng Ning

Contents

Abstract

Medical image segmentation is a key and fundamental operation in medical image analysis. Many studies have been dedicated to this field and have proposed different techniques or variations, but medical image segmentation is still a challenge due to low contrast, noise, complex shape, and so on. This chapter introduces histogram-based level set methods for medical image segmentation, which evolve level set functions by measuring the similarity of histograms. Without preprocessing, we show a comparable segmentation result on brain image using a simple gradient descent or gradient ascend method.

11.1   Introduction

Medical image analysis is a promising and fast-developing field in the interdisciplinary science of medicine and computer science in the hope of automatic diagnosis and operation. Image segmentation plays a key role in the medical image analysis and is an important preprocessing for the further operations [1–6]. In general, image segmentation is defined as "an image segmentation is the partition of an image into a set of nonoverlapping regions whose union is the entire image. The purpose of segmentation is to decompose the image into parts that are meaningful with respect to a particular application" [7]. In a specific application such as medical image analysis, image segmentation usually involves prior knowledge and semantic meaning, for example, detection and segmentation of tumor, traumatic injury, or other abnormalities for the diagnosis or measurement; annotation organs for anatomy; the preprocessing for fixing the location in robotic surgery. There are various medical images modalities, such as computed tomography (CT), magnetic resonance imaging (MRI), positron emission tomography (PET), and so on [8].

Active contour models have gained popularity a few decades ago. The idea of active contour model is to divide an image into foreground and background. An initial curve is placed on the image and it evolves according to the defined constraints or force. There are two ways to implement this curve:

1. Explicit approach: Snakes [9]
2. Implicit approach: Level set methods [10]

In this chapter, we focus on level set methods [11–13] for 2D medical image segmentation.

11.1.1   Level set method

In the level set method, the boundary of the region of interest (e.g., tumor, tissue) is represented by a curve c. One main merit of the level set method is that there is no need to parameterize the curve. The level set method uses one higher-dimension information to represent a curve implicitly. For example, the level set method imbeds a 2D curve within a surface. This makes the level set method very easy to follow the shapes that change topology, that is, merging and breaking.

Figure 11.1 illustrates how the level set method represents a curve. As shown by Figure 11.1, the red surface is defined by a function $\phi : \mathbb{R}^2 \to \mathbb{R}$, which is called a level set function. The blue plane indicates zero horizontal plane, which intersects ϕ at a curve c (the zero level set, $\phi = 0$). This curve is the boundary of the region of interest (the upper gray graphics). We denote the region of an image by Ω. The region of interest is denoted by Ω^+. If $\in \Omega^+$, $\phi(x) > 0$. Similarly, the background is denoted by $\Omega^- : \{x|\phi(x) < 0\}$. The zero level set c is denoted by $\partial\Omega$.

11.1.1.1   Signed distance functions

As shown in Figure 11.1, the red surface is smooth. The smoothness of level set function is a necessary for the stability of level set method. One reason is that a smooth level set function assures a reliable numerical approximation. For example, the curvature of the curve embedded in a surface can be calculated as,

$$k = \left(\phi_x^2 \phi_{yy} - 2\phi_x \phi_y \phi_{xy} + \phi_y^2 \phi_{xx} \right) / |\nabla\phi|^3.$$

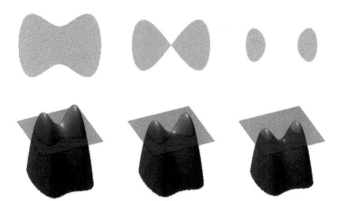

Figure 11.1 An illustration of the level set method. (Taken from Wikipedia http://en. wikipedia.org/wiki/Level_set_method.)

where ϕ_x and ϕ_{xx} are the first partial derivative and the second partial derivative of ϕ with respect to x coordinate, respectively. The other derivatives are defined in a similar manner. The numerical methods to calculate derivatives include a first-order accurate forward or backward difference, a second-order accurate central difference, or more advanced upwind differencing. And these numerical methods depend on the smoothness of function.

Signed distance functions are the good options for the level set function. Besides the smoothness, signed distance functions have the following property:

$$|\nabla \phi| = 1$$

where

$$\nabla \phi = \left(\frac{\partial \phi}{\partial x}, \frac{\partial \phi}{\partial y} \right).$$

The signed distance function is defined as follows:

$$\phi(x) = \begin{cases} d(x) & \forall x \in \Omega^+ \\ 0 & \forall x \in \partial\Omega \\ -d(x) & \forall x \in \Omega^- \end{cases},$$

$$d(x) = \min_{x_I}(\|x - x_I\|_2) \quad \forall x_I \in \partial\Omega.$$

Intuitively, $d(x)$ is the closest distance between x and x_I.

Figure 11.2 shows an example of a signed distance function. The upper image is a brain image[*] [14–17]. The zero level set is depicted by the blue curve. The level set function is shown in the lower figure. We can observe along the blue curve, the level set function equals zero. Inside the blue curve, the level set function is larger than zero. And outside the blue curve, the level set function is less than zero.

11.1.1.2 Heaviside function

As shown above, it is a key step to distinguish the foreground ($\Omega^+ : \{x | \phi(x) \geq 0\}$) and background ($\Omega^- : \{x | \phi(x) < 0\}$). In the level set method, it is convenient to introduce Heaviside

---

[*] http://www.bic.mni.mcgill.ca/brainweb/.

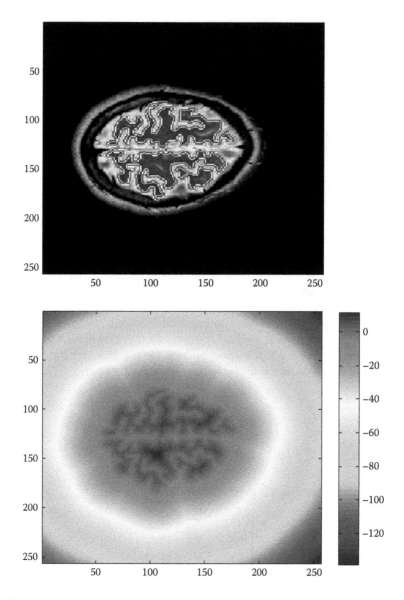

Figure 11.2 Illustration of a curve (upper) and level set function (lower).

function $H : \mathbb{R} \to \mathbb{R}$,

$$H(\phi) = \begin{cases} 1 & \phi \geq 0 \\ 0 & \phi < 0 \end{cases}.$$

The calculation can be simplified by using the Heaviside function H. For example, we can use

$$\int_{\Omega} f(x) H(\phi(x)) \, dx$$

to calculate the area (the number of pixels) of the region of interest (foreground Ω^{+}).

11.1.1.3 A simple example

Let the circle and its boundary be the region of interest Ω^+ and the zero level set, respectively. The gradient of ϕ is denoted by $\nabla\phi$, which is perpendicular to the zero level set. Because we define $\phi > 0$ in the region of interest Ω^+ and define $\phi < 0$ in the background Ω^-, the unit normal $\vec{N}$ points to Ω^+,

$$\vec{N} = \frac{\nabla\phi}{|\nabla\phi|}.$$

We show the unit normal $\vec{N}$ by the green arrows in Figure 11.3. If we use a signed distance function as the level set function, then $\vec{N}$ can be simplified as

$$\vec{N} = \nabla\phi,$$

because of $|\nabla\phi| = 1$.

Suppose the zero level set moves with a velocity $\vec{v}$, one can have

$$\phi(x, t - \nabla t) = \phi(x + \vec{v}\nabla t, t).$$

Let ∇t be sufficient small, the Taylor-expansion of both sides gives

$$\phi(x, t) - \nabla t \frac{\partial\phi(x, t)}{\partial t} \cong \phi(x, t) + \vec{v}^T \nabla t \frac{\partial\phi(x, t)}{\partial x}.$$

Finally, one can write

$$\frac{\partial\phi(x, t)}{\partial t} + \vec{v}^T \nabla\phi = 0.$$

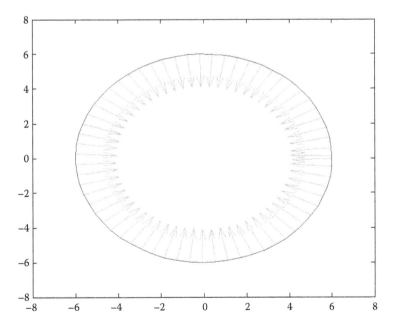

Figure 11.3 The zero level set and its normal vector.

This is called an advection equation and also referred to as the level set equation. If the zero level set has a constant motion in the normal direction $\vec{N}$, then $\vec{v}$ is defined as

$$\vec{v} = a\vec{N} = a\frac{\nabla\phi}{|\nabla\phi|}.$$

Finally, we arrive at

$$\frac{\partial\phi(x,t)}{\partial t} + a|\nabla\phi| = 0.$$

A wealth of papers in the computer vision literature address variations of level set equations. They usually propose an energy function, then calculate its gradient, and finally end up with a level set equation [18–21]. In this chapter, we mainly focus on histogram-based segmentation methods, which will be discussed in Section 11.2.

11.1.2   Prior information: Histogram

The region of interest to be segmented is characterized by a histogram over some photo-metric variable, for example, intensity, color, and texture. In the experiment of this chapter, let u be the quantified photometric variable of interest and m be the number of bins. To construct a histogram, one divides the data range in m bins. For example, if the data range is [0–255] (gray image) and $m = 16$, the interval is 16. That is, if data are in the range [0–15], they belong to the first bin; if data are in the range [16–31], they belong to the second bin and so on. We denote by $\mathbf{q}$ the histogram of the region of interest and by $\mathbf{o}$ the histogram of the background. Then we have

$$\mathbf{q} = \{q_u\}_{u=1,\ldots m} \quad \sum_{u=1}^{m} q_u = 1,$$

$$\mathbf{o} = \{o_u\}_{u=1,\ldots m} \quad \sum_{u=1}^{m} o_u = 1.$$

The region of interest is a prior input, which is usually drawn by a user. We calculate the foreground histogram $\mathbf{q}$ and background histogram $\mathbf{o}$ based on the region of interest. We take Figure 11.4 as an example. In Figure 11.4, the region enclosed by the blue curve is the foreground; the region between the blue curve and red curve is the background. Note we can decide the range of background according to the application.

Let b(x) be a function mapping x into the corresponding quantified photometric variable (the index of bin). In 2D gray image segmentation, b(x) gives the corresponding bin of an image at x. It is convenient to compute q_u and o_u by using the Heaviside function H,

$$q_u(\phi) = \frac{\iint_{\phi>-l} H(\phi(x))\delta(b(x) - u)\,dx}{\iint_{\phi>-l} H(\phi(x))dx},$$

$$o_u(\phi) = \frac{\iint_{\phi>-l} (1 - H(\phi(x)))\delta(b(x) - u)dx}{\iint_{\phi>-l} (1 - H(\phi(x)))dx},$$

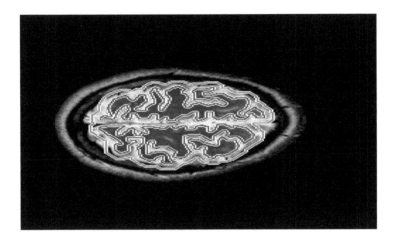

Figure 11.4 Illustration of foreground and background.

where $\delta(x) : \mathbb{R} \to \mathbb{R}$ is Kronecker delta function of x:

$$\delta(x) = \begin{cases} 1 & x = 0 \\ 0 & x \neq 0 \end{cases}.$$

In the region of interest, the level set function $\phi(\mathbf{x}) > 0$. So, the Heaviside function $H(\phi(\mathbf{x})) = 1$. In the background, the level set function $\phi(\mathbf{x}) < 0$. So, the Heaviside function $H(\phi(\mathbf{x})) = 0$. In most cases, it is not necessary to consider the complement of the region of interest as the background. As the equations above, we can only consider the background $\{\mathbf{x}| -l < \phi(\mathbf{x}) < 0\}$ and l is a tuning parameter. It is worth noting that the denominator of $q_u(\phi)$ is the area of the region of interest and the denominator of $o_u(\phi)$ is the area of the background.

11.1.2.1 Why use a prior histogram?

For the problem of medical image segmentation, prior knowledge is usually available [22,23]. Grau et al. [22] presented an improved watershed transform that enables the introduction of prior information in its calculation. This method was applied to knee cartilage segmentation and white matter–gray matter segmentation in MR brain images. Chittajallu Medical et al. [23] incorporated prior knowledge constraints into the Maximum A Posteriori (MAP) estimation of a Markov Random Field (MRF) formulation of the segmentation problem and applied it to heart segmentation.

As a kind of prior information, a histogram becomes increasingly popular [24–26]. A histogram gives an estimation of the distribution of data. In the segmentation of medical images, some medical images of different people or medical images of one person in different period do not have big difference in the histogram. Although one can construct a more precise histogram with a larger number of bins *m*, it is sensible to the noise that does not lead to a good segmentation.

11.1.3 The histogram matching criteria

This section introduces the matching criteria [27–30], which are commonly used in probability theory. To avoid confusion, the input prior histogram is denoted by **q** for foreground and **o** for background. Given the prior histogram **q** or **o**, we need to measure the similarity between the prior histogram and the predicted histogram. Let the histogram of the predicted foreground be $\mathbf{p}(\phi)$ and the histogram of its background be $\mathbf{v}(\phi)$. For the brevity of illustration, in this section, we only measure the similarity between **q** and $\mathbf{p}(\phi)$. And it is straightforward to apply the criteria to **o** and $\mathbf{v}(\phi)$.

11.1.3.1   *Kullback–Leibler divergence*

For discrete histograms **q** and $\mathbf{p}(\phi)$, the KL divergence of $\mathbf{p}(\phi)$ from **q** is defined as

$$D_{KL}(\mathbf{q}\|\mathbf{p}(\phi)) = \sum_{u=1}^{m} q_u \ln \frac{q_u}{p_u(\phi)}.$$

According to the property of logarithm, we also can write the above equation as

$$D_{KL}(\mathbf{q}\|\mathbf{p}(\phi)) = \sum_{u=1}^{m} q_u \ln(q_u) - q_u \ln(p_u(\phi)).$$

Thus, the Kullback–Leibler (KL) divergence is the expectation of the logarithm of difference between **q** and $\mathbf{p}(\phi)$ based on the probabilities **q**. It measures the information lost when the "approximation" $\mathbf{p}(\phi)$ is used to approximate the "ground truth" **q** [31]. KL divergence will be zero if $\mathbf{p}(\phi)$ is the same as **q**.

11.1.3.2   *The Bhattacharyya coefficient*

The Bhattacharyya coefficient approximately measures the amount of overlap between two statistical samples. It determines the relative closeness of the two histograms. The Bhattacharyya coefficient is defined as

$$B(\mathbf{q}, \mathbf{p}(\phi)) = \sum_{u=1}^{m} \sqrt{q_u p_u(\phi)}$$

The Bhattacharyya coefficient will be zero if there is no overlap between **q** and $\mathbf{p}(\phi)$. The more similar **q** and $\mathbf{p}(\phi)$ are, the larger Bhattacharyya coefficient is.

11.2   Histogram-based level set methods for medical image segmentation

This section introduces two histogram-based level set methods for medical image segmentation. The first method is "foreground matching with background mismatching" proposed by Zhang and Freedman [27]. The second method is "foreground and background matching" proposed by Ning et al. [28]. Both methods were originally proposed to solve the problem of tracking a nonrigid object by segmentation of each frame. They [27,28] show that the importance and robustness of using background information rather than only using the foreground matching [30]. The following sections introduce both methods [27,28] based on the calculus of variations [28,29]. Calculus of variations is a theory of finding the extrema of functionals. In the following sections, we define the functional E of the level set function ϕ. Then we derive its solution by Euler–Lagrange differential equation, which is a fundamental equation in the calculus of variations.

11.2.1   Foreground matching with background mismatching

Foreground matching with background mismatching [27] is proposed as a variation of foreground matching [30]. Given a prior histogram of the region of interest, foreground matching [30] is to find a region within an image, such that its histogram most closely matches the prior histogram. But this method can be quite sensitive to the initialization. Thus foreground matching with background mismatching [27] adds the mismatching between the prior histogram of foreground and the histogram of the predicted background. This improves the robustness. Two matching criteria (KL divergence and Bhattacharyya coefficient) are examined in Zhang and Freedman [27].

11.2.1.1   Energy based on KL divergence
The functional E is defined as,

$$E(\phi) = \lambda_1 D_{KL}(q\|p(\phi)) - \lambda_2 D_{KL}(q\|v(\phi))$$

where q is the prior histogram of the region of interest. The first term $D_{KL}(q, p(\phi))$ is the foreground matching term and the second term $-D_{KL}(q, v(\phi))$ is the background mismatching term. The coefficients $\lambda_1 > 0, \lambda_2 > 0$ tune weights of both terms. By substituting D_{KL} into $E(\phi)$, we arrive at

$$E(\phi) = \sum_{u=1}^{m} \left[\lambda_1 q_u \ln \frac{q_u}{p_u(\phi)} - \lambda_2 q_u \ln \frac{q_u}{v_u(\phi)} \right].$$

By the property of $\ln(a/b) = \ln a - \ln b$, we obtain

$$E(\phi) = \sum_{u=1}^{m} [\lambda_1 q_u (\ln q_u - \ln p_u(\phi)) - \lambda_2 q_u (\ln q_u - \ln v_u(\phi))].$$

A necessary condition for ϕ to yield the minimum of E is the variation of E, $\delta E = 0$. Note $\delta(x)$ is the Kronecker delta function of x; δE is the variation of E.

$$\delta E(\phi) = \sum_{u=1}^{m} \left[-\lambda_1 \frac{q_u}{p_u(\phi)} \delta p_u(\phi) + \lambda_2 \frac{q_u}{v_u(\phi)} \delta v_u(\phi) \right].$$

where $\delta p_u(\phi)$ is the variation of $p_u(\phi)$ and $\delta v_u(\phi)$ is the variation of $v_u(\phi)$. Refer to Appendix 11A for detail. By substituting $\delta p_u(\phi)$ and $\delta v_u(\phi)$ into $\delta E(\phi)$, we obtain

$$\delta E(\phi) = \iint_{\phi > -l} \left[\frac{\lambda_1 (p_{b(x)}(\phi) - q_{b(x)})}{N_f(\mathbf{b}(x), \phi)} + \frac{\lambda_2 (p_{b(x)}(\phi) - q_{b(x)})}{N_b(\mathbf{b}(x), \phi)} \right] \delta(\phi(x)) \, \delta\phi \, dx.$$

$\iint_{\phi>-l} H(\phi(x)) \, dx$ calculates the number of pixels in the predicted foreground and $\iint_{\phi>-l} (1 - H(\phi(x))) \, dx$ calculates the number of pixels in the corresponding background of the predicted foreground. We denoted $\iint_{\phi>-l} H(\phi(x)) \, dx$ by $A_f(\phi)$ and $\iint_{\phi>-l} (1 - H(\phi(x))) \, dx$ by $A_b(\phi)$. We denoted $p_{b(x)}(\phi) A_f(\phi)$ by $N_f(\mathbf{b}(x), \phi)$. $N_f(\mathbf{b}(x), \phi)$ is the number of pixels whose bin is $b(x)$ in the predicted foreground. Similarly, we denoted $v_{b(x)}(\phi) A_b(\phi)$ by $N_b(\mathbf{b}(x), \phi)$. Note in this chapter, we define $\phi > 0$ in the predicted foreground and $\phi < 0$ in the corresponding background. If we define $\phi < 0$ in the predicted foreground and $\phi > 0$ in the corresponding background, $\delta E(\phi)$ should be inverted to

$$
\delta E(\phi) = - \iint\limits_{\phi > -l} \left[\frac{\lambda_1(p_{b(x)}(\phi) - q_{b(x)})}{N_f(b(x), \phi)} + \frac{\lambda_2(v_{b(x)}(\phi) - q_{b(x)})}{N_b(b(x), \phi)} \right] \delta(\phi(x)) \delta\phi \, dx.
$$

Because $\delta\phi$ is the variation of the function ϕ, we obtain the Euler–Lagrange differential equation

$$
\left[\frac{\lambda_1(p_{b(x)}(\phi) - q_{b(x)})}{N_f(b(x), \phi)} + \frac{\lambda_2(v_{b(x)}(\phi) - q_{b(x)})}{N_b(b(x), \phi)} \right] \delta(\phi(x)) = 0.
$$

Thus the gradient descent with respect to the Euler–Lagrange differential yields the following evolution:

$$
\frac{\partial\phi}{\partial t} = - \left[\frac{\lambda_1(p_{b(x)}(\phi) - q_{b(x)})}{N_f(b(x), \phi)} + \frac{\lambda_2(v_{b(x)}(\phi) - q_{b(x)})}{N_b(b(x), \phi)} \right] \delta(\phi(x)).
$$

11.2.1.2   Energy based on the Bhattacharyya coefficient
The functional E is defined as

$$
E(\phi) = \lambda_1 B(q, p(\phi)) - \lambda_2 B(q, v(\phi))
$$

where q is the prior histogram of the foreground (the region of interest). The first term $B(q, p(\phi))$ is a foreground matching term and the second term $-B(q, v(\phi))$ is a background mismatching term. The coefficients $\lambda_1 > 0, \lambda_2 > 0$ tune weights of both terms. Because the more similar between q and $p(\phi)$, the larger Bhattacharyya coefficient is. Therefore gradient ascent is used to maximize $E(\phi)$. By substituting B into $E(\phi)$ we arrive at

$$
E(\phi) = \sum_{u=1}^{m} \left[\lambda_1 \sqrt{q_u p_u(\phi)} - \lambda_2 \sqrt{q_u v_u(\phi)} \right]
$$

The variation of E is

$$
\delta E(\phi) = \frac{1}{2} \sum_{u=1}^{m} \left[\lambda_1 \sqrt{\frac{q_u}{p_u(\phi)}} \delta p_u(\phi) - \lambda_2 \sqrt{\frac{q_u}{v_u(\phi)}} \delta v_u(\phi) \right].
$$

Appendix 11B describes the detailed derivation. By substituting $\delta p_u(\phi)$ and $\delta v_u(\phi)$ into $\delta E(\phi)$, we arrive at

$$
\delta E(\phi) = \frac{\lambda_1}{2A_f(\phi)} \left(\iint\limits_{\phi > -l} \left[\sqrt{\frac{q_{b(x)}}{p_{b(x)}(\phi)}} - B(q, p(\phi)) \right] \delta(\phi(x)) \, \delta\phi \, dx \right)
$$

$$
+ \frac{\lambda_2}{2A_b(\phi)} \left(\iint\limits_{\phi > -l} \left[\sqrt{\frac{q_{b(x)}}{v_{b(x)}(\phi)}} - B(q, v(\phi)) \right] \delta(\phi(x)) \, \delta\phi \, dx \right).
$$

Therefore the Euler–Lagrange differential equation is

$$\left\{\frac{\lambda_1}{2A_f(\phi)}\left[\sqrt{\frac{q_{b(x)}}{p_{b(x)}(\phi)}}-B(q,p(\phi))\right]+\frac{\lambda_2}{2A_b(\phi)}\left[\sqrt{\frac{q_{b(x)}}{v_{b(x)}(\phi)}}-B(q,v(\phi))\right]\right\}\delta(\phi(x))=0.$$

Thus the gradient ascent with respect to the Euler–Lagrange differential gives the following evolution:

$$\frac{\partial\phi}{\partial t}=\left\{\frac{\lambda_1}{2A_f(\phi)}\left[\sqrt{\frac{q_{b(x)}}{p_{b(x)}(\phi)}}-B(q,p(\phi))\right]+\frac{\lambda_2}{2A_b(\phi)}\left[\sqrt{\frac{q_{b(x)}}{v_{b(x)}(\phi)}}-B(q,v(\phi))\right]\right\}\delta(\phi(x)).$$

11.2.2 Foreground and background matching

Foreground and background matching [28] aims at finding a best candidate region whose foreground histogram and background histogram match maximally the prior foreground histogram and background separately by using Bhattacharyya coefficient. They [28] derive a level set equation.

11.2.2.1 Energy

Let the prior input histogram of the region of interest be q and the histogram of its background be o. Given an image, foreground and background matching is to find a region such that the histogram inside it is as close as to q at the same time the histogram outside it is as close as to o. Thus the energy is defined as

$$E(\phi)=B(q,p(\phi))+\alpha B(o,v(\phi))$$

where

$$B(q,p(\phi))=\sum_{u=1}^{m}\sqrt{q_u p_u(\phi)}\quad\text{and}\quad B(o,v(\phi))=\sum_{u=1}^{u=m}\sqrt{o_u v_u(\phi)}.$$

$B(q,p(\phi))$ and $B(o,v(\phi))$ are the Bhattacharyya coefficient measuring the similarity of the foreground and the background. The tuning parameter α balances the trade-off between foreground matching and background matching.

We plug $B(q,p(\phi))$ and $B(o,v(\phi))$ into $E(\phi)$ and we arrive at

$$E(\phi)=\sum_{u=1}^{m}\sqrt{q_u p_u(\phi)}+\alpha\sqrt{o_u v_u(\phi)}.$$

Thus $E(\phi)$ can be viewed as a functional of ϕ. By calculus of variations, one obtains

$$\delta E(\phi)=\frac{1}{2}\sum_{u=1}^{m}\left[\sqrt{\frac{q_u}{p_u(\phi)}}\delta p_u(\phi)+\alpha\sqrt{\frac{o_u}{v_u(\phi)}}\delta v_u(\phi)\right].$$

By the similar method as Section 11.2.1, we have

$$\delta E(\phi) = \frac{1}{2A_f(\phi)} \left(\iint\limits_{\phi > -l} \left[\sqrt{\frac{q_{b(x)}}{P_{b(x)}(\phi)}} - B(q, p(\phi)) \right] \delta(\phi(x)) \, \delta\phi \, dx \right)$$

$$- \frac{\alpha}{2A_b(\phi)} \left(\iint\limits_{\phi > -l} \left[\sqrt{\frac{o_{b(x)}}{v_{b(x)}(\phi)}} - B(o, v(\phi)) \right] \delta(\phi(x)) \, \delta\phi \, dx \right).$$

Therefore the Euler–Lagrange differential equation is

$$\left\{ \frac{1}{2A_f(\phi)} \left[\sqrt{\frac{q_{b(x)}}{P_{b(x)}(\phi)}} - B(q, p(\phi)) \right] - \frac{\alpha}{2A_b(\phi)} \left[\sqrt{\frac{o_{b(x)}}{v_{b(x)}(\phi)}} - B(o, v(\phi)) \right] \right\} \delta(\phi(x)) = 0.$$

According to the Euler–Lagrange differential equation, we obtain

$$\frac{\partial \phi}{\partial t} = \left\{ \frac{1}{2A_f(\phi)} \left[\sqrt{\frac{q_{b(x)}}{P_{b(x)}(\phi)}} - B(q, p(\phi)) \right] - \frac{\alpha}{2A_b(\phi)} \left[\sqrt{\frac{q_{b(x)}}{v_{b(x)}(\phi)}} - B(o, v(\phi)) \right] \right\} \delta(\phi(x)).$$

If we omit α, A_f, A_b, $B(q, p(\phi))$ and $B(o, v(\phi))$, then we can observe that if $\sqrt{q_{b(x)}/P_{b(x)}(\phi)}$ is large, that is the prior histogram value of $b(x)$ is larger than the histogram value of current predicted foreground by $\phi(x, t)$, then $\phi(x, t + 1)$ has a tendency to increase. This means $\phi(x, t + 1)$ is likely to become a pixel in the region of interest if $q_{b(x)} \gg p_{b(x)}(\phi)$. Similarly, if $\sqrt{o_{b(x)}/v_{b(x)}(\phi)}$ is large, then $\phi(x, t + 1)$ has a tendency to decrease. This means $\phi(x, t + 1)$ is likely to become a pixel in the background if $o_{b(x)} \gg v_{b(x)}(\phi)$.

11.3   *Result and discussion*

In this section we show the segmentation results of the histogram-based level set methods for the brain image.

We manually draw the region of interest in one brain image as shown in Figure 11.5. We calculate the histograms of the foreground and background based on the initialization. The foreground is the region inside the blue curve and the background is the region between the blue curve and red curve. The foreground histogram and the background histogram are depicted in Figures 11.6 and 11.7, respectively.

Figures 11.8 and 11.9 illustrate the segmentation results of foreground matching with background mismatching based on KL divergence and Bhattacharyya coefficient. And in Figure 11.10, we demonstrate the segmentation result of foreground and background matching based on Bhattacharyya coefficient. Although segmentation is an subjective problem, we can predict that the measure of KL divergence provides a succinct segmentation.

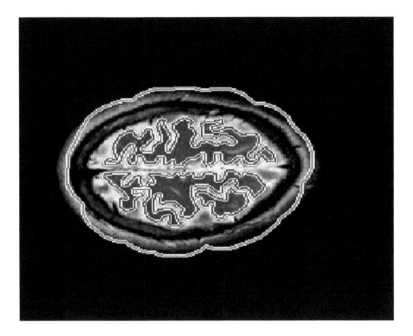

Figure 11.5 Initialization.

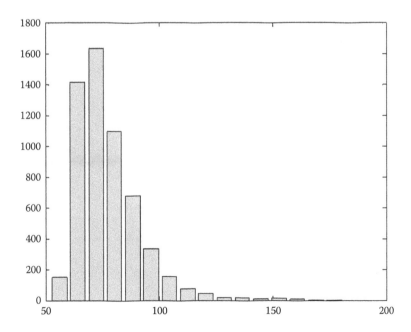

Figure 11.6 Histogram of the foreground.

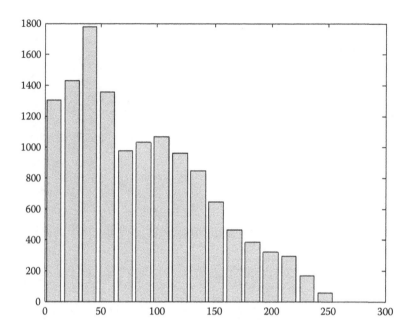

Figure 11.7 Histogram of the background.

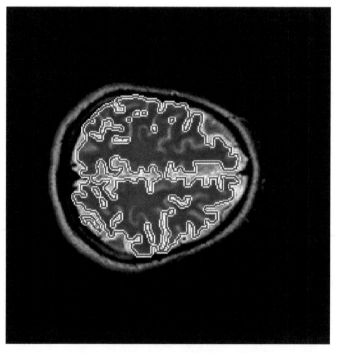

Figure 11.8 Segmentation result of foreground matching with background mismatching (KL divergence).

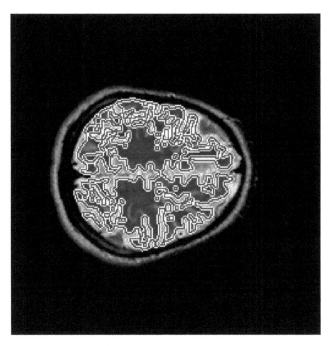

Figure 11.9 Segmentation result of foreground matching with background mismatching (Bhattacharyya coefficient).

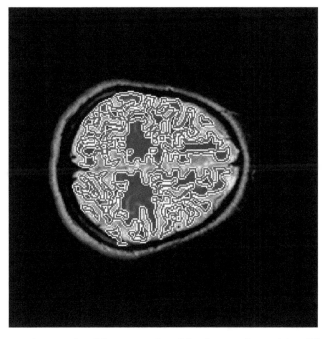

Figure 11.10 Segmentation result of foreground and background matching (Bhattacharyya coefficient).

11.4   Conclusion

The results show that histogram-based level set method can attain comparable segmentation if the prior histogram is close to the histogram of the region of interest. This kind of methods is different to the methods under the assumption of homogeneity in images. Histogram-based level set methods assume that histograms of foreground and background in a given image are similar to the prior histograms. We choose a photometric variable that can distinguish the foreground from the background. We do not consider preprocessing in this chapter, like smoothing and denoising. We suggest if the preprocessing helps to distinguish the foreground from background, then the preprocessing should be conducted. Also in this chapter we use the simple gradient descent or ascent method to calculate the solution. We suggest if we use a more advanced solver, the segmentation result would be better. For example, limited-memory Broyden–Fletcher–Goldfarb–Shanno algorithm is a popular solver. It suits the optimization problems whose value of energy and gradient of energy are available.

Appendix 11A

The variation of the energy E is,

$$\delta E(\phi) = \sum_{u=1}^{u=m} \left[-\lambda_1 \frac{q_u}{p_u(\phi)} \delta p_u(\phi) + \lambda_2 \frac{q_u}{v_u(\phi)} \delta v_u(\phi) \right].$$

where $\delta p_u(\phi)$ is the variation of $p_u(\phi)$ and $\delta v_u(\phi)$ is the variation of $v_u(\phi)$. $\iint_{\phi > -l} H(\phi(x)) \, dx$ calculates the number of pixels in the predicted foreground and $\iint_{\phi > -l} (1 - H(\phi(x))) \, dx$ calculates the number of pixels in the corresponding. We denoted $\iint_{\phi > -l} H(\phi(x)) \, dx$ by $A_f(\phi)$ and $\iint_{\phi > -l} (1 - H(\phi(x))) \, dx$ by $A_b(\phi)$.

According to the property of the variation, one obtains,

$$\delta p_u(\phi) = \frac{\iint_{\phi > -l} \delta(\phi(x)) \delta(b(x) - u) \delta\phi \, dx \, A_f(\phi)}{A_f(\phi)^2}$$

$$- \frac{\iint_{\phi > -l} \delta(\phi(x)) \delta\phi \, dx \iint_{\phi > -l} H(\phi(x)) \delta(b(x) - u) \, dx}{A_f(\phi)^2}$$

$$= \frac{\iint_{\phi > -l} \delta(\phi(x)) \delta(b(x) - u) \delta\phi \, dx}{A_f(\phi)} - \frac{\iint_{\phi > -l} \delta(\phi(x)) \delta\phi \, dx \, p_u(\phi)}{A_f(\phi)}$$

$$\delta v_u(\phi) = \frac{- \iint_{\phi > -l} \delta(\phi(x)) \delta(b(x) - u) \delta\phi \, dx \, A_b(\phi)}{A_b(\phi)^2}$$

$$+ \frac{\iint_{\phi > -l} \delta(\phi(x)) \delta\phi \, dx \iint_{\phi > -l} (1 - H(\phi(x))) \delta(b(x) - u) \, dx}{A_b(\phi)^2}$$

$$= \frac{- \iint_{\phi > -l} \delta(\phi(x)) \delta(b(x) - u) \delta\phi \, dx}{A_b(\phi)}$$

$$+ \frac{\iint_{\phi > -l} \delta(\phi(x)) \delta\phi \, dx \, v_u(\phi)}{A_b(\phi)}$$

Thus, by substituting $\delta p_u(\phi)$ and $\delta v_u(\phi)$ into δE, we arrive at,

$$\delta E(\phi) = -\lambda_1 \sum_{u=1}^{u=m} \frac{q_u}{p_u(\phi)} \left(\frac{\iint_{\phi>-l} \delta(\phi(x))\delta(b(x)-u)\delta\phi\,dx}{A_f(\phi)} - \frac{\iint_{\phi>-l} \delta(\phi(x))\delta\phi\,dx\,p_u(\phi)}{A_f(\phi)} \right)$$

$$+ \lambda_2 \sum_{u=1}^{u=m} \frac{q_u}{v_u(\phi)} \left(\frac{-\iint_{\phi>-l} \delta(\phi(x))\delta(b(x)-u)\delta\phi\,dx}{A_b(\phi)} + \frac{\iint_{\phi>-l} \delta(\phi(x))\delta\phi\,dx\,v_u(\phi)}{A_b(\phi)} \right)$$

$$= -\lambda_1 \sum_{u=1}^{u=m} \left(\frac{q_u}{p_u(\phi)} \frac{\iint_{\phi>-l} \delta(\phi(x))\delta(b(x)-u)\delta\phi\,dx}{A_f(\phi)} - \frac{q_u \iint_{\phi>-l} \delta(\phi(x))\delta\phi\,dx}{A_f(\phi)} \right)$$

$$+ \lambda_2 \sum_{u=1}^{u=m} \left(\frac{q_u}{v_u(\phi)} \frac{-\iint_{\phi>-l} \delta(\phi(x))\delta(b(x)-u)\delta\phi\,dx}{A_b(\phi)} + \frac{q_u \iint_{\phi>-l} \delta(\phi(x))\delta\phi\,dx}{A_b(\phi)} \right).$$

By changing the turn of summation and integral, we arrive at,

$$\delta E(\phi) = -\lambda_1 \left(\frac{\iint_{\phi>-l} (q_{b(x)}/p_{b(x)}(\phi))\delta(\phi(x))\delta\phi\,dx}{A_f(\phi)} - \frac{\iint_{\phi>-l} \delta(\phi(x))\delta\phi\,dx}{A_f(\phi)} \right)$$

$$+ \lambda_2 \left(\frac{-\iint_{\phi>-l} (q_{b(x)}/v_{b(x)}(\phi))\delta(\phi(x))\delta\phi\,dx}{A_b(\phi)} + \frac{\iint_{\phi>-l} \delta(\phi(x))\delta\phi\,dx}{A_b(\phi)} \right),$$

$$\delta E(\phi) = -\lambda_1 \left(\iint_{\phi>-l} \frac{q_{b(x)}}{p_{b(x)}(\phi)A_f(\phi)}\delta(\phi(x))\delta\phi dx - \frac{\iint_{\phi>-l} \delta(\phi(x))\delta\phi\,dx}{A_f(\phi)} \right)$$

$$+ \lambda_2 \left(-\iint_{\phi>-l} \frac{q_{b(x)}}{v_{b(x)}(\phi)A_b(\phi)}\delta(\phi(x))\delta\phi\,dx - \frac{\iint_{\phi>-l} \delta(\phi(x))\delta\phi\,dx}{A_b(\phi)} \right),$$

Because

$$p_{b(x)}(\phi) = \frac{\iint_{\phi>-l} H(\phi(y))\delta(b(y)-b(x))dy}{A_f(\phi)},$$

we have

$$p_{b(x)}(\phi) \iint_{\phi>-l} H(\phi(x))dx = \iint_{\phi>-l} H(\phi(y))\delta(b(y)-b(x))dy.$$

$P_{b(x)}(\phi)A_f(\phi)$ calculates the number of pixels whose bin is $b(x)$ in the predicted foreground. We denoted $P_{b(x)}(\phi)A_f(\phi)$ by $N_f(b(x))$. Similarly, we denoted $v_{b(x)}(\phi)A_b(\phi)$ by

$N_b(b(\boldsymbol{x}))$. Thus, $\delta E(\phi)$ is simplified to,

$$\delta E(\phi) = -\lambda_1 \left(\iint\limits_{\phi>-l} \frac{q_{b(x)}}{N_f(b(\boldsymbol{x}))} \delta(\phi(\boldsymbol{x}))\delta\phi \, \mathrm{d}\boldsymbol{x} - \frac{\iint_{\phi>-l} \delta(\phi(\boldsymbol{x}))\delta\phi \, \mathrm{d}\boldsymbol{x}}{A_f(\phi)} \right)$$

$$+ \lambda_2 \left(- \iint\limits_{\phi>-l} \frac{q_{b(x)}}{N_b(b(\boldsymbol{x}))} \delta(\phi(\boldsymbol{x}))\delta\phi \, \mathrm{d}\boldsymbol{x} + \frac{\iint_{\phi>-l} \delta(\phi(\boldsymbol{x}))\delta\phi \, \mathrm{d}\boldsymbol{x}}{A_b(\phi)} \right).$$

After the second term and the fourth term multiplying by $P_{b(x)}(\phi)$ and $v_{b(x)}(\phi)$ respectively, $\delta E(\phi)$ can be simplified further,

$$\delta E(\phi) = -\lambda_1 \left(\iint\limits_{\phi>-l} \frac{(q_{b(x)} - \mathrm{p}_{b(x)}(\phi))}{N_f(b(\boldsymbol{x}))} \delta(\phi(\boldsymbol{x}))\delta\phi \, \mathrm{d}\boldsymbol{x} \right)$$

$$+ \lambda_2 \left(- \iint\limits_{\phi>-l} \frac{(q_{b(x)} - v_{b(x)}(\phi))}{N_b(b(\boldsymbol{x}))} \delta(\phi(\boldsymbol{x}))\delta\phi \, \mathrm{d}\boldsymbol{x} \right),$$

$$\delta E(\phi) = \iint\limits_{\phi>-l} \left[\frac{\lambda_1(\mathrm{p}_{b(x)}(\phi) - q_{b(x)})}{N_f(b(\boldsymbol{x}))} + \frac{\lambda_2(v_{b(x)}(\phi) - q_{b(x)})}{N_b(b(\boldsymbol{x}))} \right] \delta(\phi(\boldsymbol{x}))\delta\phi \, \mathrm{d}\boldsymbol{x}.$$

Appendix 11B

The variation of the energy E is,

$$\delta E(\phi) = \frac{1}{2} \sum_{u=1}^{u=m} \left[\lambda_1 \sqrt{\frac{q_u}{\mathrm{p}_u(\phi)}} \delta\mathrm{p}_u(\phi) - \lambda_2 \sqrt{\frac{q_u}{v_u(\phi)}} \delta v_u(\phi) \right]$$

From Appendix 11A, we have,

$$\delta\mathrm{p}_u(\phi) = \frac{\iint_{\phi>-l} \delta(\phi(\boldsymbol{x}))\delta(b(\boldsymbol{x}) - u)\delta\phi \, \mathrm{d}\boldsymbol{x}}{A_f(\phi)} - \frac{\iint_{\phi>-l} \delta(\phi(\boldsymbol{x}))\delta\phi \, \mathrm{d}\boldsymbol{x} \, \mathrm{p}_u(\phi)}{A_f(\phi)},$$

$$\delta v_u(\phi) = \frac{-\iint_{\phi>-l} \delta(\phi(\boldsymbol{x}))\delta(b(\boldsymbol{x}) - u)\delta\phi \, \mathrm{d}\boldsymbol{x}}{A_b(\phi)} + \frac{\iint_{\phi>-l} \delta(\phi(\boldsymbol{x}))\delta\phi \, \mathrm{d}\boldsymbol{x} \, v_u(\phi)}{A_b(\phi)}.$$

Thus, by substituting $\delta p_u(\phi)$ and $\delta v_u(\phi)$ into δE, we arrive at

$$\delta E(\phi) = \frac{\lambda_1}{2} \sum_{u=1}^{u=m} \sqrt{\frac{q_u}{p_u(\phi)}} \left(\frac{\iint_{\phi>-l} \delta(\phi(x))\delta(b(x)-u)\delta\phi \, dx}{A_f(\phi)} - \frac{\iint_{\phi>-l} \delta(\phi(x))\delta\phi \, dx \, p_u(\phi)}{A_f(\phi)} \right)$$

$$- \frac{\lambda_2}{2} \sum_{u=1}^{u=m} \sqrt{\frac{q_u}{v_u(\phi)}} \left(\frac{-\iint_{\phi>-l} \delta(\phi(x))\delta(b(x)-u)\delta\phi \, dx}{A_b(\phi)} \right.$$

$$\left. + \frac{\iint_{\phi>-l} \delta(\phi(x))\delta\phi \, dx \, v_u(\phi)}{A_b(\phi)} \right),$$

$$\delta E(\phi) = \frac{\lambda_1}{2} \sum_{u=1}^{u=m} \left(\sqrt{\frac{q_u}{p_u(\phi)}} \frac{\iint_{\phi>-l} \delta(\phi(x))\delta(b(x)-u)\delta\phi \, dx}{A_f(\phi)} \right.$$

$$\left. - \frac{\sqrt{q_u p_u(\phi)} \iint_{\phi>-l} \delta(\phi(x))\delta\phi \, dx}{A_f(\phi)} \right)$$

$$- \frac{\lambda_2}{2} \sum_{u=1}^{u=m} \left(\sqrt{\frac{q_u}{v_u(\phi)}} \frac{-\iint_{\phi>-l} \delta(\phi(x))\delta(b(x)-u)\delta\phi \, dx}{A_b(\phi)} \right.$$

$$\left. + \frac{\sqrt{q_u v_u(\phi)} \iint_{\phi>-l} \delta(\phi(x))\delta\phi \, dx}{A_b(\phi)} \right)$$

By changing the turn of summation and integral, we arrive at

$$\delta E(\phi) = \frac{\lambda_1}{2} \left(\frac{\iint_{\phi>-l} \sqrt{(q_{b(x)}/p_{b(x)}(\phi))}\delta(\phi(x))\delta\phi \, dx}{A_f(\phi)} \right.$$

$$\left. - \frac{\iint_{\phi>-l} \sum_{u=1}^{u=m} \sqrt{q_u p_u(\phi)}\delta(\phi(x))\delta\phi \, dx}{A_f(\phi)} \right)$$

$$- \frac{\lambda_2}{2} \left(\frac{\iint_{\phi>-l} \sqrt{(q_{b(x)}/v_{b(x)}(\phi))}\delta(\phi(x))\delta\phi \, dx}{A_b(\phi)} \right.$$

$$\left. + \frac{\iint_{\phi>-l} \sum_{u=1}^{u=m} \sqrt{q_u v_u(\phi)}\delta(\phi(x))\delta\phi \, dx}{A_b(\phi)} \right)$$

We can simplify it to

$$\delta E(\phi) = \frac{\lambda_1}{2A_f(\phi)} \left(\iint_{\phi>-l} \sqrt{\frac{q_{b(x)}}{p_{b(x)}(\phi)}}\delta(\phi(x))\delta\phi \, dx - \iint_{\phi>-l} B(q, p(\phi))\delta(\phi(x))\delta\phi \, dx \right)$$

$$- \frac{\lambda_2}{2A_b(\phi)} \left(-\iint_{\phi>-l} \sqrt{\frac{q_{b(x)}}{v_{b(x)}(\phi)}}\delta(\phi(x))\delta\phi \, dx + \iint_{\phi>-l} B\left(q, v(\phi)\right)\delta(\phi(x))\delta\phi \, dx \right)$$

$\delta E(\phi)$ can be simplified further to

$$\delta E(\phi) = \frac{\lambda_1}{2A_f(\phi)} \left(\iint_{\phi > -l} \left[\sqrt{\frac{q_{b(x)}}{P_{b(x)}}}(\phi) - B(q, p(\phi)) \right] \delta(\phi(x)) \delta\phi \, dx \right)$$

$$+ \frac{\lambda_2}{2A_b(\phi)} \left(\iint_{\phi > -l} \left[\sqrt{\frac{q_{b(x)}}{v_{b(x)}}}(\phi) - B(q, v(\phi)) \right] \delta(\phi(x)) \delta\phi \, dx \right).$$

References

1. G. Läthén, Segmentation Methods for Medical Image Analysis, Doctoral dissertation, Thesis, 2010.
2. D. L. Pham, C. Xu, and J. L. Prince, Current methods in medical image segmentation 1, *Annual Review of Biomedical Engineering*, vol. 2, no. 1, pp. 315–337, 2000.
3. M. A. Balafar, A. R. Ramli, M. I. Saripan, and S. Mashohor, Review of brain MRI image segmentation methods, *Artificial Intelligence Review*, vol. 33, no. 3, pp. 261–274, 2010.
4. D. J. Withey and Z. J. Koles, Medical image segmentation: Methods and software, in *Noninvasive Functional Source Imaging of the Brain and Heart and the International Conference on Functional Biomedical Imaging, 2007, NFSI-ICFBI 2007. Joint Meeting of the 6th International Symposium on*. IEEE, Hangzhou, pp. 140–143, 2007.
5. X. Huang and G. Tsechpenakis, Medical image segmentation, *Information Discovery on Electronic Health Records*, vol. 10, pp. 251–289, 2009.
6. N. Sharma and L. M. Aggarwal, Automated medical image segmentation techniques, *Journal of medical physics/Association of Medical Physicists of India*, vol 35, no. 1, p. 3, 2010.
7. R. Haralick and L. Shapiro. *Computer and Robot Vision*. Boston, MA: Addison-Wesley, 1992.
8. D. L. Rubin, H. Greenspan, and J. F. Brinkley, Biomedical imaging informatics, *Biomedical Informatics*. London: Springer, 2014, pp. 285–327.
9. M. Kass, A. Witkin, and D. Terzopoulos, Snakes: Active contour models, *International Journal of Computer Vision*, vol. 1, no. 4, pp. 321–331, 1988.
10. S. Osher and J. A. Sethian, Fronts propagating with curvature-dependent speed: Algorithms based on Hamilton-Jacobi formulations, *Journal of Computational Physics*, vol. 79, no. 1, pp. 12–49, 1988.
11. S. Osher and R. P. Fedkiw, Level set methods: An overview and some recent results, *Journal of Computational Physics*, vol. 169, no. 2, pp. 463–502, 2001.
12. J. A. Sethian, *Level Set Methods and Fast Marching Methods: Evolving Interfaces in Computational Geometry, Fluid Mechanics, Computer Vision, and Materials Science*, Vol. 3. Cambridge: Cambridge University Press, 1999.
13. T. F. Chen, Medical image segmentation using level sets, Technical Report, University of Waterloo, Canada, 2008.
14. C. A. Cocosco, V. Kollokian, R. K.-S. Kwan, G. B. Pike, and A. C. Evans. BrainWeb: Online interface to a 3D MRI simulated brain database. *NeuroImage*, vol. 5, no. 4, 425, 1997.
15. R. K.-S. Kwan, A. C. Evans, and G. Bruce Pike, MRI simulation-based evaluation of image-processing and classification methods, *Medical Imaging, IEEE Transactions on*, vol. 18, no. 11, pp. 1085–1097, 1999.
16. R. K.-S. Kwan, A. C. Evans, and G. Bruce Pike, An extensible MRI simulator for post-processing evaluation, in *Visualization in Biomedical Computing*, Berlin: Springer, 1996.
17. Collins, D. L., A. P. Zijdenbos, V. Kollokian, J. G. Sled, N. J. Kabani, C. J. Holmes, and A. C. Evans, Design and construction of a realistic digital brain phantom, *Medical Imaging, IEEE Transactions on*, vol. 17, no. 3, pp. 463–468, 1998.

18. T. Chan and W. Zhu, Level set-based shape prior segmentation, in *Computer Vision and Pattern Recognition, 2005. CVPR 2005. IEEE Computer Society Conference on.* Vol. 2. IEEE, San Diego, CA, 2005.

19. L. A. Vese and T. F. Chan, A multiphase level set framework for image segmentation using the Mumford and Shah model, *International Journal of Computer Vision*, vol. 50, no. 3, pp. 271–293, 2002.

20. T. Brox and J. Weickert, Level set-based image segmentation with multiple regions, in *Pattern Recognition*. Berlin: Springer, 2004, pp. 415–423.

21. T. F. Chan and L. A. Vese, Active contours without edges, *Image Processing, IEEE Transactions on*, vol. 10, no. 2, pp. 266–277, 2001.

22. V. Grau, A. U. J. Mewes, M. Alcaniz, R. Kikinis, and S. K. Warfield, Improved watershed transform for medical image segmentation using prior information, *Medical Imaging, IEEE Transactions on*, vol. 23, no. 4, pp. 447–458, 2004.

23. D. R. Chittajallu et al., Fuzzy-cuts: A knowledge-driven graph-based method for medical image segmentation, in *Computer Vision and Pattern Recognition, 2009. CVPR 2009. IEEE Conference on. IEEE*, Miami Beach, FL, pp. 715–722, 2009.

24. M. Mignotte, Segmentation by fusion of histogram-based-means clusters in different color spaces, *Image Processing, IEEE Transactions on*, vol. 17, no. 5, pp. 780–787, 2008.

25. R. Yildizoglu, J.-F. Aujol, and N. Papadakis, A convex formulation for global histogram based binary segmentation, *International Conference on Energy Minimization Methods in Computer Vision and Pattern Recognition*, Lund, Sweden, 2013.

26. K. Ni, X. Bresson, T. Chan, and S. Esedoglu, Local histogram based segmentation using the Wasserstein distance, *International Journal of Computer Vision*, vol. 84, no. 1, pp. 97–111, 2009.

27. T. Zhang and D. Freedman, Improving performance of distribution tracking through background mismatch, *Pattern Analysis and Machine Intelligence, IEEE Transactions on*, vol. 27, no. 2, pp. 282–287, 2005.

28. J. Ning, W. Yu, and S. Yang, An active contour tracking method by matching foreground and background simultaneously, In: *ICIP*, Melbourne, Australia, pp. 3944–3948, 2013.

29. W. Yu, J. Ning, N. Geng, and J. Zhang, A simple derivation to implement tracking distributions, Paper presented at the meeting of the *VISAPP*, Vol. 2, 2012.

30. D. Freedman and T. Zhang, Active contours for tracking distributions, *Image Processing, IEEE Transactions on*, vol. 13, no. 4, pp. 518–526, 2004.

31. K. P. Burnham and D. R. Anderson, *Model Selection and Multimodel Inference: A Practical Information-Theoretic Approach*. Berlin: Springer, 2002.

chapter twelve

An appearance-guided deformable model for 4D kidney segmentation using diffusion MRI

Mohamed Shehata, Fahmi Khalifa, Ahmed Soliman,
Ali Taki Eldeen, Mohamed Abou El-Ghar, Tarek El-Diasty,
Ayman El-Baz, and Robert Keynton

Contents

Abstract

Early detection of acute rejection after kidney transplantation has become a focus of extensive research due to the increased demand for the donor kidneys and their limited supply. Early diagnosis of acute rejection will increases the probability of survival for both the transplanted kidney and the patient. Hence, it is imperative that a accurate, reliable and sensitive noninvasive computer-aided diagnostic (CAD) system for acute renal transplant rejection be developed. In developing the CAD system, the first key step is to segment the kidney tissue from all of the surrounding tissues. This chapter introduces a new geometric deformable model based on the use of the level sets framework for the four-dimensional segmentation of kidneys obtained from diffusion-weighted magnetic resonance imaging (DW-MRI). The evolutions of the deformable model presented are controlled by a stochastic speed relationship that depends on an adaptive shape prior, which in turn, is guided by the first- and second-order visual appearance features of the DW-MRI data. In order to enable voxel-wise guidance of the level sets, these three image features are integrated into a joint Markov–Gibbs random field (MGRF) model of the kidney and its background. The leave-one-subject-out testing method was used to evaluate the segmentation approach for 34 DW-MRI datasets acquired at different b-values ranging from 0 to 1000 s/mm^2. Then, the following three evaluation metrics—(1) the Dice similarity coefficient (DSC); (2) the 95-percentile modified Hausdorff distance (MHD); and (3) the absolute kidney volume difference (AKVD)—were used to compare the performance of the proposed segmentation approach against three other segmentation methods on the same DW-MRI data. The evaluation of the experimental results between the manually drawn and the automatically segmented contours using DSC ($91.34 \pm 3.753\%$), MHD (10.21 ± 6.18), and AKVD ($15.82 \pm 4.58\%$), strongly confirms the robustness and the accuracy of the approach presented.

12.1   Introduction

Acute renal rejection is one of the most important causes of renal dysfunction in kidney transplant patients. Clinicians have found that earlier the acute renal rejection can be diagnosed, the higher probability of survival of the transplanted kidney [1,2]. For renal functional assessment purposes, an imaging modality that has the ability to provide both anatomical and functional information is critically needed [3–7]. Diffusion-weighted magnetic resonance imaging (DW-MRI) is selected as an emerging imaging modality because it does not involve radiation exposure or the use of contrast agents like other imaging modalities (e.g., computed topography [CT] and dynamic MRI). Developing a computer-aided diagnostic (CAD) system for the early detection of renal rejection using DW-MRI essentially requires segmentation of the kidney tissue from the surrounding tissues [8–17]. However, the accurate segmentation of DW-MRI data comes with many challenges [18–24] due to similarities in intensities (i.e., gray values) for the kidney and surrounding tissues (see Figure 12.1a), interpatient anatomical differences (see Figure 12.1b), and image noise, especially at high diffusion field strengths (see Figure 12.1c). In the studies reported above [18–24], kidney segmentation from DW-MRI is rare. However, the segmentation of other anatomical structures (e.g., brain, liver, and prostate) from the same imaging modality (i.e., DW-MRI), which has been used for kidney segmentation in this chapter, has been an area of active research [25–38]; thus, we will briefly discuss some of these studies on the DW-MRI segmentation for brain, prostate, and liver applications.

In brain applications, Mujumdar et al. [25] proposed a framework for stroke lesion segmentation from DW-MR images using an automatic windowing-based technique for noise suppression of the DW-MRI data at high b-values to enhance the local contrast (LC) for candidate lesions. The optimum windowing parameters were selected based on the maximum LC of the candidate lesion. Moreover, the Chan–Vese active contour model [39] using Mumford–Shah functional was employed for the purpose of lesion segmentation. Meanwhile, Saad et al. [26] presented a fully automated region growing-based framework

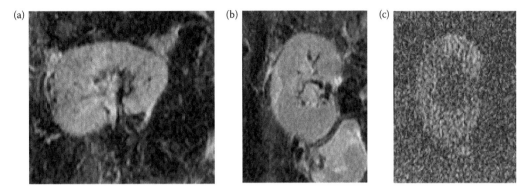

Figure 12.1 Coronal cross-sectional samples for raw DW-MRI data shows (a) similar gray level values of the kidney and surrounding tissues, (b) interpatient anatomical differences compared with (a), and (c) image noise, especially, at high diffusion field strengths (b-values).

for the segmentation of brain lesions from DW-MRI. Their framework integrated simple statistical features and homogeneity criteria that was based on the mean signal intensity and the number of pixels in a given region. However, their approach did not show an enhancement, since it was unable to fully characterize the tumor lesion as well as the semi-automated approach. Lu et al. [27] explored an automated approach to segment the brain from multidirectional DW-MRI raw data that consisted of two steps. First, segmentation was initialized by employing a hierarchical clustering (HC) technique using the minimum variance algorithm [40] to the down-sampled data. Specifically, they assumed that each tissue type and the overall distribution of the raw data were each a mixture of multivariate Gaussian functions (MoMG) [41]. This step focused on the estimation of their model parameters (i.e., meanvectors, covariance matrices of MoMG, etc.). The second segmentation was obtained using an expectation maximization (EM) algorithm, which was applied to the higher dimensional data. Another methodology created by Niethammer et al. [28], segmented near-tubular fiber bundles in the brain from DW-MR images. Segmentation was performed based on the global statistical modeling of the diffusion orientation, which utilized optimal path methods (or simple streamlining) to obtain the geometric information. In particular, a convex approximation of the probabilistic Chan–Vese energy using region-based directional statistics [39] was employed. Hevia-Montiel et al. [42] investigated segmentation of a cerebral infraction lesion from DW-MRI data that combined both region and edge information for an acute ischemic stroke. Their method consisted of three steps: (1) edge confidence map computation; (2) weighted mean shift (MS) filtering; and (3) region adjacency analysis followed by morphological operation. Li et al. [29] classified brain tissue from DW-MRI/diffusion tensor imaging (DTI) using a two-class maps approach that utilized the tissue contrast existing in the DW-MRI/DTI channels (e.g, apparent diffusion coefficient [ADC], and fractional anisotropy [FA]) to generate the two-class maps. In order to obtain the final segmentation, a multichannel fusion algorithm [43] was employed to combine these two-class maps to obtain a complete segmentation. Although this approach yielded reasonable tissue segmentation results, it has only been tested on 10 sets of brain data.

In addition to brain applications, segmentation of prostate tissue has also been investigated in a number of prostate DWI studies. For prostate cancer detection, Ozer et al. [30] presented an automated segmentation method using multispectral MRI (e.g., dynamic MRI, T2 MRI, and DW-MRI). In order to tune the support vector machines (SVMs) and relevance vector machines (RVMs), they developed threshold techniques by applying a first-order polynomial kernel for SVMs and RVMs in order to maximize accuracy. Specifically, the threshold section was obtained according to a user desired performance criterion (e.g, optimized accuracy, maximized sensitivity, etc). In addition, a comparison of their supervised (SVM, RVM) methods to an unsupervised method, based on fuzzy MRF, was conducted using their threshold scheme. Their study concluded that the developed framework improved prostate cancer segmentation; however, their method used multispectral MRI images without coregistration, which made their method prone to errors due to inter-slice variability. Liu et al. [31] proposed an unsupervised level set approach for prostate segmentation using DW-MRI that did not require training. The level set was initialized and constrained with a shape penalty term described by an elliptical deformable model that fits the prostate region. The level set results were refined using connectivity and morphological analysis. Their framework was later extended to 3D and applied to ADC images derived from DW-MRI in Liu et al. [32]. In their method, a coarse segmentation step that utilized a stack of parametric elliptic deformable models was employed to find the optimum elliptical shape to fit the prostate gland. Additionally, a weighting parameter for the shape prior (i.e., threshold) was automatically selected using Otsus method [44], and, finally, the segmentation results were obtained after a refinement step using morphological operations. An unsupervised segmentation approach using multispectral MRI prostate data (e.g., quantitative T2 MRI, DW-MRI, and dynamic MRI) was developed by Liu et al. [33]. Their framework utilized fuzzy Markov random field (MRF) modeling, in which image segmentation and the MRF parameter estimation were performed simultaneously. For early detection of prostate cancer, Firjani et al. [34] created an automated noninvasive CAD system to segment the prostate tissue using a maximum a posteriori (MAP) approach. The CAD-MAP approach incorporated three image features, namely, a prostate shape prior, voxel-wise image intensities, and the spatial interactions between prostate voxels.

In addition to the brain and prostate, the segmentation of liver tissue from DW-MRI has also been extensively studied. A fully automated algorithm for tracking liver metastatic lesions across different b-values (from 150 to 300) in echo-planner DW-MRI was developed by Krishnamurthy et al. [35]. They built their framework based on the snake-based automated segmentation algorithm [45], in which centroid tracking and block matching were combined with the active contour model to track liver lesion progression. In another study, a multiphase MRI automatic liver segmentation method based on 3D anisotropic diffusion processing was described by Platero et al. [36], in which a coarse segmentation procedure was first performed by combining multiple analysis processes, that is, edge detection techniques, histogram analysis, and binary morphological postprocessing. Then, the segmented image was refined using an active contour approach, which minimized a Mumford–Shah functional that accounted for external and internal variance in luminance between the liver and surrounding tissues. For liver applications, Veeraraghavan and Do [37] produced an automated joint segmentation and registration method using DW-MRI that computed the ADC maps for structures of interest (e.g., tumors) after a sequential alignment process using a least squares fit method. In their method, various structures were segmented in a randomly selected reference image; then, the closest image was selected using a mean shift-tracking algorithm, was registered to the reference image using a nonrigid B-spline based deformable registration technique. Once aligned, this image was selected as the new reference image, and the process was repeated for all remaining images in the sequence. To overcome the problem of nonadaptability to different DW-MRI (b-values) and segmentation of liver lesions with low contrast, an automated clustering statistical approach for liver lesion segmentation from DW-MRI was proposed by Jha et al. [38].

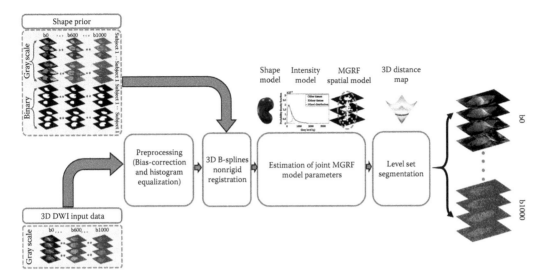

Figure 12.2 The proposed framework for 4D kidney segmentation from diffusion MRI.

They incorporated multiple image features to segment DW-MRI; in particular, the DW-MR image was modeled by a statistical finite Gaussian mixture (FGM), in which the number of classes was determined based on a histogram analysis. Also, an MRF model was used to model the spatial interactions between the DW-MRI voxels. The reader is directed to Elnakib et al. [46] for a recent survey on different image segmentation techniques.

Despite the success of the aforementioned methods in performing diffusion MRI segmentation of organs with low contrast, these methods have been limited in the application of their frameworks to kidney segmentation. Specifically, the threshold-based methods were sensitive to intensity similarities between the kidney and its background. Deformable model-based methods without adequate shape and appearance models have failed in cases of high image noise and diffused boundaries. Statistical-based methods have been based on predefined models that may not be applicable to renal applications.

To overcome these limitations, we developed a new geometric deformable model framework, shown in Figure 12.2, based on level sets for accurate 4D kidney segmentation from DW-MRI data. The proposed approach utilized a combination of both an adaptive shape prior information [47,48] and current appearance features of the DW-MRI data. The latter accounted for the first-order voxel-wise image intensity and their spatial interactions. The image features allowed us to create a more robust model for guiding the evolution of the level sets to extract the kidney borders on 4D DW-MRI data.

The rest of this chapter has been organized in the following five sections. Details of the proposed level set approach have been described in the Methods (Section 12.2). Segmentation evaluation metrics for the presented approach have been detailed in Section 12.3. Section 13.4 has described clinical images. Experimental results are given in Section 13.5, and Section 13.6 concludes the chapter.

12.1.1 Basic notations

- $\mathbf{R} = \{(x, y, z) : 0 \leq x \leq X - 1, 0 \leq y \leq Y - 1, 0 \leq z \leq Z - 1\}$ denotes a finite 3D arithmetic lattice of the size of XYZ supporting grayscale images and their region (segmentation) maps.

- $Q = \{0, 1, \ldots, Q-1\}$ denotes a finite set of Q integer gray values.
- $L = \{0, \ldots, L\}$ denotes a set of region labels L.
- $g = \{g_{x,y,z} : (x, y, z) \in R; g_{x,y,z} \in Q\}$ is a grayscale image taking values from Q, i.e., $g : R \to Q$.
- $m = \{m_{x,y,z} : (x, y, z) \in R; m_{x,y,z} \in L\}$ is a region map taking values from L, i.e., $m : R \to L$.

An input DW-MRI data, g, coaligned to the training data base, and its map, m, are described with a joint probability model: $P(g, m) = P(g|m)P(m)$, which combines a conditional distribution of the images given the map $P(g|m)$, and an unconditional probability distribution of maps $P(m) = P_{sp}(m)P_V(m)$. Here, $P_{sp}(m)$ denotes an adaptive shape prior, and $P_V(m)$ is a Gibbs probability distribution with potential V, which specifies an MGRF model of spatially homogeneous maps m. Details of the model's components are outlined below.

12.2   Methods

One of the most commonly used techniques for the segmentation of the varieties of organs from medical imaging is geometric deformable models based on level sets. These deformable model-based types have gained considerable attention for object segmentation due to their simplicity and lack of need for parametrization [49]. According to the definition of the level sets, the evolving surface at any time instant t is represented by the zero level, $\phi_n(x, y, z) = 0$, of an implicit function, namely, a distance map of the signed minimum Euclidean distance from each voxel to the surface. This formulation results in points inside the surface having negative (or positive) values and voxels outside the surface having positive (or negative) values, respectively. Mathematically, the evolution of the level set is defined by Osher and Fedkiw [50]

$$\phi_{n+1}(x, y, z) = \phi_n(x, y, z) - \tau F_n(x, y, z) |\nabla \phi_n(x, y, z)| \qquad (12.1)$$

where n indicates the time instant $t = n\tau$ (taken with a step $\tau > 0$), and $\nabla \phi_n = [\frac{\partial \phi_n}{\partial x}, \frac{\partial \phi_n}{\partial y}, \frac{\partial \phi_n}{\partial z}]$ is the gradient of $\phi_n(x, y, z)$. This evolution is guided by the speed function $F_n(x, y, z)$. The speed functions that are based on image intensities, object edges, and gradient vector flow have difficulties and problems when segmenting noisy images and those with poor object-background contrast. In this chapter, for more accurate segmentation of the kidney from DW-MRI data, a new speed function that depends on regional statistics derived from the kidney and background regions is proposed. Namely, it takes into account regional appearance, shape, and spatial features of the DW-MRI data. These features are combined using a joint Markov–Gibbs model to provide the voxel-wise guidance of the deformable model.

12.2.1   Preprocessing

The accuracy of kidney segmentation is reduced due to the illumination nonuniformity, or the bias field. Therefore, to accurately extract the kidney it is important to account for the low frequency intensity nonuniformity or heterogeneity. Here, we employed histogram equalization using the nonparametric bias correction method proposed in Tustison et al. [51]. This step is important to reduce noise effects and remove (smooth) inconsistencies of the DW-MRI data.

12.2.2   Adaptive shape model

For the variability reduction across subjects and the segmentation accuracy enhancement purposes, an adaptive shape model of the expected kidney shape is employed. In order to create the shape database, a training set of images, collected from different subjects, are coaligned using a 3D B-splines based transformation [52] using the sum of square difference (SSD) as a similarity metric. The probabilistic shape priors are spatially variant independent random fields of region labels

$$P_{sp}(\mathbf{m}) = \prod_{(x,y,z) \in R} p_{sp:x,y,z}(m_{x,y,z}) \tag{12.2}$$

where $p_{sp:x,y,z}(l)$ is the voxel-wise empirical probabilities for each label $l \in \mathbf{L}$. To segment each input DW-MRI data, an adaptive process guided by the first- and second-order visual appearance features of the input MRI data is used to construct the shape prior. This shape prior [47,48] is built at the learning stage for two labels: the kidney object, and other tissues (i.e., the background). In the training phase, 34 manually segmented datasets (b0 scans) by an MR imaging expert are used to create the probabilistic maps for the two labels. Then, for the testing phase, each DW-MRI data to be segmented is coaligned, using a 3D B-splines based registration, with one of the training sets used to create the prior kidney shapes. The reader is referred to Shehata et al. [47,48] for the basic steps of the segmentation approach.

12.2.3   Second-order appearance model

For a more accurate segmentation, spatially homogeneous 3D pairwise interactions between the region labels are additionally incorporated in our model. These interactions are calculated using the popular Potts model (i.e., an MGRF with the nearest 26-neighbors of the voxels), and analytic bivalued Gibbs potentials, which depend only on whether the nearest pairs of labels are equal or not. Let $f_{eq}(\mathbf{m})$ denote the relative frequency of equal labels in the neighboring voxel pairs $((x,y,z),(x+\xi,y+\eta,z+\zeta)) \in \mathbf{R}^2$; $(\xi,\eta,\zeta) \in \{(\pm1,0,0),(0,\pm1,0),(\pm1,\pm1,0),(\pm1,0,\pm1),(0,\pm1,\pm1),(\pm1,\pm1,\pm1)\}$. The initial region map results in an approximation with the following analytical maximum likelihood estimates of the potentials [53]:

$$v_{eq} = -v_{ne} \approx 2f_{eq}(\mathbf{m}) - 1 \tag{12.3}$$

which allows for computing the voxel-wise probabilities $p_{V:x,y,z}(m_{x,y,z} = \lambda)$ of each label; $l \in \mathbf{L}$.

12.2.4   First-order appearance model

Our approach also accounts for the visual appearance of the kidney besides the learned prior shape and the spatial model. Hence, for more accurate modeling of the current DW-MRI appearance, we use the linear combination of discrete Gaussians (LCDG) model with positive and negative discrete Gaussian (DG) components. The LCDG separates the mixed empirical 1D distribution of DW-MRI voxel intensities into two distinct components associated with each label [53]. This approximation adapts the segmentation to the changing appearance, such as nonlinear intensity variations caused by patient weight and data acquisition systems. The LCDG models the empirical distribution of the kidney labels more accurately than a conventional mixture of only positive Gaussians. This yields a better initial region map that is formed by the voxel-wise classification of the image gray values. The LCDG model is described in detail in Farag et al. [53] and El-Baz et al. [54].

As mentioned above, the proposed approach incorporates the adaptive prior shape information to two other image features (first- and second-order visual appearance models) into the level set segmentation, which in turn highlights one of the most important advantages of our framework. These features are estimated directly from the input data to be segmented, making the proposed framework an adaptive approach. These three features are used to provide the voxel-wise guidance of the level set. For each voxel (x, y, z), the speed function of Equation 12.1 as [49]:

$$F_n(x, y, z) = \kappa \vartheta(x, y, z) \tag{12.4}$$

where κ is the mean contour curvature and $\vartheta(x, y, z)$ specify the magnitude and direction of contour evolution at the voxel (x, y, z):

$$\vartheta(x, y) = \begin{cases} -P_{ob:x,y} & \text{if} P_{ob:x,y,z} > P_{bg:x,y,z} \\ P_{bg:x,y} & \text{otherwise} \end{cases} \tag{12.5}$$

where $P_{ob:x,y,z}$ and $P_{bg:x,y,z}$, are the joint MGRF probabilities for the kidney and background, respectively. $P_{ob:x,y,z} = \frac{\Omega_{ob:x,y,z}}{\Omega_{ob:x,y,z} + \Omega_{bg:x,y,z}}$ and $P_{bg:x,y,z} = \frac{\Omega_{bg:x,y,z}}{\Omega_{bg:x,y,z} + \Omega_{bg:x,y,z}} = 1 - P_{ob:x,y,z}$; where $\Omega_{ob:x,y,z} = p(q|1)p_{V:x,y,z}(1)p_{sp:x,y,z}(1)$ and $\Omega_{bg:x,y,z} = p(q|0)\left(1 - p_{V:x,y,z}(1)\right)\left(1 - p_{sp:x,y,z}(1)\right)$. Here $p(q|l)$ denote the voxel-wise probability of the intensity $q \in \mathbf{Q}$ for the LCDG model of the kidney ($l = 1$) or background ($l = 0$) appearance, $p_{V:x,y,z}(1)$ be the probability of the kidney label for the voxel (x, y, z) of the region map $\mathbf{m}$ in the MGRF spatial model; and $p_{sp:x,y,z}(1)$ is the probability of the kidney label in the adaptive shape prior $P_{sp}(\mathbf{m})$.

12.3   Segmentation evaluation

For the performance evaluation of the proposed framework, three performance metrics were used: (i) the Dice similarity coefficient (DSC) [55], (ii) the 95-percentile modified Hausdorff distance (MHD) [56], and (iii) the absolute kidney volume difference (AKVD). More details about these metrics are discussed in the following sections.

12.3.1   Dice similarity coefficient (DSC)

In order to measure the amount of overlapping between the segmented and the ground truth kidneys we use the DSC measure (as shown in Figure 12.3).

The DSC measure is described by Zou et al. [55] as:

$$\text{DSC} = \frac{2\text{TP}}{2\text{TP} + \text{FP} + \text{FN}} \tag{12.6}$$

where TP, FP, and FN denote the true-positive, false-positive, and false-negative, respectively. Better segmentation is indicated by higher DSC values, in which the segmentation results match the ground truth better than results with lower ones. If there is no overlap, DSC will be assigned a value of zero. Controversially, ideal segmentation is indicated by a DSC value of one.

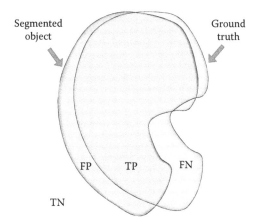

Figure 12.3 2D illustration of segmentation errors calculation between the segmented and ground truth objects for the DSC determination.

12.3.2   Modified Hausdorff distance

To measure how close the borders of the segmented kidney and the ground truth one are, that is, the distance error between the both borders, we used the MHD measure. The Hausdorff distance (HD) [56]:

$$HD(A_1, A_1) = \max_{c \in A_1}\{\min_{e \in A_2}\{d(c,e)\}\} \tag{12.7}$$

where c and e denote points of set A_1 and A_2, respectively, and $d(c,e)$ is the Euclidean distance between c and e. The bidirectional HD (HD_{Bi}) between the segmented region SR and its ground truth GT is defined as

$$HD_{Bi}(GT, SR) = max\{HD(GT, SR), HD(SR, GT)\} \tag{12.8}$$

Here, the 95-perecntile HD_{Bi} is used as a metric to measure the segmentation accuracy, termed as the modified HD (MHD). Figure 12.4 illustrates how the MHD measure is used.

12.3.3   Absolute kidney volume difference

For the third segmentation accuracy measure, the absolute kidney volume difference (AKVD) is used in addition to the DSC and the MHD. As shown in Figure 12.5, the AKVD indicates the percentage volume difference between the segmented and the ground truth kidney volumes. The AKVD is described by

$$AKVD\% = \frac{|GT| - |SR|}{|GT|} * 100 \tag{12.9}$$

where $|GT|$ and $|SR|$ indicate the total number of voxels in the ground truth and the segmented object, respectively.

12.4   Data collection

The proposed framework has been tested on 34 DW-MRI datasets that have been collected from 34 subjects at different b-values. These datasets were acquired using a scanner

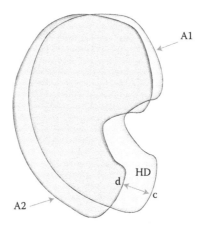

Figure 12.4 2D schematic illustration for the HD calculation.

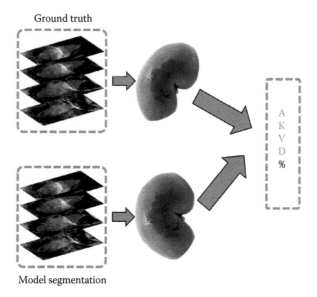

Figure 12.5 3D schematic illustration for the AKVD estimation.

(SIGNA Horizon, General Electric Medical Systems, Milwaukee, WI) with the following parameters: TR = 8000 ms; FOV = 32 cm; slice thickness = 4 mm; inter-slice gap = 0 mm; and two excitations. The DW-MRI volumes were collected with b-values ranging from 0 to 1000 s/mm^2 using a voxel size of $1.25 \times 1.25 \times 4.00$ mm^3. The ground truth segmentations used in training and verifying the segmentation results were manually created by an MR expert.

12.5   Experimental results

Since the segmentation is an important step in developing any CAD system for renal function assessment, we tested the performance of the proposed segmentation approach on the aforementioned DW-MRI data. Figure 12.6 shows some segmentation results at different

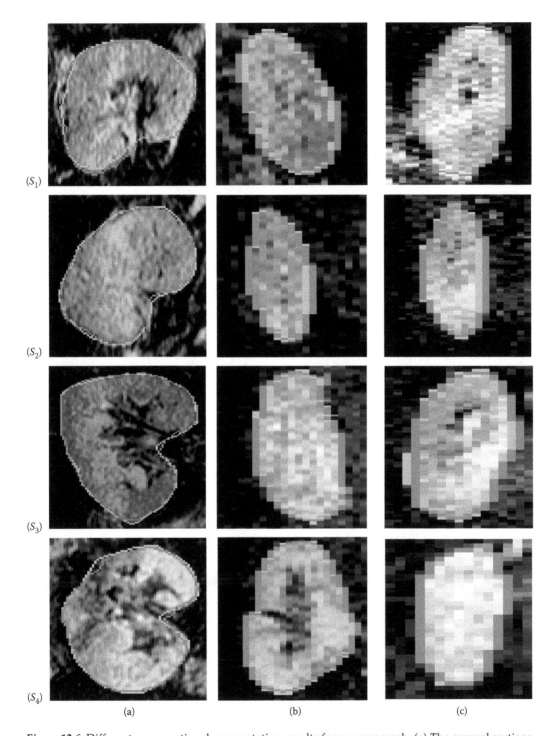

Figure 12.6 Different cross-sectional segmentation results for our approach: (a) The coronal sections, (b) the axial sections, and (c) the sagittal sections for four independent subjects (S_1, S_2, S_3, and S_4). The model segmentation is shown in red with respect to the manual ground truth (green) from an expert.

Table 12.1 Segmentation accuracy of our approach against three other level set
methods using DSC(%), MHD(mm), and AKVD(%)

| | Evaluation Metrics | | | | | |
| | DSC | | MHD | | AVKD | |
	Mean $\pm$ SD	P-value	Mean $\pm$ SD	P-value	Mean $\pm$ SD	P-value
Our	91.34 $\pm$ 3.753%	——	10.21 $\pm$ 6.18	——	15.82 $\pm$ 4.58%	——
CV [39]	69.16 $\pm$ 11.19%	< 0.0001	75.97 $\pm$ 11.96	< 0.0001	46.05 $\pm$ 13.18%	< 0.0001
I Only	54.36 $\pm$ 7.29%	< 0.0001	29.14 $\pm$ 5.34	< 0.0001	62.33 $\pm$ 7.12%	< 0.0001
I+S	63.00 $\pm$ 5.01%	< 0.0001	22.79 $\pm$ 7.36	< 0.0001	53.82 $\pm$ 5.35%	< 0.0001

Note: All metrics are represented as mean $\pm$ standard deviation (SD).

types of kidney cross-sections (i.e., axial, sagittal, and coronal) for four subjects acquired at $b0$. The accuracy of the proposed segmentation method has been evaluated using the Dice similarity coefficient (DSC) [55], the 95-percentile modified Hausdorff distance (MHD) [56], and the absolute kidney volume difference (AKVD). Metrics were computed by comparing the ground truth segmentation to results obtained by the proposed framework. The ground truth segmentations were manually created by an MR expert. Table 12.1 summarizes the DSC, MHD, and AKVD statistics for all test datasets. As shown in this figure, the proposed approach produces precise segmentation of the kidney at higher b_i values.

Moreover, the accuracy of the proposed segmentation was compared against three other methods: the level sets approach by Chan and Vese [39] (CV), the level sets guided by image intensity only, and the level sets guided by combined intensity and spatial features. Table 12.1 compares our segmentation with the other methods versus the ground truth, using the DSC, MHD, and AKVD. The comparative accuracy of the proposed approach versus the CV method on representative data at different types of kidney cross-sections (i.e., axial, sagittal, and coronal) for one selected subject acquired at $b0$ is shown in Figure 12.7. Table 12.1 shows that the advantage of our approach is statistically significant with respect to the other methods, evidenced by the P values less than 0.05, which confirms the high accuracy of the proposed segmentation techniques.

In order to assess the renal function using DW-MRI-based CAD systems, which, in turn, has gained increased attention in recent years [57], the estimation of diffusion parameters (e.g., ADC) requires the accurate segmentation of the kidney on DW-MRI data acquired at both higher and lower b-values. However, the accurate segmentation of kidney volumes at higher b-values is a challenge compared with those at lower b-values because of the decreased contrast between the object and the background. In spite of the aforementioned challenge, the proposed framework extracts accurately the kidney from diffusion data at higher b-values compared to the other three aforementioned methods as shown in Figure 12.8. In contrast to the existing DW-MRI approaches, the integration of the 3D appearance, shape, and spatial features increases the robustness of the proposed approach to overcome large image noise at higher b-values. Figure 12.8 demonstrates a sample coronal cross-section segmentation for four subjects at b-values of 300, 500, 700, and 1000 s/mm^2 for our approach and the three other approaches used before. As shown in this figure, the proposed approach produces precise segmentation of the kidney at higher b-values compared with the other methods with respect to the ground truth segmentation. Please see Figure 12.9 for more results of the proposed 3D segmentation approach.

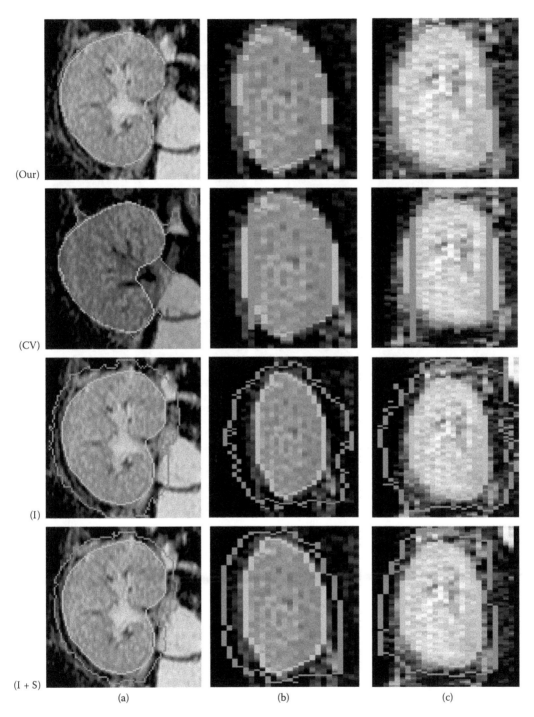

Figure 12.7 Comparative cross-sectional segmentation results for our approach, the traditional CV [39] level set, the level set guided by intensity alone, and intensity and spatial, respectively, in rows for (a) the coronal cross-section, (b) the axial cross-section, and (c) the sagittal cross-section of one subject at b_0 s/mm^2. The model segmentation is shown in red with respect to the manual ground truth (green) from an expert.

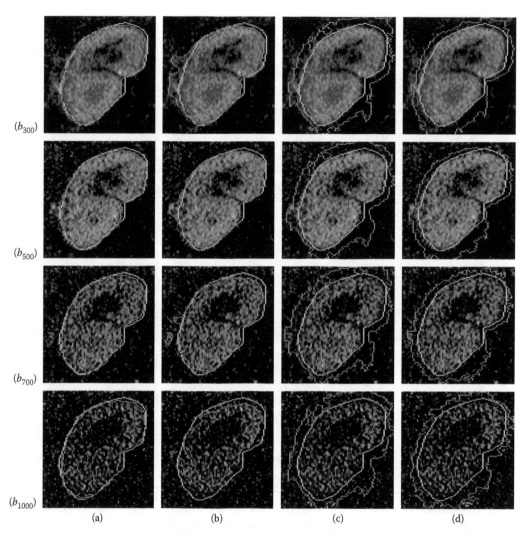

Figure 12.8 A sample coronal cross-sectional kidney segmentation for DW-MRI data acquired at b_{300} s/mm^2 (first row), b_{500} s/mm^2 (second row), b_{700} s/mm^2 (third row), and b_{1000} s/mm^2 (fourth row) for (a) the proposed approach; (b) the CV [39] approach; (c) the level set guided by intensity only; and (d) intensity and spatial.

12.6   Conclusions

To summarize, the proposed approach is a promising method for guiding a level set deformable model to segment the kidney from diffusion-weighted MRIs. Our findings confirm that combining the adaptive shape model with the first- and second-order visual appearance features makes the developed approach more accurate and robust. Compared to other level set-based methods that exploit image intensity alone, significantly, better segmentation results for the kidney using the approach described in the body of work have been shown through experimental analysis on in vivo data. Despite challenges in segmenting the kidney from DW-MRI data, such as similar intensities of the kidney and surrounding tissues, image noise, and interpatient anatomical differences, the described

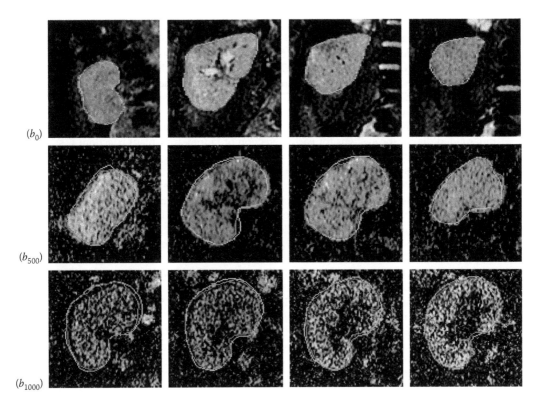

Figure 12.9 More coronal cross-sections (columns) for the proposed kidney segmentation approach for DW-MRI data acquired at different b-values s/mm^2 (rows).

approach proves that the addition of an adaptive shape model and the spatial features (i.e., spatial interactions between the DW-MRI voxels) increases robustness and accuracy, which in turn increases the reliability of this kidney segmentation method.

So far, we have developed an automated framework for 3D kidney segmentation that can be incorporated in any CAD system for renal functional assessment. We plan to test the proposed kidney segmentation approach on more subjects to increase and confirm the level of confidence of the presented framework. The promising results obtained from the presented kidney segmentation technique encourage us to utilize and extend the developed framework for the segmentation of other organs using different modalities (e.g., cardiac MR images [58–67], prostate dynamic contrast enhanced (DCE)/DW-MRI [68–74], and CT chest images [75–92]).

References

1. M. Abou-El-Ghar, T. El-Diasty, A. El-Assmy, H. Refaie, A. Refaie, and M. Ghoneim, Role of diffusion-weighted MRI in diagnosis of acute renal allograft dysfunction: A prospective preliminary study, *The British Journal of Radiology*, vol. 85, no. 1014, pp. e206–e211, 2014.
2. G. Liu, F. Han, W. Xiao, Q. Wang, Y. Xu, and J. Chen, Detection of renal allograft rejection using blood oxygen level-dependent and diffusion weighted magnetic resonance imaging: A retrospective study, *BMC Nephrology*, vol. 15, no. 1, p.158, 2014.

3. F. Khalifa, A. El-Baz, G. Gimel'farb, and M. A. El-Ghar, Non-invasive image-based approach for early detection of acute renal rejection, in *International Conference on Medical Image Computing and Computer-Assisted Intervention* (MICCAI'10), Beijing, China, September 20–24, pp. 10–18, 2010.

4. M. Mostapha, F. Khalifa, A. Alansary, A. Soliman, J. Suri, and A. El-Baz, Computer aided diagnosis systems for acute renal transplant rejection: Challenges and methodologies, in *Abdomen and Thoracic Imaging: An Engineering & Clinical Perspective*, L. S. A. El-Baz, J. Suri, Eds., vol. 1. Berlin: Springer-Verlag, 2014, pp. 1–36.

5. M. Mostapha, F. Khalifa, A. A. A. S. G. Gimel'farb, and A. El-Baz, Dynamic MRI-based computer aided diagnostic systems for early detection of kidney transplant rejection: A survey, in *Proceedings of International Symposium on Computational Models for Life Science* (CMLS'13), vol. 1559, Sydney, Australia, November 27–29, pp. 297–306, 2013.

6. F. Khalifa, G. M. Beache, M. A. El-Ghar, T. El-Diasty, G. Gimel'farb, M. Kong, and El-Baz, Dynamic contrast-enhanced MRI-based early detection of acute renal transplant rejection, *IEEE Transactions on Medical Imaging*, vol. 32, no. 10, pp. 1910–1927, 2013.

7. F. Khalifa, A. Soliman, A. El-Baz, M. A. El-Ghar, T. El-Diasty, G. Gimel'farb, R. Ouseph, and A. C. Dwyer, Models and methods for analyzing DCE-MRI: A review, *Medical Physics*, vol. 41, no. 12, p. 124301, 2014.

8. F. Khalifa, M. A. El-Ghar, B. Abdollahi, H. B. Frieboes, T. El-Diasty, and A. El-Baz, Dynamic contrast-enhanced MRI-based early detection of acute renal transplant rejection, in *2014 Annual Scientific Meeting and Educational Course Brochure of the Society of Abdominal Radiology* (SAR'14), Boca Raton, FL, March 23–28, 2014, CID: 1855912.

9. F. Khalifa, M. A. El-Ghar, B. Abdollahi, H. Frieboes, T. El-Diasty, and A. El-Baz, A comprehensive non-invasive framework for automated evaluation of acute renal transplant rejection using DCE-MRI, *NMR in Biomedicine*, vol. 26, no. 11, pp. 1460–1470, 2013.

10. L. Mackelaite, R. Ouseph, A. El-Baz, and A. Gaweda, Cortical CT perfusion of the live donor kidneys as a predictor of post transplant graft function, *American Journal of Transplantation*, vol. 12, pp. 329–329, 2012.

11. A. El-Baz, G. Gimel'farb, and M. A. El-Ghar, Image analysis approach for identification of renal transplant rejection, in *Proceedings of IAPR International Conference on Pattern Recognition* (ICPR'08), Tampa, FL, December 8–11, pp. 1–4, 2008.

12. A. El-Baz, G. Gimel'farb, and M. A. El-Ghar, A novel image analysis approach for accurate identification of acute renal rejection, in *Proceedings of IEEE International Conference on Image Processing* (ICIP'08), San Diego, CA, October 12–15, pp. 1812–1815, 2008.

13. A. El-Baz, A. A. Farag, S. E. Yuksel, M. E. A. El-Ghar, T. A. Eldiasty, and M. A. Ghoneim, Application of deformable models for the detection of acute renal rejection, In *Deformable Models*, vol. 1, in A. A. Farag and J. S. Suri, Eds., 2007, pp. 293–333.

14. A. Farag, A. El-Baz, S. Yuksel, M. A. El-Ghar, and T. Eldiasty, A framework for the detection of acute rejection with dynamic contrast enhanced magnetic resonance imaging, in *Proceedings of IEEE International Symposium on Biomedical Imaging: From Nano to Macro* (ISBI'06), Arlington, VA, April 6–9, pp. 418–421, 2006.

15. A. El-Baz, A. Farag, R. Fahmi, S. Yuksel, W. Miller, M. A. El-Ghar, T. El-Diasty, and M. Ghoneim, A new CAD system for the evaluation of kidney diseases using DCE-MRI, in *Proceedings of International Conference on Medical Image Computing and Computer-Assisted Intervention* (MICCAI'08), Copenhagen, Denmark, October 1–6, 2006, pp. 446–453.

16. A. El-Baz, A. Farag, R. Fahmi, S. Yuksel, M. A. El-Ghar, and T. Eldiasty, Image analysis of renal DCE MRI for the detection of acute renal rejection, in *Proceedings of IAPR International Conference on Pattern Recognition* (ICPR'06), Hong Kong, August 20–24, pp. 822–825, 2006.

17. S. E. Yuksel, A. El-Baz, A. A. Farag, M. E. Abo El-Ghar, T. A. Eldiasty, and M. A. Ghoneim, Automatic detection of renal rejection after kidney transplantation, in *International Congress Series*, vol. 1281, pp. 773–778, 2005.

18. A. Rudra, A. Chowdhury, A. Elnakib, F. Khalifa, A. Soliman, G. M. Beache, and A. El-Baz, Kidney segmentation using graph cuts and pixel connectivity, *Pattern Recognition Letters*, vol. 34, no. 13, pp. 1470–1475, 2013.

19. F. Khalifa, A. Elnakib, G. M. Beache, G. Gimel'farb, M. A. El-Ghar, G. Sokhadze, S. Manning, P. McClure, and A. El-Baz, 3D kidney segmentation from CT images using a level set approach guided by a novel stochastic speed function, in *Proceedings of International Conference Medical Image Computing and Computer-Assisted Intervention* (MICCAI'11), Toronto, Canada, September 18–22, pp. 587–594, 2011.

20. F. Khalifa, G. Gimel'farb, M. A. El-Ghar, G. Sokhadze, S. Manning, P. McClure, R. Ouseph, and A. El-Baz, A new deformable model-based segmentation approach for accurate extraction of the kidney from abdominal CT images, in *Proceedings of IEEE International Conference on Image Processing* (ICIP'11), Brussels, Belgium, September 11–14, pp. 3393–3396, 2011.

21. F. Khalifa, A. El-Baz, G. Gimel'farb, R. Ouseph, and M. A. El-Ghar, Shape-appearance guided level-set deformable model for image segmentation, in *Proceedings of IAPR International Conference on Pattern Recognition* (ICPR'10), Istanbul, Turkey, August 23–26, pp. 4581–4584, 2010.

22. S. E. Yuksel, A. El-Baz, A. A. Farag, M. El-Ghar, T. Eldiasty, and M. A. Ghoneim, A kidney segmentation framework for dynamic contrast enhanced magnetic resonance imaging, *Journal of Vibration and Control*, vol. 13, no. 9–10, pp. 1505–1516, 2007.

23. A. M. Ali, A. A. Farag, and A. El-Baz, Graph cuts framework for kidney segmentation with prior shape constraints, in *Proceedings of the International Conference on Medical Image Computing and Computer-Assisted Intervention* (MICCAI'07), vol. 1, Brisbane, Australia, October 29–November 2, pp. 384–392, 2007.

24. S. E. Yuksel, A. El-Baz, and A. A. Farag, A kidney segmentation framework for dynamic contrast enhanced magnetic resonance imaging, in *Proceedings of International Symposium on Mathematical Methods in Engineering* (MME'06), Ankara, Turkey, April 27–29, pp. 55–64, 2006.

25. S. Mujumdar, R. Varma, and L. Kishore, A novel framework for segmentation of stroke lesions in diffusion weighted MRI using multiple b-value data, in *21st International Conference on Pattern Recognition* (ICPR), IEEE, pp. 3762–3765, 2012.

26. M. Saad, S. Abu-Bakar, S. Muda, M. Mokji, A. Abdullah, Fully automated region growing segmentation of brain lesion in diffusion-weighted MRI, *IAENG International Journal of Computer Science*, vol. 39, no. 2, pp. 155–164, 2012.

27. C.-F. Lu, P.-S. Wang, Y.-C. Chou, H.-C. Li, B.-W. Soong, and Y.-T. Wu, Segmentation of diffusion-weighted brain images using expectation maximization algorithm initialized by hierarchical clustering, in *30th Annual International Conference of the IEEE Engineering in Medicine and Biology Society*, IEEE, pp. 5502–5505, 2008.

28. M. Niethammer, C. Zach, J. Melonakos, and A. Tannenbaum, Near-tubular fiber bundle segmentation for diffusion weighted imaging: Segmentation through frame reorientation, *NeuroImage*, vol. 45, no. 1, 2009, pp. S123–S132.

29. H. Li, T. Liu, G. Young, L. Guo, and S. T. Wong, Brain tissue segmentation based on DWI/DTI data, in *3rd IEEE International Symposium on Biomedical Imaging: Nano to Macro*, pp. 57–60, 2006.

30. S. Ozer, D. L. Langer, X. Liu, M. A. Haider, T. H. van der Kwast, A. J. Evans, Y. Yang, M. N. Wernick, and I. S. Yetik, Supervised and unsupervised methods for prostate cancer segmentation with multispectral MRI, *Medical Physics*, vol. 37, no. 4, pp. 1873–1883, 2010.

31. X. Liu, D. Langer, M. Haider, T. Van der Kwast, A. Evans, M. Wernick, and I. Yetik, Unsupervised segmentation of the prostate using MR images based on level set with a shape prior, in *International Conference of the IEEE Engineering in Medicine and Biology Society*, pp. 3613–3616, 2009.

32. X. Liu, M. A. Haider, and I. S. Yetik, Unsupervised 3D prostate segmentation based on diffusion-weighted imaging MRI using active contour models with a shape prior, *Journal of Electrical and Computer Engineering*, vol. 2011, p. 11, 2011.

33. X. Liu, D. L. Langer, M. A. Haider, Y. Yang, M. N. Wernick, and I. S. Yetik, Prostate cancer segmentation with simultaneous estimation of Markov random field parameters and class, *IEEE Transactions on Medical Imaging*, vol. 28, no. 6, pp. 906–915, 2009.

34. A. Firjani, A. Elnakib, F. Khalifa, G. Gimelfarb, M. A. El-Ghar, A. Elmaghraby, and El-Baz, A diffusion-weighted imaging based diagnostic system for early detection of prostate cancer, *Journal of Biomedical Science and Engineering*, vol. 6, no. 3, p. 346, 2013.

35. C. Krishnamurty, J. Rodriguez, N. Raghunand et al., Automatic lesion tracking in echo-planar diffusion weighted liver MRI: an active countour based approach, in *Proceeding of the International Society for Magnetic Resonance in Medicine*, vol. 13, p. 1889, 2005.

36. C. Platero, M. Gonzalez, M. Tobar, J. Poncela, J. Sanguino, G. Asensio, and E. Santos, Automatic method to segment the liver on multi-phase MRI, *Computer Assisted Radiology and Surgery 22nd International Congress and Exhibition, CARS 2008*, Barcelona, Spain, 2008.

37. H. Veeraraghavan and K. Do, Joint segmentation and sequential registration based approach for computing artifact-free ADC maps from multiple DWI-MRI sequences in liver, *Medical Physics*, vol. 40, no. 6, pp. 521–530, 2013.

38. A. K. Jha, J. J. Rodríguez, R. M. Stephen, and A. T. Stopeck, A clustering algorithm for liver lesion segmentation of diffusion-weighted MR images, in *IEEE Southwest Symposium Image Analysis and Interpretation*, IEEE, pp. 93–96, 2010.

39. T. F. Chan and L. A. Vese, Active contours without edges, *IEEE Transactions on Image Processing*, vol. 10, no. 2, pp. 266–277, 2001.

40. D. Wishart, An algorithm for hierarchical classifications, *Biometrics*, pp. 165–170, 1969.

41. Y.-T. Wu, Y.-C. Chou, W.-Y. Guo, T.-C. Yeh, and J.-C. Hsieh, Classification of spatiotemporal hemodynamics from brain perfusion MR images using expectation-maximization estimation with finite mixture of multivariate Gaussian distributions, *Magnetic Resonance in Medicine*, vol. 57, no. 1, pp. 181–191, 2007.

42. N. Hevia-Montiel, J. R. Jimenez-Alaniz, V. Medina-Banuelos, O. Yanez-Suarez, C. Rosso, Y. Samson, and S. Baillet, Robust nonparametric segmentation of infarct lesion from diffusion-weighted MR images, in *29th Annual International Conference of the IEEE Engineering in Medicine and Biology Society*, IEEE, pp. 2102–2105, 2007.

43. S. K. Warfield, K. H. Zou, and W. M. Wells, Simultaneous truth and performance level estimation (staple): An algorithm for the validation of image segmentation, *IEEE Transactions on Medical Imaging*, vol. 23, no. 7, pp. 903–921, 2004.

44. N. Otsu, A threshold selection method from gray-level histograms, *Automatica*, vol. 11, no. 285–296, pp. 23–27, 1975.

45. C. Krishnamurthy, J. Rodriguez, and R. Gillies, Snake-based liver lesion segmentation, in *6th IEEE Southwest Symposium on Image Analysis and Interpretation*, pp. 187–191, 2004.

46. A. Elnakib, G. Gimelfarb, J. S. Suri, and A. El-Baz, Medical image segmentation: A brief survey, in *Multi-Modality State-of-the-Art Medical Image Segmentation and Registration Methodologies*. Berlin: Springer, 2011, pp. 1–39.

47. M. Shehata, F. Khalifa, A. Soliman, R. Alrefai, M. A. El-Ghar, A. C. Dwyer, R. Ouseph, and A. El-Baz, A novel framework for automatic segmentation of kidney from DW-MRI, in *Proceedings of IEEE 12th International Symposium on Biomedical Imaging (ISBI), 2015*, IEEE, pp. 951–954, 2015.

48. M. Shehata, F. Khalifa, A. Soliman, R. Alrefai, M. A. El-Ghar, A. C. Dwyer, R. Ouseph, and A. El-Baz, A level set-based framework for 3D kidney segmentation from diffusion MR images, in *Proceedings of IEEE International Conference on Image Processing (ICIP'15)*, Quebec, Canada, September 27–30, IEEE, pp. 4441–4445, 2015.

49. F. Khalifa, G. M. Beache, G. Gimel'farb, G. A. Giridharan, and A. El-Baz, Accurate automatic analysis of cardiac cine images, *IEEE Transactions on Biomedical Engineering*, vol. 59, no. 2, pp. 445–455, 2012.

50. S. Osher and R. Fedkiw, *Level Set Methods and Dynamic Implicit Surfaces*. New York: Springer Verlag, 2006.

51. N. J. Tustison, B. B. Avants, P. A. Cook, Y. Zheng, A. Egan, P. A. Yushkevich, and J. C. Gee, N4ITK: Improved N3 bias correction, *IEEE Transactions on Medical Imaging*, vol. 29, no. 6, pp. 1310–1320, 2010.

52. B. Glocker, A. Sotiras, N. Komodakis, and N. Paragios, Deformable medical image registration: Setting the state of the art with discrete methods, *Annual Review of Biomedical Engineering* vol. 13, pp. 219–244, 2011.

53. A. Farag, A. El-Baz, and G. Gimelfarb, Precise segmentation of multimodal images, *IEEE Transactions on Image Processing*, vol. 15, no. 4, pp. 952–968, 2006.

54. A. El-Baz, A. Elnakib, F. Khalifa, M. A. El-Ghar, P. McClure, A. Soliman, and G. Gimel'farb, Precise segmentation of 3-D magnetic resonance angiography, *IEEE Transactions on Biomedical Engineering*, vol. 59, no. 7, pp. 2019–2029, 2012.

55. K. H. Zou, S. K. Warfield, A. Bharatha, C. M. C. Tempany, M. R. Kaus, S. J. Haker, W. M. Wells III, F. A. Jolesz, and R. Kikinis, Statistical validation of image segmentation quality based on a spatial overlap index, *Academic Radiology*, vol. 11, no. 2, pp. 178–189, 2004.

56. G. Gerig, M. Jomier, M. Chakos, Valmet: A new validation tool for assessing and improving 3D object segmentation, in *Medical Image Computing and Computer Assisted Intervention*, pp. 516–523, 2001.

57. J. Zhao, Z. Wang, M. Liu, J. Zhu, X. Zhang, T. Zhang, S. Li, and Y. Li, Assessment of renal fibrosis in chronic kidney disease using diffusion-weighted MRI, *Clinical Radiology*, vol. 69, no. 11, pp. 1117–1122, 2014.

58. A. Elnakib, G. M. Beache, G. Gimel'farb, and A. El-Baz, A new framework for automated segmentation of left ventricle wall from contrast enhanced cardiac magnetic resonance images, in *Proceedings International Conference on Image Processing* (ICIP'2011), IEEE, pp. 2289–2292, 2011.

59. F. Khalifa, G. Beache, A. El-Baz, and G. Gimel'farb, Deformable model guided by stochastic speed with application in cine images segmentation, in *Proceedings of IEEE International Conference on Image Processing* (ICIP'10), Hong Kong, September 26–29, pp. 1725–1728, 2010.

60. F. Khalifa, G. M. Beache, A. Elnakib, H. Sliman, G. Gimel'farb, K. C. Welch, and A. El-Baz, A new shape-based framework for the left ventricle wall segmentation from cardiac first-pass perfusion MRI, in *Proceedings of IEEE International Symposium on Biomedical Imaging: From Nano to Macro* (ISBI'13), San Francisco, CA, April 7–11, pp. 41–44, 2013.

61. F. Khalifa, G. M. Beache, G. Gimel'farb, and A. El-Baz, A novel approach for accurate estimation of left ventricle global indexes from short-axis cine MRI, in *Proceedings of IEEE International Conference on Image Processing* (ICIP'11), Brussels, Belgium, September 11–14, pp. 2645–2649, 2011.

62. F. Khalifa, G. M. Beache, G. Gimel'farb, G. A. Giridharan, and A. El-Baz, A new image-based framework for analyzing cine images, in *Handbook of Multi-Modality State-of-the-Art Medical Image Segmentation and Registration Methodologies*, vol. 2, A. El-Baz, U. R. Acharya, M. Mirmedhdi, J. S. Suri, Eds. New York: Springer, 2011, pp. 69–98.

63. F. Khalifa, G. M. Beache, G. G. Farb, G. Giridharan, A. El-Baz, et al., Accurate automatic analysis of cardiac cine images, *IEEE Transactions on Biomedical Engineering*, vol. 59, no. 2, pp. 445–455, 2012.

64. F. Khalifa, G. M. Beache, M. Nitzken, G. Gimel'farb, G. A. Giridharan, and A. El-Baz, Automatic analysis of left ventricle wall thickness using short-axis cine CMR images, in *Proceedings of IEEE International Symposium on Biomedical Imaging: From Nano to Macro* (ISBI'11), Chicago, IL, March 30–April 2, pp. 1306–1309, 2011.

65. H. Sliman, F. Khalifa, A. Elnakib, G. M. Beache, A. Elmaghraby, and A. El-Baz, A new segmentation-based tracking framework for extracting the left ventricle cavity from cine cardiac MRI, in *Proceedings of IEEE International Conference on Image Processing* (ICIP'13), Melbourne, Australia, September 15–18, pp. 685–689, 2013.

66. H. Sliman, F. Khalifa, A. Elnakib, A. Soliman, G. M. Beache, A. Elmaghraby, G. Gimel'farb, and A. El-Baz, Myocardial borders segmentation from cine MR images using bi-directional coupled parametric deformable models, *Medical Physics*, vol. 40, no. 9, pp. 1–13, 2013.

67. H. Sliman, F. Khalifa, A. Elnakib, A. Soliman, G. M. Beach e, G. Gimel'farb, A. Emam, A. Elmaghraby, and A. El-Baz, Accurate segmentation framework for the left ventricle wall from cardiac cine MRI, in *Proceedings of International Symposium on Computational Models for Life Science* (CMLS'13), vol. 1559, Sydney, Australia, November 27–29, pp. 287–296, 2013.

68. A. Firjani, A. Elnakib, F. Khalifa, A. El-Baz, G. Gimel'farb, M. A. El-Ghar, and A. El-maghraby, A novel 3D segmentation approach for segmenting the prostate from dynamic contrast enhanced MRI using current appearance and learned shape prior, in *Proceedings of IEEE International Symposium on Signal Processing and Information Technology* (ISSPIT'10), Luxor, Egypt, December 15–18, pp. 137–143, 2010.

69. A. Firjani, A. Elnakib, F. Khalifa, G. Gimel'farb, M. A. El-Ghar, A. Elmaghraby, and A. El-Baz, A new 3D automatic segmentation framework for accurate extraction of prostate from diffusion imaging, in *Proceedings of Biomedical Science and Engineering Conference—Image Informatics and Analytics in Biomedicine* (BSEC'11), Knoxville, TN, March 15–17, pp. 1306–1309, 2011.

70. A. Firjani, A. Elnakib, F. Khalifa, G. Gimel'farb, M. A. El-Ghar, J. Suri, A. El- maghraby, and A. El-Baz, A new 3D automatic segmentation framework for accurate extraction of prostate from DCE-MRI, in *Proceedings of IEEE International Symposium on Biomedical Imaging: From Nano to Macro* (ISBI'11), Chicago, IL, March 30–April 2, pp. 1476–1479, 2011.

71. A. Firjani, F. Khalifa, A. Elnakib, G. Gimel'farb, M. A. El-Ghar, A. Elmaghraby, and A.El-Baz, 3D automatic approach for precise segmentation of the prostate from diffusion-weighted magnetic resonance imaging, in *Proceedings of IEEE International Conference on Image Processing* (ICIP'11), Brussels, Belgium, September 11–14, pp. 2285–2288, 2011.

72. A. Firjany, A. Elnakib, A. El-Baz, G. Gimel'farb, M. El-Ghar, and A. Elmagharby, Novel stochastic framework for accurate segmentation of prostate in dynamic contrast enhanced MRI, in *Prostate Cancer Imaging. Computer-Aided Diagnosis, Prognosis, and Intervention*, vol. 6367 of Lecture Notes in Computer Science, A. Madabhushi, J. Dowling, P. Yan, A. Fenster, P. Abolmaesumi, N. Hata, Eds. Berlin: Springer, 2010, pp. 121–130.

73. A. Firjany, A. Elnakib, A. El-Baz, G. Gimelfarb, M. A. El-Ghar, and A. Elmagharby, Novel stochastic framework for accurate segmentation of prostate in dynamic contrast-enhanced MRI, in *Proceedings of the International Workshop on Prostate Cancer Imaging: Computer-Aided Diagnosis, Prognosis, and Intervention*, Beijing, China, September 24, pp. 121–130, 2010.

74. P. McClure, F. Khalifa, A. Soliman, M. Abou El-Ghar, G. Gimelfarb, A. Elma- graby, and A. El-Baz, A novel NMF guided level-set for dwi prostate segmentation, *Journal of Computer Science and Systems Biology*, vol. 7, pp. 209–216, 2014.

75. B. Abdollahi, A. C. Civelek, X.-F. Li, J. Suri, and A. El-Baz, PET/CT nodule segmentation and diagnosis: A survey, in *Multi-Detector CT Imaging*. L. Saba and J. S. Suri, Eds. New York: Taylor & Francis, 2014, pp. 639–651.

76. B. Abdollahi, A. El-Baz, and A. A. Amini, A multi-scale non-linear vessel enhancement technique, in *Engineering in Medicine and Biology Society* (EMBC), 2011 Annual International Conference of the IEEE, IEEE, pp. 3925–3929, 2011.

77. B. Abdollahi, A. Soliman, A. Civelek, X.-F. Li, G. Gimel'farb, and A. El-Baz, A novel Gaussian scale space-based joint MGRF framework for precise lung segmentation, in *Proceedings of IEEE International Conference on Image Processing* (ICIP'12), IEEE, pp. 2029–2032, 2012.

78. B. Abdollahi, A. Soliman, A. Civelek, X.-F. Li, G. Gimelfarb, and A. El-Baz, A novel 3D joint MGRF framework for precise lung segmentation, in *Machine Learning in Medical Imaging*. Berlin: Springer, 2012, pp. 86–93.

79. A. M. Ali, A. S. El-Baz, and A. A. Farag, A novel framework for accurate lung segmentation using graph cuts, in: *Proceedings of IEEE International Symposium on Biomedical Imaging: From Nano to Macro* (ISBI'07), IEEE, pp. 908–911, 2007.

80. A. El-Baz, A. Farag, G. Gimel'farb, R. Falk, M. A. El-Ghar, and T. Eldiasty, A framework for auto-matic segmentation of lung nodules from low dose chest CT scans, in *Proceedings of International Conference on Pattern Recognition* (ICPR'06), vol. 3, IEEE, pp. 611–614, 2006.

81. A. El-Baz, A. A. Farag, R. Falk, and R. La Rocca, Detection, visualization and identification of lung abnormalities in chest spiral CT scan: Phase-i, in *International Conference on Biomedical Engineering*, Cairo, Egypt, vol. 12, pp. 231–234, 2002.

82. A. El-Baz, A. A. Farag, R. Falk, and R. La Rocca, A unified approach for detection, visualiza-tion, and identification of lung abnormalities in chest spiral CT scans, in International Congress Series, vol. 1256. Amsterdam: Elsevier, 2003, pp. 998–1004.

83. A. A. Farag, A. El-Baz, G. Gimelfarb, M. A. El-Ghar, and T. Eldiasty, Quantitative nodule detec-tion in low dose chest CT scans: New template modeling and evaluation for CAD system design, in *Medical Image Computing and Computer-Assisted Intervention—MICCAI 2005*. Berlin: Springer, 2005, pp. 720–728.

84. A. El-Baz, G. Gimel'farb, and R. Falk, A novel 3D framework for automatic lung segmentation from low dose CT images, in *Lung Imaging and Computer Aided Diagnosis*, A. El-Baz and J. S. Suri, Eds. Boca Raton, FL: Taylor & Francis, 2011, pp. 1–16.

85. A. El-Baz, G. Gimelfarb, R. Falk, and M. A. El-Ghar, Automatic analysis of 3D low dose CT images for early diagnosis of lung cancer, *Pattern Recognition*, vol. 42, no. 6, pp. 1041–1051, 2009.

86. A. El-Baz, G. L. Gimel'farb, R. Falk, M. Abou El-Ghar, T. Holland, and T. Shaffer, A new stochastic framework for accurate lung segmentation, in *Proceedings of Medical Image Computing and Computer-Assisted Intervention* (MICCAI'08), pp. 322–330, 2008.

87. A. El-Baz, G. L. Gimel'farb, R. Falk, T. Holland, and T. Shaffer, A framework for unsupervised segmentation of lung tissues from low dose computed tomography images, in *Proceedings of British Machine Vision* (BMVC'08), pp. 1–10, 2008.

88. A. El-Baz, G. Gimelfarb, R. Falk, and M. A. El-Ghar, 3D MGRF-based appearance modeling for robust segmentation of pulmonary nodules in 3D LDCT chest images, in *Lung Imaging and Computer Aided Diagnosis*, Boca Raton, FL: Taylor & Francis, 2011, pp. 51–63.

89. A. A. Farag, A. El-Baz, G. Gimelfarb, R. Falk, M. A. El-Ghar, T. Eldiasty, and S. Elshazly, Appearance models for robust segmentation of pulmonary nodules in 3D LDCT chest images, in *Proceedings of Medical Image Computing and Computer-Assisted Intervention* (MICCAI), 2006. Berlin: Springer, 2006, pp. 662–670.

90. E. Hosseini-Asl, J. M. Zurada, and A. El-Baz, Lung segmentation based on nonnegative matrix factorization, in: *Image Processing* (ICIP), 2014 IEEE International Conference on, IEEE, pp. 877–881, 2014.

91. A. Soliman, F. Khalifa, A. Alansary, G. Gimel'farb, and A. El-Baz, Performance evaluation of an automatic MGRF-based lung segmentation approach, in *Proceedings of International Symposium on Computational Models for Life Sciences* (CMLS'13), vol. 1559, p. 323, 2013.

92. A. Soliman, F. Khalifa, A. Alansary, G. Gimel'farb, and A. El-Baz, Segmentation of lung region based on using parallel implementation of joint MGRF: Validation on 3D realistic lung phantoms, in *Proceedings of International Symposium on Biomedical Imaging: From Nano to Macro* (ISBI'13), IEEE, pp. 864–867, 2013.

chapter thirteen

Prostate segmentation using deformable model-based methods

A review

Islam Reda, Mohammed Elmogy, Ahmed Aboulfotouh, Marwa Ismail, Ayman El-Baz, and Robert Keynton

Contents

Abstract

Prostate cancer is the second leading cause of cancer deaths in American men. Early diagnosis of prostate cancer enhances the success rate of survival for male patients. As a result, it is critical to identify and create methods to facilitate early diagnosis of prostate cancer, especially noninvasive techniques such as medical imaging and computer-aided diagnostic (CAD) systems. In medical imaging, segmentation of tissue, such as the prostate is a critical component to improve the accuracy of image analysis and all subsequent stages, especially detection. In this chapter, the anatomy of the prostate gland will be discussed as well as the diagnostic techniques that have been traditionally used. The primary focus of this chapter will be on the application of deformable models, including both geometric and parametric models, for the prostate segmentation of images acquired from different imaging modalities, such as magnetic resonance imaging (MRI), computed tomography (CT), and ultrasound. Finally, the clinical data used in these studies will be highlighted along with a description of advantages and limitations in the performance of each segmentation algorithm.

13.1   Introduction

The prostate is a single gland that surrounds the prostatic urethra and is about the size of a golf ball [1]. The purpose of the prostate gland is to compress the urethra and secrete a fluid that sustains and protects sperm during ejaculation and while in the lower reproductive tract of females. Unfortunately, as men age, they become more susceptible to prostate cancer, which is the most common cause of cancer in men in the United States, after skin cancer, with the greatest risk factor being aging, particularly beyond age 50 [2].

The rate of prostate cancer among African American is higher than white men. The majority of prostate cancers are adenocarcinomas (cancers that commence in cells that generate and discharge mucus and other fluids). The process for determining whether cancer has spread within the prostate or to other tissues in the body is called staging and can be grouped into four stages (Figure 13.1). Specifically, in stage I, the cancer is localized in the prostate and growing at a slow rate. In stage II, the cancer is still localized in the prostate but growing at a faster rate. During stage III, cancer cells have spread to tissues surrounding the prostate gland, while in stage IV, the cancer cells have metastasized to other tissues such as lymph nodes, the rectum, etc. [3].

Several different techniques are traditionally used to diagnose prostate cancer such as a digital rectal exam (DRE) [4], prostate-specific antigen (PSA) [5], needle biopsy [6], and CAD systems. The DRE test is performed by a physician who manually checks the prostate with his fingers through the rectum to detect any abnormalities in size or hardness. While some peripheral zone tumors can be detected by the DRE test, most of the central zone and the transitional zone tumors cannot be identified as well as tumors that are too small to be palpated cannot be detected through DRE. As a result, physician experience and skill significantly influences the accuracy of this test. The PSA test has a higher sensitivity and specificity than the DRE test and is the most popular type of the blood-based tests [4]. An increased value of PSA indicates a higher probability for prostate cancer; however, elevated levels may also signify other conditions such as inflammation or enlargement of the prostate. If the blood PSA levels exceed 4 ng/mL, patients undergo additional testing, such as needle biopsy, to confirm the severity of the condition [4].

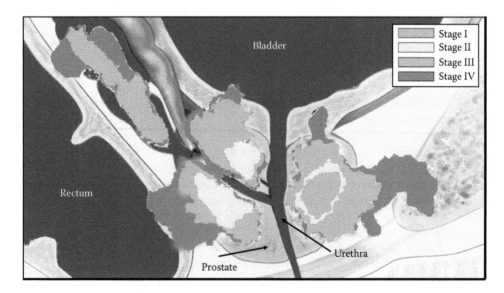

Figure 13.1 Schematic illustration of the four stages of prostate cancer.

Transrectal ultrasound (TRUS) guided needle biopsy procedures involve taking a small tissue sample from the prostate gland for histological examination. To analyze the sample, number of scoring systems have been developed, including the Gleason (1960s) [7], the modified Gleason and Mellinger (1974) [8] and the International Society of Urological Pathology (ISUP) modified Gleason system [9,10]. The ISUP modified Gleason system involves pathologist assigning a score between 1 and 5 based on the degree of each of the two tumor patterns, that is, architectural and neoplasm patterns. A score of 5 for the architectural pattern indicates that the tissue is the least differentiated typical of cancerous tissue, while a neoplasm score of 5 signifies that the tumor resembles the most prevalent neoplasm pattern. Summation of these two scores indicate the severity of the neoplasm where a score between 6 and 10 means the tumor is cancerous [11]. Although needle biopsy is the most accurate way to detect cancer and determine the aggressiveness of the cancer, it is an expensive, highly invasive, and painful procedure. Thus, it is imperative that an accurate noninvasive method with high selectivity and specificity be developed.

The field of medical imaging technology has provided excellent tools for visualizing different body structures and their associated abnormalities. Specifically, ultrasound, CT, and MRI have been used extensively to visualize the prostate to determine the severity of the disorders (Figure 13.2). Due to the limitations associated with the in vitro testing techniques described above, in vivo image-based CAD systems have been used to localize and identify the size and extent of prostate cancer. Each of the modalities mentioned above has its own advantages and disadvantages, which are discussed below.

Transrectal ultrasound (TRUS) is the most frequently used prostate imaging technique since it is used primarily in guiding needle biopsies and determining the prostate volume [12,13]. Some advantages of using TRUS in CAD systems are: its portability, low cost relative to other imaging modalities, generation of real-time imaging data, and does not involve radiation. On the other hand, its disadvantages include: produces low contrast images that contain speckles, has low signal-to-noise ratio (SNR), and generates shadow artifacts [14]. Consequently, it is difficult to detect tumors with a high level of accuracy and/or determine the stage of cancer using TRUS imaging techniques.

With regard to CT, it combines multiple x-ray projections taken from different angles to construct an image of the internal structure of the object of interest. It is used for the evaluation of the effectiveness of brachytherapy and can be used to determine the spread of the prostate cancer to bone tissues. But, it is not portable, involves radiation, has a high cost, has poor soft tissue contrast, and is not effective in detecting cancer staging.

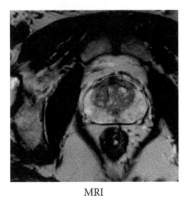 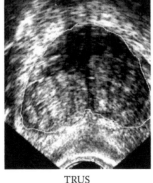 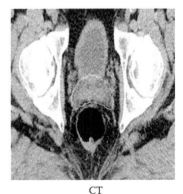

MRI   TRUS   CT

Figure 13.2 MRI, TRUS, and CT prostate images.

On the other hand, MRI provides the best contrast between soft tissues compared to other image modalities, such as CT and TRUS. MRI does not involve radiation and is useful for determining the stage of the cancer. However, MRI is not portable, is sensitive to noise and image artifacts, has difficulties to implement real-time imaging due to its relatively long and complex acquisition, and has a relatively high cost [12,15].

Several different MRI techniques have been extensively used in prostate cancer CAD systems such as T2-MRI, dynamic contrast-enhanced (DCE) MRI, and diffusion MRI. Even though T2-MRI provides good contrast between soft tissues, it lacks functional information. DCE MRI is a technique that provides detailed information on the anatomy and function of different tissues. It has gained wide attention due to the increased spatial resolution, the ability to yield information about the hemodynamics (i.e., perfusion), micro vascular permeability, and extracellular leakage space [16]. DCE MRI has been extensively used in many clinical applications [17–24] in addition to the detection of prostate cancer [25–27]. In DCE MRI, a series of MR images is taken prior to and after administering a contrast agent into the blood stream to significantly enhance the contrast between the different tissue types and ease visualization of the anatomical structures that have alternating magnetic properties in their vicinity. The acquired signal intensity is proportional to the concentration of contrast agent in each voxel. Several types of MRI contrast agents such as paramagnetic agents, superparamagnetic agents, extracellular fluid (ECF) space agents, and tissue (organ)-specific agents can be used depending on the application.

Another MRI modality is diffusion MRI, which unlike DCE MRI, does not involve the use of contrast agents and has been attracting researchers recently is based on the measurement of micromovements of water molecules inside the body [28,29]. It can be acquired in a short time and, as mentioned before, does not depend on any contrast agents. It can be classified into three major categories; diffusion-weighted imaging (DWI) [30,31], diffusion tensor imaging (DTI) [31–33], and diffusion spectrum imaging (DSI) [34,35].

Several studies have targeted early detection of prostate cancer through building CAD systems that would aid physicians in its early diagnosis, where accurate prostate segmentation is one of the main components of such CAD systems, and inaccuracies of such a process would adversely affect all the subsequent stages. This chapter focuses on the deformable model-based segmentation techniques of the prostate that have proven to be powerful in medical imaging segmentation problems. Before getting into prostate segmentation techniques, the anatomy of the prostate is briefly overviewed.

13.1.1 Prostate anatomy

The prostate gland is situated between the bladder and the penis, at the origin of the urethra, the tube that flows urine out of the body, and is in front of the rectum. It is approximately the size of a walnut and normally weighs between 20 and 30 grams. It is part of the exocrine system that secretes fluids for external functions of the body. The prostate is responsible for secreting a milky substance that protects sperm, and constitutes around 30% of semen. It also has muscles that help it squeeze to expel the sperm as semen during ejaculation.

The prostate includes branching glands, with ducts that are lined with secretory epithelial cells and basal cells, having epithelial cells as the major cell type in the gland. The epithelial cells depend on androgenic hormone for growth and produce prostatic acid phosphatase. The basal cell layer contains the stem cell population for the epithelial prostate cells. Surrounding the gland is a stroma that includes fibroblasts, smooth muscle, nerves, and lymphatics. The smooth muscle of the prostatic stroma gradually extends into

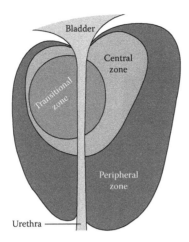

Figure 13.3 Schematic illustration of the three prostate zones.

fibrous tissue that ends in loose connective and adipose tissue. Recent research suggests that the stroma produces multiple growth factors that play a major role in the development of normal prostate and prostate cancer as well [36].

Another way to anatomically describe the prostate is the concept of anatomic zones [37]. There are three major zones within the normal prostate (Figure 13.3):

1. The peripheral zone (PZ) constitutes 70% of the prostate, and extends posterolaterally around the gland from the apex to the base. It is considered to be the most common site for developing prostate carcinomas, about 70% of cancers originate in this zone [38].
2. The central zone (CZ) constitutes 25% of the prostate, and surrounds the ejaculatory duct apparatus. It also makes up the majority of the prostatic base. Even though, only 2.5% of cancers develop in that zone [38].
3. The transition zone (TZ) constitutes 5% of the prostate, and contains two small lobules that abut the prostatic urethra and represent the region where BPH primarily originates. About 10% to 20% of cancers develop in that zone [38]. Carcinomas that originate in this zone are thought to be of lower malignant potential than they are in other zones [36].

Prostate cancer often has no early symptoms, but when it advances, it can cause men to urinate more often or have a weaker flow of urine. Also the extension of cancer outside of the prostate gland has been confirmed in many studies to be an important prognostic factor for recurrence [2].

The prostate can be affected by a number of disorders besides cancer, including prostatitis and benign prostate hyperplasia, where they all can be characterized by inflammation of the prostate. Prostatitis is a prostate infection, or it could be an inflammation though it does not carry the risk of getting prostate cancer. The primary symptom of prostatitis is repeated bladder infections, and can affect men at any age. It is considered to be chronic if it lasts for more than three months. Chronic prostatitis is related to urinary tract infections and usually follows an attack of acute prostatitis [39].

The prostate usually goes through two growth stages. The first stage occurs in puberty, where the prostate doubles in size, whereas the second stage begins at around the age of

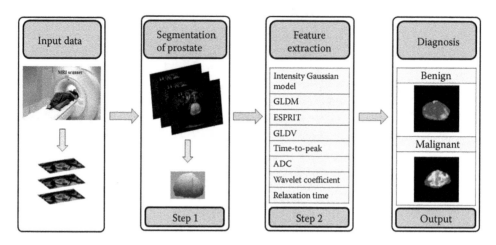

Figure 13.4 Schematic overview of a general CAD system for prostate cancer.

25 and lasts during a men's life. Benign prostate hyperplasia (BPH) is a condition that is characterized by enlargement of the prostate, yet is not cancerous. BPH usually occurs at the second growth stage [40]. As the prostate continues enlargement, the gland pinches the urethra and the bladder wall gets thicker. This might eventually cause weakening of the bladder and losing the ability to empty it completely, leaving some urine inside (urinary retention). These outcomes are strongly related to BPH [40].

The main focus of this chapter is on one of the key steps in developing any CAD system for detecting prostate cancer as shown in Figure 13.4, which is the segmentation of the prostate from medical images using deformable models.

13.2   Deformable models

Classical segmentation methods such as edge detection and thresholding do not give good results for medical images because these images are often noisy and their objects boundaries may be unclear. Deformable models (DMs), developed by Kass et al. [41] and Caselles et al. [42], are curves defined within an image domain that can evolve to delineate an object's border under the influence of internal forces that preserve smoothness of the curve during deformation, and external forces that propagate the curve toward the object boundary. Deformable models utilize mathematical, geometrical, and physical theories to constraint the curve shape, and to guide the evolution of the curve to fit the available data [43]. Different DM-based methods have been used for prostate segmentation, such as level set DMs, active shape models (ASMs), active appearance models (AAMs), and curve fitting. These methods can be classified into geometric deformable models and parametric deformable models and in each of these segmentation methods, the techniques that use the same image modality are grouped together.

13.2.1   Prostate segmentation using geometric deformable models

The level set introduced by Osher and Sethian [44–46] is a powerful technique for medical image segmentation. It has been widely used due to its adaptable evolution and lack of need for parameterization. The deformable models in this section are categorized with respect to the imaging modality used. This section focuses on TRUS, which is followed by MRI.

Wang et al. [47] proposed a fully automated method for prostate segmentation from 3D TRUS images using a level set DM guided by 3D shape and intensity priors. Their proposed method allowed the shape to propagate until the best localization was found by minimizing a region-based energy factor without particular initialization. The experimental results of testing that method on 11 ultrasound images showed that the correct segmentation rate was 0.82. Zhan et al. [48] used a level set DM guided by prostate texture and shape priors to perform 3D prostate localization. A set of Gabor-support vector machines (G-SVMs) are utilized to extract features and to distinguish between prostate and nonprostate tissues in different areas around prostate border. This method was tested on both synthesized and real data. The experimental results of testing that method on five synthesized prostate TRUS images and comparing the segmentation results to an expert ground truth showed that the mean of the surface distances was at 1.07 voxels, the mean of the overlap volume errors was 4.31%, the mean of the volume errors was 2.39% and the mean of the errors between corresponding vertices was at 2.22 voxels. The experimental results of testing that method on six real 3D TRUS images and comparing the segmentation results to the ground truth showed that the mean of the surface distances was at 1.12 voxels, the mean of the overlap volume errors was 4.16%, and the mean of the volume errors was 2.22%. Qui et al. [49] proposed a semiautomated level set-based technique constrained by shape information for prostate segmentation from 3D TRUS images. Their technique is a rotational slice-based propagation technique to overcome the problems related to handling slices near the apex and the base of the prostate. The results of validating their technique using a dataset of 20 3D TRUS images showed that the sensitivity was $94.82 \pm 2.18(\%)$, the DSC was $93.39 \pm 1.26(\%)$, and the MAD was 1.16 ± 0.34mm.

Level set DM has been applied to segment the prostate from MRI data. For example, Liu et al. [50] proposed a fully automated method for prostate segmentation from 2D DWI images. Their method implemented a level set DM guided by a shape prior and intensity information. The experimental results showed that the mean of Dice similarity coefficient (DSC) for that method was 0.91 ± 0.03. Level sets have also been used for prostate segmentation from 3D MRI, as an example the method developed by Liu et al. [51]. In their unsupervised automated method, a level set DM guided by the shape information extracted from an initial coarse segmentation was utilized. The segmentation results were refined by morphological operations. The experimental results of testing that method on data obtained from 10 subjects showed that the mean and standard deviation values of DSC, mean absolute distance (MAD), and Hausdorff distance (HD) were 0.810 ± 0.050, 2.67 ± 0.650 (mm), and 9.07 ± 1.64 (mm) respectively. In McClure et al. [52], an automated 3D framework for prostate localization was developed that integrated a level set deformable model and nonnegative matrix factorization (NMF) methods. The level set function was directed by a new speed function that was derived using NMF, which educed significant features from a large dimensional feature space. The NMF attributes were calculated from the DWI gray level, a probabilistic shape model, and the spatial interactions between prostate voxels. The shape model was built using a dataset of training prostate volumes and was then updated during the localization process using an intensity-based technique that took into account both a voxel's location and its intensity value. The spatial interactions were modeled using a second-order pairwise 3D Markov–Gibbs random field (MGRF). Table 13.1 summarizes the techniques discussed in this section.

Table 13.1 Summary of the geometric deformable model-based prostate segmentation techniques and their performance

Reference	Modality and method	Data and performance
Wang et al. [47]	• TRUS • 3D • Automated • Level set	• 11 images • ACC: 82%
Zhan et al. [48]	• TRUS • 3D • Automated • Level set	• 6 volumes • Mean surface distance: 1.12 • Mean OVE: 4.16% • AVE: 2.22%
Qui et al. [49]	• TRUS • 3D • Semiautomated • Level set	• 20 volumes • SEN: $94.82 \pm 2.18\%$ • DSC: $93.39 \pm 1.26\%$ • MAD: 1.16 ± 0.34 (mm)
Liu et al. [50]	• DWI-MRI • 2D • Automated • Level set	• DSC: 0.91 ± 0.03
Liu et al. [51]	• DWI-MRI • 3D • Automated • Level set and active contour model	• 10 subjects • DSC: 0.81 ± 0.05 • MAD: 2.67 ± 0.65 (mm) • HD: 9.07 ± 1.64 (mm)
Mcclure et al. [52]	• DWI-MRI • 3D • Automated • Level set	• 10 subjects • DSC: 0.868 ± 0.03 • HD: 5.61 ± 2.12 (mm)

ACC: Accuracy
OVE: Overlap volume error
AVE: Average volume error
SEN: Sensitivity; $\text{SEN} = \dfrac{\text{TP}}{\text{TP} + \text{FN}}$
DSC: Dice similarity coefficient: $\text{DSC} = \dfrac{2 \cdot \text{TP}}{2 \cdot \text{TP} + \text{FP} + \text{FN}}$
        where TP: true positive, FP: false positive, FN: false negative
MAD: Mean absolute distance
HD: Hausdorff distance

13.2.2   *Prostate segmentation using parametric deformable models*

13.2.2.1   *Curve fitting*

Other DMs for prostate localization include curve fitted deformable boundaries, for example, fitting the prostate boundaries to an ellipse due to its approximation of the prostates shape. TRUS is the main modality that is discussed in this section.

Gong et al. [53] proposed a semiautomated Bayesian algorithm for prostate segmentation from 2D ultrasound images that represented a prostate's edge as a deformable super ellipse. The evolution to the prostate boundaries was guided and constrained by a shape prior information. The experimental results showed that the superellipse with simple parametric deformations can efficiently represent the prostate shape with the HD error of 1.32 ± 0.62 (mm) and MAD error of 0.54 ± 0.20 (mm). This technique was tested on 125 images collected from 16 subjects and the results showed that the mean error between model-generated outlines and the manual outlines was 1.36 ± 0.58.

Saroul et al. [54] proposed a semiautomated technique for localizing the prostate from 2D TRUS images. Their technique utilized a deformable super-ellipse curve fitting guided by appearance. Also, a semiautomated technique developed by Baidiei et al. [55] used an elliptical curve fitting to outline the prostate border. They tested their technique on 17 TRUS images and the results showed the mean absolute difference was 0.67 ± 0.18 (mm), the average sensitivity was more than 97%, and the average accuracy was more than 93%.

Additionally, Mahdavi et al. [56] proposed a semiautomated method for prostate segmentation from 3D TRUS images based on ellipsoid curve fitting guided by apriori 3D shape. This method was tested on data obtained from 40 patients and the results showed that the average volume error between the volumes computed from semiautomatic contours and those computed from modified contours was 5.82 ± 4.15(%). However, ellipsoids have not been the only shapes used for 3D prostate localization. Tutar et al. [57] proposed a DM for TRUS prostate segmentation that used spherical harmonics (SHs) of degree eight to model the 3D shape of the prostate. Their method was tested on 30 volume sets and the experimental results showed that the absolute distance error between algorithm-generated boundaries and the manual boundaries was 1.26 ± 0.41 (mm) and the volume overlap was 83.5 ± 4.2(%). Table 13.2 summarizes the techniques discussed in this section and in Section 13.2.2.2.

13.2.2.2 Active shape models and active appearance models

In medical image processing, more sophisticated shape models can be integrated to provide more accurate segmentation. ASM is a statistical model developed by Cootes et al. [58] that generate a point distribution model (PDM) by using a series of manually landmarked training images then principal component analysis (PCA) is applied on that PDM to generate a statistical shape model [59]. This method has been used extensively for prostate segmentation. This section surveys the work found in the literature related to TRUS, followed by MRI, and finally the work that used the CT modality.

Shen et al. [60] proposed an automated method for prostate segmentation from 2D TRUS images using ASM guided by Gabor-based appearance features. A hierarchical deformation strategy that utilized a multiresolution technique was employed to make the segmentation method more accurate and robust. The experimental results of comparing the model-based segmentation results to the manual segmentation of eight images showed that the mean average distance was 3.2 ± 0.87 (pixels), the mean overlap area error was 3.98 ± 0.97(%), and the mean area error was 1.66 ± 1.68(%). Betrouni et al. [61] proposed an automated technique for segmenting the prostate from 2D transabdominal ultrasound images. In their technique, after applying a filter to smooth noisy regions and enhance the contours, a statistical model was optimized to segment the prostate. Comparing the segmentation results to the manual segmentation of 10 images showed that the mean distance was 3.2 ± 1.3 (pixels), the maximum distance was 6.25 ± 1.8 (pixels), and the average surface coverage index was 93 ± 9(%). Zaim and Jankun [62] proposed an automated technique for prostate segmentation from 2D TRUS images using ASM guided by extracted

Table 13.2 Summary of the parametric deformable model-based prostate
segmentation techniques and their performance

Reference	Modality and method	Data and performance
Gong et al. [53]	• TRUS • 2D • Semiautomated • Curve fitting	• 125 images (16 subjects) • HD: 1.32 ± 0.62 (mm) • MAD: 0.54 ± 0.20 (mm)
Baidiei et al. [55]	• TRUS • 2D • Semiautomated • Curve fitting	• 17 images • MAD: 0.67 ± 0.18 (mm) • SEN: 97% • ACC: 93%
Mahdavi et al. [56]	• TRUS • 3D • Semiautomated • Curve fitting	• 40 volumes • AVE: $5.82 \pm 4.15(\%)$
Tutar et al. [57]	• TRUS • 3D • Semiautomated • Spherical harmonics	• 30 volumes • Mean volume overlap: $83.5 \pm 4.2(\%)$ • MAD: 1.26 ± 0.41 (mm)
Shen et al. [60]	• TRUS • 2D • Automated • ASM	• 8 images • MAD: 3.2 ± 0.87 (pixels) • OAE: $3.98 \pm 0.97(\%)$ • Mean area error: $1.66 \pm 1.68(\%)$
Betrouni et al. [61]	• Trans-abdominal US • 2D • Automated • ASM	• 10 images • Mean distance: 3.2 ± 1.3 (pixels) • Maximum distance: 6.25 ± 1.8 (pixels)
Zaim and Jankun [62]	• TRUS • 2D • Automated • ASM	• 10 images (3 subjects) • Mean distance error: 15.3 (pixels) • OAE: 5(%) • ACC: 92(%)
Yan et al. [63]	• TRUS • 2D • Automated • ASM	• 301 images (19 subjects) • MAD: 2.01 ± 1.02 (mm)
Hodge et al. [64]	• TRUS • 3D • Semiautomated • ASM	• 36 volumes • MD: 0.12 ± 0.45 (mm) • MAD: 1.09 ± 0.49 (mm) • PVD: $0.22 \pm 4.58(\%)$ • PAVD: $3.28 \pm 3.16(\%)$
Medina et al. [65]	• TRUS • 2D • Automated • AAM	• 95 images • Overlap: 96(%)

(*Continued*)

Table 13.2 (Continued) Summary of the parametric deformable model-based prostate segmentation techniques and their performance

Reference	Modality and method	Data and performance
Zhu et al. [66]	<ul><li>T2-MRI</li><li>3D</li><li>Automated</li><li>ASM</li></ul>	<ul><li>26 volumes</li><li>RMSD: 5.48 ± 2.91 (mm)</li></ul>
Vikal et al. [67]	<ul><li>T2-MRI</li><li>3D</li><li>Semiautomated</li><li>ASM</li></ul>	<ul><li>3 datasets (39 slices)</li><li>MAD: 2 ± 0.6 (mm)</li><li>DSC: 0.93 ± 0.3</li></ul>
Gao et al. [68]	<ul><li>T2-MRI</li><li>Semiautomated</li><li>ASM</li></ul>	<ul><li>33 images</li><li>DSC: 0.84 ± 0.03</li></ul>
Toth et al. [69]	<ul><li>T2-MRI, MRS</li><li>3D</li><li>Automated</li><li>ASM</li></ul>	<ul><li>19 subjects (148 slices)</li><li>SEN: 89%</li><li>SPE: 86%</li><li>PPV: 93%</li><li>Overlap: 83%</li></ul>
Martin et al. [70]	<ul><li>T2-MRI</li><li>3D</li><li>Automated</li><li>ASM</li></ul>	<ul><li>36 volumes</li><li>Median DSC: 0.86</li><li>Mean surface error: 2.41 (mm)</li></ul>
Ghose et al. [74]	<ul><li>T2-MRI</li><li>3D</li><li>Automated</li><li>AAM</li></ul>	<ul><li>15 volumes</li><li>DSC: 0.88 ± 0.11</li><li>HD: 3.38 ± 2.81 (mm)</li></ul>
Maan et al. [75]	<ul><li>T2-MRI</li><li>3D</li><li>Automated</li><li>AAM</li></ul>	<ul><li>50 volumes</li><li>DSC: 0.78</li><li>HD: 7.32 (mm)</li></ul>
Chandra et al. [76]	<ul><li>MRI</li><li>3D</li><li>Automated</li><li>SSM</li></ul>	<ul><li>50 volumes</li><li>Mean DSC: 0.85</li><li>MASD: 1.85 (mm)</li></ul>
Makni et al. [78]	<ul><li>T2-MRI</li><li>3D</li><li>Automated</li><li>SSM</li></ul>	<ul><li>12 volumes</li><li>Mean HD: 9.94 (mm)</li><li>Overlap: 0.83%</li></ul>
Yin et al. [79]	<ul><li>MRI</li><li>3D</li><li>Automated</li><li>ASM</li></ul>	<ul><li>551 volumes</li><li>Mean DSC: 0.89</li></ul>

(Continued)

Table 13.2 (Continued) Summary of the parametric deformable model-based prostate segmentation techniques and their performance

Reference	Modality and method	Data and performance
Tnag et al. [81]	• CT • 2D • Automated • ASM	• MD: 2.44 (mm)
Feng et al. [82]	• CT • 2D • Automated • ASM	• 306 images (24 subjects) • DSC: 0.89
Costa et al. [83]	• CT • 3D • Automated • ASM	• 16 volumes • SEN: 75% • PPV: 80%

ASM:	Active shape model
AAM:	Active appearance model
HD:	Hausdorff distance
MAD:	Mean absolute distance
MASD:	Mean absolute surface distance
ACC:	Accuracy
AVE:	Average volume error
MD:	Mean distance
RMSD:	Root mean square distance
DSC:	Dice similarity coefficient: $DSC = \frac{2 \cdot TP}{2 \cdot TP + FP + FN}$
	where, TP: true positive, FP: false positive, FN: false negative
SEN:	Sensitivity; $SEN = \frac{TP}{TP + FN}$
SPE:	Specificity; $SPE = \frac{TN}{TN + FP}$; where TN: true negative
PPV:	Positive predictive value; $PPV = \frac{TP}{TP + FP}$
OAE:	Overlapping area error; $OAE = \frac{FP + FN}{TP + FN}\%$
PVD:	Percent volume difference
PAVD:	Percent absolute volume difference

image intensity features. The experimental results of comparing the model-based segmentation to the manual segmentation of 10 images from three subjects showed that the mean distance error was 15.3 (pixels), the mean overlap area error was 5(%), and the accuracy was 92(%). Additionally, Yan et al. [63] proposed an automated 2D technique for segmentation of prostate from TRUS images based on ASM guided by shape estimated from partial contours. Their technique was tested on 301 TRUS images from 19 subjects and the results showed that average mean absolute distance error was 2.01 ± 1.02 (mm). Also, Hodge et al. [64] proposed a semiautomated algorithm for 3D prostate segmentation that optimizes and extends 2D segmentations using rotational-based slicing. Their algorithm-based contours were compared to ground truth contours and the results showed that the MD was 0.12 ± 0.45 (mm), the MAD was 1.09 ± 0.49 (mm), the percent volume difference (PVD) was $0.22 \pm 4.58(\%)$ and the percent absolute volume difference (PAVD) was $3.28 \pm 3.16(\%)$. Medina et al. [65] proposed an automated technique for 2D prostate segmentation from TRUS images that used AAM guided by texture and shape information. Their algorithm was trained using a dataset of 95 TRUS images and the segmentation results showed that the algorithm-based segmentation overlaps with the manual segmentation by 96%.

Zhu et al. [66] presented a hybrid 2D + 3D ASM-based methodology to obtain a global optimal prostate segmentation of the 3D MRI data. Their idea was that 3D ASM is less robust when volumetric data in one dimension is sparse. They used a dataset of 26 male pelvis transverse MRI images of which 12 cases were used for testing their method. The results showed that the mean and the standard deviation of the root mean square distance (RMSD) between the hybrid 2D + 3D ASM-based contours and the manual contours were 5.4811 and 2.9082 respectively. Vikal et al. [67] proposed a semiautomatic prostate segmentation algorithm from 3D MRI volumes using a statistical shape model. The results of comparing the algorithm-based segmentation to the manual segmentation showed that the MAD and DSC were 2 ± 0.6 and 0.93 ± 0.3 respectively.

Gao et al. [68] proposed an algorithm that begins by registering the MR images before segmenting the prostate based on a learned shape prior. Their algorithm was evaluated by two datasets—the first one has 33 MRI images and the second one is a public available that contains 15 T2-MRI images. The results showed that the Dice coefficient was 0.84 ± 0.03 and 0.82 ± 0.05 for the first and the second datasets respectively. Toth et al. [69] proposed a multimodal automated prostate segmentation technique. Their technique consists of two main steps: (1) applying spectral clustering on magnetic resonance spectroscopy (MRS) data to separate a rectangular region that is used as initialization for the second step and (2) a trained ASM on T2 MRI images is deformed to fit the boundary points to obtain the final segmentation. To test their technique, a dataset of both MRI and MRS that contains 148 image sections from 19 patients was utilized. The results showed that the average sensitivity, specificity, positive predictive value, and overlap were 89%, 86%, 93%, and 83%, respectively. Martin et al. [70] proposed a fully automated algorithm for segmenting the prostate in 3D MRI data. Their algorithm comprises two steps: (1) registering the new image to a probabilistic atlas to get a probabilistic segmentation and (2) refining the segmentation using a spatially constrained deformable model that utilizes a statistical shape model and a feature model. Their algorithm was validated on 36 T2-MRI volumes and the results showed that the median DSC was 0.86 and the mean surface error was 2.41 mm. A combination of a 3D statistical shape model and voxel classification was utilized in the method proposed by Allen et al. [71] to segment the prostate from T2-MRI volumes. Toth et al. [72] proposed an automated ASM-based method for prostate segmentation from MRI images that utilizes a local texture model for the landmark points to overcome the restrictions related to the use of the Mahalanobis distance. Their model-based contours were compared to an expert-based contours of 230 different modality MRI images and the results showed that the mean overlap was 0.84. Their technique was utilized by Viswanath et al. [73] in developing an integrated multiparametric CAD system of prostate cancer. Ghose et al. [74] proposed an automated method for 3D prostate segmentation that used multiple AAM and a global registration for shape restriction. In their method, principle component analysis (PCA) was utilized to derive shape and appearance information. The evaluation of their method on 15 MRI volumes showed that the mean DSC and the mean HD were 0.88 ± 0.11 and 3.38 ± 2.81 (mm) respectively.

Maan et al. [75] segmented the prostate using 50 training cases using a two-step framework. First, point correspondences between the training cases is obtained using shape context based nonrigid surface registration of manually segmented images. Then, an active appearance model (AAM) is incorporated for segmentation. The integration of shape context registration and AAM enables including the texture of the prostate in the segmentation process.

Chandra et al. [76], proposed a fully automated method for segmenting the prostate along with its seminal vesicles from MRI scans. This was achieved using a deformable model that is trained on-the-fly, and was designed to be patient-specific-initialized triangulated shape and image attribute model that were trained throughout its initialization. The image attribute model was integrated to deform the initialized shape by template matching image attributes (via normalized cross-correlation) to the attributes of the scan. The resulting deformations were regularized over the shape via well-established simple shape smoothing algorithms, which were then made anatomically valid via an optimized shape model. The results of evaluating their algorithm on the Klein et al. [77] dataset that consists of 50 3T MR clinical scans showed that the mean and median of the DSCs were 0.85 and 0.87 and the MASD was 1.85 mm.

Makni et al. [78] applied a statistical shape model as a priori information for accurate contouring of the prostate, where gray level distribution was modeled by fitting histogram modes with a Gaussian mixture. Markov fields were also used to obtain information regarding neighborhoods of voxels. The final optimum labels was based on Bayesian a posteriori classification, which was estimated with the iterative conditional mode algorithm.

Yin et al. [79] proposed an automated algorithm consisting of two phases for segmenting the prostate from 3D MRI: first, the displacement and size of the prostate are detected based on the cross-correlation of the normalized gradient fields then a graph-search framework is utilized to refine the boundary. The experimental results of evaluating their approach on a dataset of 551 images showed that the mean DSC was 0.89.

A CAD system was proposed in Litjens et al. [80] for prostate cancer detection from MR images. It used a fast routine for prostate segmentation that mainly relies on anatomy features and coupled appearance models, which are mutually dependent through a probabilistic population model that restricts the size and position of the prostate based on those of other organs.

Tang et al. [81] proposed an ASM-based method to delineate the prostate and other surrounding structures, the bladder and the rectum, from CT images. The results showed that the mean distance between the model-base generated contour and the manually segmented contour and was 2.44 mm, with variance of 1.24 mm. Feng et al. [82] proposed a deformable model that was designed particularly for localizing sequential CT images of the prostate that exploited both population and patient-specific statistics, in order to precisely capture the intrapatient variation of the patient under therapy. A weighted combination of gradient and probability distribution function (PDF) features built the intensity model to guide model deformation. In order to reduce the effect of feature contradiction in the regions of gas and bone close to the prostate, the optimal profile length at each landmark was computed by statistically examining the intensity profile in the training set. Also, an online learning mechanism was used to build shape and appearance statistics for accurately capturing intra patient variation. Costa et al. [83] proposed a fully automated method for 3D segmentation of the lower abdomen structures of CT scans including the prostate and the bladder. A statistical shape prior was enforced on the prostate, along with an adaptive nonoverlapping constraint that arbitrates its evolution based on the presence of significant image data at their common boundary.

13.3   Conclusion and future trends

This chapter discussed the recent deformable model-based segmentation techniques of the prostate. Segmentation is considered to be a main key in accurate diagnosis of different abnormalities. Deformable models with their parametric and geometric techniques have revolutionized the segmentation of medical images in the past 15 years, which was the reason of focusing on such techniques in this chapter for prostate segmentation. From the survey conducted, it is shown that the deformable models have proven to be successful in segmenting prostate images, especially in two dimensions. Geometric deformable models have overcome the limitations of parametric models as curve evolution does not depend on the parameterization, yet it is still challenging to pursue the task of 3D segmentation of the prostate images from different modalities (e.g., DW MRI, CT). The MRI modality provided high accuracy in prostate segmentation (up to 90%), while CT results showed lower performance evidenced by the lower accuracy (around 80%) of segmentation.

The focus of future trends for researchers working on prostate segmentation might be the use of multiple modalities that would lead to more consistent segmentation results. Also the traditional guiding forces for the level set method might be replaced with better ones, such as integrating the edge forces (e.g., GVF), the stochastic forces (e.g., mean and variances of regions), and the prior shape (atlas) to get better convergence solution to the level set method. Another possible trend could be integrating the level sets with efficient optimization techniques, such as the global graph-based schemes (e.g., graph-cut approach).

References

1. G. J. Tortora and B. H. Derrickson, *Principles of Anatomy and Physiology*. New York: Wiley, 2011.
2. The National Cancer Institute (NCI). *Prostate Cancer* [Online]. Available. http://www. cancer.gov/types/prostate
3. The National Cancer Institute (NCI): *Prostate Cancer Treatment Stages of Prostate Cancer* [Online]. Available. http://www.cancer.gov/types/prostate/ patient/prostate-treatment-pdq#section/_120
4. K. Mistry and G. Cable, Meta-analysis of prostate-specific antigen and digital rectal examination as screening tests for prostate carcinoma, *The Journal of the American Board of Family Practice*, vol. 16, no. 2, pp. 95–101, 2003.
5. S. Dijkstra, P. Mulders, and J. Schalken, Clinical use of novel urine and blood based prostate cancer biomarkers: A review, *Clinical Biochemistry*, vol. 47, no. 10, pp. 889–896, 2014.
6. M. Davis, M. Sofer, S. S. Kim, and S. M. Soloway, The procedure of transrectal ultrasound guided biopsy of the prostate: A survey of patient preparation and biopsy technique, *The Journal of Urology*, vol. 167, no. 2, pp. 566–570, 2002.
7. D. F. Gleason, Classification of prostatic carcinomas, *Cancer Chemotherapy Reports*, Part 1, vol. 50, no. 3, 1966, pp. 125–128.
8. D. F. Gleason and G. T. Mellinger, Prediction of prognosis for prostatic adenocarcinoma by combined histological grading and clinical staging, *The Journal of Urology*, vol. 111, no. 1, pp. 58–64, 1974.
9. R. Montironi, L. Cheng, A. Lopez-Beltran, M. Scarpelli, R. Mazzucchelli, G. Mikuz, Z. Kirkali, and F. Montorsi, Original gleason system versus 2005 ISUP modified gleason system: The importance of indicating which system is used in the patient's pathology and clinical reports,. *European Urology*, vol. 58, no. 3, pp. 369–373, 2010.
10. J. I. Epstein, W. C. Allsbrook Jr, M. B. Amin, L. L. Egevad, I. G. Committee et al., The 2005 International Society of Urological Pathology (ISUP) Consensus Conference on Gleason Grading of Prostatic Carcinoma, *The American Journal of Surgical Pathology*, vol. 29, no. 9, pp. 1228–1242, 2005.
11. A. M. DeMarzo, W. G. Nelson, W. B. Isaacs, and J. I. Epstein, Pathological and molecular aspects of prostate cancer, *The Lancet*, vol. 361, no. 9361, pp. 955–964, 2003.

12. H. Hricak, P. L. Choyke, S. C. Eberhardt, S. A. Leibel, and T. P. Scardino, Imaging prostate cancer: A multidisciplinary perspective, *Radiology*, vol. 243, no. 1, pp. 28–53, 2007.

13. G. Fichtinger, A. Krieger, R. C. Susil, A. Tanacs, L. L. Whitcomb, and E. Atalar, Transrectal prostate biopsy inside closed MRI scanner with remote actuation, under real-time image guidance, in *Medical Image Computing and Computer-Assisted Intervention*, MICCAI 2002. Berlin: Springer, 2002, pp. 91–98.

14. J. C. Applewhite, B. Matlaga, D. McCullough, and M. Hall, Transrectal ultrasound and biopsy in the early diagnosis of prostate cancer, *Cancer Control: Journal of the Moffitt Cancer Center*, vol. 8, no. 2, pp. 141–150, 2000.

15. M. Fuchsja¨ger, A. Shukla-Dave, O. Akin, J. Barentsz, and H. Hricak, Prostate cancer imaging, *Acta Radiologica*, vol. 49, no. 1, pp. 107–120, 2008.

16. D. J. Collins and A. R. Padhani, Dynamic magnetic resonance imaging of tumor perfusion, *Engineering in Medicine and Biology Magazine, IEEE*, vol. 23, no. 5, pp. 65–83, 2004.

17. F. Khalifa, G. M. Beache, G. Gimel'farb, and A. El-Baz, A novel CAD system for analyzing cardiac first-pass MR images, in *Pattern Recognition* (ICPR), 2012, 21st International Conference on, IEEE, pp. 77–80, 2012.

18. A. El-Baz, A. Farag, R. Fahmi, S. Yuksela, M. El-Ghar, T. Eldisasty et al., Image analysis of renal DCE MRI for the detection of acute renal rejection, in *Pattern Recognition*, ICPR 2006, 18th International Conference on, vol. 3, IEEE, pp. 822–825, 2006.

19. A. Farag, A. El-Baz, S. E. Yuksel, M. El-Ghar, T. Eldiasty et al., A framework for the detection of acute renal rejection with dynamic contrast enhanced magnetic resonance imaging, in *Biomedical Imaging: Nano to Macro*, 2006, 3rd IEEE International Symposium on, IEEE, pp. 418–421, 2006.

20. A. El-Baz, A. A. Farag, S. E. Yuksel, M. E. El-Ghar, T. A. Eldiasty, and M. A. Ghoneim, Application of deformable models for the detection of acute renal rejection, in *Deformable Models*. Berlin: Springer, 2007, pp. 293–333.

21. A. El-Baz, G. Gimelfarb, and M. A. El-Ghar, New motion correction models for automatic identification of renal transplant rejection, in *Medical Image Computing and Computer-Assisted Intervention*—MICCAI 2007. Berlin: Springer, 2007 pp. 235–243.

22. A. El-Baz, G. Gimel'farb, M. El-Ghar et al., A novel image analysis approach for accurate identification of acute renal rejection, in *Image Processing*, 2008, ICIP 2008, 15th IEEE International Conference on, IEEE, pp. 1812–1815, 2008.

23. A. El-Baz, G. G. Farb, M. El-Ghar et al., Image analysis approach for identification of renal transplant rejection, in *Pattern Recognition*, 2008, ICPR 2008, 19th International Conference on, IEEE, pp. 1–4, 2008.

24. F. Khalifa, A. El-Baz, G. Gimelfarb, and M. A. El-Ghar, Non-invasive image-based approach for early detection of acute renal rejection, in *Medical Image Computing and Computer-Assisted Intervention*—MICCAI 2010. Berlin: Springer, 2010, pp. 10–18.

25. A. Firjani, F. Khalifa, A. Elnakib, G. Gimel'farb, M. Abou El-Ghar, A. El-maghraby, and A. El-Baz, A novel image-based approach for early detection of prostate cancer, in *Image Processing* (ICIP), 2012, 19th IEEE International Conference on, IEEE, pp. 2849–2852, 2012.

26. A. Firjani, F. Khalifa, A. Elnakib, G. Gimel'farb, M. A. El-Ghar, A. Elmaghraby, and A. El-Baz, Non-invasive image-based approach for early detection of prostate cancer, In: *Developments in E-systems Engineering* (DeSE), 2011, IEEE, 2011, pp. 172–177.

27. A. Firjani, F. Khalifa, A. Elnakib, G. Gimel'farb, M. A. El-Ghar, A. Elmaghraby, and A. El-Baz, A novel image-based approach for early detection of prostate cancer using DCE-MRI, in: *Computational Intelligence in Biomedical Imaging*. Berlin: Springer, 2014, pp. 55–82.

28. A. Firjani, A. Elnakib, F. Khalifa, G. Gimel'farb, M. A. El-Ghar, A. Elmaghraby, A. El-Baz et al., A diffusion-weighted imaging based diagnostic system for early detection of prostate cancer, *Journal of Biomedical Science and Engineering*, vol. 6, no. 3, 2013, p. 346.

29. A. Firjani, A. Elmaghraby, and A. El-Baz, MRI-based diagnostic system for early detection of prostate cancer, in *Biomedical Sciences and Engineering Conference (BSEC)*, 2013, IEEE, 2013, pp. 1–4.

30. C. Sato, S. Naganawa, T. Nakamura, H. Kumada, S. Miura, O. Takizawa, and T. Ishigaki, Differentiation of noncancerous tissue and cancer lesions by apparent diffusion coefficient values in transition and peripheral zones of the prostate, *Journal of Magnetic Resonance Imaging*, vol. 21, no. 3, pp. 258–262, 2005.

31. R. Bammer, Basic principles of diffusion-weighted imaging, *European Journal of Radiology*, vol. 45, no. 3, pp. 169–184, 2003.

32. P. Sundgren, Q. Dong, D. Gomez-Hassan, S. Mukherji, P. Maly, and R. Welsh, Diffusion tensor imaging of the brain: Review of clinical applications, *Neuroradiology*, vol. 46, no. 5, pp. 339–350, 2004.

33. F. Le Bihan, J. Mangin, C. Poupon, C. A. Clark, S. Pappata, N. Molko, and H. Chabriat, Diffusion tensor imaging: Concepts and applications, *Journal of Magnetic Resonance Imaging*, vol. 13, no. 4 pp. 534–546, 2001.

34. V. J. Wedeen, R. Wang, J. D. Schmahmann, T. Benner, W. Tseng, G. Dai, D. Pandya, P. Hagmann, H. D'Arceuil, and A. J. de Crespigny, Diffusion spectrum magnetic resonance imaging (DSI) tractography of crossing fibers, *NeuroImage*, vol. 41, no. 4, pp. 1267–1277, 2008.

35. P. Hagmann, L. Jonasson, P. Maeder, P. J. Thiran, V. J. Wedeen, and R. Meuli, Understanding diffusion MR imaging techniques: From scalar diffusion-weighted imaging to diffusion tensor imaging and beyond, *Radiographics*, vol. 26, suppl 1, pp. S205–S223, 2006.

36. D. W. Kufe, R. E. Pollock, R. R. Weichselbaum, R. C. Bast, T. S. Gansler, J. F. Holland, E. Frei, W. K. Oh, M. Hurwitz, A. V. D'Amico et al., Biology of prostate cancer, 2003.

37. J. E. McNeal, The zonal anatomy of the prostate, *The Prostate*, vol. 2, no. 1, pp. 35–49, 1981.

38. J. E. McNeal, E. A. Redwine, F. S. Freiha, and T. A. Stamey, Zonal distribution of pro-static adenocarcinoma: Correlation with histologic pattern and direction of spread, *The American Journal of Surgical Pathology*, vol. 12, no. 12, pp. 897–906, 1988.

39. WebMD, Men's Health: *Prostatitis: Causes, Symptoms, Diagnosis, Tests, and Treatment* [Online]. vailable from http://www.webmd.com/men/guide/prostatitis/

40. The National Institute of Diabetes and Digestive and Kidney Diseases (NIDDK), *Prostate Enlargement: Benign Prostatic Hyperplasia* [Online]. Available from http://www.niddk.nih.gov/health-information/health-topics/urologic-disease/benign-prostatic-hyperplasia-bph/Pages/facts.aspx

41. M. Kass, A. Witkin, and D. Terzopoulos, Snakes: Active contour models, *International Journal of Computer Vision*, vol. 1, no. 4, pp. 321–331, 1988.

42. V. Caselles, F. Catt'e, T. Coll, and F. Dibos, A geometric model for active contours in image processing, *Numerische mathematik*, vol. 66 , no. 1, pp. 1–31, 1993.

43. I. Bankman, *Handbook of Medical Image Processing and Analysis*, New York: Academic Press, 2008.

44. S. Osher and J. A. Sethian, A review of recent numerical algorithms for hypersurfaces moving with curvature dependent speed, *Journal of Differential Geometry*, vol. 31 , pp. 131–161, 1989.

45. J. A. Sethian, Fronts propagating with curvature-dependent speed: Algorithms based on Hamilton–Jacobi formulations, *Journal of Computational Physics*, vol. 79, no. 1, pp. 12–49, 1988.

46. J. A. Sethian, Curvature and the evolution of fronts, *Communications in Mathematical Physics*, vol. 101, no. 4, pp. 487–499, 1985.

47. R. Wang, J. Suri, and A. Fenster, Segmentation of prostate from 3-D ultrasound volumes using shape and intensity priors in level set framework, in *Engineering in Medicine and Biology Society*, 2006, EMBS'06, 28th Annual International Conference of the IEEE, IEEE, pp. 2341–2344, 2006.

48. Y. Zhan and D. Shen, Deformable segmentation of 3-D ultrasound prostate images using statistical texture matching method, *Medical Imaging, IEEE Transactions on*, vol. 25, no. 3, pp. 256–272, 2006.

49. W. Qiu, J. Yuan, E. Ukwatta, D. Tessier, and A. Fenster, Rotational-slice-based prostate segmentation using level set with shape constraint for 3D end-firing TRUS guided biopsy, in *Medical Image Computing and Computer-Assisted Intervention—MICCAI 2012*. Berlin: Springer, pp. 537–544, 2012.

50. X. Liu, D. Langer, M. Haider, T. Van der Kwast, A. Evans, M. Wernick, and I. Yetik, Unsupervised segmentation of the prostate using MR images based on level set with a shape prior, in

Engineering in Medicine and Biology Society, 2009, EMBC 2009. Annual International Conference of the IEEE, IEEE, pp. 3613–3616, 2009.

51. X. Liu, M. S. Haider, I. S. Yetik, Unsupervised 3D prostate segmentation based on diffusion-weighted imaging MRI using active contour models with a shape prior, *Journal of Electrical and Computer Engineering*, vol. 2011, p. 11, 2011.

52. P. McClure, F. Khalifa, A. Soliman, M. A. El-Ghar, G. Gimelfarb, A. Elmagraby, and A. El-Baz, A novel NMF guided level-set for DWI prostate segmentation, *Journal of Computer Science and System Biology*, vol. 7 , pp. 209–216, 2014.

53. L. Gong, S. D. Pathak, D. R. Haynor, P. S. Cho, and Y. Kim, Parametric shape modeling using deformable superellipses for prostate segmentation, *Medical Imaging, IEEE Transactions on*, vol. 23, no. 3, pp. 340–349, 2004.

54. L. Saroul, O. Bernard, D. Vray, and D. Friboulet, Prostate segmentation in echo-graphic images: A variational approach using deformable super-ellipse and Rayleigh distribution, in *Biomedical Imaging: From Nano to Macro*, 2008. ISBI 2008, 5th IEEE International Symposium on, IEEE, pp. 129–132, 2008.

55. S. Badiei, E. S. Salcudean, J. Varah, and W. J. Morris, Prostate segmentation in 2D ultrasound images using image warping and ellipse fitting, in *Medical Image Computing and Computer-Assisted Intervention—MICCAI 2006*. Berlin: Springer, 2006, pp. 17–24

56. S. S. Mahdavi, N. Chng, I. Spadinger, W. J. Morris, and S. E. Salcudean, Semiautomatic segmentation for prostate interventions, *Medical Image Analysis*, vol. 15, no. 2, pp. 226–237, 2011.

57. I. B. Tutar, S. D. Pathak, L. Gong, P. S. Cho, K. Wallner, and Y. Kim, Semiautomatic 3-D prostate segmentation from TRUS images using spherical harmonics, *Medical Imaging, IEEE Transactions on*, vol. 25, no. 12, pp. 1645–1654, 2006.

58. T. F. Cootes and C. J. Taylor, Active shape models smart snakes, in BMVC92. Berlin: Springer, 1992, pp. 266–275.

59. T. F. Cootes, C. J. Taylor, D. H. Cooper, and J. Graham, Active shape models-their training and application, *Computer Vision and Image Understanding*, vol. 61, no. 1, pp. 38–59, 1995.

60. D. Shen, Y. Zhan, and C. Davatzikos, Segmentation of prostate boundaries from ultrasound images using statistical shape model, *Medical Imaging, IEEE Transactions on*, vol. 22, no. 4, pp. 539–551, 2003.

61. N. Betrouni, M. Vermandel, D. Pasquier, S. Maouche, and J. Rousseau, Segmentation of abdominal ultrasound images of the prostate using a priori information and an adapted noise filter, *Computerized Medical Imaging and Graphics*, vol. 29, no. 1, pp. 43–51, 2005.

62. A. Zaim and J. Jankun, An energy-based segmentation of prostate from ultrasound images using dot-pattern select cells, in *Acoustics, Speech and Signal Processing*, 2007, ICASSP 2007, IEEE International Conference on, vol. 1, IEEE, pp. I–297, 2007.

63. P. Yan, S. Xu, B. Turkbey, and J. Kruecker, Discrete deformable model guided by partial active shape model for trus image segmentation, *Biomedical Engineering, IEEE Transactions on*, vol. 57, no. 5, pp. 1158–1166, 2010.

64. A. C. Hodge, A. Fenster, D. B. Downey, and H. M. Ladak, Prostate boundary segmentation from ultrasound images using 2D active shape models: Optimisation and extension to 3D, *Computer Methods and Programs in Biomedicine*, vol. 84, no. 2, pp. 99–113, 2006.

65. R. Medina, A. Bravo, P. Windyga, J. Toro, P. Yan, and G. Onik, A 2-D active appearance model for prostate segmentation in ultrasound images, in *Engineering in Medicine and Biology Society*, 2005. IEEE-EMBS 2005. 27th Annual International Conference of the, IEEE, pp. 3363–3366, 2006.

66. Y. Zhu, S. Williams, and R. Zwiggelaar, A hybrid ASM approach for sparse volumetric data segmentation, *Pattern Recognition and Image Analysis*, vol. 17, no. 2, pp. 252–258, 2007.

67. S. Vikal, S. Haker, C. Tempany, and G. Fichtinger, Prostate contouring in MRI guided biopsy, in *SPIE Medical Imaging*, International Society for Optics and Photonics, 2009, pp. 72594A–72594A.

68. Y. Gao, R. Sandhu, G. Fichtinger, and A. R. Tannenbaum, A coupled global registration and segmentation framework with application to magnetic resonance prostate imagery, *IEEE Transactions on*, vol. 29, no. 10, pp. 1781–1794, 2010.

69. R. Toth, P. Tiwari, M. Rosen, A. Kalyanpur, S. Pungavkar, and A. Madabhushi, A multi-modal prostate segmentation scheme by combining spectral clustering and active shape models, in *Medical Imaging, International Society for Optics and Photonics*, pp. 69144S–69144S, 2008.

70. S. Martin, J. Troccaz, and V. Daanen, Automated segmentation of the prostate in 3D MR images using a probabilistic atlas and a spatially constrained deformable model, *Medical Physics*, vol. 37, no. 4, pp. 1579–1590, 2010.

71. P. Allen, J. Graham, D. C. Williamson, and C. E. Hutchinson, Differential segmentation of the prostate in mr images using combined 3D shape modelling and voxel classification, in *3rd IEEE International Symposium on Biomedical Imaging: Nano to Macro*, 2006.

72. R. Toth, J. Chappelow, M. Rosen, S. Pungavkar, A. Kalyanpur, and A. Madabhushi, Multi-attribute non-initializing texture reconstruction based active shape model (mantra), in *Medical Image Computing and Computer-Assisted Intervention—MICCAI 2008*. Berlin: Springer, 2008, pp. 653–661.

73. S. Viswanath, B. N. Bloch, M. Rosen, J. Chappelow, R. Toth, N. Rofsky, R. Lenkinski, E. Genega, A. Kalyanpur, and A. Madabhushi, Integrating structural and functional imaging for computer assisted detection of prostate cancer on multi-protocol in vivo 3 tesla MRI, in *SPIE Medical Imaging, International Society for Optics and Photonics*, pp. 72603I–72603I, 2009.

74. S. Ghose, A. Oliver, R. Marti, X. Llad'o, J. Freixenet, J. Mitra, C. J. Vilanova, and F. Meri-audeau, A hybrid framework of multiple active appearance models and global registration for 3D prostate segmentation in MRI, in *SPIE Medical Imaging*, International Society for Optics and Photonics, pp. 83140S–83140S, 2012.

75. B. Maan and F. van der Heijden, Prostate MR image segmentation using 3D active appearance models, 2012.

76. S. S. Chandra, J. A. Dowling, K. K. Shen, P. Raniga, J. P. Pluim, P. B. Greer, O. Salvado, and J. Fripp, Patient specific prostate segmentation in 3-D magnetic resonance images, *Medical Imaging, IEEE Transactions on*, vol. 31, no. 10, pp. 1955–1964, 2012.

77. S. Klein, U. A. van der Heide, I. M. Lips, M. van Vulpen, M. Staring, and J. P. Pluim, Automatic segmentation of the prostate in 3D MR images by atlas matching using localized mutual information, *Medical Physics*, vol. 35, no. 4, pp. 1407–1417, 2008.

78. N. Makni, P. Puech, R. Lopes, A. S. Dewalle, O. Colot, and N. Betrouni, Combining a deformable model and a probabilistic framework for an automatic 3D segmentation of prostate on MRI, *International Journal of Computer Assisted Radiology and Surgery*, vol. 4, no. 2, pp. 181–188, 2009.

79. Y. Yin, S. V. Fotin, S. Periaswamy, J. Kunz, H. Haldankar, N. Muradyan, F. Cornud, B. Turkbey, and P. Choyke, Fully automated prostate segmentation in 3D MR based on normalized gradient fields cross-correlation initialization and logis-MOS refinement, in *SPIE Medical Imaging*, International Society for Optics and Photonics, pp. 831406–831406, 2012.

80. G. Litjens, P. Vos, J. Barentsz, N. Karssemeijer, and H. Huisman, Automatic computer aided detection of abnormalities in multi-parametric prostate MRI, In: *SPIE Medical Imaging*, International Society for Optics and Photonics, pp. 79630T–79630T, 2011.

81. X. Tang, Y. Jeong, J. R. Radke, and G. T. Chen, Geometric-model-based segmentation of the prostate and surrounding structures for image-guided radiotherapy, in *Electronic Imaging 2004*, International Society for Optics and Photonics, pp. 168–176, 2004.

82. Q. Feng, M. Foskey, W. Chen, and D. Shen, Segmenting CT prostate images using population and patient-specific statistics for radiotherapy, *Medical Physics*, vol. 37, no. 8, pp. 4121–4132, 2010.

83. M. J. Costa, H. Delingette, S. Novellas, and N. Ayache, Automatic segmentation of bladder and prostate using coupled 3D deformable models, in *Medical Image Computing and Computer-Assisted Intervention—MICCAI 2007*. Berlin: Springer, 2007, pp. 252–260.

chapter fourteen

A novel NMF-based CAD system for early diagnosis of prostate cancer by using 4D diffusion-weighted magnetic resonance images (DW-MRI)

Ahmed Soliman, Patrick McClure, Fahmi Khalifa, Ali Taki Eldeen, Mohamed Abou El-Ghar, Tarek El-Diasty, Jasjit S. Suri, Adel Elmaghraby, and Ayman El-Baz

Contents

Abstract

In this chapter, a computer-aided diagnostic (CAD) framework for detecting prostate cancer in DW-MRI data is proposed. The proposed CAD method consists of two major steps that use nonnegative matrix factorization (NMF) to learn meaningful features from sets of high-dimensional data. The first step, is a three-dimensional (3D) level set segmentation algorithm guided by a novel probabilistic speed function to segment the prostate region from each 3D DW-MRI for each b-value. This speed function is driven by the features learned by NMF from 3D appearance, shape, and spatial data. The second step is a probabilistic classifier that seeks to label a prostate segmented from 4-D DW-MRI data as either malignant, contain cancer, or benign, containing no cancer. This approach uses a NMF-based feature fusion to create a feature space where data classes are clustered. In addition, using DWI data acquired at a wide range of b-values (i.e., magnetic field strengths) is investigated. Experimental analysis indicates that for both of these frameworks, using NMF producing more accurate segmentation and classification results, respectively, and that combining the information from DWI data at several b-values can assist in detecting prostate cancer.

14.1   Introduction

Prostate cancer is the second most fatal cancer experienced by American males [1]. The average American male has a 16.15% chance of developing prostate cancer, which is 8.38% higher than lung cancer, the second most likely cancer [1]. Therefore, early detection of prostate cancer is crucial in decreasing prostate cancer related deaths [2]. Recent reports indicate that the mortality rate of prostate cancer has decreased by approximately 42% between 1991 and 2005 [3]. Approximately 45% of this decrease is due to the increased use of screening techniques [4]. While in vitro techniques that are based on analyzing a patient's blood, urine, or tissue samples are commonly used, they have several limitations concerning their accuracy and the invasive nature of most methods. Thus far, nonbiopsy screening techniques, predominantly prostate-specific antigen (PSA) blood-based screening [5], have a high chance of false-positive diagnosis, ranging from 28% to 58% [4]. More accurate, noninvasive diagnostic systems would aid clinicians in early detection of prostate cancer. To accomplish this, in vivo computer-aided diagnostic (CAD) systems have been developed to locate and to classify prostate tumors based on extracting information from medical images.

Recently, in vivo image-based techniques have demonstrated the proven ability to detect prostate cancer without the associated deleterious side effects of invasive techniques. These noninvasive methods for prostate cancer diagnosis are based on acquiring scans of the prostate and analyzing these scans for cancer detection. To acquire scans of the prostate, different medical imaging techniques, such as TRUS, magnetic resonance imaging (MRI), and computed tomography (CT), have been used. Each of these image modalities has its own mechanism for providing relevant physiological information of the prostate as well as its own advantages and limitations. For example, CT is currently used for posttherapy evaluation by physicians to assess the effectiveness of treatment [6]. However, it is expensive, uses radiation, and has poor contrast between soft tissues [6]. As a result, TRUS and MRI are more commonly used in CAD systems for diagnosing prostate cancer.

TRUS is the most frequently used technique for prostate imaging [6]. It is often used in planning and guiding needle biopsies [7]. In addition, TRUS is used in estimating the volume of the prostate gland, which can be used in biomarker screening [6]. TRUS is often chosen because it is relatively inexpensive and allows for real-time imaging. However, it does have several disadvantages for use in CAD systems. TRUS images have low contrast and a low signal-to-noise (SNR) ratio [8]. As a result, it can be difficult to accurately detect tumors and locate cancerous cells using TRUS images.

MRI is another widely used imaging modality for detecting prostate cancer. The main advantage of MRI is that it offers the best soft tissue contrast compared to other image modalities, such as CT and TRUS [9]. However, MRI is sensitive to noise and image artifacts, has a relatively long and complex acquisition, and has a relatively high cost [6].

Several different MRI techniques have been extensively used in prostate cancer CAD systems. T1-weighted (T1-MRI) and T2-weighted (T2-MRI) are two basic MRI techniques that measure the spin–lattice (T1) and spin–spin (T2) relaxation times to create an image [10]. Although these MRI techniques provide excellent soft tissue contrast, they lack functional information. Therefore, these MR imaging techniques have limited ability to effectively locate and classify prostate cancer [11]. Dynamic contrast-enhanced MRI (DCE-MRI) is another MR technique based on using contrast agents to provide information about the anatomy, function, and metabolism of target tissues [12]. In recent years, DCE-MRI has had considerable success in detecting and locating prostate cancer. However, intravenous administration of a contrast agent can potentially harm a patient's kidneys [13]. In addition, injecting and waiting for the contrast agent to settle in the prostate increase the time required to scan the patient. Diffusion-weighted imaging (DWI) [14] is an alternative MRI technique that avoids using contrast agents. DWI is a functional MRI technique that measures the micromovements (random, Brownian) of extracellular water molecules inside the body [15]. These movements provide indirect information about the structures surrounding these water molecules. Images collected using this modality have been shown to be useful for determining the size and shape of the prostate as well as detecting and locating cancerous tumors [14]. In several CAD systems, a combination of these MRI techniques has been used for diagnosing prostate cancer [16–22]. This is often called multiparametric imaging. These systems seek to extract different information from each type of image to detect, locate, and classify prostate tumors more accurately.

Development of CAD systems for detecting prostate cancer using these different image modalities is an ongoing area of research [23]. The success of CAD systems can be measured based on the diagnostic accuracy, speed, and automation level. A brief overview of the existing MRI-based in vivo computer-aided diagnostic (CAD) systems, which are related to the proposed MRI-based CAD system, is given below.

14.1.1 MRI-based related work

Recent research studies focus on developing CAD systems for prostate diagnosis using MRI due to its ability to offer better soft tissue contrast. These systems segment the prostate, extract features, and then perform diagnosis based on these features. In this section, the segmentation techniques, the MRI extracted features, and the MRI-based CAD systems developed are overviewed.

Prostate segmentation from in vivo *MR images*: MRI offers the best soft tissue contrast compared to the other image modalities used in prostate visualization. Therefore, the prostate can be defined more clearly in MR images than in any other imaging modalities. However, segmentation is still challenging due to patient movement, intrapatient anatomical variations of the prostate shape and appearance, noise and inhomogeneities, and discontinuities of boundaries due to occlusions and similar visual appearance of adjacent structures. To address these challenges, many techniques have been developed to extract the prostate from MR images such as deformable model-based methods and statistical-based methods.

Deformable models (DMs) have been applied extensively to segment the prostate from MRI data. For example, a hybrid 2D/3D ASM-based methodology for segmentation of the 3D MRI prostate data was proposed by Zhu et al. [24]. Toth et al. [25] presented an algorithm for the automatic segmentation of the prostate in multimodal MRI (T2-MRI and magnetic resonance spectroscopy [MRS]). Their algorithm starts by isolating the region of interest (ROI) from MRS data. Then, an ASM within the ROI is used to obtain the final segmentation. Gao et al. [26] aligned the MR images before segmenting the prostate using a level set guided by appearance information and a learned shape prior. Ghose et al. [27] used a similar approach that aligned T2-MRI data and then an AAM was used to segment the prostate. Martin et al. [28] used a probabilistic anatomical atlas to constrain a DM-based framework for segmenting the prostate from 3D MR images. Allen et al. [29] proposed a framework for 3D prostate segmentation from T2-MRI based on voxel classification and a statistical shape model. Liu et al. [30] proposed a level set technique guided by a shape prior and intensity information for 2D DWI prostate segmentation. Liu et al. [31] proposed a shape-based level set method for 3D DWI prostate segmentation guided by an initial coarse segmentation.

Statistical-based techniques have also been used to segment the prostate from MRI data such as graph-cut [32] methods, random walk classification [33], and probabilistic anatomical atlases. For example, Ghose et al. [34] proposed a probabilistic graph-cut-based framework for 3D T2-MRI prostate segmentation based on a probabilistic atlas. Firjany et al. [35] proposed a Markov random field (MRF) image model [36–50] for 2D DCE-MRI prostate segmentation that combined a graph-cut approach with a prior shape model of the prostate and the visual appearance of the prostate image, modeled using a linear combination of discrete Gaussian (LCDG) [51–62]. Their method was later extended in Firjani et al. [63,64] to allow for 3D prostate segmentation from DCE-MRI volumes. The main limitation of graph-cut techniques is that they are prone to minimizing the size of the segmented region [65].

A maximum a posteriori (MAP) [66]-based framework was proposed by Makni et al. [67] to perform automated 3D MRI prostate segmentation using a MRF model [68] and statistical shape information. Similarly, Firjani et al. used a MAP-based method that incorporated an LCDG intensity model, an MRF spatial model, and a shape prior for 3D prostate segmentation from DWI-MRI volumes [15,69,70]. Random walk classification [33] was used for MRI prostate segmentation by Khurd et al. [71]. Also, Klein et al. [72] presented an atlas-based segmentation approach to extract the prostate from MR images based on averaging the best atlases that match the image to be segmented. Another automated technique, proposed by Dowling et al. [73], used an automated atlas approach to segment the prostate region based on a selective and iterative method for performance level estimation (SIMPLE) [74]-based alignment technique. In addition to DMs and statistical-based techniques, several other methods have been proposed to segment the prostate from MR images. Flores-Tapia et al. [75] proposed a semiautomated edge detection technique for MRI prostate segmentation based on a static wavelet transform [76] to locate the prostate edges. A semiautomated approach by Vikal et al. [77] used priori knowledge of the prostate shape to detect the contour in each slice and then refined them to form a 3D prostate surface.

MRI feature extraction and diagnosis: Any MRI-based CAD system extract features in order to detect cancerous tumors. These features can be extracted from any MR image modality used in prostate CAD systems, for example, T1-MRI, T2-MRI, DCE, and DWI MRI. Several proposed CAD systems in the literature have used multiparametric MRI, a combination of multiple MRI modalities, to increase the number and quality of the features that the systems can utilize. Below, the common features extracted from each of these MRI modalities as well as the basic CAD systems developed in the last 10 years using these modalities are overviewed. T2-MRI-based diagnostic systems extract several features from T2-MRI for classifying a prostate region as cancerous or noncancerous. These features include the pixel/voxel intensity values of T2-MR images [17–19,21,22,78–83]. In addition, the 25 percentile [18], the variance and entropy of the T2-MRI intensities [19], the 2D [19], and 3D [78] intensity gradients, and the T2-MRI image texture [78] are commonly exploited as candidate features to discriminate between malignant and nonmalignant prostate tissues. In addition to pixel/voxel intensities, image filters were frequently used in order to extract features from T2-MRI. Image filtering applies a transform that maps each pixel/voxel on the image to a new value, from which new features can be extracted, such as the mean, standard deviation, average deviation, and median of the intensities of a pixel's neighbors [19,84]. Several image filters, such as the Gabor filter [85] and the Sobel filter [86], were used for feature extraction in Niaf et al. [19], Madabhushi et al. [78], Vos et al. [80], and Madabhushi et al. [82], respectively. Another T2-MRI feature is the relaxation time, the time it takes for protons to revert to their original energy state after the magnetic pulse created by an MRI machine. This feature was used in Madabhushi et al. [78] and Vos et al. [80].

Several T2-MRI CAD systems have been developed based on the extracted features from the baseline MRI methodology for prostate cancer detection (the initial image type used in prostate cancer CAD systems, i.e., T2-MRI). The main features extracted from T2-MRI images are signal intensities and texture-based features. These values have been utilized in multiple T2-MRI systems. One such semiautomated CAD system was proposed by Madabhushi et al. [78]. Pixels inside manually selected regions were labeled as tumourous or nontumourous using a Bayesian classifier. The classification was then performed using a large set of features that included: gray level statistics (intensity values, mean, and standard deviation), intensity gradient, and Gabor filter features. This pixel classification technique had a sensitivity of 42.35%, a specificity of 97.25% and a PPV of 42.85%. This system was improved in Madabhushi et al. [82]. The Bayesian classifier was replaced with a kNN classifier that was built using Bayesian learners. This modified system had an AUC of 0.957. An automated T2-MRI CAD system was developed by Lopes et al. [83]. Each pixel in the image was labeled as either cancerous or noncancerous based on their features. The fractal dimension and the multifractal spectrum calculated using a multifractional Browninan motion model were used as sources of features. Two classifiers were trained: SVM and AdaBoost [87]. The sensitivity and the specificity were 83% and 91% for SVM and 85% and 93% for AdaBoost.

DCE-MRI-based diagnostic systems were developed for prostate cancer diagnosis for several reasons. The addition of a contrast agent helps to distinguish objects of interest in MR images. In addition, the diffusion of the contrast agent can be used to add two common sources of DCE-MRI features, parametric (pharmacokinetic) and nonparametric parameters, in addition the intensity information. Pharmacokinetic parameters are measures of the kinetics of contrast agents through an organ in a DCE-MR image. The three standard pharmacokinetic parameters are the volume transfer constant (K^{trans}), the extravascular extracellular space fractional volume (v_e), and the rate constant (k_{ep}) [88]. These parameters have been used as features in several DCE-MRI prostate cancer CAD systems [80,84]. In addition, these features have also been used in many multiparametric MRI CAD systems [17–19,21,22,80,81]. Specifically, the 75 percentile K^{trans} value [18–21,80], the mean k_{ep} [17,80], the 75 percentile k_{ep} [20,89], and the 75 percentile v_e [18] have been utilized as discriminating features. In addition to the pharmacokinetic parameters, the established dynamic perfusion analysis of extracellular extravascular agents, such as gadolinium agents, have also used empirical measures, including peak signal intensity, time-to-peak, wash-in slope, wash-out slope, and area under the gadolinium curve (AUGC). The time-to-peak is defined as the time from the injection of the contrast agent until the peak intensity is observed. The wash-in rate is defined as the maximum change in intensity during the time between the start of the inflow of the contrast agent and the time where the highest signal intensity is recorded [90]. This feature was used in Peng et al. [21], Sung et al. [84], and Puech et al. [91,92]. The wash-out rate is defined as the maximum change in intensity during the time the highest signal intensity is recorded and a specified end time [93] and was used in the system proposed in Puech et al. [91,92]. The gadolinium curve is the plot of the gadolinium concentration versus time and the AUGC is the area under this curve [94]. This feature was used in the CAD system proposed in Niaf et al. [19].

Based on the extracted features from DCE-MRI, several DCE-MRI CAD systems were developed for prostate cancer diagnosis. For example, Viswanath et al. [79] proposed a semiautomated DCE-MRI-based system, where the prostate was segmented using an ASM initialized by a manually placed bounding-box and then guided by image intensity, image texture, and mutual information. To extract diagnostics features, local linear embedding (LLE) [95] was used to create a feature vector using local neighborhood intensities. K-means clustering was then used to classify the pixels within the segmented prostate as tumorous or nontumorous. Validation showed that this system had a sensitivity of 41.73%, a specificity of 84.54%, and an accuracy of 77.20%. A study by Engelbrecht et al. [96] used DCE-MRI to evaluate which MRI parameters would result in optimal discrimination of prostatic carcinoma from normal PZ and CZ of the prostate. Using the ROC curves, their study concluded that the relative peak enhancement was the most accurate perfusion parameter for cancer detection in the PZ and CZ of the gland. Additionally, a semiautomated CAD system by Kim et al. [97] demonstrated that parametric imaging of the wash-in rate was more accurate for the detection of prostate cancer in the PZ than was $T2$-MRI alone. However, they also observed a significant overlap between the wash-in rate for cancer and normal tissue in the TZ. Fütterer et al. [98] developed a CAD system to compare the accuracies of $T2$-MRI, DCE-MRI, and MRS imaging for prostate cancer localization. The results showed higher accuracy in DCE-MRI than were achieved with $T2$-MRI in prostate cancer localization. A similar study was conducted by Rouvière et al. [99] for the detection of postradiotherapy recurrence of prostate cancer. Their study also concluded that DCE-MRI possesses the ability to depict the intraprostatic distribution of recurrent cancer after therapy more accurately and with less interobserver variability than $T2$-MRI. Ocak et al. [100] developed a CAD system using PK analysis for prostate cancer diagnostics in patients with biopsy-proven lesions. In their framework, the K^{trans}, the k_{ep}, the v_e, and the area under the gadolinium concentration curve were determined and compared for cancer, inflammation, and healthy peripheral. Their results showed improvement in prostate cancer specificity using the K^{trans} and k_{ep} parameters over that obtained using conventional $T2$-MRI. Puech et al. [91,92] developed a semiautomated dynamic MRI-based CAD system for the detection of prostate cancer. Candidate lesion ROIs were selected either manually or by using a region growing technique initiated by a user-selected seed point. Lesions are classified as benign, malignant, or indeterminate based on the analysis of the median wash-in and wash-out values. Their CAD system demonstrated a sensitivity and specificity of 100% and 45% for the PZ, and sensitivity and specificity of 100% and 40% for the TZ. Sung et al. [84] proposed another semiautomated system where ROIs were manually selected. These were then classified as cancerous or noncancerous using K_{trans}, k_{ep}, v_e, wash-in rate, wash-out rate, and time-to-peak values. Testing showed that the system had a sensitivity of 90%, specificity of 77%, and accuracy of 83%. Vos et al. [89,101] proposed a semiautomated system and an automated system, respectively. In both, possible cancerous tumors in the PZ were classified as either tumorous or nontumorous. ROIs were manually selected in the first system [101] and selected using a combination of an Otsu threshold segmentation [102] and a Hessian-based blob detection method [103] in the second system [89]. In both systems, the ROIs were then classified using the pharmacokinetic parameters and an SVM classifier. The average accuracies of 88% and 80% were shown for the semiautomated and automated approaches, respectively. However, these techniques were only capable of detecting and classifying tumors in the PZ and not the rest of the prostate. Another automated DCE-MRI CAD system was proposed by Firjani et al. [104]. The first step in this system was performing probabilistic segmentation using the MAP algorithm and image intensity, spatial information modeled using an MRF, and a shape prior. The wash-in and wash-out curves were then used as sources of features for classification with a kNN classifier. This technique had an accuracy of 100% using a dataset of 21 subjects.

DWI-MRI-based diagnostic systems acquire images at varying b-values (i.e., magnetic field strengths). This allows the apparent diffusion coefficient (ADC) and other diagnostics features to be extracted. The ADC, a common intensity-based feature for DWI, is a measure of the impedance of water diffusion and is determined by evaluating the difference between two diffusion weighted images taken at different magnetic field strengths (e.g., b-values). The ADC values at each pixel/voxel are known as the ADC maps. They have been shown to be effective in differentiating between prostates containing cancerous tumors and those that do not [105]. In addition, it was shown that cancerous regions have a lower average ADC than noncancerous regions [105]. Consequently, ADC maps have been used as a source of features in several MRI prostate cancer CAD systems [15,17–21,80,81]. The mean ADC [17,18] and the median ADC value [19] are also common features for prostate cancer diagnosis. In addition, the 25 percentile ADC value [18–20], and the 10 percentile ADC value [21] are popular features. Also, a Sobel filter was applied to the ADC map to extract additional features in Niaf et al. [19]. T2 shine-through and T2 wash-out represent two additional DWI features. These features measure how much the intensity of a pixel/voxel changes between two DWI images acquired at different b-values. Typically, a b-value of 0 (i.e., T2-MRI) is used as a baseline and compared to a second, higher b-value. The intensities of these images are often referred to as S_0 and S_1, respectively. Shine-through occurs when the intensity increases drastically with an increase in b-value, whereas wash-out occurs when the intensity decreases drastically with an increase in b-value [106]. The change in the intensity has been used as a feature for CAD systems that utilize DWI [18,20]. Once a combination of these features are selected to form the feature space of a CAD system, classification can be performed. For example, Firjani et al. [15,107] developed a CAD system for prostate diagnosis using DWI-MRI. The prostate is automatically segmented based on a prior shape, spatial interactions, and appearance information. Possible tumor locations were then found using a level set DM. The average DWI intensity at b-values of 800 and 0 s/mm^2 and the mean value of the ADC map were then extracted from these locations. Finally, a kNN classifier labeled benign and malignant regions of the prostate. Validation testing showed that the system had an accuracy of 100% using a dataset of 28 subjects, 13 of which were used for training and 15 for testing.

Multiparametric-based diagnostic systems for prostate cancer use several MRI imaging modalities in conjunction as input data. This allows systems to select the most meaningful features from any of the modalities. These systems have used different combinations of MRI modalities and features. For example, T2-MRI and DCE-MRI were used as inputs in a semiautomated system proposed by Vos et al. [80]. This system classified manually delineated ROIs in the PZ as malignant or benign using T2-MRI intensities, T2-MRI relaxation time, and pharmacokinetic parameters as features. This approach showed an accuracy of 89% using an SVM classifier. Ampeliotis et al. [108] proposed another semi-automated multiparametric CAD system that used $T2$-MRI and DCE-MRI. The $T2$-MRI pixel intensities and the four low-frequency coefficients of the discrete cosine transform were used as features and probabilistic neural networks were employed as the classifier. Based on the ROC analysis (AUC of 0.898), their study concluded that the fused $T2$-MRI and dynamic MRI features outperform the use of either modality's features alone. Another semiautomated system that utilized T2-MRI and DCE-MRI as input was developed by Viswanath et al. [16]. An ASM model was initialized by a manually placed bounding-box and then guided by image intensity, image texture, and mutual information to segment the prostate region. After segmentation, prostate tissues were classified as cancerous or noncancerous using a random forest, which is made of multiple decision trees that vote on the classification. Classification integrated three features: T2 intensity, textual, and pharma-cokinetic parameters. The system validation showed that the integration of both modalities (AUC of 0.815) has a better performance of either individual modalities (0.704 for $T2$-MRI and 0.682 for DCE-MRI). Haider et al. [109] developed a semiautomated system that utilized T2-MRI and DWI MRI. T2-MRI intensities and ADC values were extracted from manually delineated ROIs. These regions were then classified using the maximum likeli-hood method assuming a bivariate Gaussian distribution for benign and malignant classes. The system showed a sensitivity of 81%, a specificity of 84%, a PPV of 75%, and an accuracy of 83%. Chan et al. [110] developed a semiautomated approach using T2-MRI, T_2-mapping, and line scan DWI to detect possible PZ prostate tumors. Both statistical maps and textural features were obtained from manually selected ROIs. Then, a SVM and a linear discrimi-nant analysis (LDA) classifiers were employed for the classification. Their systems resulted in an AUC of 0.839 ± 0.064 and 0.761 ± 0.043, respectively.

The combination of T2-MRI, DCE-MRI, and DWI MRI is a common multiparametric input. Shah et al. [22] developed an automated CAD system utilizing these modalities. In this system, prostate segmentation was performed using a k-means clustering approach based on the pixel's T2, K^{trans}, k_{ep}, and ADC values. Then, an SVM technique was imple-mented to create a cancer probability map for each prostate pixel using those features in order to perform the final classification. The system achieved a sensitivity of 90%, a speci-ficity of 90%, and a precision of 90%. Another semiautomated multiparametric system by Peng et al. [21] utilized $T2$-MRI, DCE-MRI, and DWI-MRI. Candidate features, including the $T2$-MRI intensity skew, the K^{trans}, and the average and 10th percentile ADC, were cal-culated from a manually selected ROI. Then, an LDA classifier was used to differentiate prostate cancer from normal tissue in those ROIs. Their CAD system concluded that the best diagnostic performance (AUC of 0.95 ± 0.02, sensitivity of 82.0%, and specificity of 95.3%) is obtained by combining the 10th percentile ADC, average ADC, and T2-MRI inten-sity skewness features. Another CAD system was proposed by Litjens et al. [17] using T2-MRI, DCE-MRI, and DWI MRI. The prostate is segmented using an ASM. In order to classify the segmented prostate voxels, the ADC, K^{trans}, and k_{ep} parameters were esti-mated and a SVM classifier with a radial basis function kernel was used. The validation results showed a sensitivity of 74.7% and 83.4% with seven and nine false-positives per patient, respectively. Vos et al. [18] utilized an automated CAD system for the detection of prostate cancer. Just as in Litjens et al. [17], the prostate was segmented using an ASM-based technique. Then, multiple ROIs were located within the segmented prostate using peak and mean neighborhood intensity and ADC values. These values and the differ-ences between the peak and the mean were again used as features for ROI classification. In addition, the 25 percentile T2, 25 percentile ADC, 25 percentile wash-out, 50 percentile T_1, 75 percentile K^{trans}, and 75 percentile v_e were also used as features. The resulting feature vector was classified using an LDA classifier. This system had an AUC of 0.83 ± 0.20. A maximum AUC of 0.88 was reported for high-grade tumors, but the system had difficulty classifying lower grade tumors, achieving a maximum AUC of 0.74.

In addition, several automated CAD systems that directly segment tumors have also been proposed. Liu et al. [111] proposed an automated approach that utilized fuzzy MRF modeling for prostate segmentation from multiparametric MRI (T2-MRI, DCE-MRI, and DWI MR images). Their framework exploited T2-MR image intensities, pharmacokinetic (PK) parameter k_{ep}, and apparent diffusion coefficient (ADC) values in a Bayesian approach to label prostate pixels as cancerous or noncancerous. The labeled pixels were then clustered using the k-means algorithm. The system had a specificity of 89.58%, sensitivity of 87.50%, accuracy of 89.38%, and a DSC of 62.2%. A similar approach developed by Artan et al. [112] located cancerous regions using cost-sensitive support vector machine (SVM). Prostate segmentation was performed using a conditional random field and the same three features as in Liu et al. [111] were utilized for classification. The DSC for prostate localization and segmentation was 0.46 ± 0.26, and the area under the receiver operator characteristic (ROC) curves (A_z) of the classification was 0.79 ± 0.12. Ozer et al. [81] also developed a technique that directly segmented prostate cancers using the same three features in Liu et al. [111] and Artan et al. [112]. Both the SVM and RVM [113] classifiers were used and the system showed a specificity of 0.78 and a sensitivity of 0.74 for RVM and 0.74 and 0.79 for SVM.

In summary, the CAD systems mentioned above for analyzing DWI are not sufficiently accurate and reliable for several reasons:

- The majority of the CAD systems is depending on using more than one modality (e.g., T1-MRI, T2-MRI, DCE-MRI, and DW-MRI). This makes the developed CAD system is sensitive to the accuracy of the fusion algorithm that used to fuse the extracted information from the different MRI modalities.
- The majority of these studies require user interaction to select a ROI (a small window) around the prostate.
- Automated prostate segmentation methods have one of the following limitations:
  - Deformable model-based methods without adequate appearance and shape priors fail under excessive noise, poor resolution, diffused boundaries, or occluded shapes in the images.
  - Active shape models are unsuitable for segmenting prostate objects due to a very small number of distinct landmarks.

To overcome these limitations, we propose 3D level set segmentation algorithm guided by a novel probabilistic speed function to segment the prostate region from each 3D DW-MRI for each b-value. This speed function is driven by the features learned by NMF from 3D appearance, shape, and spatial data. Followed the segmentation step, we propose to use a probabilistic classifier that seeks to label a prostate segmented from 4D DW-MRI data as either malignant, contain cancer, or benign, containing no cancer. This approach uses a NMF-based feature fusion to create a feature space where data classes are clustered.

14.2 Methods

In this chapter, a novel DW-MRI prostate CAD system (Figure 14.1) is proposed. As shown in Figure 14.1. The proposed system consists of two main steps: (i) prostate segmentation from DW-MRI data and (ii) diagnosis/classification of the segmented prostate to either

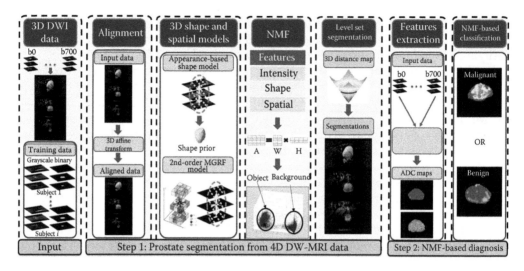

Figure 14.1 A diagram of the proposed segmentation framework.

malignant or benign based on calculating the diffusion coefficient (DC) from different b-values. We will discuss the details of each step below.

14.2.1   *3D appearance, shape, and spatial features*

Segmentation of prostate from DW-MRI data utilizes an NMF-based feature fusion approach that incorporates three features, namely DWI intensity, shape, and spatial information. The features generated by performing NMF-based feature fusion are then used to guide the evolution of a 3D level set deformable model to extract the prostate from DWI data. The definition of this level set is given below. The evolving surface of the level set at any time instant t is represented by the zero level, $\phi_{n+1}(x, y, z) = 0$, of an implicit level set function, namely a distance map of the signed minimum Euclidean distance from each voxel to the surface. This formulation results in points inside the surface having negative (or positive) values and voxels outside the surface having positive (or negative) values, respectively. Mathematically, the evolution of the level set is defined by Osher and Sethian [114]:

$$\phi_{n+1}(x, y, z) = \phi_n(x, y, z) - \tau V_n(x, y, z) |\nabla \phi_n(x, y, z)| \qquad (14.1)$$

where t is the discrete time instant $t = n\tau$ taken with a step τ, $\tau > 0$ and $\nabla = [\frac{\partial}{\partial x}, \frac{\partial}{\partial y}, \frac{\partial}{\partial z}]$ is the differential operator. This evolution is guided by the speed function $V_n(x, y, z)$ [115].

Previous speed functions that use image intensities, object edges, and gradient vector flow have had difficulty segmenting noisy images and those with poor object-background contrast. More effective speed functions have been developed by using shape priors to incorporate shape information of the object of interest. However, this has not completely overcome image inhomogeneities (e.g., large image noise and discontinuous object boundaries). In order to more accurately segment the prostate from DWI data, we propose a speed function that takes into account the 3D appearance, shape, and spatial features of the DWI data. These features are combined using an NMF-based fusion method to provide the voxelwise guidance of the deformable model.

14.2.1.1 3D appearance, shape, and spatial features

Basic Notation. Let $\mathbf{Q} = \{0, ..., Q-1\}$ and $\mathbf{L} = \{0, 1\}$ be the set of Q integer gray levels and a set of object (1) and background (0) labels, respectively. Also, let a 3D arithmetic lattice $\mathbf{R} = \{(x, y, z) : 0 \leq x \leq X - 1; 0 \leq y \leq Y - 1; 0 \leq z \leq Z - 1\}$ support the grayscale DWI data $\mathbf{g} : \mathbf{R} \to \mathbf{Q}$ and their binary region maps $\mathbf{m} : \mathbf{R} \to \mathbf{L}$. Each voxel (x, y, z) is associated with its neighbors, $\{(x + \xi, y + \eta, z + \zeta) : (x + \xi, y + \eta, z + \zeta) \in \mathbf{R}; (\xi, \eta, \zeta) \in \mathbf{N}\}$ where $\mathbf{N}$ was defined by $\xi \in \{-1, 0, 1\}$, $\eta \in \{-1, 0, 1\}$, and $\zeta \in \{-1, 0, 1\}$ (Figure 14.2).

Appearance-Based Shape Model. Most prostates have a similar near-ellipsoidal shape [116]. As a result, the inclusion of a shape prior can significantly improve the segmentation accuracy. In the proposed framework, an appearance-based shape model is built that takes into account not only a voxel's location, but also its intensity information. A shape database was constructed by coaligning training datasets using a 3D affine transformation with 12 degrees of freedom (three for the 3D translation, three for the 3D rotation, three for the 3D scaling, and three for the 3D shearing) and maximizing mutual information (MI) [117]. A shape prior is a spatially variant independent random field of region labels for the coaligned data. Mathematically, this is defined as

$$P_{\text{shape}}(\mathbf{m}) = \prod_{(x,y,z) \in \mathbf{R}} P_{\text{shape}:x,y,z}(m_{x,y,z}) \tag{14.2}$$

where $P_{\text{shape}:x,y,z}(l)$ is the voxel-wise empirical probability for label $l \in \mathbf{L}$. For each input DWI volume to be segmented, the shape prior is constructed by a process guided by the

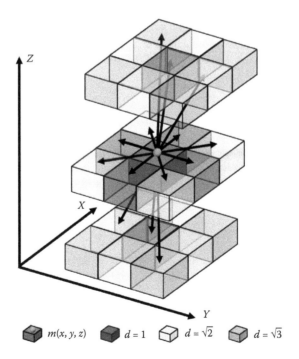

Figure 14.2 Illustration of a voxel's neighborhood.

visual appearance features of the DWI data. The appearance-based shape prior is then estimated using the method summarized in Algorithm 14.1.

ALGORITHM 14.1   Algorithm for Calculating an Appearance-Based Shape Model

Calculate the value of the shape prior probability at each voxel using the following steps:

1. Transform each test subject voxel to the shape database domain using the calculated 3D affine transformation matrix (T).
2. Initialize an $N_{1i} \times N_{2i} \times N_{3i}$ search space centered at the voxel.
3. Find voxels inside the search space with corresponding gray levels to the center voxel in all training datasets.
4. If no corresponding voxels are found, increase the search space size and repeat the previous step.
5. Calculate the label probabilities for each voxel based on the relative occurrence of each label in the search results.

Spatial Voxel Interaction Model. In addition to the prostate shape prior, analyzing the interactions of a voxel and its neighbors can improve segmentation [15,118]. In order to model these interactions, a second-order 3D MGRF model [119] is used. The MGRF model of the region map **m** is defined as

$$P_{spatial}(\mathbf{m}) = \frac{1}{Z_{\mathbf{N}}} \exp \sum_{(x,y,z) \in \mathbf{R}} \sum_{(\varepsilon,\nu,\zeta) \in \mathbf{N}} V_{eq}(m_{x,y,z}, m_{x+\varepsilon,y+\nu,z+\zeta}) \qquad (14.3)$$

where $V_{eq}(m_{x,y,z}, m_{x+\varepsilon,y+\nu,z+\zeta})$ is the Gibbs potential and Z_N is the normalization factor that can be approximated as [120]:

$$Z_N \approx \exp \sum_{(x,y,z) \in \mathbf{R}} \sum_{(\varepsilon,\nu,\zeta) \in \mathbf{N}} \sum_{l \in \mathbf{L}} V_{eq}(l, m_{x+\varepsilon,y+\nu,z+\zeta}) \qquad (14.4)$$

The MGRF used can be viewed as a 3D extension of the auto-binomial, or Potts, model with the exception that the Gibbs potential is estimated analytically. The maximum likelihood estimate of the potential is given as Farag et al. [43]:

$$V_{eq} = 2 \left(f_{eq}(\mathbf{m}) - \frac{1}{2} \right) \qquad (14.5)$$

where $f_{eq}(\mathbf{m})$ is the relative frequency of equal (eq) labels in the voxel pairs $((x,y,z), (x+\xi, y+\eta, z+\zeta))$.

14.2.1.2   *NMF-based feature fusion*

NMF is a method for extracting meaningful features from datasets for representing different categories in the data [121]. This is done by calculating a weight matrix W that transforms a vector from the input space into a new feature space (H-space) through factorizing the input matrix A so that $A \approx WH$. NMF has been applied to various data analysis problems such as document clustering [122] and facial recognition [123]. In addition, it has been used in a few segmentation systems. This includes Xie et al. [124] who used NMF to segment the spinal cord, corpus callosum, and hippocampus regions of rats from diffusion tensor imaging (DTI) by k-means clustering of the column vectors of the produced H matrix. Also, Sandler et al. [125] proposed using NMF to factorize intensity histogram data for generic image segmentation.

In this chapter, NMF is proposed to find the weights for each feature in order to create a feature space where object and background classes are better separated, dimensionality is reduced, and information from the training dataset is encoded. NMF factorizes a k by n input matrix A into a k by r weight matrix W, which contains the basis vectors of the new space as columns, and an r by n output matrix H where k is the dimensionality of the input column vectors, n is the number of input and output column vectors, and r is the dimensionality of the output column vectors [121]. Mathematically, this is defined as

$$A \approx WH \tag{14.6}$$

W and H are calculated by minimizing the Euclidean distance between A and WH with the constraint that W and H contain only nonnegative values. This results in the constrained optimization problem:

$$\underset{W,H}{\text{minimize}} \quad \frac{1}{2} \|A - WH\|^2 \tag{14.7}$$
$$\text{subject to} \quad W, H \geq 0$$

In the literature, several methods have been used to optimize this function. The most prominent methods have been multiplicative gradient descent, alternating least square (ALS), and projected gradient descent (PGD) [126]. In this chapter, the multiplicative method [127] is used because of its ease of implementation. This method iteratively updates W and H until convergence using the following rules:

$$H_{\alpha\beta} \leftarrow H_{\alpha\beta} \frac{(W^T A)_{\alpha\beta}}{(W^T WH)_{\alpha\beta}} \tag{14.8}$$

$$W_{\gamma\alpha} \leftarrow W_{\gamma\alpha} \frac{(AH^T)_{\gamma\alpha}}{(WHH^T)_{\gamma\alpha}} \tag{14.9}$$

where $\alpha : 1 \rightarrow r$, $\beta : 1 \rightarrow n$, and $\gamma : 1 \rightarrow k$.

In the proposed framework, NMF is performed on a matrix that has a kth dimensional, one dimension for each calculated feature, column vector for each voxel (x, y, z) in the training volumes. The input features are the intensity values of the voxe (x, y, z) and its neighbors, the spatial interactions between voxel (x, y, z) and its neighbors, and the value of the shape prior at (x, y, z). The resulting W is used as the basis vectors to transform new feature vectors into the new r-dimensional space (H-space). The resulting H is used to find the r-dimensional centroids corresponding to the object and background classes, C_{object} and $C_{background}$, respectively. For each voxel in a testing volume, a kth dimensional feature vector was calculated. This resulted in a k by n feature matrix B where n is the number of voxels in the volume. The new r dimensional vectors corresponding to the input voxels are calculated by multiplying B by the pseudo-inverse of W, which can be replaced by W^T assuming orthogonality of the columns of W [128]. Mathematically, this is described as

$$H_B = W^T B \tag{14.10}$$

14.2.1.3 Estimation of the stochastic speed function

In this chapter, a novel speed function to control the evolution of the level set deformable model is proposed. This speed function is derived using the NMF-based fusion of DWI features, $H_{B:x,y,z}$ for voxel (x, y, z). The proposed speed function $V_n(x, y, z)$ is defined as $V_n(x, y, z) = \kappa \vartheta(x, y, z)$, where κ is the curvature and $\vartheta(x, y, z)$ is defined as

$$\vartheta(x, y, z) = \begin{cases} -E_{1:x,y,z} & \text{if } E_{1:x,y,z} > E_{0:x,y,z} \\ E_{0:x,y,z} & \text{otherwise} \end{cases} \tag{14.11}$$

Here, $E_{1:x,y,z} = \frac{P_{nmf:x,y,z}(1) + P_{shape:x,y,z}(1) + P_{spatial:x,y,z}(1)}{3}$ where $P_{shape:x,y,z}(1)$ is the object shape prior probability and $P_{spatial:x,y,z}(1)$ is the object MGRF model probability Equation 14.3. Similarly, $E_{0:x,y,z} = \frac{P_{nmf:x,y,z}(0) + P_{shape:x,y,z}(0) + P_{spatial:x,y,z}(0)}{3}$ where $P_{shape:x,y,z}(0)$ is the background shape prior probability and $P_{spatial:x,y,z}(0)$ is the background MGRF model probability Equation 14.3. $P_{nmf:x,y,z}(1)$ and $P_{nmf:x,y,z}(0)$ are defined as:

$$P_{nmf:x,y,z}(1) = \frac{1/d_1(H_{B:x,y,z})}{1/d_1(H_{B:x,y,z}) + 1/d_1(H_{B:x,y,z})} \tag{14.12}$$

$$P_{nmf:x,y,z}(0) = \frac{1/d_0(H_{B:x,y,z})}{1/d_0(H_{B:x,y,z}) + 1/d_0(H_{B:x,y,z})} \tag{14.13}$$

where $d_1(x, y, z)$ and $d_0(x, y, z)$ are the Euclidean distances from the r-dimensional vector in H_B corresponding to the input voxel (x, y, z) to the centroids of the object and background classes, C_1 and C_0, respectively, in H-space. The overall segmentation framework is summarized by Algorithm 14.2.

ALGORITHM 14.2   Proposed Algorithm for DWI Prostate Segmentation

Segment the prostate from a DWI volume by:

1. Align the input DWI volume with the training database using the MI-based affine transformation.
2. Calculate the appearance-based shape prior using Algorithm 14.1.
3. Calculate the 3D pairwise voxel interactions (Equation 14.3).
4. Perform NMF-based feature fusion.
5. Calculate the probabilities that each voxel is object or background using the NMF-based features (Equations 14.12 and 14.13).
6. Use these probabilities to guide the evolution of a level set to segment the prostate (Equation 14.11).

14.2.2 Diagnosis/classification

In the diagnosis/classification step, we will also use NMF to reduce the estimated diffusion coefficient features and make them more separable in the feature space. As demonstrated above, the multiplicative gradient descent algorithm [127] was used to approximate a weight matrix W for an input matrix A such that $A \approx WH$. The columns of the input matrix A corresponded to the mean and maximum image intensities and ADC values at b-values of 100, 200, 300, 400, 500, 600, and 700 as well as the mean intensity at a b-value of 0. In the proposed approach, the feature vectors of both training and testing data are included in A. As in the segmentation approach proposed in the previous chapter, r, the dimensionality of the transformation space, was set to 3. Classification of a new subject was performed using the k-nearest neighbors (kNN) [129] algorithm. This method was used instead of a W^T-based approach, similar to the technique described in the previous chapter, because there was better 3D data separation in H-space versus H_A-space where $H_A = W^T A$. Once NMF was performed, the resulting H matrix was used as the input to the classification step.

Once each data sample was transformed to H-space, classification of benign and malignant subjects was performed using a probabilistic model derived using the kNN algorithm and the distances to class centroids. Each subject S_i was given a label L as benign (0) or malignant (1) per the following rule:

$$L(S_i) = \begin{cases} 1 & \text{if } P_{1:S_i} > P_{0:S_i} \\ 0 & \text{otherwise} \end{cases} \tag{14.14}$$

Here, $P_{1:S_i} = P_{knn}(1:S_i) * P_c(1:S_i)$ and $P_{0:S_i} = P_{knn}(0:S_i) * P_c(0:S_i)$ where $P_{knn}(1:S_i)$ and $P_{knn}(0:S_i)$ are the kNN-based probabilities that the subject is malignant or benign, respectively, and $P_c(1:S_i)$ and $P_c(0:S_i)$ are the centroid-based probabilities that the subject is malignant or benign, respectively. The kNN-based probabilities were calculated by finding the $k = 5$ training subjects with the smallest Euclidean distance to a test subject S_i in H-space. The number of k-nearest training points with label l is defined as n_l and is used to estimate the label probabilities as defined by

$$P_{knn}(1|S_i) = \frac{n_l}{k} \tag{14.15}$$

$$P_{knn}(0|S_i) = \frac{n_0}{k} \tag{14.16}$$

The centroid-based probabilities were calculated by finding the Euclidean distances of a test subject S_i to the centroids of the malignant and benign training subjects in H-space, d_1 and d_0, respectively. The corresponding label probabilities are defined as follows:

$$P_c(1|S_i) = \frac{\frac{1}{d_1}}{\frac{1}{d_1} + \frac{1}{d_0}} \tag{14.17}$$

$$P_c(0|S_i) = \frac{\frac{1}{d_0}}{\frac{1}{d_1} + \frac{1}{d_0}} \tag{14.18}$$

ALGORITHM 14.3   Algorithm for Refining NMF-Based Classification

Determine the label L of S_i by:

1. Calculate W and H using NMF on the training and testing data.
2. Calculate the k-means-based and the kNN-based probabilities of S_i.
3. Label S_i according to the class probabilities (Equation 14.14).
4. Repeat steps 1–3 τ times.
5. Combine the τ results using an ensemble-based method [130] to classify S_i.

Due to the random initialization of W and H, the use of gradient descent, and the low number of data points, the accuracy of classifying in H-space significantly varied when NMF was performed. In order to overcome these issues and classify more consistently, Algorithm 14.3 was used to determine the final classification of a subject.

14.3   Performance metrics for evaluating the segmentation results

The performance of the proposed segmentation framework was evaluated using two metrics: (1) Dice similarity coefficient (DSC) and (2) Hausdorff distance (HD). These metrics are detailed below.

14.3.1   Dice similarity coefficient (DSC)

Many segmentation and classification metrics are based on the determination of true-positive (TP), false-positive (FP), true-negative (TN), and false-negative (FN) values (see Figure 14.3). The TP is the number of correctly positively labeled samples; the FP is the number of incorrectly positively labeled samples; the TN is the number of correctly negatively labeled samples; and the FN is the number of incorrectly negatively labeled samples.

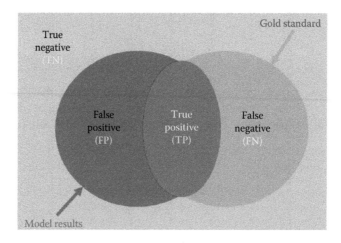

Figure 14.3 Diagram illustrating the meaning of TP, FP, TN, and FP.

These values can be used to calculate the DSC given by:

$$DSC = \frac{2TP}{2TP + FP + FN} \tag{14.19}$$

The value of the DSC ranges from 0 to 1, where 0 means that there is no similarity and 1 means that there is perfect similarity.

14.3.2 Hausdorff distance

Distance measures are another type of performance metric used for evaluating segmentation methods. The Euclidean distance is often utilized, but another common measure is the HD (see Figure 14.4). The HD from a set $\mathbf{A_1}$ to a set $\mathbf{A_2}$ is defined as the maximum distance of the set $\mathbf{A_1}$ to the nearest point in the set $\mathbf{A_2}$ [131]:

$$HD(\mathbf{A_1}, \mathbf{A_2}) = \max_{a_1 \in \mathbf{A_1}}\{\min_{a_2 \in \mathbf{A_2}}\{d(a_1, a_2)\}\} \tag{14.20}$$

where a_1 and a_2 are points of sets $\mathbf{A_1}$ and $\mathbf{A_2}$, respectively, and $d(a_1, a_2)$ is Euclidean distance between these points. The bidirectional Hausdorff distance, denoted by $HD_{Bi}(\mathbf{GT}, \mathbf{SR})$, between the segmented region ($\mathbf{SR}$) and its ground truth ($\mathbf{GT}$) is defined as:

$$HD_{Bi}(\mathbf{GT}, \mathbf{SR}) = \max\{HD(\mathbf{GT}, \mathbf{SR}), HD(\mathbf{SR}, \mathbf{GT})\} \tag{14.21}$$

The smaller the distance, the better the segmentation. The ideal case with perfect segmentation is when the bidirectional Hausdorff distance is equal to 0.

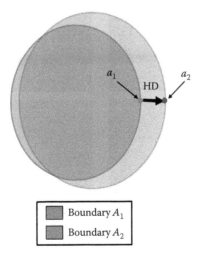

Figure 14.4 Diagram illustrating the 2D HD of boundaries A_1 and A_2 for points a_1 and a_2.

14.4 Experimental results

14.4.1 Medical images

The proposed system was tested on nine subjects, each with DWI volumes acquired at using a scanner (SIGNA Horizon, General Electric Medical Systems, Milwaukee, WI) with the following parameters: TE: 84:6 ms; TR: 8.000 ms; FOV 32 cm; slice thickness 3 mm; inter-slice gap 0 mm; and two excitations. The data was with b-values ranging of 0, 100, 200, 300, 400, 500, 600, and 700 using a voxel size of $1.25 \times 1.25 \times 3.00$ mm^3. The ground truth segmentations used in training and in verifying the segmentation results were manually created by an MR expert for each subject.

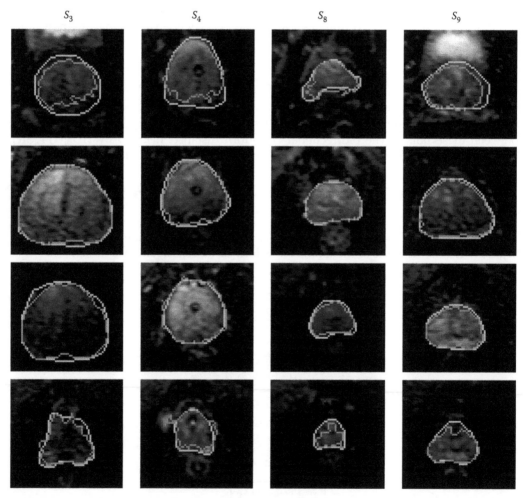

Figure 14.5 Sample segmentation results presented in 2D for visualization of the 3D segmentation performed by the proposed nonnegative matrix factorization (NMF)-based level set approach at different cross-sections for five different subjects where the green and red curves correspond to the ground truth and our segmentation, respectively.

14.4.2   Segmentation results

Evaluation of the system was done using a leave-one-out methodology, where eight subjects were used as training data and the remaining subject was used as test data. This was repeated so that each subject was tested once. Sample 2D cross-sections of the 3D segmentations generated using the proposed approach for different subjects are shown in Figure 14.5. In order to evaluate the proposed method, its performance has been compared to two different DWI prostate segmentation methods: (1) the reported results for the 3D approach developed by Liu et al. [31] and (2) a level set guided by the MAP model proposed by Osher and Fedkiw [15] that utilized the probability that a voxel was object or background based on its intensity, shape, and spatial information. Note that the MAP-based method was tested on the same data as the NMF-based approach, but the technique proposed by Liu et al. [31] was tested on a different dataset. The average DSC and HD values of the three compared methods are shown in Table 14.1. Additionally, an example is given in Figure 14.6 that contrasts the segmentations of the NMF-based and MAP-based approaches. The evaluation metrics for these two approaches corresponding to each subject are shown in Tables 14.2 and 14.3.

Table 14.1 A comparison of the average DSC and HD values over all subjects for the compared methods

Metric	NMF	MAP	Liu et al. [31]
DSC	0.870 ± 0.03	0.833 ± 0.07	0.810 ± 0.05
HD (mm^3)	5.72 ± 2.35	6.74 ± 2.04	9.07 ± 1.64

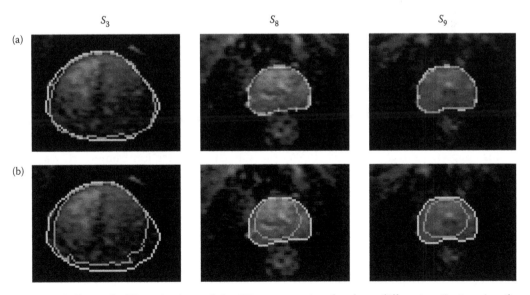

Figure 14.6 Example 2D projections of the 3D segmentation for three different patients using the (a) NMF and (b) MAP-guided level set where the green and red curves correspond to the ground truth and segmentation, respectively.

Table 14.2 The DSC segmentation performance of the NMF and MAP-guided
level set methods for each of the subjects, S_i where $i = 1 \ldots 9$

Method	S_1	S_2	S_3	S_4	S_5	S_6	S_7	S_8	S_9
NMF	0.822	0.861	0.907	0.862	0.905	0.828	0.851	0.886	0.905
MAP	0.816	0.858	0.881	0.836	0.900	0.827	0.849	0.647	0.880

Table 14.3 The HD segmentation performance of the NMF and
MAP-guided level set methods for each of the subjects, S_i where
$i = 1 \ldots 9$

Method	S_1	S_2	S_3	S_4	S_5	S_6	S_7	S_8	S_9
NMF	5.30	3.00	6.00	6.00	5.96	8.72	9.75	3.49	3.25
MAP	5.30	3.00	6.34	6.00	6.93	8.75	9.08	9.27	6.00

Table 14.4 A comparison of the accuracies of the kNN
classifier without NMF and the NMF-based method with
refinement (NMF+R)

Method	ACC	Range
kNN	0.667	–
NMF+R	0.833 ± 0.078	0.667–0.917

14.4.3   Diagnostic results

Testing was performed using a leave-one-out methodology and nine subjects, each with a
DWI scan at b-values ranging from 0 to 700. Six of the subjects were malignant and six were
benign. The above approach was tested with a refinement using $\tau = 10$. For comparison,
kNN classification without NMF-based feature fusion was performed using only the input
data, similar to the approach proposed by Firjani et al. [15]. The accuracies of these methods
are shown in Table 14.4. It may be noted that the minimum accuracy of this approach is
equivalent to the accuracy of the kNN method. In addition, the mode accuracy of the NMF
approach was 0.917, occurring in four of the 10 runs.

14.5   Conclusions and future work

In this chapter, a novel NMF-based DWI prostate cancer detection framework was proposed. It has been demonstrated that using 3D intensity, shape, and spatial features
combined with NMF-based feature fusion is significantly better at guiding a level set for
DWI prostate segmentation than either using MAP with the same input information or
intensity and shape information alone. The addition of NMF-based feature fusion allows
the proposed method to perform robust prostate segmentation despite image noise, interpatient anatomical differences, and the similar intensities of the prostate and surrounding
tissues. In addition, it is shown that the use of NMF leads to better clustering of malignant
and benign data points allowing for increased classification accuracy. Also, our classification approach shows that the fusion of DWI features from multiple b-values can be used
for detecting prostate cancer. To further test and validate this approach, it should be tested
on larger datasets.

In addition, several possibilities for future work relating to and extending this work are: (i) testing the proposed segmentation and classification frameworks on larger datasets, with a wider range of b-values, and using a variety of method parameters; (ii) integrating the proposed NMF-based frameworks into a contiguous CAD system for prostate cancer and testing this system; and (iii) applying these NMF-based frameworks to other medical image analysis applications such as dyslexia [132–140], autism [141–152], acute renal rejection [37,38,56,153–170], and lung cancer [119,171–200].

References

1. R. Siegel, D. Naishadham, and A. Jemal, Cancer statistics 2013, *CA—Cancer Journal of Clinics*, vol. 63, no. 1, pp. 11–30, 2013.
2. P. Vineis and C. P. Wild, Global cancer patterns: Causes and prevention, *Lancet*, 2013.
3. M. S. Wachtel, T. Nelius, A. L. Haynes, S. Dahlbeck, and W. de Riese, PSA screening and deaths from prostate cancer after diagnosis: a population based analysis, *Prostate*, vol. 73, no. 12, pp. 1365–1369, 2013.
4. R. Etzioni, R. Gulati, M. Cooperberg, D. Penson, N. Weiss, and I. Thompson, Limitations of basing screening policies on screening trials: The U.S. Preventive Services Task Force and Prostate Cancer Screening, *Medical Care*, vol. 51, no. 4, pp. 295–300, 2013.
5. M. J. Barry, Prostate-specific–antigen testing for early diagnosis of prostate cancer, *New England Journal of Medicine*, vol. 344, no. 18, pp. 1373–1377, 2001.
6. H. Hricak, P. L. Choyke, S. C. Eberhardt, S. A. Leibel, and P. T. Scardino, Imaging prostate cancer: A multidisciplinary perspective, *Radiology*, vol. 243, no. 1, pp. 28–53, 2007.
7. G. Fichtinger, A. Krieger, R. C. Susil, A. Tanacs, L. L. Whitcomb, and E. Atalar, Transrectal prostate biopsy inside closed MRI scanner with remote actuation, under real-time image guidance, in *Proceedings of the International Conference on Medical Image Computing and Computer-Assisted Intervention (MICCAI'02)*. Tokyo, Japan: Springer, September 25–28, 2002, pp. 91–98.
8. J. C. Applewhite, B. Matlaga, D. McCullough, M. Hall et al., Transrectal ultrasound and biopsy in the early diagnosis of prostate cancer. *Cancer Control*, vol. 8, no. 2, p. 141, 2001.
9. M. Fuchsjäger, A. Shukla-Dave, O. Akin, J. Barentsz, and H. Hricak, Prostate cancer imaging, *Acta Radiologica*, vol. 49, no. 1, pp. 107–120, 2008.
10. S. C. Bushong, *Magnetic Resonance Imaging*. Amsterdam: Elsevier Health Sciences, 2003.
11. M. Seitz, A. Shukla-Dave, A. Bjartell, K. Touijer, A. Sciarra, P. J. Bastian, C. Stief, H. Hricak, and A. Graser, Functional magnetic resonance imaging in prostate cancer, *European Urology*, vol. 55, no. 4, pp. 801–814, 2009.
12. S. Punwani, M. Emberton, M. Walkden, A. Sohaib, A. Freeman, H. Ahmed, C. Allen, and A. Kirkham, Prostatic cancer surveillance following whole-gland high-intensity focused ultrasound: comparison of MRI and prostate-specific antigen for detection of residual or recurrent disease, *British Journal of Radiology*, vol. 85, no. 1014, pp. 720–728, 2012.
13. H. Kajihara, Y. Hayashida, R. Murakami, K. Katahira, R. Nishimura, Y. Hamada, K. Kitani et al., Usefulness of diffusion-weighted imaging in the localization of prostate cancer, *International Journal of Radiation, Oncology and Biolocgial Physics*, vol. 74, no. 2, pp. 399–403, 2009.
14. K. K. Yu and H. Hricak, Imaging prostate cancer, *Radiology Clinics of North America*, vol. 38, no. 1, pp. 59–85, 2000.
15. A. Firjani, A. Elnakib, F. Khalifa, G. Gimmel'farb, M. A. El-Ghar, A. Elmaghraby, and A. El-Baz, A diffusion-weighted imaging based diagnostic system for early detection of prostate cancer, *Journal of Biomedical Science and Engineering*, vol. 6, no. 3, pp. 346–356, 2013.
16. S. Viswanath, B. N. Bloch, M. Rosen, J. Chappelow, R. Toth, N. Rofsky, R. Lenkinski, E. Genega, A. Kalyanpur, and A. Madabhushi, Integrating structural and functional imaging for computer assisted detection of prostate cancer on multi-protocol in vivo 3 Tesla MRI, in *Proceedings of the SPIE Conference on Medical Imaging 2009*. San Diego, CA: International Society for Optics and Photonics, February 7–12, p. 72603I, 2009.

17. G. Litjens, P. Vos, J. Barentsz, N. Karssemeijer, and H. Huisman, Automatic computer aided detection of abnormalities in multi-parametric prostate MRI, in *Proceedings of the SPIE Conference on Medical Imaging 2011*, International Society for Optics and Photonics, pp. 79 630T–79 630T, 2011.

18. P. Vos, J. Barentsz, N. Karssemeijer, and H. Huisman, Automatic computer-aided detection of prostate cancer based on multiparametric magnetic resonance image analysis, *Physical and Medical Biology*, vol. 57, no. 6, p. 1527, 2012.

19. E. Niaf, O. Rouvie're, F. Me'ge-Lechevallier, F. Bratan, and C. Lartizien, Computer-aided diagnosis of prostate cancer in the peripheral zone using multiparametric MRI, *Physical and Medical Biology*, vol. 57, no. 12, p. 3833, 2012.

20. T. Hambrock, P. C. Vos, C. A. Hulsbergen-van de Kaa, J. O. Barentsz, and H. J. Huisman, Prostate cancer: Computer-aided diagnosis with multiparametric 3-T MR imaging—Effect on observer performance, *Radiology*, vol. 266, no. 2, pp. 521–530, 2013.

21. Y. Peng, Y. Jiang, C. Yang, J. B. Brown, T. Antic, I. Sethi, C. Schmid-Tannwald, M. L. Giger, S. E. Eggener, and A. Oto, Quantitative analysis of multiparametric prostate MR images: Differentiation between prostate cancer and normal tissue and correlation with Gleason score, *Radiology*, vol. 267, no. 3, pp. 787–796, 2013.

22. V. Shah, B. Turkbey, H. Mani, Y. Pang, T. Pohida, M. J. Merino, P. A. Pinto, P. L. Choyke, and M. Bernardo, Decision support system for localizing prostate cancer based on multiparametric magnetic resonance imaging, *Medical Physics*, vol. 39, p. 4093, 2012.

23. A. Jemal, R. Siegel, E. Ward, Y. Hao, J. Xu, T. Murray, and M. J. Thun, Cancer statistics, 2008, *CA—Cancer Journal of Clinics*, vol. 58, no. 2, pp. 71–96, 2008.

24. Y. Zhu, S. Williams, and R. Zwiggelaar, A hybrid ASM approach for sparse volumetric data segmentation, *Pattern Recognition and Image Analysis*, vol. 17, no. 2, pp. 252–258, 2007.

25. R. Toth, P. Tiwari, M. Rosen, A. Kalyanpur, S. Pungavkar, and A. Madabhushi, A multimodal prostate segmentation scheme by combining spectral clustering and active shape models, in *Proceedings of the SPIE Conference on Medical Imaging 2008*, San Diego, CA, February 16–21, pp. 1–12, 2008.

26. Y. Gao, R. Sandhu, G. Fichtinger, and A. R. Tannenbaum, A coupled global registration and segmentation framework with application to magnetic resonance prostate imagery, *IEEE Transactions on Medical Imaging*, vol. 29, no. 10, pp. 1781–1794, 2010.

27. S. Ghose, A. Oliver, R. Mart'i, X. Llado', J. Freixenet, J. Mitra, J. C. Vilanova, and F. Meriaudeau, A hybrid framework of multiple active appearance models and global registration for 3D prostate segmentation in MRI, in *Proceedings of the SPIE Conference on Medical Imaging 2012*, February 4–9, p. 83140S, 2012.

28. S. Martin, J. Troccaz, and V. Daanen, Automated segmentation of the prostate in 3D MR images using a probabilistic atlas and a spatially constrained deformable model, *Medical Physics*, vol. 37, p. 1579, 2010.

29. P. D. Allen, J. Graham, D. C. Williamson, and C. E. Hutchinson, Differential segmentation of the prostate in MR images using combined 3D shape modelling and voxel classification, in *Proceedings of the 3rd IEEE International Symposium on Biomedical Imaging: (ISBI'06)*. Arlington, VA: IEEE, April 6–9, pp. 410–413, 2006.

30. X. Liu, D. Langer, M. Haider, T. Van der Kwast, A. Evans, M. Wernick, and I. Yetik, Unsupervised segmentation of the prostate using MR images based on level set with a shape prior, in *Proceedings of the Annual International Conference of the IEEE Engineering in Medicine and Biology Society (EMBC'09)*. Minneapolis, MN: IEEE, September 2–6, pp. 3613–3616, 2009.

31. X. Liu, M. A. Haider, and I. S. Yetik, Unsupervised 3D prostate segmentation based on diffusion-weighted imaging MRI using active contour models with a shape prior, *Journal of Electrical And Computing Engineering*, vol. 2011, p. 11, 2011.

32. Y. Boykov and O. Veksler, Graph cuts in vision and graphics: Theories and applications, in *Handbook of Mathematical Models in Computer Vision*. Berlin: Springer, 2006, pp. 79–96.

33. L. Grady, Random walks for image segmentation, *IEEE Transactions on Pattern Analysis and Machine Intelligence*, vol. 28, no. 11, pp. 1768–1783, 2006.

34. S. Ghose, J. Mitra, A. Oliver, R. Marti, X. Llado, J. Freixenet, J. C. Vilanova, D. Sidibé, and F. Mériaudeau, Graph cut energy minimization in a probabilistic learning framework for 3D prostate segmentation in MRI, in *Proceedings of the 21st International Conference on Pattern Recognition (ICPR'12)*. Tsukuba Science City, Japan: IEEE, November 11–15, pp. 125–128, 2012.

35. A. Firjany, A. Elnakib, A. El-Baz, G. Gimel'farb, M. El-Ghar, and A. Elmagharby, Novel stochiastic framework for accurate segmentation of prostate in dynamic contrast enhanced MRI, in *Proceedings of the First International Workshop on Prostate Cancer Imaging: Computer-Aided Diagnosis, Prognosis, and Intervention*, vol. 1, Beijing, China, September 24, pp. 123–130, 2010.

36. A. Alansary, A. Soliman, F. Khalifa, A. Elnakib, M. Mostapha, M. Nitzken, M. Casanova, and A. El-Baz, MAP-based framework for segmentation of MR brain images based on visual appearance and prior shape, *MIDAS Journal*, vol. 1, pp. 1–13, 2013.

37. F. Khalifa, M. A. El-Ghar, B. Abdollahi, H. Frieboes, T. El-Diasty, and A. El-Baz, A comprehensive non-invasive framework for automated evaluation of acute renal transplant rejection using DCE-MRI, *NMR Biomedicine*, vol. 26, no. 11, pp. 1460–1470, 2013.

38. F. Khalifa, G. M. Beache, M. A. El-Ghar, T. El-Diasty, G. Gimel'farb, M. Kong, and A. El-Baz, Dynamic contrast-enhanced MRI- based early detection of acute renal transplant rejection, *IEEE Transactions on Medical Imaging*, vol. 32, no. 10, pp. 1910–1927, 2013.

39. H. Sliman, F. Khalifa, A. Elnakib, A. Soliman, A. El-Baz, G. M. Beache, A. Elmaghraby, and G. Gimel'farb, Myocardial borders segmentation from cine MR images using bidirectional coupled parametric deformable models, *Medical Physics*, vol. 40, no. 9, pp. 1–13, 2013.

40. F. Khalifa, G. M. Beache, G. Gimel'farb, G. A. Giridharan, and A. El-Baz, Accurate automatic analysis of cardiac cine images, *IEEE Transactions on Biomedical Engineering*, vol. 59, no. 2, pp. 445–455, 2012.

41. A. Elnakib, G. M. Beache, G. Gimel'farb, and A. El-Baz, New automated Markov–Gibbs random field based framework for myocardial wall viability quantification on agent enhanced cardiac magnetic resonance images, *International Journal of Cardiovascular Imaging*, vol. 28, no. 7, pp. 1683–1698, 2012.

42. A. El-Baz, G. Gimel'farb, R. Falk, and M. A. El-Ghar, Automatic analysis of 3D low dose CT images for early diagnosis of lung cancer, *Pattern Recognition*, vol. 42, no. 6, pp. 1041–1051, 2009.

43. A. A. Farag, A. S. El-Baz, and G. Gimel'farb, Precise segmentation of multimodal images, *IEEE Transactions on Image Processing*, vol. 15, no. 4, pp. 952–968, 2006.

44. H. Sliman, F. Khalifa, A. Elnakib, A. Soliman, G. Beache, A. Elmaghraby, and A. El-Baz, A new segmentation-based tracking framework for extracting the left ventricle cavity from cine cardiac MRI, in *Proceedings of the IEEE Conference on Image Processing (ICIP'13)*. Melbourne, Australia: IEEE, September 15–18, pp. 685–689, 2013.

45. A. Elnakib, G. M. Beache, M. Nitzken, G. Gimel'farb, and A. El-Baz, A new framework for automated identification of pathological tissues in contrast enhanced cardiac magnetic resonance images, in *Proceedings of the IEEE International Symposium on Biomedical Imaging: From Nano to Macro (ISBI'11)*. Chicago, IL: IEEE, March 30–April 2, pp. 1272–1275, 2011.

46. A. El-Baz, G. Gimel'farb, R. Falk, M. A. El-Ghar, V. Kumar, and D. Heredia, A novel 3D joint Markov–Gibbs model for extracting blood vessels from PC-MRA images, in *Proceedings of the International Conference on Medical Image Computing and Computer-Assisted Intervention (MICCAI'09)*, London, UK, September 20–24, pp. 943–950, 2009.

47. A. El-Baz and G. Gimel'farb, Robust image segmentation using learned priors, in *Proceedings of the International Conference on Computer Vision (ICCV'09)*. Kyoto, Japan: IEEE, September 27–October 4, pp. 857–864, 2009.

48. A. El-Baz and G. Gimel'farb, Robust medical images segmentation using learned shape and appearance models, in *Proceedings of the International Conference on Medical Image Computing and Computer Assisted Intervention (MICCAI'09)*. London, UK: Springer, September 20–24, pp. 281–288, 2009.

49. A. El-Baz, A. Farag, and G. Gimel'farb, MGRF controlled stochastic deformable model, in *Proceedings of the Scandinavian Conference on Image Analysis (SCIA'05)*. Joensuu, Finland: Springer, June 19–22, pp. 1138–1147, 2005,.

50. A. El-Baz and A. Farag, Image segmentation using GMRF models: parameters estimation and applications, in *Proceedings of the 20th International Conference on Image Processing (ICIP'03)*, vol. 2, Barcelona, Catalonia, Spain, September 14–18, pp. 177–180, 2003.

51. A. El-Baz and G. Gimel'farb, EM based approximation of empirical distributions with linear combinations of discrete Gaussians, in *Proceedings of the International Conference on Image Processing (ICIP'07)*. San Antonio, TX: IEEE, September 16–19, pp. 373–376, 2007.

52. A. A. Farag, A. S. El-Baz, and G. Gimel'farb, Precise segmentation of multi-modal images, *IEEE Transactions on Image Processing*, vol. 15, no. 4, pp. 952–968, 2006.

53. A. El-Baz, Novel stochastic models for medical image analysis, Ph.D. dissertation, University of Louisville, Louisville, KY, 2006.

54. A. El-Baz, A. Elnakib, F. Khalifa, M. A. El-Ghar, R. Falk, and G. Gimel'farb, Precise segmentation of 3-D magnetic resonance angiography, *IEEE Transactions on Biomedical Engineering*, vol. 59, no. 7, pp. 2019–2029, 2012.

55. A. Elnakib, G. Gimel'farb, T. Inanc, and A. El-Baz, Modified Akaike information criterion for estimating the number of components in a probability mixture model, in *Proceedings of the IEEE International Conference on Image Processing (ICIP'12)*, Orlando, FL, September 30–October 3, pp. 2497–2500, 2013.

56. F. Khalifa, G. Gimel'farb, M. El-Ghar, G. Sokhadze, S. Manning, P. McClure, R. Ouseph, and A. El-Baz, A new deformable model-based segmentation approach for accurate extraction of the kidney from abdominal CT images, in *Proceedings of the IEEE International Conference on Image Processing (ICIP'11)*, Brussels, Belgium, September 11–14, pp. 3393–3396, 2011.

57. A. A. Farag, A. El-Baz, and G. Gimel'farb, Density estimation using modified expectation-maximization algorithm for a linear combination of Gaussians, in *Proceedings of the International Conference on Image Processing (ICIP'04)*, vol. 3. Singapore: IEEE, October 24–27, pp. 1871–1874, 2004.

58. A. Farag, A. El-Baz, and G. Gimel'farb, Precise image segmentation by iterative EM-based approximation of empirical grey level distributions with linear combinations of Gaussians, in *Proceedings of the IEEE Computer Vision and Pattern Recognition Workshop (CVPRW'04)*. Washington, DC: IEEE, June 27–July 2, pp. 121–129, 2004.

59. G. Gimel'farb, A. Farag, and A. El-Baz, Expectation–maximization for a linear combination of Gaussians, in *Proceedings of the International Conference on Pattern Recognition (ICPR'2004)*, Cambridge, UK, August 23–26, pp. 422–425, 2004.

60. A. A. Farag, A. El-Baz, and R. M. Mohamed, Density estimation using generalized linear model and a linear combination of Gaussians, *International Journal of Signal Processing*, vol. 1, pp. 76–79, 2005.

61. A. El-Baz, R. M. Mohamed, A. A. Farag, and G. Gimel'farb, Unsupervised segmentation of multi-modal images by a precise approximation of individual modes with linear combinations of discrete Gaussians, in *Proceedings of the IEEE Computer Society Conference on Computer Vision and Pattern Recognition-Workshops (CVPRW'05)*. San Diego, CA: IEEE, June 20–26, 2005, pp. 54–54.

62. A. El-Baz, A. A. Farag, and G. Gimel'farb, Iterative approximation of empirical grey-level distributions for precise segmentation of multimodal images, *EURASIP Journal of Applied Signal Processing*, vol. 2005, pp. 1969–1983, 2005.

63. A. Firjani, A. Elnakib, F. Khalifa, G. Gimmel'farb, M. Abo El-Ghar, J. Suri, A. Elmagharby, and A. El-Baz, A new 3D automatic segmentation framework for accurate segmentation of prostate from DCE-MRI, in *Proceedings of the IEEE International Conference on Image Processing (ICIP'11)*, Brussels, Belgium, September 11–14, 2011.

64. A. Firjani, A. Elnakib, F. Khalifa, G. Gimel'farb, M. Abo El-Ghar, J. Suri, A. Elmaghraby, and A. El-Baz, A new 3D automatic segmentation framework for accurate segmentation of

prostate from DCE-MRI, in *Proceedings of the IEEE International Symposium on Biomedical Imaging (ISBI'11)*. Chicago, IL: IEEE, March 40–April 2, pp. 1476–1479, 2011.

65. J. Shi and J. Malik, Normalized cuts and image segmentation, *IEEE Transactions on Pattern Analysis and Machine Intelligence*, vol. 22, no. 8, pp. 888–905, 2000.

66. B. L. Mark and W. Turin, *Probability, Random Processes, and Statistical Analysis*. Cambridge: Cambridge University Press Textbooks, 2011.

67. N. Makni, P. Puech, R. Lopes, A.-S. Dewalle, O. Colot, and N. Betrouni, Combining a deformable model and a probabilistic framework for an automatic 3D segmentation of prostate on MRI, *International Journal of Computer Assisted Radiology and Surgery*, vol. 4, no. 2, pp. 181–188, 2009.

68. S. Z. Li and S. Singh, *Markov Random Field Modeling in Image Analysis*, vol. 3. Berlin: Springer, 2009.

69. A. Firjani, F. Khalifa, A. Elnakib, G. Gimmel'farb, M. Abo El-Ghar, A. Elmagharby, and A. El-Baz, 3D automatic approach for precise segmentation of the prostate from diffusion-weighted magnetic resonance imaging, in *Proceedings of the IEEE International Conference on Image Processing (ICIP'11)*, Brussels, Belgium, September 11–14, 2011.

70. A. Firjani, A. Elnakib, F. Khalifa, G. Gimel'farb, M. Abo El-Ghar, A. Elmaghraby, and A. El-Baz, A new 3D automatic segmentation framework for accurate extraction of prostate from diffusion imaging, in *Proceedings of the Biomedical Sciences and Engineering Conference (BSEC'11)*, Knoxville, TN, March 15–17, pp. 1–4, 2011.

71. P. Khurd, L. Grady, K. Gajera, M. Diallo, P. Gall, M. Requardt, B. Kiefer, C. Weiss, and A. Kamen, Facilitating 3D spectroscopic imaging through automatic prostate localization in MR images using random walker segmentation initialized via boosted classifiers, in *Prostate Cancer Imaging*. Berlin: Springer, 2011, pp. 47–56.

72. S. Klein, U. A. van der Heide, I. M. Lips, M. van Vulpen, M. Staring, and J. P. Pluim, Automatic segmentation of the prostate in 3D MR images by atlas matching using localized mutual information, *Medical Physics*, vol. 35, p. 1407, 2008.

73. J. A. Dowling, J. Fripp, S. Chandra, J. P. W. Pluim, J. Lambert, J. Parker, J. Denham, P. B. Greer, and O. Salvado, Fast automatic multi-atlas segmentation of the prostate from 3D MR images, in *Prostate Cancer Imaging*. Berlin: Springer, 2011, pp. 10–21.

74. T. R. Langerak, U. A. van der Heide, A. N. Kotte, M. A. Viergever, M. van Vulpen, and J. P. Pluim, Label fusion in atlas-based segmentation using a selective and iterative method for performance level estimation (SIMPLE), *IEEE Transactions on Medical Imaging*, vol. 29, no. 12, pp. 2000–2008, 2010.

75. D. Flores-Tapia, G. Thomas, N. Venugopal, B. McCurdy, and S. Pistorius, Semiautomatic MRI prostate segmentation based on wavelet multiscale products, in *Proceedings of the 30th Annual International Conference of the IEEE Engineering in Medicine and Biology Society (EMBS'08)*. Vancouver, British Columbia, Canada: IEEE, August 20–25, pp. 3020–3023, 2008.

76. J.-C. Pesquet, H. Krim, and H. Carfantan, Time-invariant orthonormal wavelet representations, *IEEE Transactions on Signal Processing*, vol. 44, no. 8, pp. 1964–1970, 1996.

77. S. Vikal, S. Haker, C. Tempany, and G. Fichtinger, Prostate contouring in MRI guided biopsy, in *Proceedings of SPIE Medical Imaging: Image Processing*, 2009, pp. 1–11.

78. A. Madabhushi, M. D. Feldman, D. N. Metaxas, J. Tomaszeweski, and D. Chute, Automated detection of prostatic adenocarcinoma from high-resolution ex vivo MRI, *IEEE Transactions on Medical Imaging*, vol. 24, no. 12, pp. 1611–1625, 2005.

79. S. Viswanath, B. N. Bloch, E. Genega, N. Rofsky, R. Lenkinski, J. Chappelow, R. Toth, and A. Madabhushi, A comprehensive segmentation, registration, and cancer detection scheme on 3 Tesla in vivo prostate DCE-MRI, in *Proceedings of the Conference on Medical Image Computing and Computer-Assisted Intervention (MICCAI'08)*, New York, NY, September 6–10, pp. 662–669, 2008.

80. P. C. Vos, T. Hambrock, J. O. Barenstz, and H. J. Huisman, Computer-assisted analysis of peripheral zone prostate lesions using T2-weighted and dynamic contrast enhanced T1-weighted MRI, *Physical and Medical Biology*, vol. 55, no. 6, p. 1719, 2010.

81. S. Ozer, M. A. Haider, D. L. Langer, T. H. van der Kwast, A. J. Evans, M. N. Wernick, J. Trachtenberg, and I. S. Yetik, Prostate cancer localization with multispectral MRI based on relevance vector machines, in *IEEE International Symposium on Biomedical Imaging: From Nano to Macro (ISBI'2009)*. Boston, MA: IEEE, June 28–July 1, pp. 73–76, 2009.

82. A. Madabhushi, J. Shi, M. Feldman, M. Rosen, and J. Tomaszewski, Comparing ensembles of learners: Detecting prostate cancer from high-resolution MRI, in *Computer Vision Approaches to Medical Image Analysis*. Berlin: Springer, 2006, pp. 25–36.

83. R. Lopes, A. Ayache, N. Makni, P. Puech, A. Villers, S. Mordon, and N. Betrouni, Prostate cancer characterization on MR images using fractal features, *Medical Physics*, vol. 38, p. 83, 2011.

84. Y. S. Sung, H.-J. Kwon, B.-W. Park, G. Cho, C. K. Lee, K.-S. Cho, and J. K. Kim, Prostate cancer detection on dynamic contrast- enhanced MRI: Computer-aided diagnosis versus single perfusion parameter maps, *American Journal of Roentgenology*, vol. 197, no. 5, pp. 1122–1129, 2011.

85. D. Gabor, Theory of communication, *Journal of Institute of Electrical Engineering*, vol. 93, no. 26, pp. 429–441, 1946.

86. K. Engel, M. Hadwiger, J. M. Kniss, C. Rezk-Salama, and D. Weiskopf, *Real-Time Volume Graphics*. AK Peters Limited, 2006.

87. Y. Freund and R. E. Schapire, Experiments with a new boosting algorithm, in *Proceedings of the International Conference on Machine Learning (ICM9̂6)*, Bari, Italy, July 3–6, 1996, pp. 148–156.

88. P. S. Tofts, G. Brix, D. L. Buckley, J. L. Evelhoch, E. Henderson, M. V. Knopp, H. B. Larsson et al., Estimating kinetic parameters from dynamic contrast-enhanced T1-weighted MRI of a diffusable tracer: Standardized quantities and symbols, *Journal of Magnetic Resonance Imaging*, vol. 10, no. 3, pp. 223–232, 1999.

89. P. C. Vos, T. Hambrock, J. O. Barenstz, and H. J. Huisman, Automated calibration for computerized analysis of prostate lesions using pharmacokinetic magnetic resonance images, in *Proceedings of the International Conference on Medical Image Computing and Computer-Assisted Intervention (MICCAI'09)*, London, UK, September 20–24, pp. 836–843, 2009.

90. J. K. Kim, S. S. Hong, Y. J. Choi, S. H. Park, H. Ahn, C.-S. Kim, and K.-S. Cho, Wash-in rate on the basis of dynamic contrast- enhanced MRI: Usefulness for prostate cancer detection and localization, *Journal of Magnetic Resonance Imaging*, vol. 22, no. 5, pp. 639–646, 2005.

91. P. Puech, N. Betrouni, R. Viard, A. Villers, X. Leroy, and L. Lemaitre, Prostate cancer computer-assisted diagnosis software using dynamic contrast-enhanced MRI, in *Proceedings of the 29th Annual International Conference of the IEEE Engineering in Medicine and Biology Society (EMBS'07)*. Lyon, France: IEEE, August 23–26, pp. 5567–5570, 2007.

92. P. Puech, N. Betrouni, N. Makni, A.-S. Dewalle, A. Villers, and L. Lemaitre, Computer-assisted diagnosis of prostate cancer using DCE-MRI data: Design, implementation and preliminary results, *International Journal of Computed Assisted Radiology and Surgery*, vol. 4, no. 1, pp. 1–10, 2009.

93. J. Veltman, R. Mann, T. Kok, I. Obdeijn, N. Hoogerbrugge, J. Blickman, and C. Boetes, Breast tumor characteristics of BRCA1 and BRCA2 gene mutation carriers on MRI, *European Radiology*, vol. 18, no. 5, pp. 931–938, 2008.

94. I. Ocak, M. Bernardo, G. Metzger, T. Barrett, P. Pinto, P. S. Albert, and P. L. Choyke, Dynamic contrast-enhanced MRI of prostate cancer at 3 T: A study of pharmacokinetic parameters, *American Journal of Roentgenology*, vol. 189, no. 4, pp. 192–201, 2007.

95. S. T. Roweis and L. K. Saul, Nonlinear dimensionality reduction by locally linear embedding, *Science*, vol. 290, no. 5500, pp. 2323–2326, 2000.

96. M. R. Engelbrecht, H. J. Huisman, R. J. Laheij, G. J. Jager, G. J. van Leenders, C. A. Hulsbergen-Van De Kaa, J. J. de la Rosette, J. G. Blickman, and J. O. Barentsz, Discrimination of prostate cancer from normal peripheral zone and central gland tissue by using dynamic contrast-enhanced MR imaging, *Radiology*, vol. 229, no. 1, pp. 248–254, 2003.

97. J. K. Kim, S. S. Hong, Y. J. Choi, S. H. Park, H. Ahn, C.-S. Kim, and K.-S. Cho, Wash-in rate on the basis of dynamic contrast-enhanced MRI: Usefulness for prostate cancer detection and localization, *Journal of Magnetic Resonance Imaging*, vol. 22, no. 5, pp. 639–646, 2005.

98. J. J. Fu¨tterer, S. W. T. P. J. Heijmink, T. W. J. Scheenen, J. Veltman, H. J. Huisman, P. Vos, C. A. Hulsbergen-Van de Kaa, J. A. Witjes, P. F. M. Krabbe, A. Heerschap, and J. O. Barentsz, Prostate cancer localization with dynamic contrast-enhanced MR imaging and proton MR spectroscopic imaging, *Radiology*, vol. 241, no. 2, pp. 449–458, 2006.

99. O. Rouvie're, O. Valette, S. Grivolat, C. Colin-Pangaud, R. Bouvier, J. Y. Chapelon, A. Gelet, and D. Lyonnet, Recurrent prostate cancer after external beam radiotherapy: Value of contrast-enhanced dynamic MRI in localizing intraprostatic tumorcorrelation with biopsy findings, *Urology*, vol. 63, no. 5, pp. 922–927, 2004.

100. I. Ocak, M. Bernardo, G. Metzger, T. Barrett, P. Pinto, P. S. Albert, and P. L. Choyke, Dynamic contrast-enhanced MRI of prostate cancer at 3T: A study of pharmacokinetic parameters, *American Journal of Roentgenology*, vol. 189, no. 4, pp. W192–W201, 2007.

101. P. C. Vos, T. Hambrock, J. J. Fu¨tterer, C. Hulsbergen-Van De Kaa, J. Barentsz, and H. H. Huisman, Effect of calibration on computerized analysis of prostate lesions using quantitative dynamic contrast-enhanced magnetic resonance imaging, in *Proceedings of the SPIE Conference on Medical Imaging*. International Society for Optics and Photonics, 2007, pp. 65 140U–65 140U.

102. N. Otsu, A threshold selection method from gray-level histograms, *Automatica*, vol. 11, no. 285–296, pp. 23–27, 1975.

103. A. F. Frangi, W. J. Niessen, K. L. Vincken, and M. A. Viergever, Multiscale vessel enhancement filtering, in *Proceedings of the Conference on Medical Image Computing and Computer-Assisted Intervention (MICCAI'98)*. Cambridge, MA: Springer, October 11–13, pp. 130–137, 1998.

104. A. Firjani, F. Khalifa, A. Elnakib, G. Gimel'farb, M. A. El-Ghar, A. Elmaghraby, and A. El-Baz, Non-invasive image-based approach for early detection of prostate cancer, in *Developments in E-systems Engineering (DeSE'11)*. Dubai, United Arab Emirates: IEEE, December 6–8, pp. 172–177, 2011.

105. T. Tamada, T. Sone, Y. Jo, S. Toshimitsu, T. Yamashita, A. Yamamoto, D. Tanimoto, and K. Ito, Apparent diffusion coefficient values in peripheral and transition zones of the prostate: Comparison between normal and malignant prostatic tissues and correlation with histologic grade, *Journal of Magnetic Resonance Imaging*, vol. 28, no. 3, pp. 720–726, 2008.

106. L. C. Maas and P. Mukherjee, Diffusion MRI: Overview and clinical applications in neuroradiology, *Applied Radiology*, vol. 34, no. 11, p. 44, 2005.

107. A. Firjani, F. Khalifa, A. Elnakib, G. Gimel'farb, M. Abou El-Ghar, A. Elmaghraby, and A. El-Baz, A novel image-based approach for early detection of prostate cancer, in *Proceedings of the IEEE International Conference on Image Processing (ICIP'12)*, Orlando, FL, September 30–October 3, pp. 2849–2852, 2012.

108. D. Ampeliotis, A. Antonakoudi, K. Berberidis, E. Psarakis, and A. Kounoudes, A computer-aided system for the detection of prostate cancer based on magnetic resonance image analysis, in *Proceedings of the 3rd International Symposium on Communications, Control and Signal Processing (ISCCSP'08)*. St. Julians, Malta: IEEE, March 12–14, pp. 1372–1377, 2008.

109. M. A. Haider, T. H. van der Kwast, J. Tanguay, A. J. Evans, A.-T. Hashmi, G. Lockwood, and J. Trachtenberg, Combined T2-weighted and diffusion-weighted MRI for localization of prostate cancer, *American Journal of Roentgenology*, vol. 189, no. 2, pp. 323–328, 2007.

110. I. Chan, W. Wells III, R. V. Mulkern, S. Haker, J. Zhang, K. H. Zou, S. E. Maier, and C. M. Tempany, Detection of prostate cancer by integration of line-scan diffusion, T2-mapping and T2-weighted magnetic resonance imaging; a multichannel statistical classifier, *Medical Physics*, vol. 30, p. 2390, 2003.

111. X. Liu, D. L. Langer, M. A. Haider, Y. Yang, M. N. Wernick, and I. S. Yetik, Prostate cancer segmentation with simultaneous estimation of Markov random field parameters and class, *IEEE Transactions on Medical Imaging*, vol. 28, no. 6, pp. 906–915, 2009.

112. Y. Artan, M. A. Haider, D. L. Langer, T. H. van der Kwast, A. J. Evans, Y. Yang, M. N. Wernick, J. Trachtenberg, and I. S. Yetik, Prostate cancer localization with multispectral MRI using cost-sensitive support vector machines and conditional random fields, *IEEE Transactions on Image Processing*, vol. 19, no. 9, pp. 2444–2455, 2010.

113. M. E. Tipping, Sparse Bayesian learning and the relevance vector machine, *Journal of Machine Learning Research*, vol. 1, pp. 211–244, 2010.

114. S. Osher and J. A. Sethian, Fronts propagating with curvature-dependent speed: Algorithms based on Hamilton-Jacobi formulations, *Journal of Computational Physics*, vol. 79, no. 1, pp. 12–49, 1988.

115. S. Osher and R. Fedkiw, *Level Set Methods and Dynamic Implicit Surfaces*. New York: Springer-Verlag, 2006.

116. D. Shier, J. Butler, and R. Lewis, *Hole's Essentials of Human Anatomy and Physiology*. New York: McGraw-Hill, 2006.

117. P. A. Viola and W. M. Wells III, Alignment by maximization of mutual information, *International Journal of Computer Vision*, vol. 24, no. 2, pp. 137–154, 1997.

118. F. Khalifa, A. El-Baz, G. Gimel'farb, R. Ouseph, and M. El-Ghar, Shape-appearance guided level-set deformable model for image segmentation, in *Proceedings of the 20th International Conference on Pattern Recognition (ICPR'10)*, Istanbul, Turkey, August 23–26, 2010.

119. A. El-Baz, A. Soliman, P. McClure, G. Gimel'farb, M. A. El-Ghar, and R. Falk, Early assessment of malignant lung nodules based on the spatial analysis of detected lung nodules, in *Proceedings of the IEEE International Symposioum on Biomedical Imaging: From Nana to Macro (ISBI'12)*. IEEE, pp. 1463–1466, 2012.

120. J. Besag, Spatial interaction and the statistical analysis of lattice systems, *Journal of the Royal Statistical Society. Series B (Methodological)*, pp. 192–236, 1974.

121. D. D. Lee and H. S. Seung, Learning the parts of objects by non-negative matrix factorization, *Nature*, vol. 401, no. 6755, pp. 788–791, 1999.

122. F. Shahnaz, M. W. Berry, V. P. Pauca, and R. J. Plemmons, Document clustering using non-negative matrix factorization, *Information Processing Management*, vol. 42, no. 2, pp. 373–386, 2006.

123. S. Zafeiriou, A. Tefas, I. Buciu, and I. Pitas, Exploiting discriminant information in nonnegative matrix factorization with application to frontal face verification, *IEEE Transactions on Neural Networks*, vol. 17, no. 3, pp. 683–695, 2006.

124. Y. Xie, J. Ho, and B. C. Vemuri, Nonnegative factorization of diffusion tensor images and its applications, in *Information Processing Medical Imaging*. Berlin: Springer, 2011, pp. 550–561.

125. R. Sandler and M. Lindenbaum, Nonnegative matrix factorization with earth mover's distance metric for image analysis, *IEEE Transactions on Pattern Analysis*, vol. 33, no. 8, pp. 1590–1602, 2011.

126. M. W. Berry, M. Browne, A. N. Langville, V. P. Pauca, and R. J. Plemmons, Algorithms and applications for approximate nonnegative matrix factorization, *Computatational Statistics Data Analysis*, vol. 52, no. 1, pp. 155–173, 2007.

127. D. D. Lee and H. S. Seung, Algorithms for non-negative matrix factorization, in *Advances in Neural Information Processing Systems*, 2000, pp. 556–562.

128. A. Hyva¨rinen, Sparse code shrinkage: Denoising of nongaussian data by maximum likelihood estimation, *Neural Computing*, vol. 11, no. 7, pp. 1739–1768, 1999.

129. R. O. Duda, P. E. Hart, and D. G. Stork, *Pattern Classification*. New York: Wiley, 2012.

130. R. Polikar, Ensemble based systems in decision making, *IEEE Circuits Systems Magazine*, vol. 6, no. 3, pp. 21–45, 2006.

131. K. O. Babalola, B. Patenaude, P. Aljabar, J. Schnabel, D. Kennedy, W. Crum, S. Smith, T. Cootes, M. Jenkinson, and D. Rueckert, An evaluation of four automatic methods of segmenting the subcortical structures in the brain, *NeuroImage*, vol. 47, no. 4, pp. 1435–1447, 2009.

132. A. El-Baz, M. Casanova, G. Gimel'farb, M. Mott, A. Switala, E. Vanbogaert, and R. McCracken, Dyslexia diagnostics by 3D texture analysis of cerebral white matter gyrifications, in *Proceedings*

of the International Conference on Pattern Recognition (ICPR'08). Tampa, FL: IEEE, December 8–11, pp. 1–4, 2008.

133. A. El-Baz, M. Casanova, G. Gimel'farb, M. Mott, and A. Switala, An MRI-based diagnostic framework for early diagnosis of dyslexia, *International Journal of Computer Assisted Radiological Surgery*, vol. 3, no. 3–4, pp. 181–189, 2008.

134. A. Elnakib, M. F. Casanova, G. Gimel'farb, A. E. Switala, and A. El-Baz, Dyslexia diagnostics by 3-D shape analysis of the corpus callosum, *IEEE Transactions on Information Technology in Biomedicine*, vol. 16, no. 4, pp. 700–708, 2012.

135. E. L. Williams, A. El-Baz, M. Nitzken, A. E. Switala, and M. F. Casanova, Spherical harmonic analysis of cortical complexity in autism and dyslexia, *Translations in Neuroscience*, vol. 3, no. 1, pp. 36–40, 2012.

136. M. Nitzken, M. F. Casanova, G. Gimel'farb, A. Elnakib, F. Khalifa, A. Switala, and A. El-Baz, 3D shape analysis of the brain cortex with application to dyslexia, in *Proceedings of the IEEE International Conference on Image Processing (ICIP'11)*, 2011, pp. 2657–2660.

137. M. F. Casanova, A. El-Baz, A. Elnakib, J. Giedd, J. M. Rumsey, E. L. Williams, and A. E. Switala, Corpus callosum shape analysis with application to dyslexia, *Translations on Neuroscience*, vol. 1, no. 2, pp. 124–130, 2010.

138. A. Elnakib, A. El-Baz, M. F. Casanova, G. Gimel'farb, and A. E. Switala, Image-based detection of corpus callosum variability for more accurate discrimination between dyslexic and normal brains, in *Proceedings of the IEEE International Symposium on Biomedical Imaging: From Nano to Macro, (ISBI'10)*, pp. 109–112, 2010.

139. A. Elnakib, A. El-Baz, M. F. Casanova, and A. E. Switala, Dyslexia diagnostics by centerline-based shape analysis of the corpus callosum, in *Proceedings of the International Conference on Pattern Recognition (ICPR'10)*, pp. 261–264, 2010.

140. A. El-Baz, M. Casanova, G. Gimel'farb, M. Mott, A. Switala, E. Vanbogaert, and R. McCracken, Dyslexia diagnostics by 3D texture analysis of cerebral white matter gyrifications, in *Proceedings of the International Conference on Pattern Recognition (ICPR'08)*, pp. 1–4, 2008.

141. A. El-Baz, M. F. Casanova, G. Gimelfarb, M. Mott, and A. E. Switala, Autism diagnostics by 3D texture analysis of cerebral white matter gyrifications, in *Proceedings of the International Conference on Medical Image Computing and Computer-Assisted Intervention (MICCAI'07)*, Brisbane, Australia, October 29–November 2, pp. 882–890, 2007.

142. A. El-Baz, A. Elnakib, M. F. Casanova, G. Gimelfarb, A. E. Switala, D. Jordan, and S. Rainey, Accurate automated detection of autism related corpus callosum abnormalities, *Journal of Medical Systems*, vol. 35, no. 5, pp. 929–939, 2011.

143. M. Nitzken, M. F. Casanova, F. Khalifa, G. Sokhadze, and A. El-Baz, Shape-based detection of cortex variability for more accurate discrimination between autistic and normal brains, in *Handbook of Multi-Modality State-of-the-Art Medical Image Segmentation and Registration Methodologies*, A. El-Baz, R. Acharya, A. Laine, and J. Suri, Eds. Berlin: Springer, 2011, ch. 7, pp. 161–185.

144. A. Elnakib, M. F. Casanova, G. Gimel'farb, A. E. Switala, and A. El-Baz, Autism diagnostics by centerline-based shape analysis of the corpus callosum, in *Proceedings of the IEEE International Symposium on Biomedical Imaging: From Nano to Macro, (ISBI'11)*, 2011, pp. 1843–1846.

145. A. El-Baz, A. Elnakib, M. F. Casanova, G. Gimel'farb, A. E. Switala, D. Jordan, and S. Rainey, Accurate automated detection of autism related corpus callosum abnormalities, *Journal of Medical Systems*, vol. 35, no. 5, pp. 929–939, 2011.

146. M. F. Casanova, A. El-Baz, A. Elnakib, A. E. Switala, E. L. Williams, D. L. Williams, N. J. Minshew, and T. E. Conturo, Quantitative analysis of the shape of the corpus callosum in patients with autism and comparison individuals, *Autism*, vol. 15, no. 2, pp. 223–238, 2011.

147. M. Nitzken, M. F. Casanova, G. Gimel'farb, F. Khalifa, A. Elnakib, A. E. Switala, and A. El-Baz, 3D shape analysis of the brain cortex with application to autism, in *Proceedings of the IEEE International Symposium on Biomedical Imaging: From Nano to Macro, (ISBI'11)*, pp. 1847–1850, 2011.

148. M. F. Casanova, B. Dombroski, and A. E. Switala, *Imaging and the Corpus Callosum in Patients with Autism*. Berlin: Springer, 2014.

149. M. F. Casanova, A. S. El-Baz, and J. S. Suri, *Imaging the Brain in Autism*. Berlin: Springer, 2013.

150. B. Dombroski, M. Nitzken, A. Elnakib, F. Khalifa, A. El-Baz, and M. F. Casanova, Cortical surface complexity in a population-based normative sample, *Translations on Neuroscience*, vol. 5, no. 1, pp. 1–8, 2014.

151. M. F. Casanova, A. El-Baz, S. S. Kamat, B. A. Dombroski, F. Khalifa, A. Elnakib, A. Soliman, A. Allison-McNutt, and A. E. Switala, Focal cortical dysplasias in autism spectrum disorders, *Acta Neuropathologica Communications*, vol. 1, no. 1, p. 67, 2013.

152. A. Elnakib, M. F. Casanova, G. Gimel'farb, and A. El-Baz, Autism diagnostics by 3D shape analysis of the corpus callosum, in *Machine Learning in Computer-aided Diagnosis: Medical Imaging Intelligence and Analysis*, K. Suzuki, Ed. Berlin: IGI Global, 2012, ch. 15, pp. 315–335.

153. M. Mostapha, F. Khalifa, A. Alansary, A. Soliman, J. Suri, and A. El-Baz, Computer-aided diagnosis systems for acute renal transplant rejection: Challenges and methodologies, in *Abdomen and Thoracic Imaging*, A. El-Baz, L. Saba, and J. Suri, Eds. Berlin: Springer, 2014, pp. 1–35.

154. S. E. Yuksel, A. El-Baz, A. A. Farag, M. El-Ghar, T. Eldiasty, and M. A. Ghoneim, A kidney segmentation framework for dynamic contrast enhanced magnetic resonance imaging, *Journal of Vibrational Control*, vol. 13, no. 9–10, pp. 1505–1516, 2007.

155. A. Rudra, A. Chowdhury, A. Elnakib, F. Khalifa, A. Soliman, G. M. Beache, and A. El-Baz, Kidney segmentation using graph cuts and pixel connectivity, *Pattern Recognition Letters*, vol. 34, no. 13, pp. 1470–1475, 2013.

156. F. Khalifa, A. Elnakib, G. M. Beache, G. Gimel'farb, M. A. El-Ghar, G. Sokhadze, S. Manning, P. McClure, and A. El-Baz, 3D kidney segmentation from CT images using a level set approach guided by a novel stochastic speed function, in *Proceedings of the Medical Image Computing and Computer-Assisted Intervention (MICCAI'11)*, Toronto, Canada, September 18–22, pp. 587–594, 2011.

157. F. Khalifa, A. El-Baz, G. Gimel'farb, and M. Abo El-Ghar, Non-invasive image-based approach for early detection of acute renal rejection, in *Proceedings of the Medical Image Computing and Computer-Assisted Intervention (MICCAI'10)*, pp. 10–18, 2010.

158. F. Khalifa, A. El-Baz, G. Gimel'farb, R. Ouseph, and M. A. El-Ghar, Shape-appearance guided level-set deformable model for image segmentation, in *Proceedings of the International Conference on Pattern Recognition (ICPR'10)*, 2010, pp. 4581–4584.

159. A. El-Baz and G. Gimel'farb, Robust medical images segmentation using learned shape and appearance models, in *Proceedings of the International Conference on Medical Image Computing and Computer-Assisted Intervention (MICCAI'09)*. London, UK: Springer, September 20–24, pp. 281–288, 2009.

160. A. El-Baz, G. Gimel'farb, and M. Abo El-Ghar, A novel image analysis approach for accurate identification of acute renal rejection, in *Proceedings of the IEEE International Conference on Image Processing (ICIP'08)*, San Diego, CA, October 12–15, pp. 1812–1815, 2008.

161. A. El-Baz, G. Gimel'farb, and M. A. El-Ghar, Image analysis approach for identification of renal transplant rejection, in *Proceedings of the IEEE International Conference on Pattern Recognition (ICPR'08)*, San Diego, CA, October 12–15, pp. 1–4, 2008.

162. A. El-Baz and G. Gimel'farb, Image segmentation with a parametric deformable model using shape and appearance priors, in *Proceedings of the IEEE International Conference on Computer Vision and Pattern Recognition (CVPR'08)*, Anchorage, AK, June 24–26, pp. 1–8, 2008.

163. A. El-Baz, A. A. Farag, S. E. Yuksel, M. E. A. El-Ghar, T. A. Eldiasty, and M. A. Ghoneim, Application of deformable models for the detection of acute renal rejection, in *Deformable Models*, A. A. Farag and J. S. Suri, Eds., 2007, vol. 1, ch. 10, pp. 293–333.

164. A. El-Baz, G. Gimel'farb, and M. Abou El-Ghar, New motion correction models for automatic identification of renal transplant rejection, in *Proceedings of the Medical Image Computing and Computer-Assisted Intervention (MICCAI'07)*, Brisbane, Australia, October 29–November 2, pp. 235–243, 2007.

165. A. M. Ali, A. A. Farag, and A. El-Baz, Graph cuts framework for kidney segmentation with prior shape constraints, in *Proceedings of the Medical Image Computing and Computer-Assisted Intervention (MICCAI'07)*, vol. 1, Brisbane, Australia, October 29–November 2, pp. 384–392, 2007.

166. A. El-Baz, A. Farag, R. Fahmi, S. Yuksel, W. Miller, M. Abou El-Ghar, T. El-Diasty, and M. Ghoneim, A new CAD system for the evaluation of kidney diseases using DCE-MRI, in *Proceedings of the Medical Image Computing and Computer-Assisted Intervention (MICCAI'08)*, New York, NY, September 6–10, pp. 446–453, 2006.

167. A. El-Baz, A. Farag, R. Fahmi, S. Yuksel, M. Abo El-Ghar, and T. Eldiasty, Image analysis of renal DCE MRI for the detection of acute renal rejection, in *Proceedings of the IEEE International Conference on Pattern Recognition (ICPR'06)*, Arlington, VA, April 6–9, pp. 822–825, 2006.

168. A. Farag, A. El-Baz, S. Yuksel, M. Abou El-Ghar, and T. Eldiasty, A framework for the detection of acute rejection with dynamic contrast enhanced magnetic resonance imaging, in *Proceedings of the IEEE International Symposium on Biomedical Imaging: From Nano to Macro (ISBI'06)*, Arlington, VA, April 6–9, pp. 418–421, 2006.

169. S. E. Yuksel, A. El-Baz, and A. A. Farag, A kidney segmentation framework for dynamic contrast enhanced magnetic resonance imaging, in *Proceedings of the International Symposium on Mathematical Methods in Engineering (MME'06)*, pp. 55–64, 2006.

170. S. E. Yuksel, A. El-Baz, A. A. Farag, M. E. Abo El-Ghar, T. A. Eldiasty, and M. A. Ghoneim, Automatic detection of renal rejection after kidney transplantation, in *International Congress Series*, vol. 1281, pp. 773–778, 2005.

171. A. El-Baz, A. A. Farag, R. Falk, and R. La Rocca, Automatic identification of lung abnormalities in chest spiral CT scans, in *Proceedings of the IEEE International Conference on Acoustic, Speech, and Signal Processing (ICASSP'03)*, vol. 2, Hong Kong, Hong Kong, April 6–10, pp. 261–264, 2003.

172. A. El-Baz, A. A. Farag, R. Falk, and R. L. Rocca, A unified approach for detection, visualization, and identification of lung abnormalities in chest spiral CT scans, in *International Congress Series*, vol. 1256, pp. 998–1004, 2003.

173. A. El-Baz, A. A. Farag, R. Falk, and R. La Rocca, Detection, visualization and identification of lung abnormalities in chest spiral CT scan: Phase-I, in *Proceedings of the International Conference on Biomedical Engineering*, pp. 38–42, 2002.

174. A. A. Farag, A. El-Baz, G. Gimel'farb, and R. Falk, Detection and recognition of lung abnormalities using deformable templates, in *Proceedings of the International Conference on Pattern Recognition (ICPR'04)*, vol. 3, Cambridge, UK, August 23–26, pp. 738–741, 2004.

175. A. A. Farag, A. El-Baz, G. G. Gimelfarb, R. Falk, and S. G. Hushek, Automatic detection and recognition of lung abnormalities in helical CT images using deformable templates, in *Proceedings of the Medical Image Computing and Computer-Assisted Intervention (MICCAI'04)*, Sint-Malo, France, September 26–29, pp. 856–864, 2004.

176. A. El-Baz, S. E. Yuksel, S. Elshazly, and A. A. Farag, Non-rigid registration techniques for automatic follow-up of lung nodules, in *Proceedings of the Conference on Computer Assisted Radiology and Surgery (CARS'05)*, vol. 1281, Berlin, Germany, June 22–25, pp. 1115–1120, 2005.

177. A. A. Farag, A. El-Baz, G. Gimelfarb, M. A. El-Ghar, and T. Eldiasty, Quantitative nodule detection in low dose chest CT scans: new template modeling and evaluation for cad system design, in *Proceedings of the Medical Image Computing and Computer-Assisted Intervention (MICCAI'05)*, Palm Springs, CA, October 26–29, pp. 720–728, 2005.

178. A. El-Baz, A. Farag, G. Gimel'farb, R. Falk, M. A. El-Ghar, and T. Eldiasty, A framework for automatic segmentation of lung nodules from low dose chest CT scans, in *Proceedings of the International Conference on Pattern Recognition (ICPR'06)*, pp. 611–614, 2006.

179. A. M. Ali, A. S. El-Baz, and A. A. Farag, A novel framework for accurate lung segmentation using graph cuts, in *Proceedings of the IEEE International Symposium on Biomedical Imaging: From Nano to Macro (ISBI'07)*, Washington, DC, April 12–15, pp. 908–911, 2007.

180. A. El-Baz, G. Gimel'farb, R. Falk, and M. A. El-Ghar, A novel approach for automatic follow-up of detected lung nodules, in *Proceedings of the IEEE International Conference on Image Processing (ICIP'07)*, vol. 5, San Antonio, TX, September 16–19, pp. 501–504, 2007.

181. A. A. Farag, A. El-Baz, G. Gimelfarb, R. Falk, M. A. El-Ghar, T. Eldiasty, and S. Elshazly, Appearance models for robust segmentation of pulmonary nodules in 3D LDCT chest images, in *Proceedings of the International Conference on Medical Image Computing and Computer-Assisted Intervention (MICCAI'06)*, Copenhagen, Denmark, October 1–6, pp. 662–670, 2006.

182. A. M. Ali and A. A. Farag, Automatic lung segmentation of volumetric low-dose CT scans using graph cuts, in *Advances in Visual Computing*, pp. 258–267, 2008.

183. A. El-Baz, G. L. Gimel'farb, R. Falk, M. Abou El-Ghar, T. Holland, and T. Shaffer, A new stochastic framework for accurate lung segmentation, in *Proceedings of Medical Image Computing Computer-Assisted Interviews (MICCAI'08)*, 2008, pp. 322–330.

184. A. El-Baz, G. L. Gimel'farb, R. Falk, D. Heredis, and M. Abou El-Ghar, A novel approach for accurate estimation of the growth rate of the detected lung nodules, in *Proceedings of the International Workshop Pulmonary Image Analysis*, pp. 33–42, 2008.

185. A. El-Baz, G. L. Gimel'farb, R. Falk, T. Holland, and T. Shaffer, A framework for unsupervised segmentation of lung tissues from low dose computed tomography images. in *Proceedings of the British Machine Vision Conference (BMVC'08)*, M. Everingham, C. J. Needham, and R. Fraile, Eds. Leeds, UK: British Machine Vision Association, September 1–4, 2008.

186. A. El-Baz, G. Gimel'farb, R. Falk, T. Holland, and T. Shaffer, A new stochastic framework for accurate lung segmentation, in *Proceedings of the International Conference on Medical Image Computing and Computer-Assisted Intervention (MICCAI'08)*, New York, NY, September 6–10, 2008.

187. A. El-Baz, G. Gimel'farb, R. Falk, M. A. El-Ghar, and H. Refaie, Promising results for early diagnosis of lung cancer, in *Proceedings of the IEEE International Symposium on Biomedical Imaging: From Nano to Macro (ISBI'08)*, Paris, France, May 14–17, pp. 1151–1154, 2008.

188. A. El-Baz, G. Gimel'farb, R. Falk, and M. Abo El-Ghar, Automatic analysis of 3D low dose CT images for early diagnosis of lung cancer, *Pattern Recognition*, vol. 42, no. 6, pp. 1041–1051, 2009.

189. A. El-Baz, G. Gimel'farb, R. Falk, M. A. El-Ghar, S. Rainey, D. Heredia, and T. Shaffer, Toward early diagnosis of lung cancer, in *Proceedings of the International Conference on Medical Image Computing and Computer-Assisted Intervention (MICCAI'09)*, London, UK, September 20–24, pp. 682–689, 2009.

190. A. El-Baz, G. Gimel'farb, R. Falk, and M. El-Ghar, Appearance analysis for diagnosing malignant lung nodules, in *Proceedings of the IEEE International Symposium on Biomedical Imaging: From Nano to Macro (ISBI'10)*, Rotterdam, The Netherlands, April 14–17, pp. 193–196, 2010.

191. A. El-Baz, P. Sethu, G. Gimel'farb, F. Khalifa, A. Elnakib, R. Falk, and M. A. El-Ghar, Elastic phantoms generated by microfluidics technology: Validation of an imaged-based approach for accurate measurement of the growth rate of lung nodules, *Biotechnology Journal*, vol. 6, no. 2, pp. 195–203, 2011.

192. A. El-Baz, G. Gimel'farb, R. Falk, M. A. El-Ghar, and J. Suri, Appearance analysis for the early assessment of detected lung nodules, in *Lung Imaging and Computer Aided Diagnosis*, 2011, ch. 17, pp. 395–404.

193. A. El-Baz, P. Sethu, G. Gimelfarb, F. Khalifa, A. Elnakib, R. Falk, M. A. El-Ghar, and J. Suri, Validation of a new imaged-based approach for the accurate estimating of the growth rate of detected lung nodules using real computed tomography images and elastic phantoms generated by state-of-theart microfluidics technology, in *Lung Imaging and Computer Aided Diagnosis*, 2011, ch. 18, pp. 405–420.

194. A. El-Baz, M. Nitzken, G. Gimelfarb, E. Van Bogaert, R. Falk, M. A. El-Ghar, and J. Suri, Three-dimensional shape analysis using spherical harmonics for early assessment of detected lung nodules, in *Lung Imaging and Computer Aided Diagnosis*, 2011, ch. 19, pp. 421–438.

195. A. El-Baz, M. Nitzken, F. Khalifa, A. Elnakib, G. Gimel'farb, R. Falk, and M. A. El-Ghar, 3D shape analysis for early diagnosis of malignant lung nodules, in *Proceedings of the Conference on Information Processing in Medical Imaging, (IPMI'11)*, pp. 772–783, 2011.

196. B. Abdollahi, A. Soliman, A. Civelek, X.-F. Li, G. Gimelfarb, and A. El-Baz, A novel 3D joint MGRF framework for precise lung segmentation, in *Machine Learning in Medical Imaging*, pp. 86–93, 2012.
197. A. El-Baz, F. Khalifa, A. Elnakib, M. Nitzken, A. Soliman, P. McClure, M. A. El-Ghar, and G. Gimelfarb, A novel approach for global lung registration using 3D Markov-Gibbs appearance model, in *Proceedings of the International Conference on Medical Image Computing and Computer-Assisted Intervention (MICCAI'12)*, Nice, France, October 1–5, pp. 114–121, 2012,
198. A. El-Baz, G. Gimel'farb, M. Abou El-Ghar, and R. Falk, Appearance-based diagnostic system for early assessment of malignant lung nodules, in *Proceedings of the IEEE International Conference on Image Processing (ICIP'12)*, Orlando, FL, September 30–October 3, pp. 533–536, 2012.
199. A. El-Baz, A. Elnakib, M. Abou El-Ghar, G. Gimel'farb, R. Falk, and A. Farag, Automatic detection of 2D and 3D lung nodules in chest spiral CT scans, *International Journal of Biomedical Imaging*, vol. 2013, 2013.
200. A. Elnakib, G. Gimelfarb, J. S. Suri, and A. El-Baz, Medical image segmentation: A brief survey, in *Multi Modality State-of-the-Art Medical Image Segmentation and Registration Methodologies*. Berlin: Springer, 2011, pp. 1–39.

chapter fifteen

Distance regularized level sets for segmentation of the left and right ventricles

Yu Liu, Shaoxiang Zhang, Xiaoping Yang, Jia Wu, and Chunming Li

Contents

Abstract

In this chapter, we present a novel active contour method, called the distance regularized two-layer level set (DR2LS) algorithm to automatically segment both the left and right ventricles. The DR2LS approach fuses the strengths from two of our previous works, including the region-scalable fitting (RSF) model in Li et al. [1] and the distance regularized level set evolution (DRLSE) method in Li et al. [2], both proposed by Li et al. We first review the frameworks of the RSF and DRLSE models, and then we describe how to combine them efficiently into DR2LS model and the application of this combined model toward the left and right ventricle segmentation. In the combined level set algorithm, named DR2LS, we use the 0-level and k-level contours of a level set function to mathematically represent the endocardial and epicardial surfaces of both ventricles. In order to combine the strengths from our previous works, we update the formulate of level set accordingly, with the data term from the RSF model adopted for the detection of endocardium and epicardium, and the distance regularization term in the DRLSE framework to regularize the distance between the 0-level and k-level contours, and a commonly used arc-length term to regularize the 0-level and k-level contours. Lastly, we provide some preliminary segmentation results of the left and right ventricles by initializing the boundaries with the standard edge-based DRLSE model and then implementing the DR2LS model to extract both endocardium and epicardium. Experimental results have demonstrated the effectiveness of the proposed two-step level set approach to segment cardiac left and right ventricles simultaneously.

15.1   Introduction

Active contour models have been widely implemented to segment different biological structures from medical images [3–6]. Several desirable advantages exist for active contour models over other classical image segmentation methods, such as thresholding, edge detection, and region grow. First, active contour models have capable of achieving subpixel accuracy of object boundaries. Second, these models can be easily formulated in a principled energy minimization framework and facilitate incorporation of various prior knowledge, such as shape or intensity distribution, for robust image segmentation [7,8]. Third, active contour models can provide smooth and closed contours as segmentation outcomes, which are essential for segmenting most of the biological structures and can be readily used for further applications, such as shape analysis and recognition [9–11].

Existing active contour models can be mainly categorized into two groups: edge-based models [5,6,12–17] and region-based models [3,18–22]. Edge-based models depend on local edge information to draw the active contour toward the object boundaries. In contrast, region-based models target to detect each region of interest via a certain region descriptor to guide the motion of the active contour. However, popular region-based active contour models [3,18–20] are very likely to rely on intensity homogeneity within the interested regions for further segmentation. In fact, intensity distribution is often inhomogeneity within real medical images from different modalities. This inhomogeneity is usually due to artifacts introduced by the object being imaged or inevitable technical limitations. In particular, the inhomogeneity phenomenon in magnetic resonance (MR) images arises from the nonuniformly distributed magnetic fields produced by variations in object susceptibility as well as by radio-frequency coils. Segmentation of such MR images usually requires an intensity inhomogeneity correction as a preprocessing step [23].

In this chapter, we briefly review some of our previous works and discuss how they help to support the whole area [1,2,24–27]. In an early study [1], we proposed a region-based active contour model in a variational level set formulation. First, we defined a region-scalable fitting (RSF) energy functional in terms of a contour as well as two fitting functions that locally estimate the image intensities on the both sides of the predefined contour. Additionally, the optimum fitting functions are proven to be the averaged local intensities on both sides of the contour, and the region-scalability of the RSF energy is related to the kernel function of a scale parameter, which allows the use of intensity information in regions at a controllable scale, ranging from small neighborhoods to the entire image domain. Then, this RSF energy functional is assembled into a variational level set formulation by a level set regularization term. In the following curve evolution aiming at minimizing the related energy functional, intensity information in local areas at a certain scale is applied to calculate the two fitting functions and, thus, guide the motion of the contour toward the object boundaries. As a result, the proposed model can be used to segment images with intensity inhomogeneity. However, the practical implementation of this proposed algorithm have been plagued with the irregularities of the RSF that are developed during the level set evolution, which produced numerical errors and eventually destroy the stability of the level set evolution. To defeat this challenge, a numerical remedy, commonly known as reinitialization [28,29], was introduced to restore the regularity of the RSF and maintain a stable level set evolution. In general, the whole idea of reinitialization is based on periodically stopping the evolution and reshaping the degraded RSF as a signed distance function [29,30]. However, the practice of reinitialization not only raises severe questions, like when and how it should be executed, but also affects numerical accuracy in an undesirable way. Therefore, in a later study [2], we proposed a revised variational level set formulation in which the regularity of the level set function is intrinsically conserved during the level set evolution. The level set evolution is obtained as the gradient flow that minimizes an energy functional with a distance regularization term and an external energy that moves the motion of the zero level set toward desired locations. The distance regularization term is defined with a potential function such that the derived level set evolution has a distinctive forward-and-backward (FAB) diffusion effect, which is capable of preserving a wanted shape of the level set function, particularly a signed distance profile near the zero level set. This yields another type of level set evolution known as distance regularized level set evolution (DRLSE).

Segmentation of the left ventricle (LV) and the right ventricle (RV) is becoming increasingly important for noninvasively assessing cardiac functions, which is especially useful in diagnosing and treating various cardiovascular disease [31–38]. Recently, cine magnetic resonance imaging (cine MRI) has been proven to be a both precise and informative modality for quantitative evaluation of biventricular function [18,32,39–47]. The clinical measurements include ventricular volume, mass, and cavity ejection fraction (EF), which provide fundamental and significant characteristics of the heart function, can be accurately derived from the segmentation results of both endocardial and epicardial boundaries via various segmentation techniques [31,32]. Even though a lot of methods have been proposed to segment the cardiac structure, primarily focused on LV [48–56], the LV and RV automated segmentation is still an open challenge because of the poor image contrast across the desired ventricle boundaries. In order to segment the inner and outer surfaces of both ventricles from cine MRI, we propose a novel two-layer level set approach, named distance regularized two-layer level set (DR2LS), which fuses the strengths from two of our previous works, including the distance regularized level set evolution (DRLSE) method in Li et al. [2] and the region-scalable fitting (RSF) model in Li et al. [1]. In this new method, endocardial and epicardial surfaces are mathematically represented by two specified level contours of a level set function. Biventricular segmentation is expressed as an optimization problem of the level set function such that both level set contours best capture the biological structures of epicardium and endocardium. A distance regularization (DR) constraint term is presented to maintain the smoothly varying distance between the level contours that represent the inner and outer surfaces. As shown later in the result section, this DR constraint leads to a desirable interaction between the level contours, which contributes to maintaining the anatomical geometry of the endocardial and epicardial surfaces. The negative influence of intensity inhomogeneities on image segmentation are solved by using a data term derived from a local intensity clustering property, which can robustly segment the desired ventricular surfaces even with the presence of intensity inhomogeneities [1].

The chapter is further structured as follows: Section 15.2 outlines two existing level set algorithms, Section 15.3 describes the details of DR2LS algorithm, Section 15.4 proposes a two-step approach for segmentation of left and right ventricles, and Section 15.5 presents the implementation details as well as segmentation results, which is followed by the concluding remarks in Section 15.6.

15.2   Review of two level set methods

In this section, we first review two level set formulations proposed by Li et al., known as DRLSE model [2] and RSF model [1], which will be used in our DR2LS model for cardiac left and right ventricle segmentation in Section 15.3.

15.2.1   Distance regularized level set evolution (DRLSE) model

Let I be an image on a domain Ω, we define an edge indicator function g by

$$g \triangleq \frac{1}{1 + |\nabla G_\sigma * I|^2} \tag{15.1}$$

where G_δ is a Gaussian kernel with a standard deviation δ. The convolution in Equation 15.1 is used to smooth the image to reduce the noise. This function g usually takes smaller values at object boundaries than at other locations.

For a level set function (LSF) $\phi : \Omega \to R$, we define an energy functional $\mathcal{E}(\phi)$ by

$$\mathcal{E}(\phi) = \mu \mathcal{R}_p(\phi) + \lambda \mathcal{L}_g(\phi) + \alpha \mathcal{A}_g(\phi) \tag{15.2}$$

where $\mu > 0$, $\lambda > 0$ and $\alpha \in R$ are the coefficients of the energy functionals $\mathcal{R}_p(\phi)$, $\mathcal{L}_g(\phi)$, and $\mathcal{A}_g(\phi)$, which are defined by

$$\mathcal{R}_p(\phi) \triangleq \int_\Omega p(|\nabla \phi|) \, d\mathbf{x} \tag{15.3}$$

$$\mathcal{L}_g(\phi) \triangleq \int_\Omega g \delta(\phi) |\nabla \phi| \, d\mathbf{x} \tag{15.4}$$

and

$$\mathcal{A}_g(\phi) \triangleq \int_\Omega g H(-\phi) \, d\mathbf{x} \tag{15.5}$$

where p is a potential function $p : [0, \infty) \to R$, and H, δ are the the Heaviside function and Dirac delta function, respectively. In practice, the Heaviside function H is approximated by the following smooth function H_ϵ defined as

$$H_\epsilon(y) = \begin{cases} \frac{1}{2}\left[1 + \frac{y}{\epsilon} + \frac{1}{\pi}\sin\left(\frac{\pi y}{\epsilon}\right)\right], & \text{if } |x| \leq \epsilon \\ 1, & \text{if } x > \epsilon \\ 0, & \text{if } x < -\epsilon \end{cases} \tag{15.6}$$

and δ_ϵ is the derivative of H_ϵ as

$$\delta_\epsilon(y) = \begin{cases} \frac{1}{2\epsilon}\left[1 + \cos\left(\frac{\pi y}{\epsilon}\right)\right], & \text{if } |x| \leq \epsilon \\ 0, & \text{if } |x| > \epsilon. \end{cases} \tag{15.7}$$

A naive choice of the potential function is $p(s) = s^2$ for the regularization term $\mathcal{R}_p$, which forces $|\nabla\phi|$ to be zero. Such a level set regularization term has a strong smoothing effect, but it tends to flatten the LSF and finally make the zero level contour disappear. In fact, the purpose of imposing the level set regularization term is not only to smooth the LSF ϕ, but also to maintain the signed distance property $|\nabla\phi| = 1$, at least in a vicinity of the zero level set, in order to ensure accurate computation for curve evolution. This goal can be achieved by using a potential function $p(s)$ with a minimum point $s = 1$, such that the level set regularization term $\mathcal{R}_p(\phi)$ is minimized when $|\nabla\phi| = 1$. Therefore, the potential function $p(s)$ should have a minimum point at $s = 1$ (it may have other minimum points). The corresponding level set regularization term $\mathcal{R}_p(\phi)$ is referred to as a distance regularization term for its role of maintaining the signed distance property of the LSF. A simple and straightforward definition of the potential p for distance regularization is

$$p = p_1(s) \triangleq \frac{1}{2}(s - 1)^2 \tag{15.8}$$

which has $s = 1$ as the unique minimum point. With this potential $p = p_1(s)$, the level set regularization term $\mathcal{R}_p(\phi)$ can be explicitly expressed as

$$\mathcal{P}(\phi) = \frac{1}{2}\int_\Omega (|\nabla\phi| - 1)^2 \, d\mathbf{x} \tag{15.9}$$

which characterizes the deviation of ϕ from a signed distance function.

A preferable potential function p for the distance regularization term $\mathcal{R}_p$ is a double-well potential. Here, we provide a specific construction of the double-well potential $p_2(s)$ as

$$p_2(s) = \begin{cases} \frac{1}{(2\pi)^2}(1 - \cos(2\pi s)), & \text{if } s \leq 1 \\ \frac{1}{2}(s - 1)^2, & \text{if } s \geq 1. \end{cases} \tag{15.10}$$

This potential $p_2(s)$ has two minimum points at $s = 0$ and $s = 1$. It is easy to verify that p_2 is twice differentiable in $[0, \infty)$, with the first and second derivatives given by

$$p_2'(s) = \begin{cases} \dfrac{1}{2\pi} \sin(2\pi s), & \text{if } s \leq 1 \\ s - 1, & \text{if } s \geq 1 \end{cases} \tag{15.11}$$

and

$$p_2''(s) = \begin{cases} \cos(2\pi s), & \text{if } s \leq 1 \\ 1, & \text{if } s \geq 1. \end{cases} \tag{15.12}$$

It is easy to verify that the function $d_p(s) = p_2'(s)/s$ satisfies

$$|d_p(s)| < 1, \quad \text{for all } s \in (0, \infty) \tag{15.13}$$

and

$$\lim_{s \to 0} d_p(s) = \lim_{s \to \infty} d_p(s) = 1. \tag{15.14}$$

Therefore, we have

$$|\mu d_p(|\nabla \phi|)| \leq \mu \tag{15.15}$$

which verifies the boundedness of the diffusion rate for the potential $p = p_2$.

The sign of the function $d_p(s)$ for $p = p_2(s)$ indicates the property of the FAB diffusion in the following three cases: (1) for $|\nabla \phi| > 1$, the diffusion rate $\mu d_p(|\nabla \phi|)$ is positive, and the diffusion is forward, which decreases $|\nabla \phi|$; (2) for $(1/2) < |\nabla \phi| < 1$, the diffusion rate $\mu d_p(|\nabla \phi|)$ is negative, and the diffusion becomes backward, which increases $|\nabla \phi|$; (3) for $|\nabla \phi| < (1/2)$, the diffusion rate $\mu d_p(|\nabla \phi|)$ is positive, and diffusion is forward, which further decrease $|\nabla \phi|$ down to zero. The key differences between the FAB diffusions with potentials p_1 and p_2 are the boundedness of the corresponding diffusion rate and the diffusion behavior for the case $|\nabla \phi| < (1/2)$, as can be seen from the former descriptions for both cases.

With the Dirac delta function δ, the energy $\mathcal{L}_g(\phi)$ computes the line integral of the function g along the zero level contour of ϕ. By means of parameterizing the zero level set of ϕ as a contour $C : [0, 1] \to \Omega$, the energy $\mathcal{L}_g(\phi)$ can be expressed as a line integral $\int_0^1 g(C(s))|C'(s)| \, ds$. Moreover, the energy $\mathcal{L}_g(\phi)$ is minimized when the zero level contour of ϕ is located at the object boundaries. Note that the line integral $\int_0^1 g(C(s))|C'(s)| \, ds$ was first introduced by Caselles et al. as an energy of a parameterized contour C in their proposed geodesic active contour model [12].

The energy functional $\mathcal{A}_g(\phi)$ calculates a weighted area of the region $\Omega_\phi^- \triangleq \{x : \phi(x) < 0\}$. For the special case $g = 1$, this energy is precisely the area of the region Ω_ϕ^-. This energy $\mathcal{A}_g(\phi)$ is introduced to speed up the motion of the zero level contour in the level set evolution procedure, which is essential when the initial contour is positioned far away from the desired object boundaries. In this chapter, we customize LSFs in a way that take positive values outside the zero level contour and negative values inside. Therefore, if the initial contour is placed inside the object, the coefficient α should take negative value to expand the contour, and if the initial contour is placed outside the object, the coefficient α in the weighted area term should be positive, so that the zero level contour can shrink in the level set evolution. From the level set evolution given in Equation 15.17, we can see that the role of g in this energy term A_g is to decelerate of the zero level contour when it arrives at object boundaries where g takes smaller values.

The energy functional $\mathcal{E}(\phi)$ is then approximated by

$$\mathcal{E}_\varepsilon(\phi) = \mu \int_\Omega p(|\nabla\phi|)\,\mathrm{d}\mathbf{x} + \lambda \int_\Omega g\delta_\varepsilon(\phi)|\nabla\phi|\,\mathrm{d}\mathbf{x} + \alpha \int_\Omega gH_\varepsilon(-\phi)\,\mathrm{d}\mathbf{x}. \tag{15.16}$$

where H_ε and δ_ε are defined in Equations 15.23 and 15.24 respectively.

This energy functional can be minimized by solving the following gradient flow:

$$\frac{\partial\phi}{\partial t} = \mu\,\mathrm{div}(d_p(|\nabla\phi|)\nabla\phi) + \lambda\delta_\varepsilon(\phi)\mathrm{div}\left(g\frac{\nabla\phi}{|\nabla\phi|}\right) + \alpha g\delta_\varepsilon(\phi) \tag{15.17}$$

15.2.2   Region-scalable fitting (RSF) model

15.2.2.1   Region-scalable fitting energy

In this section, we review a region-based model using intensity information in local regions at a controllable scale. We first introduce a nonnegative kernel function $K : R^n \to [0, +\infty)$, which has the following properties:

1. $K(-u) = K(u)$;

2. $K(u) \geq K(v)$, if $|u| < |v|$, and $\lim_{|u| to\infty} K(u) = 0$;

3. $\int K(\mathbf{y})\,\mathrm{d}\mathbf{y} = 1$.

Consider a given vector-valued image $I : \Omega \to R^d$, where $\Omega \subset R^n$ is the complete image domain, and $d \geq 1$ is the dimensionality of the vector $I(\mathbf{y})$. In particular, $d = 1$ for gray-level images, while $d = 3$ for RGB color images. Let C be a closed outline in the image domain Ω, which separates the complete image Ω into two areas: $\Omega_1 = outside(C)$ and $\Omega_2 = inside(C)$. For any given point $\mathbf{y} \in \Omega$, we define the following local intensity fitting energy:

$$\mathcal{E}_\mathbf{y}^{Fit}(C, f_1(\mathbf{y}), f_2(\mathbf{y})) = \sum_{i=1}^{2}\lambda_i \int_{\Omega_i} K(\mathbf{y} - \mathbf{x})\left|I(\mathbf{x}) - f_i(\mathbf{y})\right|^2\,\mathrm{d}\mathbf{x} \tag{15.18}$$

where λ_1 and λ_2 are positive constants, and $f_1(\mathbf{y})$ and $f_2(\mathbf{y})$ are two values to estimate image intensities in two divided regions Ω_1 and Ω_2, respectively.

The choice of the kernel function K is very flexible, as long as it satisfies the above three basic properties. In the previous work, we chose it as a Gaussian kernel

$$K_\sigma(u) = \frac{1}{(2\pi)^{\frac{n}{2}}\sigma^n}e^{-\frac{|u|^2}{2\sigma^2}} \tag{15.19}$$

with a scale parameter $\sigma > 0$.

With a given center point $\mathbf{y}$, the fitting energy $\mathcal{E}_{\mathbf{y}}^{Fit}$ can be minimized when the contour C is exactly overlapped with the object boundary and the fitting values f_1 and f_2 optimally approximate the local image intensities on both sides of C. To obtain the entire object boundary, we must find a contour C that minimizes the energy $\mathcal{E}_{\mathbf{y}}^{Fit}$ for all $\mathbf{y}$ in the image domain Ω. This can be achieved by minimizing the integral of $\mathcal{E}_{\mathbf{y}}^{Fit}$ over all the center points $\mathbf{y}$ in the image domain Ω, namely, $\int \mathcal{E}_{\mathbf{y}}^{Fit}(C, f_1(\mathbf{y}), f_2(\mathbf{y}))\, d\mathbf{y}$. In addition, it is essential to smooth the contour C by penalizing its length $|C|$, as proposed in most of active contour models. Therefore, we define the following energy functional:

$$\mathcal{E}(C, f_1(\mathbf{y}), f_2(\mathbf{y})) = \int \mathcal{E}_{\mathbf{y}}^{Fit}(C, f_1(\mathbf{y}), f_2(\mathbf{y}))\, d\mathbf{y} + v|C|. \tag{15.20}$$

This energy functional is defined for a contour C. In order to handle topological changes, we will transform it to a level set formulation in the following section.

15.2.2.2 Level set formulation

In level set methods [57], a contour $C \subset \Omega$ is represented by the zero level set of a Lipschitz function $\phi : \Omega \rightarrow \mathcal{R}$, which is called a level set function. In our work, we allow the level set function ϕ to take positive and negative values outside and inside the contour C, respectively. Let H be the Heaviside function, then the energy functional $\mathcal{E}_{\mathbf{y}}^{Fit}(C, f_1(\mathbf{y}), f_2(\mathbf{y}))$ can be expressed as

$$\mathcal{E}_{\mathbf{y}}^{Fit}(\phi, f_1(\mathbf{y}), f_2(\mathbf{y})) = \sum_{i=1}^{2} \int K_\sigma(\mathbf{y} - \mathbf{x}) |I(\mathbf{x}) - f_i(\mathbf{y})|^2 M_i(\phi(\mathbf{x}))\, d\mathbf{x} \tag{15.21}$$

where $M_1(\phi) = H(\phi)$ and $M_2(\phi) = 1 - H(\phi)$. Thus, the energy $\mathcal{E}$ in Equation 15.20 can be written as

$$\mathcal{E}(\phi, f_1, f_2) = \sum_{i=1}^{2} \lambda_i \int \left(\int K_\sigma(\mathbf{y} - \mathbf{x}) |I(\mathbf{x}) - f_i(\mathbf{y})|^2 M_i(\phi(\mathbf{x}))\, d\mathbf{x} \right) d\mathbf{y}$$

$$+ v \int |\nabla H(\phi(\mathbf{y}))|\, d\mathbf{y} \tag{15.22}$$

where the last term $\int |\nabla H(\phi(\mathbf{y}))|\, d\mathbf{y}$ computes the length of the zero level contour of ϕ.

In practice, the Heaviside function H in the above energy functionals is approximated by a smooth function H_ϵ defined as

$$H_\epsilon(y) = \frac{1}{2} \left[1 + \frac{2}{\pi} arctan\left(\frac{y}{\epsilon} \right) \right]. \tag{15.23}$$

The derivative of H_ϵ is

$$\delta_\epsilon(y) = H_\epsilon'(y) = \frac{1}{\pi} \frac{\epsilon}{\epsilon^2 + y^2}. \tag{15.24}$$

where $M_1^\epsilon(\phi) = H_\epsilon(\phi)$ and $M_2^\epsilon(\phi) = 1 - H_\epsilon(\phi)$.

In order to preserve the regularity of the level set function ϕ, which is crucial for accurate computation and stable level set evolution, we introduce a level set regularization term in our variational level set formulation. As proposed in Li et al. [15], we define the level set regularization term as

$$P(\phi) = \int \frac{1}{2}(|\nabla\phi(\mathbf{y})| - 1)^2 \, d\mathbf{y} \tag{15.25}$$

which characterizes the deviation of the function ϕ from a signed distance function. Therefore, we propose to minimize the energy functional

$$\mathcal{F}(\phi, f_1, f_2) = \mathcal{E}_\epsilon(\phi, f_1, f_2) + \mu P(\phi) \tag{15.26}$$

where μ is a positive constant. To minimize this energy functional, its gradient flow is used as the level set evolution equation in the proposed method.

15.2.2.3   Energy minimization

We use the standard gradient descent (or steepest descent) method to minimize the energy functional (15.26). For a fixed level set function ϕ, we minimize the functional $\mathcal{F}(\phi, f_1, f_2)$ with respect to the functions $f_1(\mathbf{y})$ and $f_2(\mathbf{y})$. By calculus of variations, it can be shown that the functions $f_1(\mathbf{y})$ and $f_2(\mathbf{y})$ that minimize $\mathcal{F}(\phi, f_1, f_2)$ satisfy the following Euler–Lagrange equations:

$$\int K_\sigma(\mathbf{y} - \mathbf{x}) M_i^\epsilon(\phi(\mathbf{x}))(I(\mathbf{x}) - f_i(\mathbf{y})) \, d\mathbf{x} = 0, \quad i = 1, 2. \tag{15.27}$$

From Equation 15.27, we obtain

$$f_i(\mathbf{y}) = \frac{K_\sigma(\mathbf{y}) * [M_i^\epsilon(\phi(\mathbf{y}))I(\mathbf{y})]}{K_\sigma(\mathbf{y}) * M_i^\epsilon(\phi(\mathbf{y}))}, \quad i = 1, 2 \tag{15.28}$$

Keeping f_1 and f_2 fixed, we minimize the energy functional $\mathcal{F}(\phi, f_1, f_2)$ with respect to ϕ using the standard gradient descent method by solving the gradient flow equation as follows:

$$\frac{\partial\phi}{\partial t} = -\delta_\epsilon(\phi)(\lambda_1 e_1 - \lambda_2 e_2) + v\delta_\epsilon(\phi)\mathrm{div}\left(\frac{\nabla\phi}{|\nabla\phi|}\right) + \mu\left(\nabla^2\phi - \mathrm{div}\left(\frac{\Delta\phi}{|\nabla\phi|}\right)\right) \tag{15.29}$$

where δ_ϵ is the smoothed Dirac delta function given by Equation 15.24, and e_1 and e_2 are the functions

$$e_i(\mathbf{y}) = \int K_\sigma(\mathbf{x} - \mathbf{y})|I(\mathbf{y}) - f_i(\mathbf{x})|^2 \, d\mathbf{x}, \quad i = 1, 2 \tag{15.30}$$

where f_1 and f_2 are given by Equation 15.28.

15.3   Distance regularized two-layer level set (DR2LS) method

15.3.1   Anatomical knowledge for left and right ventricle segmentation

In order to facilitate cardiac function analysis [58,59], it is highly desirable to automatically extract the epicardial and endocardial surfaces of the left and right ventricles from cardiac images. However, the previously proposed RSF and DRLSE models can only take account of one-layer segmentation, which fail to obtain the inner and outer surfaces of both ventricles simultaneously. Therefore, in this section, we are going to develop a new algorithm, named as distance regularized two-layer level set (DR2LS) model. This method fuses the strengths from two of our previous works, including the region-scalable fitting (RSF) model and the distance regularized level set evolution (DRLSE) method, and is capable of efficiently segmenting the cardiac endocardium and epicardium at the same time.

First, we take account of the anatomy of the both ventricles for the development of DR2LS model. As presented in Figure 15.1, endocardium is the innermost surface of the ventricle, which is a smooth membrane of endothelial cells that lines the cavities of the heart and the valves [60]. Myocardium is a thick layer of cardiac muscle, which is responsible for the contraction and relaxation of the ventricles and atria, and this layer is composed almost completely of cardiomyocytes [32]. The outside of the myocardium is covered with a thin layer called the epicardium, which consists mostly of connective tissue and fat [32,60].

Based on several informative observations of the cardiac anatomy, the desired segmentation outputs should fulfill the following two criteria: first, the endocardial and epicardial surfaces should be smooth contours and second, the interval between endocardial and epicardial surfaces should vary smoothly. Figure 15.1 demonstrates a typical example of the desired LV and RV segmentation results, which satisfy the predefined two criteria.

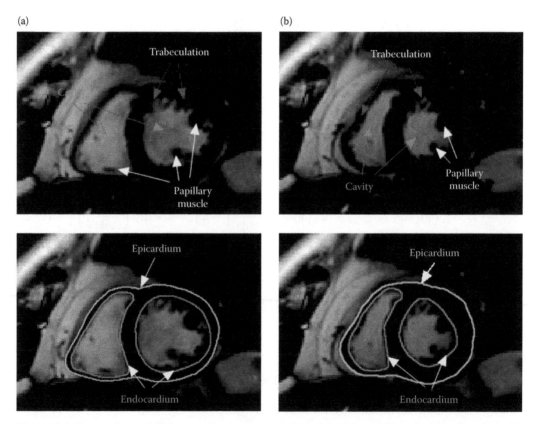

Figure 15.1 Short-axis cine MRI view of one representative patient at end-diastole (a) and end-systole (b) respectively, including the anatomical explanation of both left and right ventricles (top row) as well as the desired epicardial contours (green) and endocardial contours (red) from both ventricles.

Both criteria will be incorporated into the formulation of DR2LS model for LV and RV segmentation. In particular, the first criterion will be introduced to smooth the epicardial and endocardial surfaces individually, while the second criterion will be introduced to provide an interaction between the two surfaces such that the distance between them is gradually varying.

Figure 15.1a,b presents the examples of short-axis images from cine MRI at end-diastole and end-systole respectively. From these images, it is easy to find out that left and right ventricular cavity appears brighter than its surrounding tissues, including myocardium, papillary muscles, and trabeculae. Papillary muscles and trabeculae locate between myocardium and the cavity, and they seem to have similar intensity value in comparison to the myocardium. Therefore, a direct implementation of certain intensity-based segmentation methods will mislabel papillary muscles and trabeculae as myocardium [61,62]. Consequently, the obtained endocardial contour would not be smooth because of the irregular shape of papillary muscles and trabeculae, and accordingly, the distance between the endocardial and epicardial contours will fluctuate significantly. These undesirable and irregular segmentation results can be avoided by maintaining the predefined two criteria of endocardial and epicardial contours.

15.3.2   General framework

We denote an image I as a function $I : \Omega \to \Re$ that is defined on a continuous domain Ω. Let $\phi : \Omega \to \Re$ be a level set function. We use C_0 and C_k to indicate the 0-level and the k-level contours of ϕ, that is, $C_0 \triangleq \{x : \phi(x) = 0\}$ and $C_k \triangleq \{x : \phi(x) = k\}$. We consider the contours C_0 and C_k to represent the endocardium and epicardium individually. The contours C_0 and C_k separate the image domain Ω into three regions: $\Omega_1 \triangleq \{x : \phi(x) < 0\}$, $\Omega_2 \triangleq \{x : 0 < \phi(x) < k\}$, and $\Omega_3 \triangleq \{x : \phi(x) > k\}$, as shown in Figure 15.2, which represent the cavity, myocardium, respectively, and Ω_3 is the region outside the epicardium. Let H be the Heaviside function, then the membership functions of Ω_1, Ω_2, and Ω_3 can be expressed as

$$M_1(\phi(x)) = 1 - H(\phi(x)), \tag{15.31}$$

$$M_2(\phi(x)) = H(\phi(x)) - H(\phi(x) - k), \tag{15.32}$$

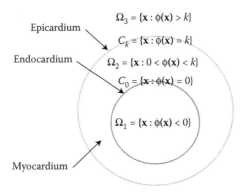

Figure 15.2 The level set representation of endocardium and epicardium as proposed in the DR2LS method.

and

$$M_3(\phi(\mathbf{x})) = H(\phi(\mathbf{x}) - k) \tag{15.33}$$

with $M_i(\phi(\mathbf{x})) = 1$ for $\mathbf{x} \in \Omega_i$ and $M_i(\phi(\mathbf{x})) = 0$ for $\mathbf{x} \notin \Omega_i$, which can be described as

$$M_i(\phi(\mathbf{x})) = \begin{cases} 1, & \mathbf{x} \in \Omega_i \\ 0, & \mathbf{x} \notin \Omega_i. \end{cases} \tag{15.34}$$

With the above two-layer level set representation of endocardium and epicardium, we formulate the segmentation of both ventricles as an optimal problem of seeking for a level set function such that its 0-level and k-level contours best fit the epicardial and endocardial surfaces respectively inside the images. Meanwhile, according to the anatomical properties of endocardium and epicardium, as discussed in Section 15.3.1, the optimal level set function should satisfy the following two properties: first the 0-level and k-level contours are smooth, and second the distance between the 0-level and k-level contours is smoothly changing. All in all, we propose an updated framework with an energy functional in the following form:

$$\mathcal{F} = \mathcal{D} + \mathcal{E} + \mathcal{L} \tag{15.35}$$

where $\mathcal{D}$ is the distance regularization term, which ensures the distance between the 0-level contour and k-level contour is close to a constant; $\mathcal{E}$ is the data term, from the region-scalable fitting (RSF) model proposed in Li et al. [1], which is able to capture object boundaries in the presence of intensity inhomogeneities and $\mathcal{L}$ is the contour regularization term, which is introduced to smooth the 0-level and k-level contours. We name the proposed formulation as distance regularized two-layer level set (DR2LS) model. These three terms in the DR2LS formulation will be elaborated in the following.

15.3.3 Distance regularization

According to the anatomy of the both ventricles, the endocardial and epicardial surfaces are smooth and the distance between them is smoothly changing, as presented in Figure 15.1. We will incorporate this property into our level set model formulation. First, let's consider an ideal case where the depth of the myocardium is strictly a constant. In this case, the distance between the 0-level contour and the k-level contour of the level set function ϕ is also a constant. This property can be characterized by

$$|\nabla\phi(\mathbf{x})| = \alpha, \tag{15.36}$$

which can be used as a *hard constraint* on the level set function ϕ to ensure the constant distance between the 0-level contour and the k-level contour. While in the actual anatomy of the heart, the thickness of the myocardium is never strictly a constant. In this case, we should not apply the hard constraint as defined in Equation 15.36 to force the gradient magnitude $|\nabla\phi(\mathbf{x})|$ to be a constant. Therefore, in the general framework described in Equation 15.35, this distance regularization term $\mathcal{D}$ will be defined by

$$\mathcal{D}(\phi) = \mu \int \frac{1}{2}(|\nabla\phi(\mathbf{x})| - \alpha)^2 d\mathbf{x} \tag{15.37}$$

where $\mu > 0$ is the weighting coefficient. In the evolution of the level set function, $\mathcal{D}(\phi)$, as a soft constraint, tends to force $|\nabla\phi(\mathbf{x})|$ to be close to a constant α. Thus, the distance between the 0-level contour (endocardial contour) and the k-level contour (epicardial contour) of the optimized level set function will be close to a constant.

The energy $\mathcal{D}(\phi, \alpha)$ is used as the distance regularization term in conjunction with a data term and a contour regularization term in the proposed framework. It is worth noting that this distance regularization term with $\alpha = 1$ was originally used by Li et al. [15] to force the level set function to be close to a signed distance function, thereby eliminating the need for reinitialization in conventional level set methods. Here, the distance regularization term is used for a different purpose, that is, to maintain a smoothly varying distance between two level contours.

Moreover, the distance between the 0-level and k-level contours depends on the values of k and $|\nabla\phi|$. For any given value of k, the values of $|\nabla\phi|$ is able to adaptively change in the energy minimization process, such that the distance between the 0-level and k-level contours, can optimally represent the actual distance between the endocardium and epicardium. Additionally, the choice of the level k is flexible, and moreover the result of the proposed level set method is not sensitive to the choice of k.

In order to account for theoretical completeness, we further generalize the constant α as a smooth function $\alpha(\mathbf{x})$, and accordingly define an energy functional by

$$\mathcal{D}(\phi, \alpha) = \mu \int \frac{1}{2}(|\nabla\phi(\mathbf{x})| - \alpha(\mathbf{x}))^2 d\mathbf{x} + \omega \int |\nabla\alpha(\mathbf{x})|^2 d\mathbf{x}, \tag{15.38}$$

where $\mu > 0$, $\omega > 0$ are the weighting coefficients. The first term forces $|\nabla\phi|$ to be a smooth function $\alpha(\mathbf{x})$, and the second term ensure the smoothness of the function $\alpha(\mathbf{x})$.

15.3.4 Region-scalable fitting in two-layer level set formulation

Because of the intensity inhomogeneities in cine MRI, the distributions of the intensities in the regions Ω_1, Ω_2, and Ω_3 often overlap, which causes a major challenge when using certain intensity-based segmentation methods. In order to overcome this challenge, we propose to exploit the property of intensities within a relatively small circular neighborhood, in which the slowly varying bias can be ignored as shown in Figure 15.3. Given a point $\mathbf{y} \in \Omega$, pixels in its neighborhood with radius ρ can be defined by $\mathcal{O}_\mathbf{y} \triangleq \{\mathbf{x} : |\mathbf{x} - \mathbf{y}| \le \rho\}$. The partition $\{\Omega_i\}_{i=1}^3$ of the entire domain Ω induces a partition of the neighborhood $\mathcal{O}_\mathbf{y}$, that is, $\{\mathcal{O}_\mathbf{y} \cap \Omega_i\}_{i=1}^3$ forms a partition of $\mathcal{O}_\mathbf{y}$ as shown in Figure 15.3. For the slowly varying bias field, image intensities at $\mathbf{x}$ in $\mathcal{O}_\mathbf{y} \cap \Omega_1$, $\mathcal{O}_\mathbf{y} \cap \Omega_2$, and $\mathcal{O}_\mathbf{y} \cap \Omega_3$ can be approximated by

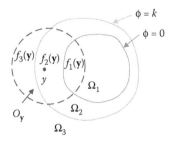

Figure 15.3 Illustration of region-scalable fitting in two-layer level set formulation.

three constants, denoted by $f_1(\mathbf{y})$, $f_2(\mathbf{y})$, and $f_3(\mathbf{y})$. Therefore, the intensities in the set

$$\mathbf{I}_i^{\mathbf{y}} = \{I(\mathbf{x}) : \mathbf{x} \in \mathcal{O}_y \cap \Omega_i\}$$

form a cluster with cluster center $m_i \approx f_i(\mathbf{y})$, $i = 1, 2, 3$. These three clusters $\mathbf{I}_1^{\mathbf{y}}$, $\mathbf{I}_2^{\mathbf{y}}$, and $\mathbf{I}_3^{\mathbf{y}}$, are well-separated, with individual cluster centers $m_i \approx f_i(\mathbf{y})$, $i = 1, 2, 3$. This local intensity clustering property is used to formulate the proposed method for segmenting both ventricles from cine MRI.

The above-described local intensity clustering property indicates that the intensities in the neighborhood $\mathcal{O}_y$ can be classified into three clusters, with centers $m_i \approx f_i(\mathbf{y})$, $i = 1, 2, 3$. This allows us to apply the standard K-means clustering to classify these local intensities. Therefore, the same as defined in Li et al. [1], we define a clustering criterion for classifying the intensities in $\mathcal{O}_y$ as follows:

$$\mathcal{E}_{\mathbf{y}} = \sum_{i=1}^{3} \lambda_i \int_{\mathcal{O}_y \cap \Omega_i} K_\rho(\mathbf{x} - \mathbf{y}) |I(\mathbf{x}) - f_i(\mathbf{y})|^2 d\mathbf{x} \qquad (15.39)$$

where λ_1, λ_2, and λ_3 are the weighting coefficients and K_ρ is a nonnegative kernel function $K_\rho : \Re^n \rightarrow [0, +\infty)$, defined by

$$K_\rho(\mathbf{u}) = \begin{cases} a, & \text{for } |\mathbf{u}| \leq \rho \\ 0, & \text{for } |\mathbf{u}| > \rho \end{cases} \qquad (15.40)$$

where $a > 0$ is a normalization factor such that $\int_{|\mathbf{u}| \leq \rho} K_\rho(\mathbf{u}) = 1$. Since $K_\rho(\mathbf{x} - \mathbf{y}) = 0$ for $\mathbf{x} \notin \mathcal{O}_y$, we can rewrite $\mathcal{E}_{\mathbf{y}}$ as

$$\mathcal{E}_{\mathbf{y}} = \sum_{i=1}^{3} \lambda_i \int_{\Omega_i} K_\rho(\mathbf{x} - \mathbf{y}) |I(\mathbf{x}) - f_i(\mathbf{y})|^2 d\mathbf{x}. \qquad (15.41)$$

Using the membership functions $M_1(\phi(\mathbf{x}))$, $M_2(\phi(\mathbf{x}))$, and $M_3(\phi(\mathbf{x}))$ defined earlier, $\mathcal{E}_{\mathbf{y}}$ can be expressed as

$$\mathcal{E}_{\mathbf{y}} = \sum_{i=1}^{3} \lambda_i \int K_\rho(\mathbf{x} - \mathbf{y}) |I(\mathbf{x}) - f_i(\mathbf{y})|^2 M_i(\phi(\mathbf{x})) d\mathbf{x}. \qquad (15.42)$$

The energy functional $\mathcal{E}_{\mathbf{y}}$ should be minimized for all $\mathbf{y} \in \Omega$. This can be achieved by minimizing the integral of $\mathcal{E}_{\mathbf{y}}$, with respect to the neighborhood center $\mathbf{y}$, which is the energy functional defined by

$$\mathcal{E}(\phi, f_1, f_2, f_3) = \int_{\Omega} \mathcal{E}_{\mathbf{y}} d\mathbf{y}$$

$$= \sum_{i=1}^{3} \lambda_i \int \left(\int K_\rho(\mathbf{x} - \mathbf{y}) |I(\mathbf{x}) - f_i(\mathbf{y})|^2 M_i(\phi(\mathbf{x})) d\mathbf{x} \right) d\mathbf{y}. \qquad (15.43)$$

This data term can be used to robustly segment the LV and RV from cine cine MRI even with the presence of intensity inhomogeneities. For more information on the original formulation of the RSF model, please refer to Li et al. [1,27].

15.3.5 Contour regularization

Similar to most of other active contour models, we will smooth the endocardial and epicardial contours by penalizing their arc lengths with the following contour regularization term:

$$\mathcal{L}(\phi) = \nu_1 \int |\nabla H(\phi(\mathbf{x}))| d\mathbf{x} + \nu_2 \int |\nabla H(\phi(\mathbf{x}) - k)| d\mathbf{x} \qquad (15.44)$$

where the first term and the second term calculate the arc lengths of the 0-level and k-level contours, respectively.

15.3.6 Energy minimization

With the energy terms including $\mathcal{D}(\phi, \alpha)$, $\mathcal{E}(\phi, f_1, f_2, f_3)$, and $\mathcal{L}(\phi)$ defined above, we propose to minimize the following energy functional:

$$\mathcal{F}(\phi, \alpha, f_1, f_2, f_3) = \mathcal{D}(\phi, \alpha) + \mathcal{E}(\phi, f_1, f_2, f_3) + \mathcal{L}(\phi). \qquad (15.45)$$

This energy functional can be minimized by alternately minimizing $\mathcal{F}$ with respect to each of its variables. The energy minimization process starts with an initialization of the level set function ϕ and the smooth function α.

For fixed f_1, f_2, f_3, and α, we minimize the energy functional $\mathcal{F}$ with respect to ϕ using the standard gradient descent method and obtain

$$\begin{aligned} \frac{\partial \phi(\mathbf{x})}{\partial t} = {} & \lambda_1 e_1(\mathbf{x}) \delta(\phi(\mathbf{x})) \\ & - \lambda_2 e_2(\mathbf{x})(\delta(\phi(\mathbf{x})) - \delta(\phi(\mathbf{x}) - k)) \\ & - \lambda_3 e_3(\mathbf{x}) \delta(\phi(\mathbf{x}) - k) \\ & + (\nu_1 \delta(\phi(\mathbf{x})) + \nu_2 \delta(\phi(\mathbf{x}) - k)) \operatorname{div}\left(\frac{\nabla \phi(\mathbf{x})}{|\nabla \phi(\mathbf{x})|}\right) \\ & + \mu \left(\nabla^2 \phi(\mathbf{x}) - \alpha(\mathbf{x}) \operatorname{div}\left(\frac{\nabla \phi(\mathbf{x})}{|\nabla \phi(\mathbf{x})|}\right)\right) \end{aligned} \qquad (15.46)$$

where

$$e_i(\mathbf{x}) = \int K_\rho(\mathbf{y} - \mathbf{x}) |I(\mathbf{x}) - f_i(\mathbf{y})|^2 d\mathbf{y}, \quad i = 1, 2, 3. \qquad (15.47)$$

The function e_i can be written into $e_i = [K_\rho * 1]I^2 - 2K_\rho * [If_i] + K_\rho * f_i^2$.

For fixed level set function ϕ and α, we minimize $\mathcal{F}(\phi, \alpha, f_1, f_2, f_3)$ with respect to f_1, f_2, and f_3. It can be shown that the energy $\mathcal{F}(\phi, \alpha, f_1, f_2, f_3)$ is minimized when f_1, f_2, and f_3 are given by

$$f_1 = \frac{K_\rho * (I - H(\phi)I)}{K_\rho * (1 - H(\phi))}, \qquad (15.48)$$

$$f_2 = \frac{K_\rho * (H(\phi)I - H(\phi - k)I)}{K_\rho * (H(\phi) - H(\phi - k))}, \qquad (15.49)$$

$$f_3 = \frac{K_\rho * [H(\phi - k)I]}{K_\rho * H(\phi - k)}. \qquad (15.50)$$

For the generalized distance regularization term defined by Equation 15.38, we also need to minimize the energy $\mathcal{D}(\phi, \alpha)$ with respect to the function α. This can be achieved by solving the gradient flow equation derived from the energy $\mathcal{D}(\phi, \alpha)$ in Equation 15.38, which is a standard heat equation as follows:

$$\frac{\partial \alpha(\mathbf{x})}{\partial t} = \mu \left(|\nabla \phi(\mathbf{x})| - \alpha(\mathbf{x}) \right) + 2\omega \nabla^2 \alpha(\mathbf{x}). \tag{15.51}$$

The heat equation Equation 15.51 can be approximately solved by a convolution of the function $|\nabla \phi|$ with a Gaussian kernel.

In each iteration, f_i and e_i, $i = 1, 2, 3$ are first updated. Then, the values of level set function and function α are updated using partial differential equation in Equations 15.46 and 15.51 by the finite difference method, respectively. In practice, the Heaviside function H in the above energy functionals is approximated by a smooth function H_ϵ with $\epsilon = 1$, defined by Equation 15.23 and the derivative of H_ϵ is used to approximate the Dirac delta function δ as in Li et al. [1], defined by Equation 15.24.

15.4   Application of DR2LS to segmentation of left and right ventricles

In this section, we describe a two-step approach for segmentation of LV and RV. In the first step, we use the DRLSE to perform a preliminary segmentation of LV and RV to roughly locate the endocardial contours of the LV and RV. The level set function obtained in the first step is used as the initial level set function of the DR2LS in the second step, with the 0-level and k-level contours representing the initial endocardial and epicardial contours, respectively. The final endocardial and epicardial contours of LV and RV is then obtained as the result of the level set evolution in the DR2LS model. The details of this two-step approach are described below.

15.4.1   Roughly locate endocardial contours of LV and RV using DRLSE

In the first step, we use distance regularized level set evolution (DRLSE) model to obtain a preliminary segmentation of left and right ventricles, which is then applied to define the initial level set function for the distance regularized two-layer level set (DR2LS) model described in Section 15.3.

Figure 15.4 illustrates the complete process of preliminary segmentation from cardiac images, which includes manual initialization as well as final contours resulted from the DRLSE model, respectively. First, we manually place two square blocks inside cavities of the left and the right ventricle for the initialization of the DRLSE model. Then the final zero level contour in DRLSE is evolved to capture the inner surfaces of both LV and RV. The final contours of the DRLSE model are going to be used as the initial endocardial contours in the following segmentation step. Given the segmented left and right ventricles obtained in the first step, denoted by V_{left} and V_{right}, we constructed the initial level set function for the second step as:

$$\phi_0(\mathbf{x}) = \begin{cases} c & \mathbf{x} \in V_{left} \cup V_{right} \\ -c & else \end{cases} \tag{15.52}$$

where c is a positive constant.

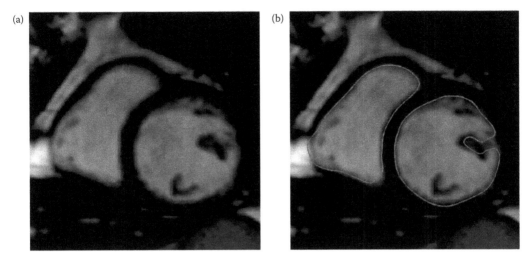

Figure 15.4 Roughly locate the endocardial contours of the LV and RV using the distance regularized level set evolution (DRLSE) model: (a) initialization for DRLSE, (b) final zero level of DRLSE used as the initialization of a two-layer level set function.

15.4.2   Extraction of both endocardial and epicardial contours using DR2LS

The second step of our method aims to accurately capture both the endocardial contours as well as the epicardial contours of both LV and RV at the same time, based on the previously initialized results. In this step, we incorporate the anatomical knowledge of the heart as shown in Figure 15.1 into our two-layer level set formulation, where the endocardial and epicardial contours are represented by two specified level contours from one-level set function. With the above two-layer level set representation of endocardial and epicardial contours, we implement the mathematical model discussed in Section 15.3 to accurately segment left and right ventricles from cine MRI based on previously initialized contours from DRLSE method.

In details, the preliminary segmentation of inner surfaces of left and right ventricles from DRLSE as well as selected different level contours from the same level set function are used to initialize the endocardial contour and the epicardial contour separately in DR2LS model, which are labeled as the zero level contour and the k-level contour. Both level sets are optimized by an energy minimization process as proposed in Section 15.3.6 to best estimate the actual endocardium and epicardium of LV and RV from cardiac images. In order to ensure smoothly varying distance between the two level contours, we introduce a distance regularization constraint as discussed in Section 15.3.3 in the energy function. Additionally, with the introducing of region-scalable fitting (RSF) energy as the data term as show in Section 15.3.4, the DR2LS model has capable to deal with intensity inhomogeneities in the cardiac images, which is the main source of challenge for image segmentation. In the following section, we are going to demonstrate the implementation details as well as the segmentation results from the proposed two-step method.

15.5   Results of left and right ventricle segmentation

In this section, we will demonstrate the implementation details as well as the segmentation results of the proposed two-step approach with the application to segment both left and right ventricles from cardiac cine MRI data, where the data are obtained from MICCAI 2009 challenge on left ventricle segmentation and MICCAI 2012 right ventricle segmentation challenge.

15.5.1 Parameters selection

In first step, we set the parameters for the DRLSE model with $\Delta t = 1$, $\mu = 0.2$, and $\lambda = 10$. In the second step, we numerically solve the level set evolution equation of the DR2LS model presented in Equation 15.46 by following a standard finite difference scheme proposed in Li et al. [1]. The details of the selected parameters for the DR2LS model are given in the following. The time step Δt used in the approximation of temporal derivative is set to $\Delta t = 0.1$ in our implementation. For the datasets used in this chapter, we set the other parameters $\rho = 3$, $\mu = 1$, $\omega = 0.5$, $\lambda_1 = 0.002$, $\lambda_2 = 0.05$, $\lambda_3 = 0.0015$, and $\nu_1 = 0.001 \times 255 \times 255$, $\nu_2 = 0.001 \times 255 \times 255$. The choice of the level $k = 30$. The smooth function α can be initialized as a constant $c > 0$ (we set $c = 1$ in this chapter). The function f_i and e_i, $i = 1, 2, 3$ are updated at each time step before the update of the level set function ϕ.

15.5.2 Segmentation results

Our two-step approach has been tested on the dataset of MICCAI 2009 challenge on left ventricle segmentation as well as the dataset of MICCAI 2012 right ventricle segmentation challenge (both available from the following link: http://www.litislab.eu/rvsc), and this two-step approach has already showed the promising capability over other existing segmentation algorithms.

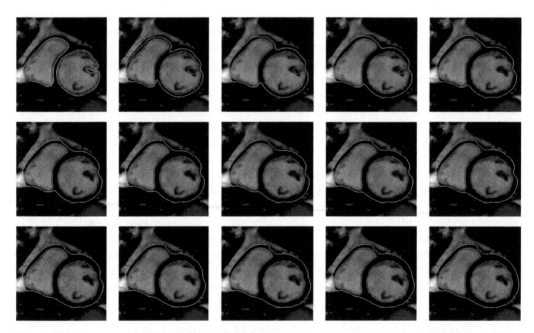

Figure 15.5 Process of implementing a distance regularized two-layer level set (DR2LS) model to segment both LV and RV from a selected patient's cine MRI. Note, the iteration starts from left to right and from top to bottom.

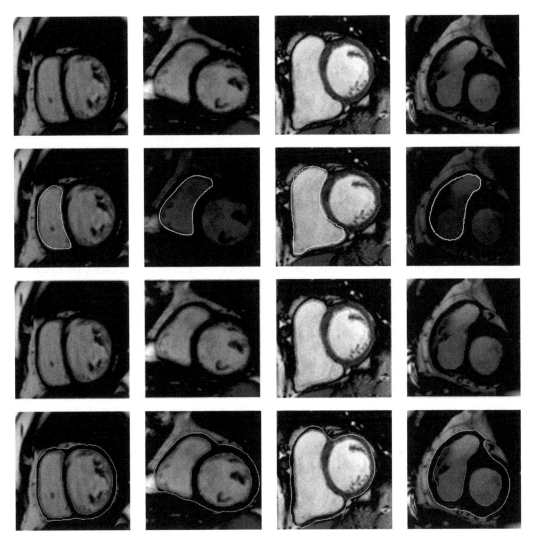

Figure 15.6 Results of our proposed LV and RV segmentation framework. Row 1: Original cardiac MR images. Row 2: Ground truth. Row 3: Initial segmentation results of DRLSE model. Row 4: Final segmentation results of the proposed DR2LS method.

Figure 15.5 shows the illustrative segmentation results of both left and right ventricles from a selected patient cine MRI using distance regularized two-layer level set (DR2LS) method after applying DRLSE initialization, where each of these figures corresponds to one of the middle steps within iteration (iterates from left to right and from top to bottom). It is easy to find out the output of the proposed DR2LS segmentation model (as shown in the bottom right figure in Figure 15.5) is capable of accurately capturing both the endocardial and epicardial contours, even in presence of the intensity inhomogeneity and image noises.

Figure 15.6 presents the segmentation results of both left and right ventricles from cardiac cine MR short-axis images for various patients. In Figure 15.6, four different patients cardiac MR images are displayed in different columns. Rows 1 and 2 are the original images as well as the ground truth segmented by experienced radiologists, separately. Row

3 shows the preliminary segmentation results with first-step DRLSE method, which is then used as initialization of the second step. Row 4 is the final segmentation results of our DR2LS method. Note that we use results in Row 3 as initialization of endocardial contour and choose $k = 30$ as the epicardial contour for our experiments, and then obtain final endocardial and epicardial contours. From experimental results, we can see that the two contours of our proposed algorithm can optimally fit endocardium and epicardium of the cardiac ventricles.

15.6   Conclusions

In this chapter, we present the development of a new segmentation framework for left and right ventricles from cardiac MR short-axis images. This framework contains two key steps: first, we apply the DRLSE method as initialization of endocardial contour and then we use the DR2LS model to accurately capture both endocardial and epicardial contours for LV and RV, simultaneously. Moreover, this proposed DR2LS approach fuses the strengths from two of our previous works, including the region-scalable fitting (RSF) model in Li et al. [1] and the distance regularized level set evolution (DRLSE) method in Li et al. [1]. Also, within the DR2LS model, the distance between the two-level contours, which represent endocardium and epicardium can be kept smoothly varying due to the proposed distance regularization term. Experimental results have demonstrated the effectiveness of this proposed two-step level set approach for segmenting cardiac left and right ventricles from cine MRI, which can facilitate the future analysis of cardiac shape and function for cardiovascular diseases [9].

References

1. C. Li, C. Kao, J. C. Gore, and Z. Ding, Minimization of region-scalable fitting energy for image segmentation, *IEEE Transactions on Image Processing*, vol. 17, no. 10, pp. 1940–1949, 2008.
2. C. Li, C. Xu, C. Gui, and M. D. Fox, Distance regularized level set evolution and its application to image segmentation, *IEEE Transactions on Image Processing*, vol. 19, no. 12, pp. 3243–3254, 2010.
3. T. Chan and L. Vese, Active contours without edges, *Image Processing, IEEE Transactions on*, vol. 10, no. 2, pp. 266–277, 2001.
4. L. Cohen and I. Cohen, Finite-element methods for active contour models and balloons for 2-D and 3-D images, *Pattern Analysis and Machine Intelligence, IEEE Transactions on*, vol. 15, no. 11, pp. 1131–1147, 1993.
5. M. Kass, A. Witkin, and D. Terzopoulos, Snakes: Active contour models, *International Journal of Computer Vision*, vol. 1, no. 4, pp. 321–331, 1988.
6. R. Malladi, J. Sethian, and B. Vemuri, Shape modeling with front propagation: A level set approach, *Pattern Analysis and Machine Intelligence, IEEE Transactions on*, vol. 17, no. 2, pp. 158–175, 1995.
7. Y. Chen, H. D. Tagare, S. Thiruvenkadam, F. Huang, D. Wilson, K. S. Gopinath, R. W. Briggs, and E. A. Geiser, Using prior shapes in geometric active contours in a variational framework, *International Journal of Computer Vision*, vol. 50, pp. 315–328, 2002.
8. M. Leventon, W. Grimson, and O. Faugeras, Statistical shape influence in geodesic active contours, in *Computer Vision and Pattern Recognition, 2000. Proceedings. IEEE Conference on*, vol. 1, pp. 316–323, 2000.
9. J. Wu, Y. Wang, M. A. Simon, and J. C. Brigham, A new approach to kinematic feature extraction from the human right ventricle for classification of hypertension: A feasibility study, *Physics in Medicine and Biology*, vol. 57, no. 23, p. 7905, 2012.

10. J. Wu and J. C. Brigham, Computational techniques for analysis of shape and kinematics of biological structures, in *Image-Based Geometric Modeling and Mesh Generation*. Berlin: Springer, pp. 251–269, 2013.

11. J. Wu, K. G. Brigham, M. A. Simon, and J. C. Brigham, An implementation of independent component analysis for 3D statistical shape analysis, *Biomedical Signal Processing and Control*, vol. 13, pp. 345–356, 2014.

12. V. Caselles, R. Kimmel, and G. Sapiro, Geodesic active contours, *International Journal of Computer Vision*, vol. 22, no. 1, pp. 61–79, 1997.

13. S. Kichenassamy, A. Kumar, P. Olver, A. Tannenbaum, and A. Yezzi, Gradient flows and geometric active contour models, in *Computer Vision, 1995. Proceedings, Fifth International Conference on*, pp. 810–815, 1995.

14. R. Kimmel, A. Amir, and A. Bruckstein, Finding shortest paths on surfaces using level sets propagation, *Pattern Analysis and Machine Intelligence, IEEE Transactions on*, vol. 17, no. 6, pp. 635–640, 1995.

15. C. Li, C. Xu, C. Gui, and M. D. Fox, Level set evolution without re-initialization: a new variational formulation, in *IEEE Conference on Computer Vision and Pattern Recognition (CVPR)*, pp. 430–436, 2005.

16. A. Vasilevskiy and K. Siddiqi, Flux maximizing geometric flows, *Pattern Analysis and Machine Intelligence, IEEE Transactions on*, vol. 24, no. 12, pp. 1565–1578, 2002.

17. C. Xu and J. Prince, Snakes, shapes, and gradient vector flow, *Image Processing, IEEE Transactions on*, vol. 7, no. 3, pp. 359–369, Mar 1998.

18. N. Paragios, A variational approach for the segmentation of the left ventricle in cardiac image analysis, *International Journal of Computer Vision*, vol. 50, no. 3, pp. 345–362, 2002.

19. R. Ronfard, Region-based strategies for active contour models, *International Journal of Computer Vision*, vol. 13, no. 2, pp. 229–251, 1994.

20. C. Samson, L. Blanc-Feraud, G. Aubert, and J. Zerubia, A variational model for image classification and restoration, *Pattern Analysis and Machine Intelligence, IEEE Transactions on*, vol. 22, no. 5, pp. 460–472, May 2000.

21. A. Tsai, J. Yezzi, A., and A. Willsky, Curve evolution implementation of the Mumford–Shah functional for image segmentation, denoising, interpolation, and magnification, *Image Processing, IEEE Transactions on*, vol. 10, no. 8, pp. 1169–1186, 2001.

22. L. Vese and T. Chan, A multiphase level set framework for image segmentation using the Mumford and Shah model, *International Journal of Computer Vision*, vol. 50, no. 3, pp. 271–293, 2002.

23. Z. Hou, A review on MR image intensity inhomogeneity correction, *International Journal of Biomedical Imaging*, vol. 2006, pp. 1–11, 2006.

24. Y. Liu, G. Captur, J. C. Moon, S. Guo, X. Yang, S. Zhang, and C. Li, Distance regularized two level sets for segmentation of left and right ventricles from cine MRI, *Magnetic Resonance Imaging*, vol. 34, no. 5, pp. 699–706, 2015.

25. C. Li, J. C. Gore, and C. Davatzikos, Multiplicative intrinsic component optimization (mico) for MRI bias field estimation and tissue segmentation, *Magnetic Resonance Imaging*, vol. 32, no. 7, pp. 913–923, 2014.

26. Y. Liu, C. Li, S. Guo, Y. Song, and Y. Zhao, A novel level set method for segmentation of left and right ventricles from cardiac MR images, in *Engineering in Medicine and Biology Society (EMBC), 2014 36th Annual International Conference of the IEEE*. IEEE, pp. 4719–4722, 2014.

27. C. Li, R. Huang, Z. Ding, J. C. Gatenby, D. N. Metaxas, and J. C. Gore, A level set method for image segmentation in the presence of intensity inhomogeneities with application to MRI, *IEEE Transactions on Image Processing*, vol. 20, no. 7, pp. 2007–2016, 2011.

28. J. A. Sethian, *Level Set Methods and Fast Marching Methods*. Cambridge: Cambridge University Press, 1999.

29. F. R. Osher, Stanley, *Level Set Methods and Dynamic Implicit Surfaces*. New York: Spinger, 2002.

30. S. O. Mark Sussman and P. Smereka, A level set approach for computing solutions to incompressible two-phase flow, *Journal of Computational Physics*, vol. 114, no. 4, pp. 146–159, 1994.

31. A. F. Frangi, W. J. Niessen, and M. A. Viergever, Three-dimensional modelling for functional analysis of cardiac images: A review, *IEEE Transactions on Medical Imaging*, vol. 20, no. 1, pp. 2–5, 2001.

32. C. Petitjean and J. N. Dacher, A review of segmentation methods in short axis cardiac MR images, *Medical Image Analysis*, vol. 15, no. 2, pp. 169–184, 2011.

33. G. Carneiro, J. C. Nascimento, and A. Freitas, The segmentation of the left ventricle of the heart from ultrasound data using deep learning architectures and derivative-based search methods, *IEEE Transactions on Image Processing*, vol. 21, no. 3, pp. 968–982, 2012.

34. X. Huang, D. P. Dione, C. B. Compas, X. Papademetris, B. A. Lin, A. Bregasi, A. J. Sinusas, L. H. Staib, and J. S. Duncan, Contour tracking in echocardiographic sequences via sparse representation and dictionary learning, *Medical Image Analysis*, vol. 18, no. 2, pp. 253–271, 2014.

35. M. Pereanez, K. Lekadir, C. Butakoff, C. Hoogendoorn, and A. F. Frangi, A framework for the merging of pre-existing and correspondenceless 3D statistical shape models, *Med Image Analysis*, vol. 18, no. 7, pp. 1044–1058, 2014.

36. J. Montagnat, M. Sermesant, H. Delingette, G. Malandain, and N. Ayache, Anisotropic filtering for model-based segmentation of 4D cylindrical echocardiographic images, *Pattern Recognition Letters*, vol. 24, no. 4–5, pp. 815–828, 2003.

37. C. Y. Ahn, Y. M. Jung, and J. K. S. O. I. Kwonb, Fast segmentation of ultrasound images using robust Rayleigh distribution decomposition, *Pattern Recognition*, vol. 45, no. 9, pp. 3490–3500, 2012.

38. L. Dornheim, K. D. Tönnies, and K. Dixon, Automatic segmentation of the left ventricle in 3D SPECT data by registration with a dynamic anatomic model, *Medical Image Computing and Computing-Assisted Intervention (MICCAI)*, vol. 8, no. 1, pp. 335–342, 2005.

39. M. Lorenzo-Valde's, G. I. Sanchez-Ortiz, A. G. Elkington, R. H. Mohiaddin, and D. Rueckert, Segmentation of 4D cardiac MR images using a probabilistic atlas and the EM algorithm, *Medical Image Analysis*, vol. 8, no. 3, pp. 255–265, 2004.

40. M. Lynch, O. Ghita, and P. F. Whelan, Left-ventricle myocardium segmentation using a coupled level-set with a priori knowledge, *Computerized Medical Imaging and Graphics*, vol. 30, no. 4, pp. 255–262, 2006.

41. X. Zeng, L. H. Staib, R. T. Schultz, and J. S. Duncan, Volumetric layer segmentation using coupled surfaces propagation, in *IEEE Conference on Computer Vision and Pattern Recognition (CVPR)*, pp. 708–715, 1998.

42. G. I. Sanchez-Ortiz, D. Rueckert, and P. Burger, Knowledge-based tensor anisotropic diffusion of cardiac magnetic resonance images, *Medical Image Analysis*, vol. 3, no. 1, pp. 245–254, 1993.

43. U. Kurkure, A. Pednekar, R. Muthupillai, S. D. Flamm, and I. A. Kakadiaris, Localization and segmentation of left ventricle in cardiac cine-MR images, *IEEE Transactions on Biomedical Engineering*, vol. 56, no. 5, pp. 1360–1370, 2009.

44. S. Queiro's, D. Barbosa, B. Heyde, P. Morais, J. L. Vilaa, D. Friboulet, O. Bernard, and J. Dhooge, Fast automatic myocardial segmentation in 4D cine CMR datasets, *Medical Image Analysis*, vol. 18, no. 7, pp. 1115–1131, 2014.

45. D. Wei, Y. Sun, S.-H. Ong, P. Chai, L. L. Teo, and A. F. Low, Three-dimensional segmentation of the left ventricle in late gadolinium enhanced MR images of chronic infarction combining long- and short-axis information, *Medical Image Analysis*, vol. 17, no. 6, pp. 685–697, 2013.

46. A. Eslami, A. Karamalis, A. Katouzian, and N. Navab, Segmentation by retrieval with guided random walks: Application to left ventricle segmentation in MRI, *Medical Image Analysis*, vol. 17, no. 2, pp. 236–253, 2013.

47. C. M. S. Nambakhsh, J. Yuan, K. Punithakumar, A. Goela, M. Rajchl, T. M. Peters, and I. B. Ayed, Left ventricle segmentation in MRI via convex relaxed distribution matching, *Medical Image Analysis*, vol. 17, no. 8, pp. 1010–1024, 2013.

48. M. Lorenzo-Valde's, G. I. Sanchez-Ortiz, A. G. Elkington, R. H. Mohiaddin, and D. Rueckert, Segmentation of 4D cardiac MR images using a probabilistic atlas and the em algorithm, *Medical Image Analysis*, vol. 8, no. 3, pp. 255–265, 2004.

49. M. Lynch, O. Ghita, and P. F. Whelan, Left-ventricle myocardium segmentation using a coupled level-set with a priori knowledge, *Computerized Medical Imaging and Graphics*, vol. 30, no. 4, pp. 255–262, 2006.

50. H. Zhang, A. Wahle, R. K. Johnson, T. D. Scholz, and M. Sonka, 4-D cardiac MR image analysis: Left and right ventricular morphology and function, *Medical Imaging, IEEE Transactions on*, vol. 29, no. 2, pp. 350–364, 2010.

51. I. B. Ayed, H.-M. Chen, K. Punithakumar, I. Ross, and S. Li, Max-flow segmentation of the left ventricle by recovering subject-specific distributions via a bound of the bhattacharyya measure, *Medical Image Analysis*, vol. 16, no. 1, pp. 87–100, 2012.

52. K. Rajpoot, V. Grau, J. A. Noble, H. Becher, and C. Szmigielski, The evaluation of single-view and multi-view fusion 3D echocardiography using image-driven segmentation and tracking, *Medical Image Analysis*, vol. 15, no. 4, pp. 514–528, 2011.

53. S. K. Zhou, Shape regression machine and efficient segmentation of left ventricle endocardium from 2D b-mode echocardiogram, *Medical Image Analysis*, vol. 14, no. 4, pp. 563–581, 2010.

54. M. Ma, M. van Stralen, J. H. Reiber, J. G. Bosch, and B. P. Lelieveldt, Model driven quantification of left ventricular function from sparse single-beat 3D echocardiography, *Medical Image Analysis*, vol. 14, no. 4, pp. 582–593, 2010.

55. Y. Zhu, X. Papademetris, A. J. Sinusas, and J. S. Duncan, A coupled deformable model for tracking myocardial borders from real-time echocardiography using an incompressibility constraint, *Medical Image Analysis*, vol. 14, no. 3, pp. 429–448, 2010.

56. H. Hu, H. Liu, Z. Gao, and L. Huang, Hybrid segmentation of left ventricle in cardiac MRI using Gaussian-mixture model and region restricted dynamic programming, *Magnetic Resonance Imaging*, vol. 31, no. 4, pp. 575–584, 2013.

57. J. A. S. Stanley Osher, Fronts propagating with curvature-dependent speed: Algorithms based on Hamilton–Jacobi formulations, *Journal of Computational Physics*, vol. 79, pp. 12–49, 1988.

58. J. Wu, Y. Wang, M. A. Simon, M. S. Sacks, and J. C. Brigham, A new computational framework for anatomically consistent 3D statistical shape analysis with clinical imaging applications, *Computer Methods in Biomechanics and Biomedical Engineering: Imaging and Visualization*, vol. 1, no. 1, pp. 13–27, 2013.

59. J. Xu, J. Wu, B. Notghi, M. Simon, and J. C. Brigham, A feasibility study on kinematic feature extraction from the human interventricular septum toward hypertension classification, in *Computational Modeling of Objects Presented in Images: Fundamentals, Methods, and Applications*. Berlin: Springer, pp. 36–47, 2014.

60. M. Jolly, Automatic segmentation of the left ventricle in cardiac MR and CT images, *International Journal of Computer Vision*, vol. 70, no. 2, pp. 151–163, 2006.

61. S. Kirschbaum, J. P. Aben, T. Baks, A. M. K. Gruszczynska, G. P. Krestin, W. J. van der Giessen, D. J. Duncker, P. J. de Feyter, and R. J. van Geuns, Accurate automatic papillary muscle identification for quantitative left ventricle mass measurements in cardiac magnetic resonance imaging, *Academy of Radiology*, vol. 15, no. 10, pp. 1227–1233, 2008.

62. B. Sievers, S. Kirchberg, A. Bakan, U. Franken, and H. J. Trappe, Impact of papillary muscles in ventricular volume and ejection fraction assessment by cardiovascular magnetic resonance, *Journal of Cardiovascular Magnetic Resonance*, vol. 6, no. 1, pp. 9–16, 2004.

chapter sixteen

Salient object segmentation with a shape-constrained level set

*Bin Wang, Xinbo Gao, Dacheng Tao, Xuelong Li,
and Souleymane Balla-Arabé*

Contents

Abstract

A novel salient object segmentation based on the level set method with shape constraint is proposed. Given an image, this method first initializes the curve according to the saliency map which is subsequently combined into evolution in a multi-channel manner, and then rebuilds an energy functional with shape constraint. In such a way, the salient objects with a specified shape can be de-parted out automatically. The proposed one has some advantages as follows. First, the saliency map is taken as a considerable clue into LSMs to eliminate manual interaction and realize an automatic segmentation. Second, the saliency map is involved into curve's evolution which contributes to accelerating the evolution. Finally, shape priors are utilized to constrain the shape of curve which endow LSMs with a capability of handing broken or occluded objects. We respectively applied the proposed method to synthetic, medical, and natural images and obtained promising results.

16.1 Introduction

Image segmentation is a traditional task in computer vision and pattern recognition and the most of segmentation methods aim at finding the similar pixels and taking them as the interested object, or finding the discontinuity of features and taking them as the edges of the objects. This difference results in categorizing the published literatures into two groups, that is, the region-based and the edge-based segmentation methods. Numerous studies have explored the pros and cons of these two categories, which are well known and need not be repeated here. In general, neither of these two categories is well developed and the latest trend is incorporating some external knowledge or priors to guide segmentation.

As a prevalent branch of segmentation methods, active contour models (ACMs) possess a wide application in the relevant fields. ACMs derived from Snake model [1–3] and were extended by Sethian and Osher via introducing a zero level set to implicitly describe the evolving curves [4]. It is the zero level set, a signed distance function (i.e., the level set function, LSF) defined in high-dimensional space, which makes the planar curve capable of changing its topology very easily and elegantly [5,6]. That is actually why this implicit ACMs are also called level set methods (LSMs). The early LSMs [1,2,4,6–9] realize image segmentation by numerically resolving a partial differential equation (PDE) designed in advance, and an edge indicator function of this PDE could enforce the evolving curve move toward image edges. Although, having many different variants [10,11], the definitions of these edge indicator functions depend on the image gradient or the mutation of features in principle. This dependence results that the edge-based LSMs are not robust against noise as well as the initial curve, although some improved edge indicator function is designed [12].

The CV model introduced by Chan and Vese simplifies the Mumford–Shah model [13], and applies a 2D piecewise constant function to approximate the given image [14]. The fitting error between the image and its approximation is utilized to build an energy functional which will be optimally minimized to realize segmentation. The CV model does not include the edge indicator function based on image gradient, and is more robust against noise and initialization. However, disregarding the local mutational clues of image as well as the strong assumption about the piecewise constant function lead it to the undesired performance on inhomogeneous objects. Although CV model achieves great success in this manner, and inspires many subsequent works, for example, Chan et al. extended it to multi-channel images [15], Vese et al. enhanced it to be multiple phase LSF [16], Wang et al. and Vemuri et al. extended it to the tensor-diffusion MRI images [17] and tensor field [18], Tsai et al. proposed a piecewise smooth model [19] which provides a more accurate approximation to image. Additionally, Li et al. proposed a local LSM over-performing the piecewise smooth model in terms of computational efficiency [20].

Both the edge-based and region-based LSMs mentioned above basically design the external force (or called external energy term in energy functional) on some low-level clues, for example, image grayscale, gradient, etc. The performance on the real images with noise and complex background is usually undesired. To overcome this shortcoming, shape priors as a reasonable solution are introduced into LSMs. Under the constraint of shape priors, the evolving curve could keep similar shape to the shape priors in the period of evolution. To some extent, shape priors restrict the topological flexibility, but they endow LSMs with the capability of handling the segmentation of the objects seriously disturbed by noise or in a complex background. Numerous studies on this topic have been published as follows. Tsai et al. applied principal component analysis (PCA) to extract the eigen shapes whose linear combination is used to approximate the current shapes [21]. Cremers et al. utilized image moments to align shape priors, and then employed kernel density estimation (KDE) to model the distribution of shape priors [22]. Dambreville et al. employed kernel principal component analysis (KPCA) to extract eigen shapes [23]. Wang et al. alternatively employed locality preserving projections (LPP) [24] to expand a subspace in which the associative energy term is built [25].

In recent years, the saliency map of image widely attracts the attention of scholars since it provides a reasonable visual clue for further processing. The earliest work about saliency map could be tracked back to 1985 in which Koch and Ullman proposed a biologically inspired model and gave a specified definition of saliency map [26]. Subsequently, Itti et al. implemented and verified this model [27]. A graph-based visual saliency (GBVS) model was proposed by Harel et al. based on Markov chain theory to accelerate Itti et al.'s model [28]. Gopalakrishnan extended this model by using local and global random walk matrix [29]. Hou et al. [30] proposed a fast and effective model based on spatial frequency domain analysis. Achanta et al. created saliency map by the comparison of local region and the associative surrounding region [31]. Goferman et al. exploited the local low-level features, the global considerations, the visual organization rules as well as the high-level components to propose a context-aware based saliency detection model [32]. Cheng et al. proposed a regional contrast based saliency extraction algorithm which takes both global contrast differences and spatial coherence into consideration [33].

The traditional LSMs depend on the edge indicator to find image edges, and they tend to find the near and sharp edges. The region-based LSMs derive the PDEs from some associated concave energy functional, which results in the problem of local extreme. For some methods [34–36] possessing a convex energy functional, an initialization far away from the global optimal extreme will take a long time to converge. These facts suggest that LSMs are sensitive to the initialization of the evolving curve. A reasonable estimation of initialization is crucially important to accelerate segmentation based on LSMs. Considering that visually salient regions are usually is or include the objects of interest, we proposed a salient object segmentation method based on a LSM with shape priors. The proposed method first initializes the evolving curve according to a saliency map built by GBVS [28], and then incorporates the saliency map into the curve's evolution in a multi-channel manner. Second, shape priors are projected onto a low-dimensional subspace in which a regularized energy term is designed to keep the shape of curve similar to the applied shape priors [23]. The main contributions of this paper are as follows: (1) introducing saliency map into LSMs to guide the initialization, accelerate the evolution of curve, and consequently improve the effectiveness and efficiency of LSMs and (2) shape priors being involved into the energy functional contributes to handling some objects with blur boundary and specified shape. Compared to the representative LSMs, our proposed method is more efficient, practical, and targeted.

The rest of this paper is organized as follows: Section 16.2 will revisit the related work and develop the relationship with our paper; Section 16.3 will introduce the proposed method, including saliency map based curve initialization and evolution, LSM with shape priors and the entire energy functional; Section 16.4 will present the comparison experimental results, and finally the conclusion will be given in Section 16.5.

16.2   Related works

In this section, we revisit an early outstanding work of LSMs and a novel method for creating visual saliency map.

16.2.1   The CV model

Chan and Vese proposed a method, that is, CV model, by simplifying Mumford-Shah model to well handle the segmentation of objects with weak boundaries and noise. This model employs a fitting error between the image and its approximation of a binary piece-wise constant function to build a variational LSM instead of the aforementioned edge indicator function.

Let $I : \Omega \to R$ be a given image, where $\Omega \subset R^2$ and denotes the image domain. The closed curve $C \subset \Omega$, and is implicitly represented by the zero level set of a Lipschitz function $\phi : \Omega \to R$, that is, $C = \{(x, y) | \phi(x, y) = 0\}$. The associated energy functional is defined by

$$
\begin{aligned}
E &= E_{curve}^{cv} + E_{data}^{cv} \\
&= \mu \int_{\Omega} \delta(\phi) |\nabla H(\phi)| \, dx \, dy \\
&\quad + \lambda_1 \int_{\Omega} |I(x, y) - c_1|^2 \phi(x, y) \, dx \, dy \\
&\quad + \lambda_2 \int_{\Omega} |I(x, y) - c_2|^2 (1 - \phi(x, y)) \, dx \, dy,
\end{aligned}
\tag{16.1}
$$

where the parameters μ, v, λ_1, and λ_2 are the adjustable positive weighting factors. E_{curve}^{cv} denotes the circumference of the region enclosed by the evolving curve, and it plays a role of making curve smooth in energy functional. The LSF ϕ is initialized as

$$
\phi_0 = \begin{cases} d(x, y) \in \omega_0 \\ 0(x, y) \in C_0 \\ -d(x, y) \in \Omega - \omega_0 - C_0, \end{cases}
\tag{16.2}
$$

where C_0 is the initial curve, and ω_0 is the region enclosed by C_0. d is a positive constant. The averages inside and outside of the curve C could be computed and updated as following

$$
c_1 = \frac{\int_{\Omega} I H(\phi) \, dx \, dy}{\int_{\Omega} H(\phi) \, dx \, dy}, \quad c_2 = \frac{\int_{\Omega} I(1 - H(\phi)) \, dx \, dy}{\int_{v} (1 - H(\phi)) \, dx \, dy},
\tag{16.3}
$$

where $H(\cdot)$ is a Heaviside function, and plays a role of indicating the region ω_0 enclosed by a curve C_0. Once the Euler–Lagrange equation of the energy functional, that is, Equation 16.1, is deduced out, some numerical scheme could be used to resolve these PDEs and consequently realize image segmentation.

16.2.2   Graph-based visual saliency

As a typical bottom-up visual saliency model, graph-based visual saliency, that is, GBVS, could be divided into three stages. First, GBVS extracts the similar features to Itti's model from the given image, that is, color histogram, orientation, etc. These features form the different channels. Second, GBVS creates the activation maps on certain feature channels.

Given a feature map $M : R^2 \to R$, a location $(x, y) \in R^2$ which is somehow unusual in its neighborhood should take a high value in activation map $A : R^2 \to R$. So a dissimilarity of $M(i, j)$ and $M(p, q)$ is defined as

$$d\left((i, j) \parallel (p, q)\right) \triangleq \left| \log \frac{M(i, j)}{M(p, q)} \right|. \tag{16.4}$$

A fully connected directed graph G_A is built by connecting every node of M with a weight of the edge, and the weight from node (i, j) to node (p, q) of the lattice M is defined as

$$w\left((i, j) \parallel (p, q)\right) \triangleq d\left((i, j) \parallel (p, q)\right) \cdot F\left(i - p, j - q\right), \tag{16.5}$$

where $F(a, b) \triangleq \exp(-(a^2 + b^2)/(2\sigma^2))$, σ is a free parameter.

The last step, that is, normalization, is to concentrate activation into a few key locations. Given an activation map $A : R^2 \to R$, a graph G_N is built by connecting all nodes in A. For each node (i, j) and every node (p, q) to which it is connected, a weight is defined as

$$w_2((i, j) \parallel (p, q)) \triangleq A(p, q) \cdot F(i - p, j - q). \tag{16.6}$$

Once the equilibrium distribution is obtained, the normalization is finished, and the saliency map is built. The saliency map responds the extent of human's visual concentration, and it could be taken as a reasonable clue to guide segmentation.

16.2.3   The locality persevering projections

In general, the number of shape priors is usually limited and the dimensionality of shape priors is very high, which result in the shape priors getting distributed sparsely into a high dimensional space. This sparseness is not conducive to an accurate statistical model. To overcome it, locality preserving projections, that is, LPP, is employed to project these shape priors from the high dimensional space onto a low dimensional subspace [23]. LPP accomplishes dimensionality reduction by minimizing an objective function [24], that is,

$$\sum_{i,j} \left(\psi'_i - \psi'_j\right)^2 W_{i,j}, \tag{16.7}$$

where ψ'_i and ψ'_j are the projections in subspace corresponding to the aligned shape priors ψ_i and ψ_j in high dimensional space, respectively; $W_{i,j}$ is a weighting matrix to keep the neighborhood in observation space being still together in subspace. This minimization problem could be solved by

$$\Psi L \Psi^T a_i = \lambda \Psi D \Psi^T a_i, \tag{16.8}$$

where $\Psi = [\psi_1, \psi_1, \dots, \psi_N]$, that is, the i-th column of Ψ is ψ_i, and α_i is the solution of Equation 16.8; L is a Laplacian matrix and is built by $L = D - W$, where D is a diagonal matrix whose diagonal entry is defined as

$$D_{ii} = \sum_j W_{ij}. \tag{16.9}$$

Let $\alpha_0, \alpha_2, \ldots, \alpha_{l-1}$ be the solutions of Equation 16.8, the embedding is as follows:

$$\psi_i \rightarrow \tilde{\psi}_i = A^T \psi_i, \tag{16.10}$$

where $A = [\alpha_0, \alpha_2, K, \alpha_{l-1}]$, and is a $n \times l$ matrix, $\tilde{\psi}_i$ is a l-dimensional vector.

It is worth noting that although LPP is a linear operation, it possesses many data representation properties of nonlinear techniques.

16.3   *The salient object segmentation by LSM with shape priors*

This section first presents the curve's initialization according to saliency map and the evolution in the manner of multiple channel in which the saliency map is involved. Second, it comprehensively describes shape alignment and the design of energy regularization term of shape priors in a low-dimensional subspace. Finally, the whole energy functional is presented and numerically resolved.

16.3.1   *The initialization of curve and data-driven energy term*

For LSMs, a reasonable initial value close to the global extreme minimum contributes to obtaining a stable solution in a fewer iterations. A saliency map presents a visual guide for segmentation illustrated by a binary image as follows.

A saliency map utilizes a score value ranged in $[0, 1]$ to depict the visual attention. Figure 16.1 shows that the salient map of a binary image with an airplane. The different contour lines of a saliency map could depict the outline of a salient object. Inspired by this, a simple way based on threshold could be employed to guide the curve's initialization. Taking the salient score as a probability of the pixel belonging object, we just assume that the ε-level set of saliency map is the outline of the object to be segmented. This could be formulated as

$$C_0 = \left\{ (x, y) \mid S(x, y) = \varepsilon \right\}, \tag{16.11}$$

where ε is an adjustable constant controlling the area of salient region. In such way, the initial curve C_0 is placed around the salient object which will avoid manual initialization, and accelerate the evolution of curve. Once the planar initial curve is determined, we can initialize the LSF according to C_0 according to Equation 16.2.

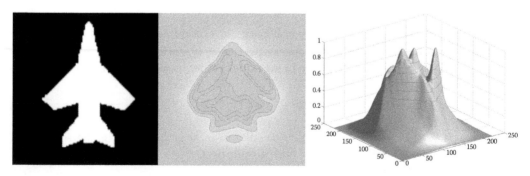

Figure 16.1 An initialization of curve according to saliency map. The left one is the shape encoded by binary image; the middle one is its saliency map with contour map; and the right one is the one in 3D space.

Considering that the initialization based on saliency map cannot guarantee the curve move to the salient object, we subsequently incorporate the saliency map into the curve's evolution by

$$E_{saln} = \lambda_1 \int_{\Omega} \left| S(x,y) - c_1^{saln} \right|^2 H(\phi) \, dx \, dy \tag{16.12}$$

$$+ \lambda_2 \int_{\Omega} \left| S(x,y) - c_2^{saln} \right|^2 (1 - H(\phi)) \, dx \, dy,$$

where c_1^{saln} and c_2^{saln} are the means inside and outside of the curve C on the saliency map S, and computed respectively as

$$c_1^{saln} = \frac{\int_{\Omega} SH() \phi \, dx \, dy}{\int_{\Omega} H(\phi) \, dx \, dy}, \quad c_2^{saln} = \frac{\int_{\Omega} S(1 - H(\phi)) \, dx \, dy}{\int_{\Omega} (1 - H(\phi)) \, dx \, dy}. \tag{16.13}$$

Combining E_{saln} with the energy term E_{data}^{cv} which is the fitting error between the image and it's piecewise constant approximation, we redesign the data-driven energy term as

$$E_{data} = E_{saln} + E_{data}^{cv}. \tag{16.14}$$

Rewriting the above equation in a vector form, we can obtain

$$E_{data} = \vec{\lambda}_1^T \int_{\Omega} |[I,S]^T - \vec{c}_1|^2 H(\phi) dx \, dy$$

$$+ \vec{\lambda}_2^T \int_{\Omega} |[I,S]^T - \vec{c}_2|^2 (1 - H(\phi)) \, dx \, dy, \tag{16.15}$$

where $[S,I]$ is the abbreviation of $[S(x,y), I(x,y)]$ which is a row vector, $\vec{c}_i$ and $\vec{\lambda}_i$ are the abbreviations of the column vector $[c_i, c_i^{saln}]^T$ and $[\lambda_i, \lambda_i^{saln}]^T$, respectively. Thus, the saliency map is incorporated into curve's evolution in the manner of multiple channels to drive the curve move to the salient object.

16.3.2 The energy term with shape priors

Due to the presence of noise and occlusion, LSMs without external constraint usually could not produce the desired result on the objects with weak boundaries and in the noisy complex background. Shape priors as a reasonable external constraint are introduced by many studies. Here, we involve constraint of shape priors by an energy term designed in subspace [23]. The specified process can be divided into two steps as follows.

16.3.2.1 Step 1: The shape prior alignment
Image moments are applied to intrinsically describe the segmented objects which are usually presented by a binary image. Considering the shape prior is encoded by a binary image

too, here, image moments are utilized for the shape alignment. A general definition of moments is

$$M_{p,q} = \sum_x \sum_y x^p y^q I(x,y).$$ (16.16)

Then, the center of object is

$$\begin{cases} x_0 = \dfrac{M_{10}}{M_{00}} \\[2mm] y_0 = \dfrac{M_{01}}{M_{00}}, \end{cases}$$ (16.17)

which could be used to make a translation transformation. When $I(x,y)$ is a binary image, the 0-order moment M_{00} equals the area of the interested object. Thus, we employ it for aligning the shape prior into a same scale. The scale ratio is

$$s_i = \frac{M_{00}^{base}}{M_{00}^{s_i}}$$ (16.18)

where M_{00}^{base} is the 0-order moment of a randomly selected benchmark shape prior with which all priors will be aligned, and $M_{00}^{s_i}$ is the 0-order moment of the i-th shape prior. The principle orientation of the i-th shape prior is computed as

$$\theta_i = \frac{1}{2} \arctan\left(\frac{2M_{11}}{M_{20} - M_{02}}\right).$$ (16.19)

Once the orientation is known, these shape priors can be aligned in term of angle by rotating a certain angle, that is,

$$\nabla\theta_i = \theta_i - \theta_{base}.$$ (16.20)

To put it briefly, before projected onto the low-dimensional subspace, the shape priors should be aligned by an affine transformation including translation (Equation 16.17), rotation (Equation 16.20), and scale (Equation 16.18).

16.3.2.2   Step 2: The energy term design

To avoid modeling energy term in a high-dimensional observation space, shape priors are usually projected onto a low dimensional subspace expanded by some leading eigenvectors. This procedure is finished by using Equation 16.10. After that, the associated energy term could be designed. We focus on a general case, that is, the multiple shape priors. Inspired by Cremers et al. [22], here we employed Kernel density estimation (KDE) to model the distribution in subspace. The Heaviside function $H(\cdot)$ truncates the LSF ϕ and concentrates on the shape of curve rather than the LSF. Consequently, instead of LSF ϕ we employ $H(\phi)$ to make a comparison between the shape of current curve and the shapes priors. The energy term associated with shape constraint is defined as

$$E_{shape} = -\ln\left(\frac{1}{N}\sum_{i=1}^{N}\exp\left(-\frac{d^2(H(\phi)', H(\tilde{\psi})_i')}{2\sigma^2}\right)\right)$$ (16.21)

where $H(\phi)$ is the current LSF ϕ applied Heaviside function, and $H(\psi)_i$ is actually the i-th LSF $\tilde{\psi}_i$ (i.e., shape prior encoded by LSF) applied Heaviside function. $H(\phi)'$ and $H(\tilde{\psi})'_i$ are the projection of $H(\phi)$ and $H(\tilde{\psi})_i$ respectively in observation space. $d(\cdot)$ is a Euclidean distance function measuring the similarity of two shapes encoded by LSF.

16.3.3   The energy functional

After the energy terms discussed above are obtained, we combine these energy terms with E_{curve} to build a whole energy functional. The proposed energy functional is conceptually defined as

$$E = \frac{1}{\beta}(E_{curve} + E_{data}) + E_{shape} \tag{16.22}$$

where $E_{curve} = E_{curve}^{cv}$ in Equation 16.1. Substituting Equations 16.15 and 16.21 into Equation 16.22, we could obtain the following equation:

$$
\begin{aligned}
E = \frac{1}{\beta}\Bigg\{ & \delta(\phi)\,|\nabla\phi| + \vec{\lambda}_1^T \int_\Omega \left\| [I,S]^T - \vec{c}_1 \right\|^2 H(\phi)\,dx\,dy \\
& + \vec{\lambda}_2^T \int_\Omega \left\| [I,S]^T - \vec{c}_2 \right\|^2 (1 - H(\phi))\,dx\,dy \Bigg\} \\
& + \ln\left(\frac{1}{N}\sum_{i=1}^N \exp\left(-\frac{d^2\left(H(\phi)',H(\tilde{\psi})'_i\right)}{2\sigma^2} \right) \right),
\end{aligned}
\tag{16.23}
$$

where

$$\sigma^2 = \frac{1}{N}\sum_{i=1}^N \min_{j\neq i} d^2(H(\tilde{\psi})'_i, H(\tilde{\psi})'_j). \tag{16.24}$$

Applying Euler–Lagrange equation, we could deduce the evolution equation as follows:

$$
\begin{aligned}
\frac{\partial\phi}{\partial t} = \frac{1}{\beta}\delta(\phi)&\left[div\left(\frac{\nabla\phi}{|\nabla\phi|} \right) - \vec{\lambda}_1^T |[I,S]^T - \vec{c}_1|^2 + \vec{\lambda}_2^T |[I,S]^T - \vec{c}_2|^2 \right] \\
& + \frac{\sum_{i=1}^N b_i(H(\phi)' - H(\tilde{\psi})'_i)A^T\delta(\phi)}{2\sigma^2\sum_{i=1}^N b_i},
\end{aligned}
\tag{16.25}
$$

where

$$b_i = \exp\left(-\frac{d^2\left(H(\phi)',H(\tilde{\psi})'_i\right)}{2\sigma^2} \right). \tag{16.26}$$

Thus far, we have designed the entire energy functional and deduced the relevant PDE. This PDE is numerically resolved to realize salient object segmentation by LSM with shape priors.

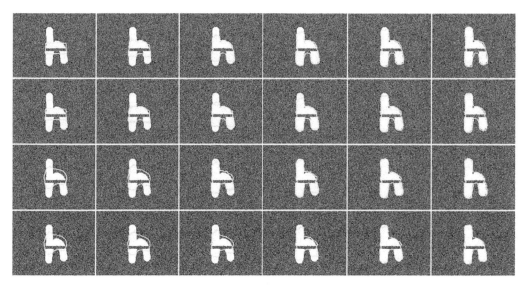

Figure 16.2 The comparison on a synthetic image. The segmentation procedures of M1, M2, M3, and M4 are ordered from the top row to the bottom one.

16.4   Experiments

To verify the performance of the proposed method, we compare it with Cremer's method [22] and one of our previous work [25] on synthetic, natural and healthcare images. These two methods are denoted by M1 and M2, respectively. Additionally, the proposed method excluding saliency map from evolution is also involved into the comparison for verifying the effect of saliency map for evolution, and it is denoted by M3. Four experiments on seven images are presented to illustrate the performance qualitatively and quantitatively. To facilitate writing and reading, the above algorithms and our method are denoted by M1, M2, M3, and M4.

The parameters of the proposed method are empirically assigned as follows. ε controls the degree of saliency, and its value is chosen from the range of $[0.5, 0.8]$; β in Equation 16.23 could adjust the weighting of the energy term of data, and its value fall into the range of $[0.9, 1.1]$. In all experiments, the initial curves of M1 and M2 are manually set, and the ones of M3 and M4 are automatically created according to saliency map.

Experiment 1 executes the four methods on a synthetic image where an English character "h" is broken and noised by Gaussian noise shown in Figure 16.2. Here, nine shape priors are incorporated into the curve's evolution. The four methods are basically used to obtain the similar segmentation results in conformity with their original intention of design.

In experiment 2, the four methods are applied to two medical images, that is, mammogram. The mass in the mammogram of Figure 16.3 has a very blur edge and share the common density with the adjacent tissues; the mass in Figure 16.4 possesses a radial shape without clear boundary. These make the segmentation a challenging task. M3 and M4 could correctly find the position of the masses and place the initial curve. Additionally, M3 and M4 depart a bigger region than M1 and M2 do since saliency map is involved into curve's evolution.

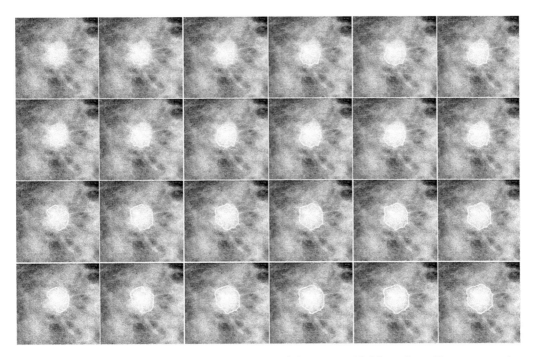

Figure 16.3 The comparison on the mammogram of the mass with blur edges. The segmentation procedures of M1, M2, M3, and M4 are ordered from the top row to the bottom one.

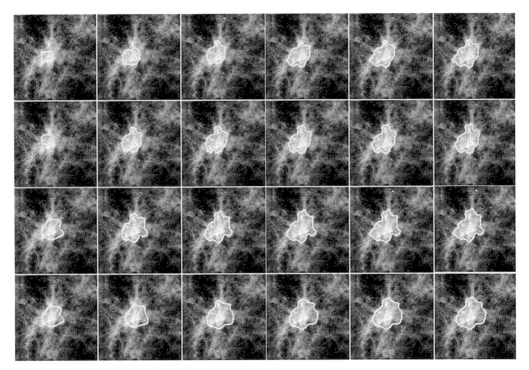

Figure 16.4 The comparison on the mammogram of radial mass. The segmentation procedures of M1, M2, M3, and M4 are ordered from the top row to the bottom one.

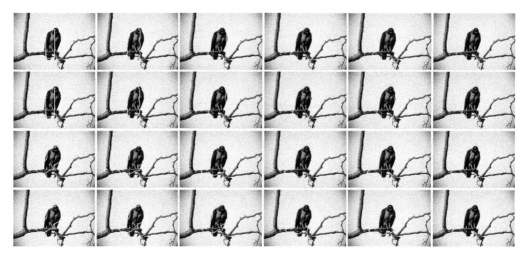

Figure 16.5 The comparison on the natural image of a bird on a tree. The segmentation procedures of M1, M2, M3, and M4 are ordered from the top row to the bottom one.

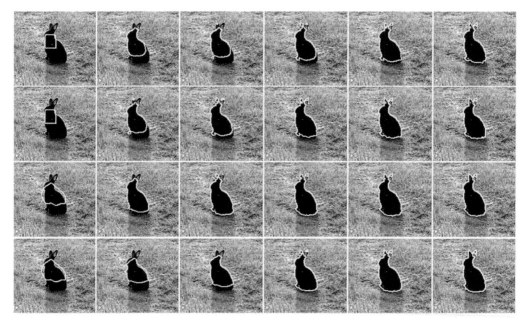

Figure 16.6 The comparison on the natural image of a rabbit on grass. The segmentation procedures of M1, M2, M3, and M4 are ordered from the top row to the bottom one.

Experiment 3 feeds four natural images to the four methods for an assessment of the performance on natural images. The results, shown in Figures 16.5 through 16.8, suggest that the proposed one could obtain the similar or better performance on these four natural images.

A form of execution time (i.e., CPU time and the number of iteration) on the aforementioned seven images is presented in experiment 4 for a quantitative comparison. The

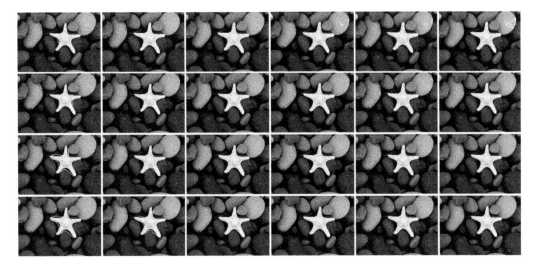

Figure 16.7 The comparison on the natural images of starfish on rocks. The segmentation procedures of M1, M2, M3, and M4 are ordered from the top row to the bottom one.

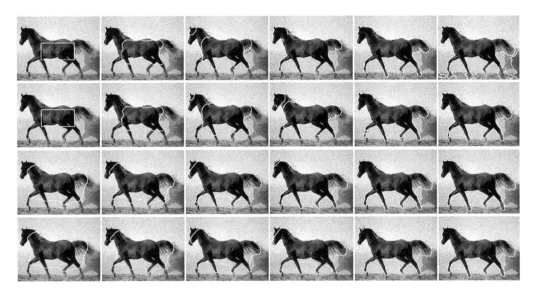

Figure 16.8 The comparison on the natural image of horses. The segmentation procedures of M1, M2, M3, and M4 are ordered from the top row to the bottom one.

quantities in Table 16.1 suggests that the proposed method achieves the shortest computational time of the four methods for segmentation. M2 projects shape priors onto a subspace, which leads to more computational time compared to M1; M3 utilizes the saliency map initialization curve around the salient object which shortens the convergence time of M2; besides the curve's initialization, M4 also involves the saliency map into evolution as an additional channel compared to M3, which further shortens the computational cost of M3.

In summary, the comparison results show that the proposed method could obtain similar or better performance compared with the representative or latest LSMs with shape priors, meanwhile, it costs the shorter computation time.

Table 16.1 Comparison of execution time

Method image	M1		M2		M3		M4	
	CPU-T	ITER	CPU-T	ITER	CPU-T	ITER	CPU-T	ITER
Figure 16.2 (200 × 150)	35.8	100	52.2	100	45.3	80	29.6	60
Figure 16.3 (170 × 160)	104.4	300	113.3	250	70.1	160	39.8	80
Figure 16.4 (128 × 128)	84.0	300	109.3	240	67.4	150	37.8	70
Figure 16.5 (240 × 160)	36.1	100	67.9	120	38.0	50	17.5	30
Figure 16.6 (151 × 130)	90.6	200	120.2	280	74.8	160	30.9	60
Figure 16.7 (335 × 233)	106.1	200	140.0	200	78.1	120	66.6	80
Figure 16.8 (232 × 174)	57.8	150	82.0	150	71.8	120	58.0	90

16.5   Conclusion

In this chapter, we presented a novel salient object segmentation by LSM with shape priors. The major works are as follows. First, saliency map could guide LSM to initialize the curve, and consequently eliminate the manual initialization to realize an automatically segmentation of salient objects. Second, a shape-based energy term, which is designed in the subspace spanned by the leading vectors of LPP, is incorporated into the entire energy functional to constraint curve's evolution. Finally, the entire energy functional is presented and numerically solved. The experiments show that the proposed method could obtain the promising result with the shorter computational time.

References

1. C. Chesnaud, P. Refregier, and V. Boulet, Statistical region snake-based segmentation adapted to different noise models, *IEEE Transactions on Pattern Analysis and Machine Intelligence*, vol. 21, no. 11, pp. 1145–1157, 1999.
2. M. Kass, A. Witkin, and D. Terzopoulos, Snakes: Active contour models, *International Journal of Computer Vision*, vol. 1, no. 4, pp. 321–331, 1988.
3. C. Xu and J. L. Prince, Snake, shapes, and gradient vector flow, *IEEE Transactions on Image Processing*, vol. 7, no. 3, pp. 359–369, 1998.
4. S. Osher and J. A. Sethian, Fronts propagating with curvature-dependent speed: Algorithms based on Hamilton-Jacobi formulation, *Journal of Computational Physics*, vol. 79, no. 1, pp. 12–49, 1988.
5. J. S. Suri, K. Liu, S. Singh, S. N. Laxminarayan, X. Zeng, and L. Reden, Shape recovery algorithms using level sets in 2D/3D medical imagery: A state-of-the-art review, *IEEE Transactions on Information Technology in Biomedicine*, vol. 6, no. 1, pp. 8–28, 2002.
6. S. Osher and R. Fedkiw, *Level Set Methods and Dynamics Implicit Surfaces*. Berlin: Springer, 2003.
7. C. Li, C. Xu, C. Gui, and M. D. Fox, Level set evolution without re-initialization: A new variational formulation, *IEEE Conference on Computer Vision Pattern Recognition*, vol. 1, pp. 430–436, 2005.
8. R. Malladi, J. A. Sethian, and B. C. Vemuri, Shape modeling with front propagation: A level set approach, *IEEE Transactions on Pattern Analysis and Machine Intelligence*, vol. 17, no. 2, pp. 158–175, 1995.
9. D. Peng, B. Merriman, S. Osher, H. K. Zhao, and M. Kang, A PDE based fast local level set method, *Journal of Computational Physics*, vol. 155, no. 2, pp. 410–438, 1999.
10. X. Gao, B. Wang, D. Tao, and X. Li, A relay level set method for automatic image segmentation, *IEEE Transactions on Systems, Management, Cybernetics B: Cybernetics*, vol. 41, no. 2, pp. 518–525, 2011.

11. C. Li, C. Xu, C. Gui, and M. D. Fox, Distance regularized level set evolution and its application to image segmentation, *IEEE Transactions on Image Processing*, vol. 19, no. 12, pp. 3243–3254, 2010.

12. B. Wang, X. Gao, D. Tao, and X. Li, A nonlinear adaptive level set for image segmentation, *IEEE Transactions on Cybernetics*, vol. 44, no. 3, pp. 418–428, 2014.

13. D. Mumford and J. Shah, Optimal approximations by piecewise smooth functions and associated variational problems, *Communications of Pure Applied Mathematics*, vol. 42, no. 5, pp. 577–685, 1989.

14. T. F. Chan and L. A. Vese, Active contours without edges, *IEEE Transactions on Image Processing*, vol. 10, no. 2, pp. 266–277, 2001.

15. T. F. Chan, B. Y. Sandberg, and L. A. Vese, Active contours without edges for vector-valued images, *Journal of Visual Communication and Image Representation*, vol. 11, no. 2, pp. 130–141, 2000.

16. L. A. Vese and T. F. Chan, A multiphase level set framework for image segmentation using the Mumford and Shah model, *International Journal of Computer Vision*, vol. 50, no. 3, pp. 271–293, 2002.

17. Z. Wang and B. C. Vemuri, DTI segmentation using an information theoretic tensor dissimilarity measure, *IEEE Transactions on Medical Imaging*, vol. 24, no. 10, pp. 1267–1277, 2005.

18. B. Wang, X. Gao, D. Tao, and X. Li, A unified tensor level set for image segmentation, *IEEE Transactions on Systems, Management, and Cybernetics B: Cybernetics*, vol. 40, no. 3, pp. 857–867, 2010.

19. A. Tsai, A. Yezzi, and A. S. Willsky, Curve evolution implementation of the Mumford–Shah functional for image segmentation, denoising, interpolation, and magnification, *IEEE Transactions on Image Processing*, vol. 10, pp. 1169–1186, 2001.

20. C. Li, R. Huang, J. C. Gatenby, D. N. Metaxas, and J. C. Gore, A level set method for image segmentation in the presence of intensity inhomogeneities with application to MRI, *IEEE Transactions on Image Processing*, vol. 20, no. 7, pp. 2007–2016, 2011.

21. A. Tsai, A. Yezzi, W. Wells, C. Tempany, D. Tucker, A. Fan, W. E. Grimson, and A. Willsky, A shape-based approach to the segmentation of medical imagery using level sets, *IEEE Transactions on Medical Imaging*, vol. 22, no. 2, pp. 137–154, 2003.

22. D. Cremers, S. J. Osher, and S. Soatto, Kernel density estimation and intrinsic alignment for shape priors in level set segmentation, *International Journal of Computer Vision*, vol. 69, no. 3, pp. 335–351, 2006.

23. S. Dambreville, Y. Rathi, and A. Tannenbaum, A framework for image segmentation using shape models and kernel space shape priors, *IEEE Transactions on Pattern Analysis and Machine Intelligence*, vol. 30, no. 8, pp. 1385–1399, 2008.

24. He, X. and P. Niyogi, The LPP algorithm, *Advances in Neural Information Processing Systems 16 (NIPS)*, vol. 1, pp. 153–160, 2003.

25. B. Wang, X. Gao, J. Li, X. Li, and D. Tao, A level set with shape priors using moment-based alignment and locality preserving projections, *Proceedings of the 2013 International Conference on Intelligence Science and Big Data Engineering (IScIDE 2013)*, LNCS 8261, pp. 697–704, 2013.

26. C. Koch and S. Ullman, Shifts in selective visual attention: Towards the underlying neural circuitry, *Human Neurobiology*, vol. 4, no. 4, pp. 219–227, 1985.

27. L. Itti, C. Koch, and E. Niebur, A model of saliency-based visual attention for rapid scene analysis, *IEEE Transactions on Pattern Analysis and Machine Intelligence*, vol. 20, no. 11, pp. 1254–1259, 1998.

28. J. Harel, C. Koch, and P. Perona, Graph-based visual saliency, *Advances in Neural Information Processing Systems*, pp. 545–552, 2007.

29. V. Gopalakrishnan, Y. Hu, and D. Rajan, Random walks on graphs to model saliency in images, *IEEE Conference on Computer Vision and Pattern Recognition*, pp. 1698–1705, 2009.

30. X. Hou and L. Zhang, Saliency detection: A spectral residual approach, *IEEE Conference on Computer Vision and Pattern Recognition*, pp. 1–8, 2007.

31. R. Achanta, F. Estrada, P. Wils, and S. Susstrunk, Salient region detection and segmentation, *International Conference on Computer Vision Systems*, pp. 66–75, 2008.
32. S. Goferman, L. Zelnik-Manor, and A. Tal, Context-aware saliency detection, *IEEE Conference on Computer Vision and Pattern Recognition*, pp. 2376–2383, 2010.
33. M. Cheng, G. Zhang, and N. Mitra, Global contrast based salient region detection, *IEEE Conference on Computer Vision and Pattern Recognition*, pp. 409–416, 2011.
34. L. Cohen, Global minimum for active contour models: A minimal path approach, *International Journal of Computer Vision*, vol. 24, no. 1, pp. 57–778, 1997.
35. S. Lee and J. Seo, Level set-based bimodal segmentation with stationary global minimum, *IEEE Transactions on Image Processing*, vol. 15, no. 9, pp. 2843–2852, 2006.
36. K. Zhang, L. Zhang, H. Song, and W. Zhou, Active contours with selective local or global segmentation: A new formulation and level set method, *Image Vision computing*, vol. 28, no. 4, pp. 668–676, 2010.

chapter seventeen

Tracking and segmentation of the endocardium of the left ventricle in a 2D ultrasound using deep learning architectures and Monte Carlo sampling

Jacinto C. Nascimento, Gustavo Carneiro, and António Freitas

Contents

Abstract

The tracking and segmentation of the left ventricle (LV) of the heart from ultrasound data still deserves the attention in medical image community, being a commonly used method in practical clinical setup nowadays. The goal above stated can be formulated as a sequential state estimation problem, which is essential to the study of linear and nonlinear dynamical systems. In this work, we present a particle filter-based approach, rooted in Bayesian estimation and Monte Carlo procedures, for tracking and segmenting the LV. Two main ingredients characterize this formalism: the prediction that models the dynamic of the object in consecutive frames and filtering that collects information in the present frame. This methodology allows the computation of the expected segmentation value at the current time instant of the object, given all previous and current observations. Although the probability values of the filtering distribution can be straightforwardly computed, sampling from it is challenging, so this means that a *proposal* distribution is needed since it provides an easier way for sampling the filtering distribution. In this work, we present an algorithm for tracking and segmenting the LV in 2D ultrasound data based on the observations made above. The contributions are as follows: (i) a new transition model (prediction) that combines different motion regimes presented in the systole and diastole phases of the cardiac cycle, (ii) a new observation model (filtering) built with a deep neural network, and (iii) a new proposal distribution for efficient sampling mechanism. The usefulness of our approach is evaluated using a database of disease cases and another dataset of normal cases, where both datasets present long axis views of the left ventricle. Using a training set comprising diseased and healthy cases, we show that our approach produces accurate results for tracking the endocardium. Also, we show that our method correlates well with interuser statistics produced by four cardiologists.

17.1 Introduction

Automatic tracking and segmentation of the left ventricle (LV) endocardium of the heart is an important step toward the estimation of the heart condition, since its quantitative measurement is used as a crucial indicator of the cardiac health. Such tool is able to provide useful information to improve the workflow by increasing the patient throughput and decreasing the interuser variability. Moreover, it constitutes a way of measuring the dynamic behavior of the human heart, where the regional characterization of the heart wall motion is necessary to isolate the severity and extent of diseases such as ischemia. Other features, such as the ejection fraction of the left ventricle, the left ventricle mass of the myocardium and wall thickness and thickening constitute important information that can be accessed with such automatic procedure.

This is, however, a difficult problem to be fully solved. Indeed, when developing an algorithm for tracking and segmenting the LV, several problems are encountered in ultrasound data. This usually comprises: (i) fast motion during systole (contraction) phase, (ii) low signal-to-noise ratio, (iii) edge dropout caused by motion, (iv) presence of shadows produced by the dense muscles, (v) specific properties and settings of the ultrasound machine, as well as (vi) anisotropy of the ultrasonic image formation [1]. In ultrasound images, the LV appearance is characterized by a dark region, representing the blood pool inside the chamber, enclosed by the endocardium, myocardium, and epicardium, which are roughly depicted by a brighter region. Also note that specific spatial texture and gray value distribution of each region vary substantially among different cases and even within each case. All the above mentioned issues impose obstacles when developing an automatic procedure for the LV segmentation in ultrasound data.

Most of the current methodologies formulate the problem of tracking as a state estimation problem, in which the expected segmentation is computed taking into account the previous and current observations over the space of segmentation parameters [2]. Under this formalism, the segmentation parameters constitute the state vector while the image represents the observations. The expected segmentation described above is computed using the filtering distribution, which calculates the probability of a possible segmentation given the previous and current observations. The computation of this expected value is not possible to be obtained analytically, given the high number of dimensions of the space of segmentation parameters and the non-Gaussianity of the distribution. As such, it is common to approximate this expected value using sequential Monte Carlo (SMC) sampling techniques, meaning that only a few weighted samples (each sample representing a segmentation of the object) are needed to produce the expected value. The weights in the samples are computed using the observation and transition models, while the samples are obtained from sampling the filtering distribution [3]. Another usual problem is the difficulty in sampling this filtering distribution, which is solved by sampling another distribution, called the proposal distribution, that provides a reasonable approximation to the filtering distribution, but being much simpler to sample. Then the probability of the proposal distribution has to be taken into account when calculating the sample weights. Finally, using the samples and their respective weights, it is possible to compute the expected segmentation mentioned above.

17.2   Related work

Several trends characterize the related work for object segmentation. One such trend is represented by the active contours [4] whose geometry allows a broad shape coverage by employing a geometric representation that involves many degrees of freedom. The deformable model designation stems from the use of elasticity theory at the physical level within a Lagrangian dynamics setting. In particular, deformable model acts as an elastic body that responds to applied forces and constraints, and coupled with it an energy is associated and modified as the deformable model moves in the image domain. In the Lagrangian setting, the deformation energy is associated to elastic forces that are internal to the model, which are called internal forces (i.e., the prior). Under physics perspective, the external potential energy functions are defined in terms of data of interest in the image (e.g., boundary of the object to be segmented). These potential energies are associated to the external forces that are able to deform the model to fit the desired data. The energy of the deformable model is supposed to be minimal when the deformable model is located at boundary of interest (external energy) and has a shape that is supposed to be relevant considering the shape of the sought object (internal energy).

Though successful at several tasks [5,6], problems regarding the initialization, as well as the presence of outliers in the image motivated the development of level set methods [7]. Level set theory aims to exchange the Lagrangian formalization (used in active contours) and replace it with a Eulerian form. In this class of approaches, the initial valued partial differential equations control the front (i.e., boundary of the object) evolution, representing the boundary as the zero level set instance. For the level set class of approaches, the LV contour is represented by the zero-level in the signed distance function. In general the level set-based approaches can provide higher robustness against the initialization [6,8–16] and robustness to sharp corners and cusps. Although, level sets have shown outstanding results in medical image applications, they face limitations when dealing with the prior knowledge defined in the optimization function regarding the LV boundary, shape, and texture distribution.

The above issues motivated another line of research, namely the pattern recognition methods that involve the use of a database of annotated LV images (i.e., a training set) to automatically build a model of the LV shape and appearance. One of the first examples of pattern recognition models is the active shape and appearance model [1,17–19]. There are a few issues that affect these approaches: (1) need of large annotated training set, (2) during inference, the initialization must be close to a local optimum, and (3) the Gaussian distribution assumption for the shape and appearance models constrain their capacity. The initialization problem has been successfully handled [20,21], but the large training set is still an issue in the field.

Though receiving less attention, the transition model plays an important role in the computation of the filtering distribution, since it conveys information about the dynamics. The most usual transition model is the prediction estimated from the Kalman filtering [22]. However, the Gaussian assumption of the Kalman filter is not realistic, given the complex motion patterns of the heart that violates such assumption. More interesting transition models are built when providing more degrees of freedom to explain those motion patterns that are more likely to happen in practice. For instance, Sun et al. [23] introduce a transition model that is learned from training data using an information-theoretic criterion, but the lack of a prior distribution in the model imposes the need of a large training set to provide a reliable transition model. A related approach is proposed by Yang et al. [24] consisting of a transition model that depends not only on the previous state vector, but also on all state vectors up to current time instant. As previously, this model is also automatically learned from training data and consists of a manifold describing the motion pattern of the heart. Models based solely on prior information [25] also seem inadequate given that there might be information present in training data that may not have been captured by the prior. The transition model proposed by Nascimento [26] consisting of a mixture of two models (one for systole and another for diastole) seems more adequate, and inspired us to implement our transition model. The main difference is that we use both a prior information on the motion patterns, assuming the existence of two cardiac cycles (i.e., systole and diastole), and a learned model from data instead of a transition model containing only prior distributions [26].

Concerning now the tracking methods based on SMC sampling techniques, it is necessary to use a proposal distribution that approximates the filtering distribution reasonably well [3]. Sénégas et al. [25] propose an SMC sampling method using a proposal distribution based only on the observation model, which does not take into consideration the transition model. Sun et al. [23] introduce a proposal distribution based only on the transition model, which also presents a limitation given that the observation model is not considered. The work that inspired our model was proposed by Okuma et al. [27], who proposed a tracking algorithm (i.e., not LV tracking) combining discriminative classifier detections and particle filtering to track multitarget nonrigid objects. Notice, however, that the work presented herein contrasts with Okuma et al. [27] in sense that we are now concerned with the precision of the segmentation, which is a mandatory requirement concerning the segmentation of the LV.

17.3 Contributions

In this chapter, we propose a new LV tracking algorithm based on SMC methods. See Figure 17.1 for an illustration of the proposal. Our main contributions are the following:

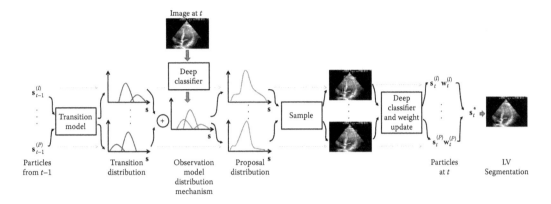

Figure 17.1 Block diagram containing all steps of the tracking algorithm proposed in this chapter.

1. *New transition model*: The transition model proposed in this chapter makes use of the prior information that at each time instant, the heart is either expanding (diastole) or contracting (systole). The deformation caused by these motion patterns is described by a linear transform, whose parameters are learned from the training data.

2. *New observation model*: The model is built with deep learning architectures, which involves a statistical pattern recognition model, where we address the robustness to imaging conditions unseen in training data. In order to handle the robustness to imaging conditions, we move away from the use of boosting classifiers [21], and rely on the use of deep neural network classifiers [28]. The main advantage of deep neural networks is its ability to produce more abstract feature spaces for classification and to automatically generate optimum feature spaces directly from image data.

3. *New proposal distribution*: The proposal is inspired by the work of Okuma et al. [27], which combines the detection results from the deep learning architecture with the transition model. This combination provides precise segmentation, and robustness to imaging conditions and drifting.

17.4 Statistical model of the segmentation algorithm

We assume a non-Gaussian state-space model, where the state sequence is a process represented by $\{k_t, \mathbf{s}_t | t \in \mathbb{N}\}$, where $k \in \{\text{systole}, \text{diastole}\}$ is a (discrete) label indicating the cardiac phase at t-th time instant, and $\mathbf{s} \in \mathbb{R}^{2N}$ denotes the contour representation with N key points. The above hybrid state is assumed to be an unobserved (hidden) Markov process with the initial state distribution represented by $p(k_0, \mathbf{s}_0)$ and the transition distribution that takes into consideration the previous cardiac phase and contour representation with $p(k_t, \mathbf{s}_t | k_{t-1}, \mathbf{s}_{t-1})$. The observations consist of the images $\{I_t | t \in \mathbb{N}^*\}$, which are conditionally independent given the process $\{k_t, \mathbf{s}_t | t \in \mathbb{N}\}$, with marginal distribution $p(I_t | k_t, \mathbf{s}_t)$. Also, we assume the existence of a training set $\mathcal{D} = \{(I, \theta, \mathbf{s}, k)_j\}_{j=1}^{M}$ containing M training images I of the ultrasound imaging of LV, the parameters of a rigid transformation $\theta = [\mathbf{x}, \gamma, \sigma] \in \mathbb{R}^5$ (position $\mathbf{x} \in \mathbb{R}^2$, orientation $\gamma \in [-\pi, \pi]$, and scale $\sigma \in \mathbb{R}^2$) that aligns rigidly the annotation points to a canonical coordinate system (see Figure 17.2), a respective

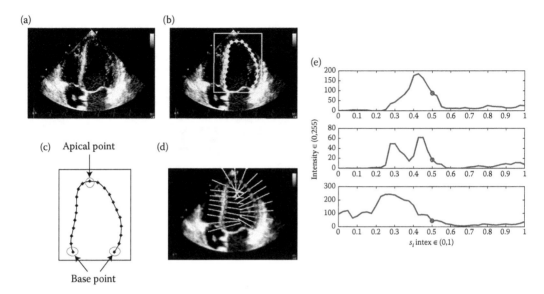

Figure 17.2 (a) Original training image; (b) manual segmentation of the LV in yellow dots inside the rectangular patch (yellow lines); (c) representation of the canonical coordinate system for LV contour with the base and apical points highlighted and located at their canonical locations within the patch delimited in (b); (d) orthogonal lines radiating from the points depicted in (b); (e) intensity profiles in three lines.

manual annotation $\mathbf{s} \in \mathbb{R}^{2N}$ in this canonical coordinate system (this means that the contour has N two-dimensional points), and $k \in \{\text{systole,diastole}\}$, which denotes the phase of the cardiac cycle.

17.4.1   An overview of the method

The goal of the algorithm proposed herein is to produce a segmentation $\mathbf{s}_t$ for each frame I_t, where $t \in \{1, ..., T\}$ represents the time variable with T denoting the number of frames in the sequence. The optimal contour at each time instant t is produced as follows:

$$\mathbf{s}_t^* = \int_{\mathbf{s}_t} \mathbf{s}_t p(\mathbf{s}_t | I_{1:t}) d\mathbf{s}_t, \tag{17.1}$$

The above integral is difficult to compute given the high space dimensionality of $\mathbf{s}$. Thus, we resort to use the sequential importance resampling (SIR) algorithm [3] to estimate it. With SIR, the filtering distribution $p(\mathbf{s}_t | I_{1:t})$ is approximated with a set of P weights and particles $\{w_t^{(l)}, \mathbf{s}_t^{(l)}\}_{l=1}^{P}$, which can approximate the segmentation as illustrated by Doucet et al. [2]:

$$\mathbf{s}_t^* \approx \sum_{l=1}^{P} \mathbf{s}_t^{(l)} w_t^{(l)}, \tag{17.2}$$

with $w_t^{(l)} \approx p(\mathbf{s}_t^{(l)} | I_{1:t})$ and $\sum_{l=1}^{P} w_t^{(l)} = 1$. The main steps of the SIR method are listed in Algorithm 17.1

ALGORITHM 17.1 SIR Algorithm

1: **for** $t = 1$ to T **do**
2: sample $\{k_t^{(l)}, \mathbf{s}_t^{(l)}\}_{l=1}^{P}$
3: Update sample weights $\{\tilde{w}_t^{(l)}\}_{l=1}^{P}$
4: Normalize sample weights: $w_t^{(l)} = \dfrac{\tilde{w}_t^{(l)}}{\sum_l \tilde{w}_t^{(l)}}$ for $l \in \{1, ..., P\}$;
5: Compute effective number of particles $N_{eff} = 1/\sum_l (w_t^{(l)})^2$;
6: **if** $N_{eff} < K_{Neff} \times P$ **then**
7:    resample by drawing P particles from current particle set proportionally to weight and replace particle, and set $w_t^{(l)} = 1/P$ for $l \in \{1, ..., P\}$
8: **end if**
9: Compute LV segmentation for I_t, i.e., how it is computed $\mathbf{s}_t^*$ in Equation 17.2
10: **end for**

One of the issues of the SIR algorithm is that while it is easy to compute $p(\mathbf{s}_t^{(l)}|I_{1:t})$ for a contour $\mathbf{s}_t^{(l)}$, it is hard to sample from this distribution, so it is necessary to have a proposal distribution that approximates well this filtering distribution, and from which is relatively simple to sample. In the next sections we describe the main components of the proposed model comprising the transition model, the observation model and the proposal detailing precisely how do we compute the steps 2, 3, and 9 shown in Algorithm 17.1.

17.4.2 Transition model

One of our contributions is the definition of the transition model. The main assumptions are: the current cardiac phase k_t only depends on the previous cardiac phase k_{t-1} and the current LV contour $\mathbf{s}_t$ depends on the previous contour $\mathbf{s}_{t-1}$ as well as the previous cardiac phase k_{t-1}. Based on these assumptions, the transition model becomes:

$$p(k_t, \mathbf{s}_t|k_{t-1}, \mathbf{s}_{t-1}) = p(k_t|k_{t-1})p(\mathbf{s}_t|k_{t-1}, \mathbf{s}_{t-1}), \tag{17.3}$$

where $p(k_t|k_{t-1})$ stands for the switching/staying of the cardiac phases at each time step. The second term in Equation 17.3, is given as

$$p(\mathbf{s}_t|k_{t-1}, \mathbf{s}_{t-1}) = g(\mathbf{s}_t|f(\mathbf{s}_{t-1}, \mathbf{M}(k_{t-1})), \Sigma_\mathbf{s}), \tag{17.4}$$

where $g(.)$ represents a multivariate Gaussian density function, the function $f(.)$ produces an affine transformation of the contour $\mathbf{s}_{t-1}$; $\mathbf{M}(k_{t-1})$ is a linear transform of the contour $\mathbf{s}_{t-1}$ learned from the training data that allows an expansion (or contraction) according to the phase k_{t-1}; and $\Sigma_\mathbf{s}$ is the covariance of the annotations obtained during the training phase.

17.4.3 Observation model

The observation model is defined as the process of image formation assumed to be

$$p(I_t|k_t, \mathbf{s}_t) \propto p(k_t, \mathbf{s}_t|I_t)p(I_t), \tag{17.5}$$

where $p(I_t)$ is constant and the first term expanded as follows

$$p(k_t, \mathbf{s}_t | I_t) = \int_\theta p(k_t | \theta, I_t) p(\mathbf{s}_t | \theta, k_t, I_t) p(\theta | I_t) d\theta. \qquad (17.6)$$

Equation 17.6 contains three terms: the rigid (affine) detection contained in $p(k_t | \theta, I_t)$, the nonrigid segmentation in $p(\mathbf{s}_t | \theta, k_t, I_t)$, and the prior distribution of the rigid detection $p(\theta | I_t)$.

The first term in Equation 17.6 represents the rigid detection that is computed using discriminative classifier. The classifier receives as input an image patch extracted from image I_t using θ and outputs the probability of $k_t \in \{\text{systole, diastole}\}$. Figure 17.2b,c illustrates how the image patch is extracted given the aligned base and apical points. The second term in Equation 17.6, represents the nonrigid segmentation that is defined as follows:

$$p(\mathbf{s}_t | \theta, k_t, I_t) = \prod_{i=1}^{N} p(\mathbf{s}_t(i) | \theta, k_t, I_t), \qquad (17.7)$$

where $p(\mathbf{s}_t(i) | \theta, k_t, I_t)$ represents the probability that the *ith* contour keypoint $\mathbf{s}_t(i) \in \mathbb{R}^2$ is located at the LV contour. Figure 17.2d shows that for each $i \in \{1, ..., N\}$ the possible $\mathbf{s}_t(i)$ is confined to points lying on a line orthogonal to the LV contour.

Finally, the third term in Equation 17.16 is defined as $p(\theta | I_t) = g(\theta | \bar{\theta}, \Sigma_\theta)$, where $\bar{\theta}$ and Σ_θ are the mean and covariance values of the training set values for θ, and $g(.)$ denotes the multivariate Gaussian density function.

17.4.4   The filtering distribution

From the transition model defined in Section 17.4.2, and the observation model detailed in Section 17.4.3 we can now derive the solution to the filtering problem. Denoting the state and observation vectors up to time instant t as $\mathbf{s}_{0:t} \triangleq \{\mathbf{s}_0, ..., \mathbf{s}_t\}$ (similarly for $k_{0:t}$ and $I_{1:t}$), the solution is given by the following Bayesian recursion [2]:

$$
\begin{aligned}
p(k_t, \mathbf{s}_t | I_{1:t}) &= \frac{p(I_t | k_t, \mathbf{s}_t) p(k_t, \mathbf{s}_t | I_{1:t-1})}{p(I_t | I_{1:t-1})} \\
&= \frac{p(I_t | k_t, \mathbf{s}_t) \sum_{k_{t-1}} \int p(k_t, \mathbf{s}_t | k_{t-1}, \mathbf{s}_{t-1}) p(k_{t-1}, \mathbf{s}_{t-1} | I_{1:t-1}) d\mathbf{s}_{t-1}}{\sum_{k_t} \int p(I_t | k_t, \mathbf{s}_t) p(k_t, \mathbf{s}_t | I_{1:t-1}) d\mathbf{s}_t},
\end{aligned}
\qquad (17.8)
$$

where $p(k_t, \mathbf{s}_t | I_{1:t-1}) = \sum_{k_t} \int p(k_t, \mathbf{s}_t | k_{t-1}, \mathbf{s}_{t-1}) p(k_{t-1}, \mathbf{s}_{t-1} | I_{1:t-1}) d\mathbf{s}_{t-1}$. The first term (in the numerator of Equation 17.8) is the observation model given in Equation 17.5, the second is the transition model (see Equation 17.3), whilst the third is the available estimate at the previous time step.

Notice that Equation 17.8 computes the distribution of cardiac phases and LV contours at every single time instant without taking any option regarding the cardiac phases or contour values. This is an important issue, since it endows a robustness in the algorithm.

17.4.5 Deep particle filtering

In the particle filtering setup, the posterior $p(k_t, \mathbf{s}_t | I_{1:t})$ in Equation 17.8 is approximated with a finite set of P particles, as follows:

$$p(k_t, \mathbf{s}_t | I_{1:t}) \approx \sum_{l=1}^{P} w_t^{(l)} \delta(k_t - k_t^{(l)}) \delta(\mathbf{s}_t - \mathbf{s}_t^{(l)}), \tag{17.9}$$

where $\delta(.)$ is the delta function. The particles $\{k_t^{(l)}, \mathbf{s}_t^{(l)}\}_{l=1}^{P}$ are sampled from a proposal distribution $q(.)$ with $(k_t^{(l)}, \mathbf{s}_t^{(l)}) \sim q(k_t, \mathbf{s}_t | k_{0:t-1}^{(l)}, \mathbf{s}_{0:t-1}^{(l)}, I_{1:t})$, where each particle is expressed as

$$\tilde{w}_t^{(l)} = w_{t-1}^{(l)} \frac{p(I_t | k_t^{(l)} \mathbf{s}_t^{(l)}) p(k_t^{(l)}, \mathbf{s}_t^{(l)} | k_{t-1}^{(l)} \mathbf{s}_{t-1}^{(l)})}{q(k_t^{(l)}, \mathbf{s}_t^{(l)} | k_{0:t-1}^{(l)} \mathbf{s}_{0:t-1}^{(l)}, I_{1:t})}, \tag{17.10}$$

where $\tilde{w}_t^{(l)}$ and $w_t^{(l)}$ represent the un-normalized and normalized weights, respectively.

In this work, the proposal distribution combines both prediction and filtering distributions as in Okuma et al. [27]. The key difference is that we accomplish this task differently. More specifically, the proposal distribution takes into account a transition model (see Equation 17.3) for each particle and a detection provided by a discriminative classifier based on a deep belief network (DBN). This, of course, results in a mixture of Gaussians as follows

$$q(k_t, \mathbf{s}_t | k_{0:t-1}^{(l)}, \mathbf{s}_{0:t-1}^{(l)}, I_{1:t}) = q(k_t, \mathbf{s}_t | k_{t-1}^{(l)} \mathbf{s}_{t-1}^{(l)}, I_t)$$

$$= \alpha q_{DBN}(k_t, \mathbf{s}_t | I_t) + (1 - \alpha) p(k_t, \mathbf{s}_t | k_{t-1}^{(l)}, \mathbf{s}_{t-1}^{(l)}) \tag{17.11}$$

with the detection term (first term in Equation 17.11) given by

$$q_{DBN}(k_t, \mathbf{s}_t | I_t) = \sum_{\{\tilde{k}_t, \tilde{\mathbf{s}}_t\}} p(\tilde{k}_t, \tilde{\mathbf{s}}_t | I_t) g(\mathbf{s}_t | \tilde{\mathbf{s}}_t, \Sigma_{\mathbf{s}}) p(k_t | \tilde{k}_t) \tag{17.12}$$

where $\{\tilde{k}_t, \tilde{\mathbf{s}}_t\}$ stands for the top detections, that is, the local maxima of the observation distribution defined in Equation 17.6, $g(.)$ is the multivariate Gaussian density function with mean $\tilde{\mathbf{s}}_t$ and covariance $\Sigma_{\mathbf{s}}$, and $p(k_t | \tilde{k}_t)$ is the transition between cardiac phases defined in Equation 17.3. The parameter $\alpha \in [0, 1]$ in Equation 17.11 is used to weight the contribution of the observation and transition models. Note that $\alpha = 0$ represents a distribution that takes into account only the transition model, while $\alpha = 1$ denotes a proposal distribution built based on the observation model only.

Note that the main advantage of this proposal distribution is that when the motion model fails, the observation model has a chance to recover the boundary based on the observations computed from the current image. For the LV tracking this is important because it is hard to obtain a faithful model of the LV motion. Nevertheless, the presence of the transition model is still quite important to deal with the detection and segmentation failures of the observation model.

17.4.6   Segmentation of the left ventricle

Using the particle filter setup in Equation 17.9 for the filtering distribution, we estimate the values for the state variables at each time step t as follows:

$$\mathbf{k}_t^* = \arg \max_{k \in \{systole, diastole\}} E_{p(k_t, \mathbf{s}_t | I_{1:t})}[k], \qquad (17.13)$$

where $E_{p(k_t, \mathbf{s}_t | I_{1:t})}[k] \approx \sum_{l=1}^{P} w_t^{(l)} \delta(k - k_t^{(l)})$, and

$$\mathbf{s}_t^* = E_{p(k_t, \mathbf{s}_t | I_{1:t})}[\mathbf{s}_t | k_t^*] \approx \frac{1}{\sum_{l=1}^{P} w_t^{(l)} \delta(k_t - k_t^*)} \sum_{l=1}^{P} w_t^{(l)} \mathbf{s}_t^{(l)} \delta(k_t - k_t^*). \qquad (17.14)$$

Given all the main ingredients of the statistical model in Sections 17.4.2 through 17.4.6, we can now provide more details about the SIR in Algorithm 17.1. Thus, the sampling in step §2 is done by using Equation 17.11; the weights update in step §3 is accomplished using Equation 17.10, and finally the segmentation in step §9, is performed using Equations 17.13 and 17.14, to update k_t^* and $\mathbf{s}_t^*$, respectively.

In the following section we provide details concerning the training and inference of the Deep belief network, for the rigid and nonrigid classifiers (Equation 17.6) in the observation model in Equation 17.5.

17.5   Training and inference on deep belief networks

Deep belief networks (DBN) are artificial networks containing a large number of hidden layers and nodes, which allows the construction of models of large capability. However, the backpropagation algorithm for estimating the classifier parameters is limited, in sense that it only provides reliable estimates when the initial guess is close enough of the local optimum of the objective function to be minimized. Hinton et al. [28] found an efficient mechanism to surpass this difficulty using unsupervised training of multiple layers of restricted Boltzmann machines (RBM), which are represented by a hidden and a visible layer of stochastic binary units with connections only between layers (i.e., no connections within layers).

After the parameters of several layers of RBMs are learned, the whole network is trained using backpropagation to adjust the weights to a local maximum for the regressor and classifier functions. The use of deep learning is grounded on the two following main ideas [29]:

§1 An unsupervised generative model learns the process of the LV image generation
§2 A discriminative model that is trained on the above generative model

17.5.1   Training the DBN

The training stage of the DBN comprises both the training of the rigid and nonrigid classifiers (see Equation 17.6). For training the rigid classifier (first term in Equation 17.6) we follow the strategy proposed by Carneiro et al. [30]. Basically, this method builds an image scale space $L(\mathbf{x}, \sigma) = G(\mathbf{x}, \sigma) * I(\mathbf{x})$, where $G(\mathbf{x}, \sigma)$ is a Gaussian kernel, and $*$ is the convolution operator, and $I(\mathbf{x})$ is the input image, σ is the image scale parameter. In this methodology we have to define a set of images scales, say $\{\sigma_1, ..., \sigma_Q\}$. More specifically, in the present approach we have three scales, that is, $\sigma = \{4, 8, 16\}$, $(Q = 3)$ and we train three classifiers separately. For training each classifier we generate a set of positive and negative training sets, that are defined based on a scale-dependent margin m_σ. The generation process of each training sample (positive or negative), can be viewed as function $\varphi(.)$ that receives a triplet containing the jth image I_j, scale σ_q and a set of affine parameter θ, and outputs the image patch $\mathcal{P}_{n_q \times n_q}$ of size $n_q \times n_q$ containing the LV, that is, formally $\mathcal{P}_{n_q \times n_q} = \varphi(I_j, \sigma_q, \theta)$. Basically, the function $\varphi(.)$ comprises a scale operation on image I with σ_q and then perturbing by an affine transformation in $\theta \in \mathbb{R}^5$. This produces a patch of size $n_q \times n_q$, where n is a vector indexed by $q \in \{1, .., Q\}$. After this process, we finally subtract each patch pixel with its mean. This contrast normalization provides more robustness against brightness variations.

The difference between the generation positives and negatives are the ranges in which the affine transformation parameters in θ are defined. Thus, for positive samples, denoted herein as $\mathcal{P}os(k, q, j)$, and considering a training image I_j, an image scale σ, and a cardiac phase $k \in \{\text{diastole, systole}\}$, the samples are randomly generated inside the following range

$$\mathcal{P}os(k, q, j) = \{\mathcal{P}_{n_q \times n_q} | \theta \sim \text{Dist}(\mathcal{R}(\theta)), |\theta - \theta_j| < m_p, k_j = k\} \tag{17.15}$$

where Dist(.) is an uniform distribution, over the range $\mathcal{R}(\theta) = [\max(\{\theta_j\}_{j=1,..,M}) - \min(\{\theta_j\}_{j=1,..,M})] \in \mathbb{R}^5$

For the negative samples the range of parameters $\mathcal{R}$ is now larger and becomes as

$$\mathcal{N}eg(q, j) = \{\mathcal{P}_{n_q \times n_q} | \theta \sim \text{Dist}(\mathcal{R}(\theta)), |\theta - \theta_j| > 2m_p\} \tag{17.16}$$

where m_p in Equations 17.15 and 17.16 is the margin between positive and negative samples that facilitates the training process by avoiding similar examples with opposite labels. This avoids overtraining in the classifiers.

Notice that, with the above procedure, we are able to train the rigid (affine) DBN. To accomplish this, we stack several hidden layers to reconstruct the input patches in the $\mathcal{P}os$ and $\mathcal{N}eg$ sets. This corresponds to unsupervised training (issue § 1 above). After this, three nodes are added to the top layer of the DBN to account for: (1) $p(k = \text{systole}|I, \theta)$, (2) $p(k = \text{diastole}|I, \theta)$, and (3) the formed patch $\mathcal{P}_{n_q \times n_q}$ does not contain the LV. Finally, the discriminative training on the generative model is to find the appropriate weights of the DBN (issue § 2 above).

The nonrigid regressor is trained only at the finest scale $\sigma = 4$ (second term in Equation 17.6). In the training process we build an orthogonal line radiating from each contour sample (see Figure 17.2d). This allows us to define the ith sample of the jth contour point $s_j(i)$. The input of the regressor is the profile (gray levels) of the orthogonal line (see Figure 17.2d for an illustration), and returns the location in each normal line that is closest to the LV boundary.

17.6 Experimental evaluation

In this section we first examine the data used for the experimental evaluation, the annotation procedure and the team involved. We next describe the learned configurations of the deep belief networks, for both rigid and nonrigid classifiers. Finally we perform a interuser statistics study comprising the *modified Williams index* the *Bland–Altman* and *Scatter plots* and a comparison with the state of the art.

17.6.1   Datasets and manual annotations

The dataset used for the experiments comprises 20 sequences for training and testing (20 sequences from 20 subjects with no overlap), from which 16 present some kind of cardiopathy. According to the cardiologist's report,[*] the following cardiopathies/abnormalities are considered:

§1. Dilation of the LV. The dilation can be classified in mild, moderate, or severe.
§2. Presence of hypertrophy of the LV. The hypertrophy can also be classified into mild, moderate, or severe.
§3. Wall motion abnormalities. The abnormalities can be classified as global (affecting all the LV segments), or localized (affecting some of the LV segments).
§4. Function of the LV. The function may be preserved, mild, depressed, or severe (i.e., dysfunction of the LV).
§5. Presence of valvular heart disease.
§6. Presence of a pacemaker device.

The dataset is divided into two sets: T_1 and T_2. The set T_1 contains 16 sequences presenting some cardiopathy as mentioned above and other two sequences from healthy subjects, we term these sequences as $T_{1_{A...R}}$. The other set comprises two healthy sequences $T_{2_{A,B}}$.

We worked with four members of the cardiology services from Hospital Fernando Fonseca[†] who annotated five sequences in T_1, they annotated roughly 20 frames in each sequence; one annotation in the systole and in diastole phases of the cardiac cycle. In the set $T_{2_{A,B}}$ the head of the team provides us 40 annotations (20 for each sequence in T_2). We access how the results of the proposed algorithm correlate with interuser variation in the set T_1. Also, we perform a quantitative comparison between the estimates obtained in T_2, thus, the results reported in five sequences of the LV.

17.6.2   Training of the DBN

This section describes the two training phases of the DBN, comprising the affine (rigid) and nonrigid stages. For training the rigid classifier, three separate classifiers are trained, each one at different scale, that is, $q \in \{1, \ldots, Q\}$. To accomplish this, we generated 100 positive and 500 negative patches that will integrate the sets Pos and Neg, respectively (see Equation 17.15). This initial training set, is further, divided 80% in Pos and Neg for training and validation sets. The multiscale strategy mentioned in Section 17.5.1 is used in training and segmentation purposes at three different scales; $\sigma = \{16, 8, 4\}$. The dimension of the patches depends on the scale used. Thus, the original patch size is 56×56, but it decreases as the scale increases. More specifically, we used patches of dimension, 4×4, 7×7, and 14×14, for scales $16, 8$, and 4, respectively. The validation set, is used to estimate the parameters of the DBN, namely: (i) number of visible, hidden, and output layers; (ii) number of nodes for the visible, hidden, and output layers. These sets of parameters are shown in Table 17.1 for both rigid and nonrigid classifiers. This was achieved using the annotations dataset contained in T_1.

---

[*] This was done in collaboration with Dr. António Freitas from Hospital Fernando Fonseca who detailed each of the sequences.
[†] The annotations were possible thanks to the collaboration with the cardiology service in Hospital Fernando Fonseca headed by Dr. António Freitas.

Table 17.1 Learned configuration for the deep belief networks

σ	Visible layer	Hidden layer 1	Hidden layer 2	Hidden layer 3	Hidden layer 4	Output layer
			Affine classifier			
4	196 (14 × 14 pix.)	100	100	200	200	3
8	49 (7 × 7 pix.)	50	100	–	–	3
16	16 (4 × 4 pix.)	100	50	–	–	3
			Nonrigid classifier			
4	41	50	50	–	–	1

The nonrigid classifier (see Equation 17.7 and Figure 17.2d,e) is trained with the approach described in Section 17.5.1. Each normal line has 41 pixel-length. In this training stage we also use the same positive set $\mathcal{P}os$, 80 samples for training and 20 for validation.

17.6.3   Error measures

To perform a quantitative assessment we use several error mesures that compute the mismatch between the estimated LV and the ground truth contours. Among possible choices for the quantitative study, we will use metrics that are common and widely known in the literature. More specifically, we use the Jaccard distance (JCD) [31], average error (AV) [26], mean absolute distance (MAD) [32], and average perpendicular error (AVP) between the estimated and ground truth contours, (see Nascimento and Marques [26] and Carneiro and Nascimento [33] for a complete definition of these measures).

17.6.4   Comparison with inter-user statistics

The robustness of the proposed approach against the interuser variability is assessed following the works of Chalana et al. [34] and Lopez et al. [35]. The measures used are the following: (i) *Modified William index*, (ii) *Bland–Altman plot* [36], and (iii) *Scatter plot*. These comparisons are performed on the diseased sets contained in $\mathcal{T}_{1,\{A,B,C\}}$, for which we have four LV manual annotations per image delineated by four different Cardiologists (Section 17.5.1).

Figure 17.3 illustrates the inter-variance of the delineations given by the four cardiologists. This figure shows that indeed the delineation of the LV contour is somehow subjective. Parts of the contour belonging to the apex and the right lateral part are the regions in which the discrepancy is larger.

For each sequence we have about 17 expertise annotations. Considering four cardiologists, this gives 51 manual annotation for each sequence, resulting in a total amount of 204 annotations in $\mathcal{T}_1$

In order to have a fair comparison, we train three separate DBN classifiers using the following training sets: (1) $\mathcal{T}_1 \setminus \mathcal{T}_{1,A}$, (2) $\mathcal{T}_1 \setminus \mathcal{T}_{1,B}$, and (3) $\mathcal{T}_1 \setminus \mathcal{T}_{1,C}$, where \ represents the set difference operator. These three classifiers are necessary because when testing any image

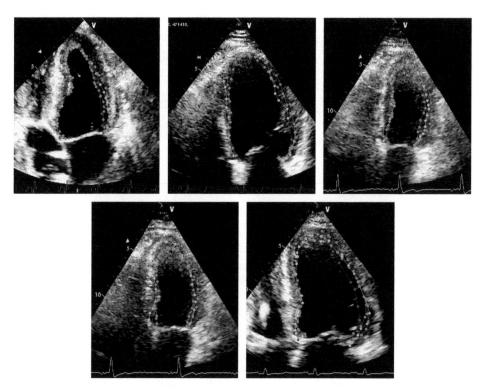

Figure 17.3 In each image, four manual delineations of the LV contour are shown, where each color refers to the annotation of an expert.

inside each one of these three sequences, we cannot use any image of that same sequence in the training process.

17.6.4.1 Modified Williams index

To provide the results concerning the modified Williams index, we start by considering the set $\{\mathbf{s}_{j,k}\}$, where $j \in \{1..M\}$ indexes the testing images, and $k \in \{0..U\}$ indexes the manual annotations, where the index $k = 0$ denotes the computer-generated contour (i.e., each one of the M images has U manual annotations). The function $D_{k,k'}$ measures the mismatch or disagreement between users k and k', which is defined as

$$D_{k,k'} = \frac{1}{M} \sum_{j=1}^{M} d_-(\mathbf{s}_{j,k}, \mathbf{s}_{j,k'}),\tag{17.17}$$

where $d_-(.,.)$ is an error measure between two annotations $\mathbf{s}_{j,k}$, $\mathbf{s}_{j,k'}$. The measure can be, for instance, the average distance between the estimated contour and the ground truth contour. The modified Williams index is defined as

$$I' = \frac{\frac{1}{U} \sum_{k=1}^{U} \frac{1}{D_{0,k}}}{\frac{2}{U(U-1)} \sum_{k} \sum_{k':k' \neq k} \frac{1}{D_{k,k'}}}.\tag{17.18}$$

A confidence interval (CI) is estimated using a jackknife (leave one out) nonparametric sampling strategy [34] as follows:

$$I'_{(.)} \pm z_{0.95} se, \tag{17.19}$$

where $z_{0.95} = 1.96$ represents 95th percentile of the standard normal distribution, and

$$se = \left\{ \frac{1}{M-1} \sum_{j=1}^{M} [I'_{(j)} - I'_{(.)}] \right\} \tag{17.20}$$

with $I'_{(.)} = \frac{1}{M} \sum_{j=1}^{M} I'_{(j)}$, and $I'_{(j)}$ is the Williams index (17.18) calculated by leaving image j out of computation of $D_{k,k'}$. A successful measurement for the Williams index is to have the average and confidence interval (17.19) close to one.

17.6.4.2   Bland–Altman and scatter plots

In this section, we provide experimental evaluation concerning the Bland–Altman [36] and scatter plots, from which we compute the correlation coefficient and the p-value. To accomplish this, we have: (i) the gold standard LV volume computed via an iterative process using the manual annotations [34]; (ii) the Cardiologists' LV volumes, and (iii) the computer generated LV volume. To estimate the LV volume from 2-D contour annotation we use the area-length equation [37,38] with $V = \frac{8A^2}{3\pi L}$, where A denotes the projected surface area, L is the distance from upper aortic valve point to apex, and V is expressed in cubic pixels. The p-values are computed as follows: (1) compute several independent p-values from 3 samples, each taken from separate sequence; and then (2) combine the p-values using the Fisher's method into a single result by assuming independence among the p-values [39].

17.6.5   Experimental results

Figure 17.4 shows the qualitative performance of the proposed approach at segmenting the LV. In green contour it is displayed the expertise annotation superimposed with the estimated contour in red. Each row corresponds to a different cardiac sequence, and all the sequences are contained in the set $T_{1,\{A,B,C\}}$. It is seen that the proposed approach exhibits quite remarkable segmentations in these sequences.

We show a comparison with the state of the art in Table 17.2 using the error metrics Jaccard (JCD), average (Aver.), and Hausdorff (Hausd.). In this study, we used the two test sequences $T_{2_{A,B}}$ and compared with our previous methods [26,40]. The approach in Carneiro et al. [40] only contains the observation model, which means that does not contain any dynamic model, only the static segmentation. In Nascimento and Marques [26], a deformable based approach is proposed, which contains a transition model that is based on a switching mechanism. More specifically, at each time instant (each frame) the deformable model is able to switch between the two phases (i.e., $k = \{$systole,diastole$\}$).

In terms of inter-user statistics, Table 17.3 shows the mean values, as well as and confidence intervals of the Williams index defined in Equations 17.18 and 17.19. This is done for all ultrasound sequences considered for the comparison with inter-user statistics. Figure 17.5 shows the scatter and Bland–Altman plots. Concerning the scatter plot, the correlation coefficient between the users and gold standard is 0.99 with p-value = 3.11×10^{-68} (left images in the figure) and for the gold standard versus computer the correlation is 0.95 with p-value= 1.9×10^{-4} (right image in the figure). In the Bland–Altman plots, the

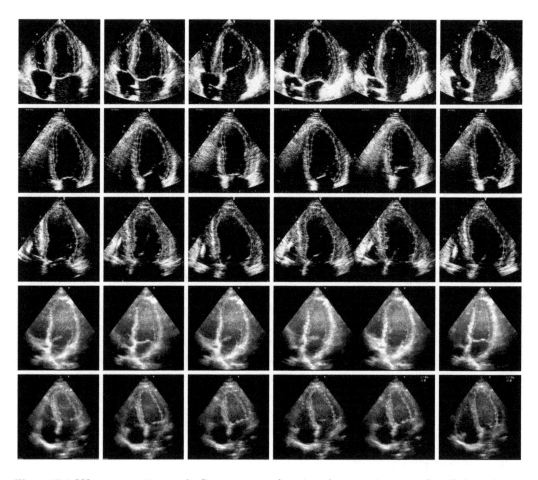

Figure 17.4 LV contour estimates (red) are compared against the expertise ground truth (green).

Table 17.2 Comparisons in the sequences

Approach	JCD	Aver.	Hausd.
	Sequence one		
Proposal	**0.17(0.04)**	3.3(0.8)	**19.1(2.2)**
[40]	0.18(0.06)	**3.2(0.8)**	20.0(2.6)
[26]	0.24(0.03)	4.8(0.9)	22.4(2.1)
	Sequence two		
Proposal	**0.15(0.03)**	**2.9(0.5)**	**19.4(1.4)**
[40]	0.17(0.02)	3.0(0.5)	19.8(1.1)
[26]	0.24(0.03)	4.8(0.7)	20.2(1.4)

Note: Each cell shows the mean value and the standard deviation in parentheses.

Table 17.3 Comparison of the computer-generated curves to the users' curves with respect to all the error measures for three sequences using the average and 0.95% confidence interval (in parentheses) of the Williams index

Measure	d_{HMD}	d_{AV}	d_{MAD}	d_{AVP}
Average (CI)	0.83 (0.82, 0.84)	0.91 (0.90, 0.92)	0.94 (0.93, 0.95)	0.83 (0.82, 0.84)

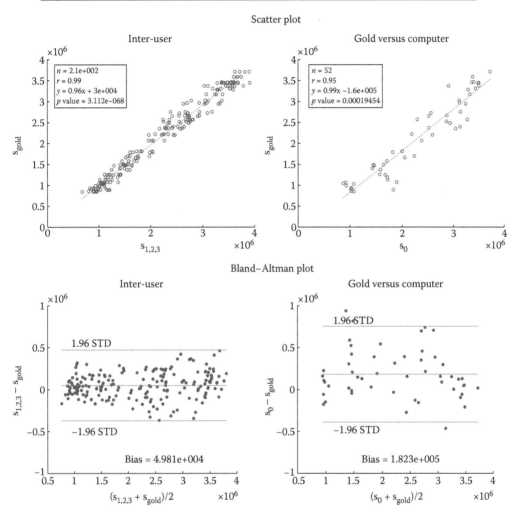

Figure 17.5 Scatter plots with linear regression and Bland–Altman bias plots.

Inter-user plot produced a bias of 4.9×10^4 with confidence interval of $[-5 \times 10^5, 5 \times 10^5]$, while the Gold vs Computer plot shows a bias of 1.8×10^5 and confidence interval of $[-4 \times 10^5, 7 \times 10^5]$.

17.7   Conclusions and further work

We have described an automatic algorithm for the segmentation and tracking of the LV in 2D ultrasound data. The contribution presented herein resides in the ability to combine deep learning architectures with sampling importance resampling (SIR) techniques incorporating dynamical model. Under this framework, a novel transition and observation models are presented. In the dynamical model, there is no commitment to a specific heart dynamical regime, instead it combines the transition and observation results. Notice however, that there are some limitations concerning the training sets used. In particular, the present framework is still dependent on a rich training dataset, being preferable to have several frames from distinct patients rather several frames from the same patient. Also, when generating the positive and negatives samples (in Section 17.5.1 Equations 17.15 and 17.16) that are estimated from the training set, the range may not be enough to robustly represent all the variation that can happen with the left ventricle. In further work we plan to address the above issues by developing a semi-supervised based techniques to reduce such dependence. We also plan to apply this approach to other anatomies and other medical imaging techniques.

References

1. J. Bosch, S. Mitchell, B. Lelieveldt, F. Nijland, O. Kamp, M. Sonka, and J. Reiber, Automatic segmentation of echocardiographic sequences by active appearance motion models, *IEEE Transactions on Medical Imaging*, vol. 21, no. 11, pp. 1374–1383, 2002.

2. A. Doucet, N. de Freitas, N. Gordon, and A. Smith, *Sequential Monte Carlo Methods in Practice*. Berlin: Springer-Verlag, 2001.

3. M. Arulampalam, S. Maskell, N. Gordon, and T. Clapp, A tutorial on particle filters for online nonlinear/non-Gaussian Bayesian tracking, *IEEE Transactions on Signal Processing*, vol. 50, no. 2, pp. 174–188, 2002.

4. M. Kass, A. Witkin, and D. Terzopoulos, Snakes: Active contour models, *International Journal of Computer Vision*, vol. 4, no. 1, pp. 321–331, 1987.

5. T. F. Cootes, G. J. Edwards, and C. J. Taylor, Active appearance models, in *European Conference on Computer Vision*, 1998, pp. 484–498.

6. N. Paragios, A level set approach for shape-driven segmentation and tracking of the left ventricle, *IEEE Transactions on Medical Imaging*, vol. 21, no. 9, pp. 773–776, 2003.

7. R. Malladi, J. Sethian, and B. Vemuri, Shape modeling with front propagation: A level set approach, *IEEE Transactions on Pattern Analysis and Machine Intelligence*, vol. 17, pp. 158–175, 1995.

8. O. Bernard, D. Friboulet, P. Thevenaz, and M. Unser, Variational B-spline level-set: A linear filtering approach for fast deformable model evolution, *IEEE Transactions on Imaging Processing*, vol. 18, no. 6, pp. 1179–1991, 2009.

9. C. Corsi, G. Saracino, A. Sarti, and C. Lamberti, Left ventricular volume estimation for real-time three-dimensional echocardiography, *IEEE Transactions on Medical Imaging*, vol. 21, no. 9, pp. 1202–1208, 2002.

10. D. Cremers, S. Osher, and S. Soatto, Kernel density estimation and intrinsic alignment for shape priors in level set segmentation, *International Journal of Computer Vision*, vol. 69, no. 3, pp. 335–351, 2006.

11. E. Debreuve, M. Barlaud, G. Aubert, I. Laurette, and J. Darcourt, Space-time segmentation using level set active contours applied to myocardial gated SPECT, *IEEE Transactions on Medical Imaging*, vol. 20, no. 7, pp. 643–659, 2001.

12. Q. Duan, E. D. Angelini, and A. Laine, Real time segmentation by active geometric functions, *Computational Methods Programs in Biomedicine*, vol. 98, no. 3, pp. 223–230, 2010.

13. N. Lin, W. Yu, and J. Duncan, Combinative multi-scale level set framework for echocardiographic image segmentation, *Medical Image Analysis*, vol. 7, no. 4, pp. 529–537, 2003.

14. M. Lynch, O. Ghita, and P. Whelan, Segmentation of the left ventricle of the heart in 3-D+T MRI data using an optimized nonrigid temporal model, *IEEE Transactions on Medical Imaging*, vol. 27, no. 2, pp. 195–203, 2008.

15. N. Paragios and R. Deriche, Geodesic active regions and level set methods for supervised texture segmentation, *International Journal of Computer Vision*, vol. 46, no. 3, pp. 223–247, 2002.

16. A. Sarti, C. Corsi, E. Mazzini, and C. Lamberti, Maximum likelihood segmentation of ultrasound images with Rayleigh distribution, *IEEE Transactions on Ultrasonics, Ferroelectrics, Frequency Control*, vol. 52, no. 6, pp. 947–960, 2005.

17. T. Cootes, C. Taylor, D. Cooper, and J. Graham, Active shape models—their training and application, *Computational Vision Image Understanding*, vol. 61, no. 1, pp. 38–59, 1995.

18. T. Cootes, C. Beeston, G. Edwards, and C. Taylor, A unified framework for atlas matching using active appearance models, in *Information Processing in Medical Imaging*, 1999, pp. 322–333.

19. S. Mitchell, B. Lelieveldt, R. van der Geest, H. Bosch, J. Reiber, and M. Sonka, Multistage hybrid active appearance model matching: Segmentation of left and right ventricles in cardiac MR images, *IEEE Transactions on Medical Imaging*, vol. 20, no. 5, pp. 415–423, 2001.

20. D. Comaniciu, X. Zhou, and S. Krishnan, Robust real-time myocardial border tracking for echocardiography: An information fusion approach, *IEEE Transactions on Medical Imaging*, vol. 23, no. 7, pp. 849–860, 2004.

21. B. Georgescu, X. S. Zhou, D. Comaniciu, and A. Gupta, Databased-guided segmentation of anatomical structures with complex appearance, in *Conference on Computer Vision and Pattern Recording (CVPR)*, 2005.

22. D. Terzopoulos and R. Szeliski, *Tracking with Kalman Snakes*. Cambridge, MA: MIT Press, 1993.

23. W. Sun, M. Cetin, R. Chan, V. Reddy, G. Holmvang, V. Chandar, and A. Willsky, Segmenting and tracking the left ventricle by learning the dynamics in cardiac images, *Information on Processing Medical Imaging*, vol. 19, pp. 553–565, 2005.

24. L. Yang, B. Georgescu, Y. Zheng, P. Meer, and D. Comaniciu, 3D ultrasound tracking of the left ventricle using one-step forward prediction and data fusion of collaborative trackers, in *Conference on Computer Vision and Pattern Recording (CVPR)*, 2008.

25. J. Se'ne'gas, T. Netsch, C. Cocosco, G. Lund, and A. Stork, Segmentation of medical images with a shape and motion model: A Bayesian perspective, in *ECCV Workshops CVAMIA and MMBIA*, 2004, pp. 157–168.

26. J. C. Nascimento and J. S. Marques, Robust shape tracking with multiple models in ultrasound images, *IEEE Transactions on Image Processing*, vol. 17, no. 3, pp. 392–406, 2008.

27. K. Okuma, A. Taleghani, N. de Freitas, J. Little, and D. Lowe, A boosted particle filter: Multitarget detection and tracking, in *ECCV*, 2004.

28. R. Salakhutdinov and G. Hinton, Learning a non-linear embedding by preserving class neighbourhood structure, in *Artificial Imaging and Statistics*, 2007.

29. G. Hinton. http://videolectures.net/nips09-hinton-dlmi/.

30. G. Carneiro, B. Georgescu, S. Good, and D. Comaniciu, Detection and measurement of fetal anatomies from ultrasound images using a constrained probabilistic boosting tree, *IEEE Transactions on Medical Imaging*, vol. 27, no. 9, pp. 1342–1355, 2008.

31. A. Hammoude, Computer-assited endocardial border identification from a sequence of two-dimensional echocardiographic images, Ph.D. dissertation, University Washington, 1988.

32. X. S. Zhou, D. Comaniciu, and A. Gupta, An information fusion framework for robust shape tracking, *IEEE Transactions on Pattern Analysis and Machine Intelligence*, vol. 27, no. 1, pp. 115–129, 2005.

33. G. Carneiro and J. C. Nascimento, Combining multiple dynamic models and deep learning architectures for tracking the left ventricle endocardium in ultrasound data, *IEEE Transactions on Pattern Analysis on Machine Intelligence*, vol. 35, no. 11, pp. 2592–2607, 2013.

34. V. Chalana and Y. Kim, A methodology for evaluation of boundary detection algorithms on medical images, *IEEE Transactions on Medical Imaging*, vol. 16, no. 10, 1997.

35. C. Alberola-Lopez, M. Martin-Fernandez, and J. Ruiz-Alzola, Comments on: A methodology for evaluation of boundary detection algorithms on medical images, *IEEE Transactions on Medical Imaging*, vol. 23, no. 5, pp. 658–660, 2004.

36. J. Bland and A. Altman, Statistical methods for assessing agreement between two methods of clinical measurement, *Lancet*, vol. 1, no. 8476, pp. 307–310, 1986.

37. J. C. Reiber, A. R. Viddeleer, G. Koning, M. J. Schalij, and P. E. Lange, Left ventricular regression equations from single plane cine and digital X-ray ventriculograms revisited, *Clinical Cardiology*, vol. 12, no. 2, pp. 69–78, 1996.

38. H. Sandler and H. T. Dodge, The use of single plane angiocardiograms for the calculation of left ventricular volume in man, *American Heart Journal*, vol. 75, no. 3, pp. 325–334, 1968.

39. R. Fisher, Questions and answers number 14, *The American Statistician*, vol. 2, no. 5, pp. 30–31, 1948.

40. G. Carneiro, J. C. Nascimento, and A. Freitas, Robust left ventricle segmentation from ultrasound data using deep neural networks and efficient search methods, in *IEEE International Symposium on Biomedical Imaging, From Nano to Macro (ISBI)*, 2010, pp. 1085–1088.

chapter eighteen

A shortest path approach to interactive medical image segmentation

Jonathan-Lee Jones, Xianghua Xie, and Ehab Essa

Contents

Abstract

In this chapter, we discuss using a shortest path methodology combined with a region-based selection, for a user assisted segmentation, as either an enclosed object or as an open curve. We will investigate this method of image segmentation in specific medical applications (user-assisted segmentation of the media adventitia border in intravascular ultrasound [IVUS] images, and lumen border in optical coherence tomography [OCT] images), and then demonstrate the method with generic medical and real-world images to show how it could be utilized in various other types of medical image, and is not limited to the applications described.

Our method combines point-based soft constraints, to detect object boundary and a stroke-based regional constraint. The user points act as attraction points and are treated as soft constraints, penalizing the segmentation based on distance of the boundary from this point; rather than hard constraints that the segmented boundary has to pass through. This gives an accurate result while not insisting on precise and time-consuming input from the user. In this way, we hope to increase efficiency while still allowing the experienced user to control the process. This edge-based boundary constraint is imposed through searching the shortest path in a three-dimensional graph, derived from a multilayer image representation.

The user can also specify areas to be considered as foreground. The probabilities of belonging to the foreground areas for each pixel are then calculated and their discontinuity is used to indicate object boundary, fitting well into the multilayer approach. The combinations of different types of user constraints and image features allow flexible and robust segmentation, which is formulated as an energy minimization problem on a multilayered graph and is solved using a shortest path search algorithm. We show that this combinatorial approach allows efficient and effective interactive segmentation, which can be used with both open and closed curves to segment a variety of images in different ways. Using two medical applications (IVUS and OCT), we look at the efficacy of the technique both quantitatively and qualitatively, comparing to other methods available. In both these modalities, image artifacts such as acoustic shadow, stent reflections, and calcification are commonplace and thus user guidance is desirable. We further demonstrate the method in a series of other images, both medical and real-world images.

18.1   Introduction

Image segmentation is of great importance and commonly used in various medical applications [1]. There are two broad categories of techniques: automatic and interactive, each with many different approaches. Automated techniques (such as in Essa et al. [2] shown in Figure 18.1) are appealing in terms of efficiency, as they do not require extra work from the user. More often than not, however, prior knowledge about object appearance and/or shape is necessary to achieve meaningful results; and in the medical idiom, any training or prior knowledge would have to be such that it was enough to deal with unexpected

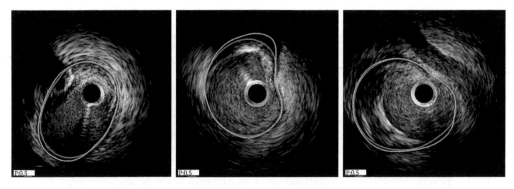

Figure 18.1 An example of automated segmentation of media–adventitia border in IVUS images [2]. Both appearance and shape priors are necessary to constrain the segmentation. The results are shown in red and the manual labeling is shown in green.

variations and nonstandard data. The situation is further complicated by problems that are inherent to most medical imaging modalities, such as noise and artifacts. It is, therefore, not always practical, or even possible, to obtain comprehensive prior information and a sufficiently robust learning algorithm to deal with large and sometimes unpredictable variations that occur in medical images. An alternative approach to automated segmentation is to allow and encourage user input and provide interactive segmentation results to suffice user demand. This has the advantage of being able to use expert user knowledge to avoid problems, and to inform the segmentation. This, however, leads to a dilemma; as the increase in the amount and precision of user input, while improving the segmentation is many cases, takes time and is less efficient and optimum for the user. The goal is to balance user involvement and interaction flexibility, particularly given the ubiquitous imaging device and ever increasing amount of images in modern age. To effectively and efficiently capture user intent is vitally important, allowing the expertise of the user to be used, without the system being too labor-intensive for the user, or so inflexible that it cannot adapt to extreme cases.

The ability to segment both closed region and open contour is also important. Hence, methods that are capable of both may have a wider appeal in medical applications than those, for instance, can only partition images into disjoint and self-enclosed regions.

The user interaction is conventionally made either by simple mouse click or drag operations on the region of interest, or on the object boundary—mechanisms that are familiar to the user, without specialist hardware and training. For example, in Intelligent Paint [3], which is a simple interactive method that allows the user to identify all the regions inside an object. The object region is interactively expanded by a simple click and drag operation. Then a homogeneous area that has the same intensity profile is selected, which is very similar to those techniques adopted in commercial software. Similarly, with Magic Wand, for example, in Adobe Photoshop, a user can highlight all the homogeneous area that has the same intensity profile by simple mouse clicks. The intelligent scissors [4], shown in Figure 18.2, and live wire [5], shown in Figure 18.3 methods are among early methods to perform on-the-fly segmentation by allowing the user to follow the object boundary, instead of region, through a few mouse clicks. These methods are based on well-known shortest path algorithms, such as Dijkstra's method, to find the optimal shortest path between two user points. Shortest path methods have an advantage of segmenting both open and closed objects. However, often only edge-based features are used to find the shortest path, and more importantly usually those user points are treated as anchor points that the segmented path has to go through.

Another method of segmentation that is commonly used is active contour model (or snake). Active contour models provide a good quality segmentation, but many suffer from initialization dependency problems. Typically, this is tackled by adding a prior to the model to give the segmentation a better initial state or an overall constraint, which may not be always practical. There are various solutions proposed to alleviate this problem, such as in Humnabadkar et al. [6] that uses another automatic segmentation method on a coarse down-sampled image to provide the initialization for their active contour model, and Li et al. [7] that uses coarse results extracted by spatial fuzzy C-means clustering (see example results in Figure 18.4). There are, however, other methods that attempt to achieve global minima, either through global minimization or through deriving external force field that is initialization independent. For example, in Xie and Mirmehdi [8,9], the authors show that even using conventional gradient-based boundary description, it is possible to achieve global minima with gradient descent. Its force field is computed based on global interaction of image gradient vectors and its force is always perpendicular to the evolving contour.

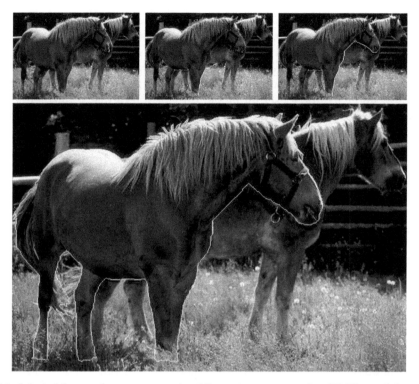

Figure 18.2 Selected frames from an example of live-wire segmentation [4]. The red dots show the seed points; the green crosshair is the free point; the blue contour segments correspond to portions of the set boundary; and the yellow contour segment is the live-wire boundary segment. Top row (left to right) shows selected frames from the interactive segmentation process and the main image shows the result.

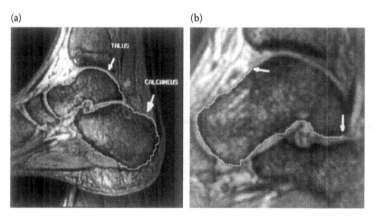

Figure 18.3 Live Lane segmentation example from Falco et al. [5]. (a) An MRI slice of the foot of a subject showing the bones talus and calcaneus (marked). (b) A zoomed-in image of a tracing on the boundary of the talus.

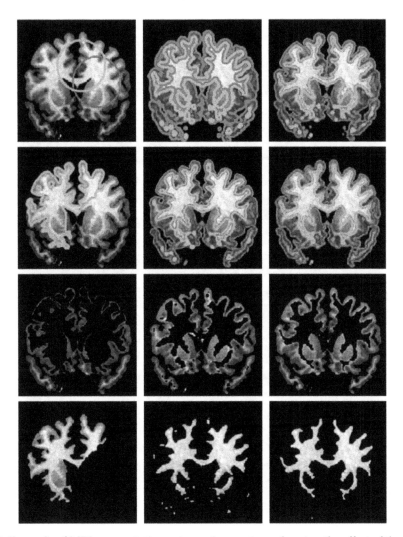

Figure 18.4 Example of MRI segmentation using active contour, showing the effect of three different initialization methods [7]. The top row shows the initial curves. The second row shows the stable curves obtained from the method. The last two rows show the segmented gray and white matter, respectively. The first column shows manual initialization, which gives unsatisfactory convergence. The center column uses a threshold method based on coarse segmentation and the right-hand column uses preprocessing as suggested by Li et al. [7].

Figure 18.5 provides a comparative example of classical gradient-based methods and the magnetostatic active contour (MAC) model [9].

With the help of powerful optimization techniques, the method of user interaction has been expanded, for example, adding object/background strokes, at the same time simplify user involvement compared to painstakingly tracing the object boundary [5,15–20]. For example, the user can simply draw multiple strokes inside and outside the object and then the segmentation model can learn the distribution of pixel intensities for both object and background. These techniques usually are more suited for segmenting closed objects, but not for open curve segmentation, but in the proposed method, we adapt the method so that it can be used with both open and closed objects.

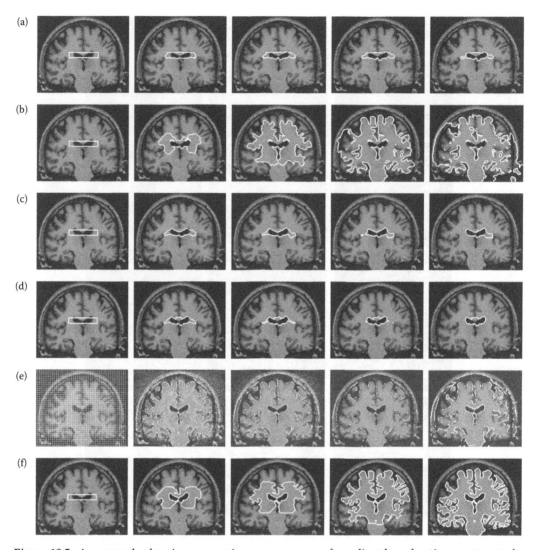

Figure 18.5 An example showing comparison among several gradient-based active contour techniques that are popular in interactive segmentation. User interaction, however, is simplistic and generally limited to initialization. Results by row: (a) DVF [10], (b) Geodesic [11], (c) GGVF [12], (d) GeoGGVF [13], (e) CPM [14], (f) MAC [9].

In terms of optimization technique, graph-cut and shortest path search are two of the most common categories of methods of interactive segmentation. Graph-cut algorithms are widely used to find optimal solution in interactive segmentation at polynomial time complexity and are most usually used for segmenting closed objects. Boykov and Jolly [15] (shown in Figure 18.6) introduced a graph-cut-based interactive segmentation method by defining unary and pairwise costs of each pixels. The unary cost is inversely proportional with the probability of each pixel to be in the object or in the background while the pairwise cost is based on the intensity difference between two neighboring pixels.

Many methods have been introduced to extend this method, such as to combine shape prior with user initialization [21] (shown in Figure 18.7), Grab Cut [16] and Lazy

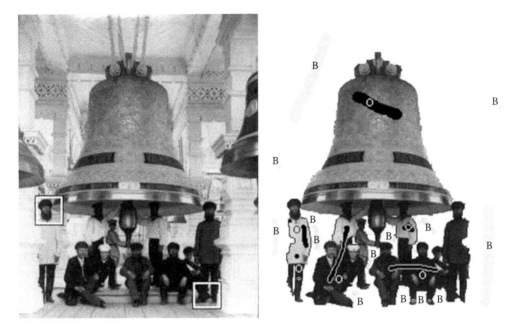

Figure 18.6 An example of graph-cut segmentation using s-t cut [15]. The original image is on the left, and the results are shown on the right. The results are marked "O" for object and "B" for background.

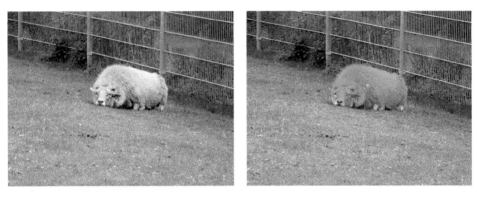

Figure 18.7 Automatic segmentation with minimal user input (green point marking the center of an object) [21].

Snapping [22], shown in Figure 18.8. In Grab Cut, the authors proposed to use a Gaussian mixture model to build a local color model to build the unary cost. It reduces the user intervention by allowing the user to define a rectangular window surrounding the object, and also allows iterative interaction to refined the result. Lazy Snapping is also based on graph-cut over a presegmented image using a watershed algorithm. K-means is used to cluster the foreground/background colors and assign each pixel to the nearest cluster. The method also has a boundary editing tool to refine the result. However, this method usually needs multiple user interventions to correctly cut out the object, due to the simplicity in its cost function.

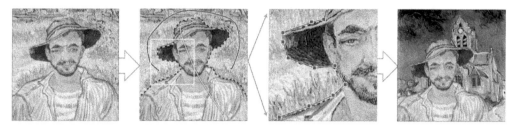

Figure 18.8 Lazy Snapping [22] is an interactive image cutout system, consisting of two stages: first, an object marking stage and second boundary editing. In the second picture, the two user selections (yellow to indicate the foreground, blue background) are drawn. The box represents the zoomed section in the next image. In the third (zoomed) image, the segmentation is shown, with control points. The final image shows the cut out is superimposed onto another Van Gogh painting.

Shortest path is another optimization technique that has been used in interactive segmentation, for example, Mortensen and Barrett [4], Falco et al. [5], and Windheuser et al. [20]. These methods place the emphasis on boundary-based features; edge-based features are used to define the cost between pixels, and can be used on both open and closed segmentations. The user interactively identifies a starting point of the path and iteratively adds more seeds around the outline of the object. On the other hand, the intelligent paint method [3] allows the user to identify regions inside the object instead of the boundary. The region is interactively expanded by simple click and dragging operations. Shortest path has an advantage of segmenting both open and close end objects, however many of them only use edge-based features to find the shortest path and the user points are generally treated as hard constraints.

Incorporating shape prior into graph-based segmentation has also shown improving the segmentation result [2,18,23–25]. Veksler [18] introduced a star shape prior to graph-cut, also through user interaction. User is required to specify the center of region of interest (ROI) as the star point, and hence all boundary points of ROI lie on the radial spikes from the star point. Additional points, specifying foreground and background, are often necessary. A ballooning term is also used to discourage bias toward small segment. However, the method can only segment the convex shapes. Gulshan et al. [26] have extended the method to multiple stars by using geodesic paths instead of Euclidean rays. Other interactive segmentation methods such as a transductive framework of Laplacian graph regularizer [27] have been also introduced.

In this chapter, we look at an approach combining two different types of user interactions, that is, boundary-based interaction (utilizing the user input control points) and region-based stroke interaction, to segment the image. Unlike previously discussed edge-based methods, we utilize a series of soft constraints to guide the image segmentation. By switching to soft constraint, imprecise user input is allowed; without adversely affecting the segmentation. To further augment this edge-based approach, we allow the user to select regions for foreground interest with strokes; this allows effective combination of boundary and region-based features in a wide variety of image modalities. The user points give the user control over the segmentation process, allowing errors in segmentation to be easily prevented and a more desirable result to be obtained (see Figure 18.9).

We investigate two medical applications for our proposed method; intravascular ultrasound (IVUS) imaging and optical coherence tomography (OCT) doing a full comparison of the method in both cases; we will then, afterwards look at some examples from other imaging methods, and real-world images). Both of these modalities are catheter based and

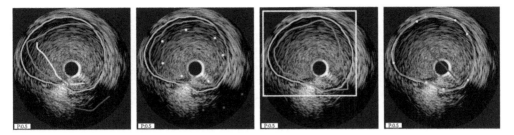

Figure 18.9 Examples of different segmentation methods on an IVUS image. From left: Graph-cut [15], seeded star graph-cut [18], Grab Cut [16], and proposed method. Red curve shows the segmentation result, blue or yellow for user points, background/foreground selections, and the initial window of the Grab Cut. Green shows the ground truth from manually labeled image.

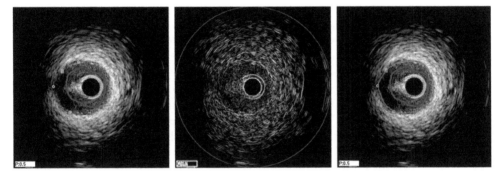

Figure 18.10 Edge-based detection in IVUS images. From left to right, initial image with user selections added, resultant edge map obtained, the segmentation produced (shown in red).

used in cardiology diagnosis, with IVUS being more commonplace. These catheter-based approaches can be used to assess the severity of any stenoses present, and to categorize their morphology; give the clinician tools to measure the vessel diameter allowing the severity of any occlusions to be assessed, and the location of any lesions to be identified, as well as many other clinical and therapeutic studies [28]. In most IVUS B-mode images, a cross-section of the arterial wall is proceeded, with three regions: the lumen, the vessel (made up of the intima and media layers), and the adventitia surrounding the vessel wall (see Figure 18.10). The media–adventitia border is the dividing layer representing the outer arterial wall. In IVUS images, the media can be seen as a dark band, with no other distinct features. It is encapsulated by the adventitia, which is a wide layer of fibrous connective tissue. IVUS segmentation as a cost function minimization problem has been a popular approach to solve this problem. OCT images are segmented to reveal the lumen border. This is clearly visible for the most part, but in a similar fashion to IVUS images there are a number of artifacts present. These are reflections/shadows caused by the guide wire, reflections/shadows caused by stents, and other anomalies such as shearing (sew-up errors), presence of blood in lumen, etc. See Figure 18.11 for some examples.

Due to the nature of these artifacts, automatic methods employed in these applications require a significant amount of preprocessing [29,30]; a large dataset for training set [31], or a method to remove the artifacts [32]. Our proposed method, by giving the user control to help the process, removes the need for extensive preprocessing or large datasets for training, allowing user guidance to avoid pitfalls used by image quality or artifacts present.

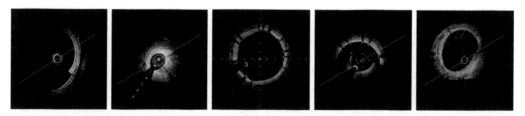

Figure 18.11 Examples of artifacts in OCT images. These are (from left to right) sew-up (shearing) error, guide-wire reflection/shadow, stents, swirls, and speckles caused by blood in lumen occluding the light source.

The nature of the IVUS and OCT images, with very pronounced artifacts, lend themselves well to this semiautomatic approach, with most parts of the image being such that the automatic process will be suitable, but by allowing user input, the difficult regions (such as shadows and various artifacts) can be accommodated easily. Interactive segmentation that can efficiently and effectively transfer user knowledge to the segmentation is thus highly desirable in this application. It also allows us quantitatively evaluate our method, including both efficiency and accuracy.

The rest of the chapter is organized as follows: Section 18.2 presents the proposed method, including user input, superpixel segmentation, and multilayered graph segmentation, as well as an overview of the cost terms and minimization method. Experimental results from segmenting medical datasets with ground truth are presented in Section 18.3. These show the results for IVUS and OCT images, and quantitative data obtained from these datasets, demonstrating the effectiveness of the technique compared to other methodologies. We show a selection of examples from other medical imaging modalities to demonstrate that the method can be used for other image types and then show results for generic images, further demonstrating the versatility and robustness of the method. Section 18.4 concludes the work.

18.2   Proposed method

The proposed method involves the user selecting a series of user control points on the image. These represent the start and the end point for the segmentation, and the user-selected points act as the attraction points in the shortest path search, which results in the segmentation. These user-selected points act in a fashion similar to an elastic band, pulling the segmentation toward them. In this way, it is possible for the user to influence the segmentation process allowing them to preferentially select features that they want. In order to enhance the image segmentation, the user can also select areas for foreground using strokes.

An energy function is then formulated based on the combination of the attraction force, which is computed using distance transform, and the discontinuity in foreground probability. By assuming the user points are in a sequential order (as without this the problem will be NP-hard and computationally intensive), we construct a multilayer graph with each layer encapsulating a single individual user point. Effectively, we create multiple identical layers, all made up of duplicates of the image, for each user point added. The segmentation problem is then transformed into searching the shortest path in this layered graph, which is the resulting segmentation is obtained through searching a minimum path in this stack of layers in a manner similar to a 3D object.

Another effect caused by the creation of layers is that order is forced onto the problem. With no sequential order to the points, the problem becomes that of the traveling salesman, and becomes NP-hard. By using the layered approach, which ensures sequential transition between layers, the segmentation can be carried out in polynomial time, instead of an NP-hard optimization problem, at the same time achieving global minima.

18.2.1   User input

The proposed method allows two different types of user input: attraction points to indicate the edge of the desired object and strokes to indicate region of interest. Figure 18.10 provides an example of segmentation using the proposed method. Conventionally, user input to segmentation is focused on foreground and background specification [15–18]. For example, in Blake et al. [16], the user interaction consists of dragging a rectangle around the object of interest and in doing so the user specifies a region of background that is modeled in separating the foreground object. Several other methods require user to specify points on the object boundaries instead [5,19,20]. Examples of these methods are shown in Figure 18.9. However, more often than not, these boundary-based user points are treated as anchor points and the segmentation path has to go through them. This kind of hard constraint is not always desirable. It does not allow imprecise user input, and it can lead to difficulties in combining region-based and boundary-based approaches as discrepancy between different object descriptions is generally expected. Notably, in Windheuser et al. [20] the authors introduced soft constraint user point by embedding the user constraint in distance functions. The segmentation result is considered to be the shortest path to loosely connect the user points. However, it is known to be a NP-hard problem. Hence, it is assumed that the user points are placed in a sequential order and such a constraint reduced the computational complexity to polynomial time. This user input constraint can be seen to be generally acceptable as it is intuitive to follow the outline of an object, rather than skipping around. In this work, we follow this approach to treat boundary-based user points. However, we also allow user to place region-based strokes. These strokes are used to model foreground probability, and the discontinuity in foreground probability indicates the presence of object boundary. We combine these two types of user input with image features in an energy functional, which is then optimized using graph partitioning through finding the shortest path from the first to last user points. Moreover, we apply a superpixel segmentation in order to generate a much coarser, but irregular, multilayer graph so that the computational cost is drastically reduced. It also provides a regional support at a low level for the shortest path search in the graph.

18.2.2   Superpixel segmentation

Efficient search for the shortest path, for instance, using Dijkstra's algorithm on a multidimensional graph is not a trivial task. Many researchers attempted to speed up the Dijkstra's algorithm by, for example, using multilevel scaling [33] or restricting the search space [34] by deciding whether or not the edge will be considered during the searching process. One mechanism that can be used to minimize the amount of nodes on the graph is superpixel segmentation. Superpixel segmentation is a process that groups a set of homogeneous neighboring pixels together to reduce the complexity of solving further image processing such as segmentation [3,22] and object localization [35]. Superpixel segmentation algorithms vary from graph based [36,37] to gradient descent methods [38,39].

In this chapter, we speed up the Dijkstra's algorithm by using the mean shift method to oversegment the image, and thus create the superpixels. This oversegmented image is then used to create the graph, by only considering the boundary of the superpixel regions as a potential paths that can be used to find the shortest path between two points, and the whole process is thus far more efficient. Additionally, this superpixel segmentation provides low-level regional information to the graph search, which relies significantly on edge information.

Mean shift algorithm [38] is a nonparametric gradient descent method that iteratively shifts the mean of the region toward the local maxima of the density for a given set of samples. Mean shift method is suitable for clustering data without any assumption of the cluster shape. It has been widely used in many applications, such as segmentation [38] and tracking [40]. Given n data points (pixels) of x_i in the d-dimensional space R^d, the nonparametric probability function is defined by kernel density estimator (KDE) as the following:

$$f(x) = \frac{1}{nh^d} \sum_{i=1}^{n} K\left(\frac{x - x_i}{h}\right) \tag{18.1}$$

where h is the bandwidth parameter and K is the radially symmetric kernel such as Gaussian kernel $K(x) = (2\pi)^{-d/2} \exp(-\frac{1}{2}\|x\|^2)$. The local maxima of density is located among the zeros of the gradient $\|\nabla f(x)\| \cong 0$. So the mean shift can be derived as the following:

$$m_{h,G(x)}(x) = \frac{\sum_{i=1}^{n} x_i G\left(\left\|\frac{x-x_i}{h}\right\|^2\right)}{\sum_{i=1}^{n} G\left(\left\|\frac{x-x_i}{h}\right\|^2\right)} - x \tag{18.2}$$

where $G(x) = -K'(x)$ and $m_{h,G(x)}(x)$ is the difference between the weighted mean, using kernel G, and x, the center of the kernel. The mean shift vector points toward the maximum increase of the density and it converges at a nearby point where the density estimate has zero gradient.

Figure 18.12 provides an example of the mean shift segmentation. Mean shift is preserving the edge features in the image. The black region, shown in the rightmost of the figure, represents areas on or close to edges in the superpixel segmentation, and are used

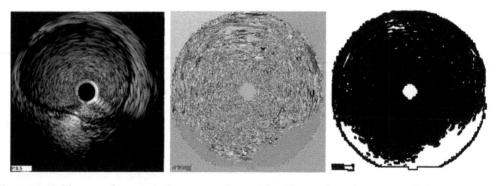

Figure 18.12 The use of superpixel segmentation to identify graph nodes in a single layer in a IVUS image. From left to right, initial image, superpixel segmentation, binary representation of graph nodes.

to construct the graph as it is discussed in the next section. In order to prevent the segmentation being too jagged in IVUS images, it was necessary to increase the amount of segmentation obtained in this stage.

18.2.3 Layered graph construction

In order to impose a soft constraint for a user point, we follow the approach proposed in Windheuser et al. [20] to construct a layered graph so that given a set of attraction points we fit a curve to follow the edges in the image and pass through the vicinity of the given points. The user points are assumed to be placed in a sequential order, which is acceptable in most applications. The computational complexity, however, is reduced from being NP-hard to polynomial time.

For each user point, $X_i, i \in \{1, 2, \ldots, k\}$, we create a new layer of directed graph. This is a copy of the image layer, with the same edge-based weighting. In that way, we have a series of layers equal to the number of user points n, plus an additional layer in order for the weighting of the last user point to be used, as shown in Figure 18.13. This results in a multilayer directed graph, $G = (V, E)$, where V is the set of vertices, and E the set of weighted edges. For each pixel p, there exits an edge e to each of its neighboring pixels on the same layer, providing that they are on the boundaries of the superpixels. Therefore, a pair of neighboring pixels $(p, q) \in V$ with a corresponding edge $e = (v_p, v_q)$ also have an edge to the corresponding point on the superseding layer $e = (v_{p_i}, v_{p_{i+1}})$, where i represents the current layer of the image. For each edge, we assign a weight w to build a weighted graph (V, E). These weights are calculated based on whether the edge is internal to a layer (w_i) or translayer (w_x). By creating the graph in this way, an order is established with the user points, yet allowing for a global minimum to be found, rather than a series of pairwise local minima. Edges of zero weight are added from the start node s to each pixel in the first

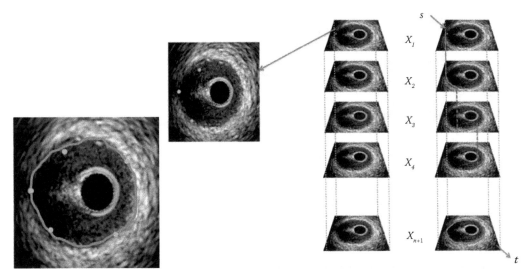

Figure 18.13 Example of 3D graph traversal. The stack of images on the right show how the graph is constructed out of a number of layers corresponding to the number of user points $n + 1$. The algorithm finds the shortest path through the layers, minimizing the costs of edges, boundaries, and distance from user points. The final result of the segmentation is shown on the left.

layer, and from the last layer $k + 1$ to the terminal node t. This has the effect of making the first and the last user points elastic and not hard constraints. For example, if the first user point X_1 is not located on an edge, then in the overall minimization, it would be of lower cost to enter the first layer at the nearest point to X_1 on a strong edge. In this way, all user points act as soft constraints.

If P is the set of pixels in the image, P_s is therefore the subset of pixels that also fall on the boundaries of our superpixels, and p_i and q_i are pixels in layer i giving v_{p_i} as the vertex p in layer i, we can define the set of nodes V as

$$V = \{s, t\} \cup \{p_i \in P_s \wedge 1 \leq i \leq k + 1\} \tag{18.3}$$

and thusly the set of edges as

$$E = \begin{cases} (s, v_{p_1}) | p \in P_s & \cup \\ (v_{p_{k+1}}, t) | p \in P_s & \cup \\ (v_{p_i}, v_{q_i}) | (p, q) \in N \wedge 1 \leq i \leq k + 1 & \cup \\ (v_{p_i}, v_{p_{i+1}}) | p \in P_s \wedge 1 \leq i \leq k + 1. \end{cases} \tag{18.4}$$

The segmentation is thus to find the shortest path from the start point s to the end point t. See Figure 18.13 across the 3D graph.

The edges on the directed layered graph are categorized as internal edges w_i within individual layers and interlayer edges w_x. The weighting for these two types of edges is assigned differently. The internal edges are assigned with two types of weights, that is, boundary-based edge weights and region-based edge weights. The boundary-based edge weights are calculated based on the magnitude of image gradients, created for example with a Sobel filter, that is, using an edge detection function $g_e = 1/(1 + \nabla I)$ where I denotes the image or its smoothed version using, for instance, Gaussian filtering. Hence, for any given edge between neighboring pixels (v_p, v_q), we assign a weight (w_e) according to

$$w_e((v_p, v_q)) := \frac{1}{2} \|p - q\| (g_e(p) + g_e(q)). \tag{18.5}$$

The region-based edge weights are computed from foreground probabilities. The user strokes placed in the foreground provide an estimation for foreground intensity distribution, which is then used to evaluate each pixel in the image. The discontinuity in this generated probability map is then used to compute the region-based edge weight in the similar fashion to image intensity, that is,

$$w_f((v_p, v_q)) := \frac{1}{2} \|p - q\| (g_f(p) + g_f(q)) \tag{18.6}$$

where g_f is the edge detection function based on probability values.

By combining in a weight derived from this discontinuity map, we add an extra level of robustness to the method. As regions not selected as foreground will have an increased cost, if there exists strong edges that may cause errors in our segmentation, but are not selected as foreground then the likelihood of the segmentation following these edges is greatly reduced.

The internal edge weight is thus the linear combination of the boundary-based weight and region-based weight:

$$w_i = w_e + w_f \tag{18.7}$$

The attraction force imposed by user points is materialized through the interlayer edge weights w_x. We apply distance transform to the user points in each layer of the graph, and the interlayer edge weight is assigned as $w_x = d(v_{p_i}, v_{p_j})$ where d denotes the distance transform function. This distance weighting produces isolinear bands of weight around the user point, with increasing weight to go through to the next layer as the distance from the user point increases.

18.2.4 Energy minimization

The energy function for any curve C in our method is a combination of three terms, that is, for any arc C between two points p_i and q_j where the points are

$$C(p, q) = w_x + w_i \tag{18.8}$$

as w_x can be written as

$$\alpha \sum_{i=1}^{k} ||C(s_i) - X_i|| \tag{18.9}$$

and likewise w_i can be written as:

$$\beta \int_0^{L(C)} g(C(s))ds + \int_0^{L(C)} g_f(C(s))ds, \tag{18.10}$$

This is all providing that the points are treated as being in a sequential order, and that the interconnections between layers are unidirectional. The overall energy function can then be expressed as:

$$\mathcal{E}(C, s_1, ..., s_k) = \alpha \sum_{i=1}^{k} ||C(s_i) - X_i|| + \beta \int_0^{L(C)} g(C(s))ds + \int_0^{L(C)} g_f(C(s))ds, \tag{18.11}$$

$$s.t. \quad s_i < s_j, \forall i < j.$$

where α and β are real constants used to weigh the effects of the edge- and distance-based terms, respectively. Figure 18.14 shows how changing the ratio of these constants can be used to put more or less emphasis on the control points (even going so far as to remove the elastic property when the ratio is skewed largely in favor of α.

The first term is used to enforce the soft constraint by the user points, and it penalizes the paths further away from the user points. The second term is the boundary-based data term that prefers the path passing through strong edges, while the last term is the region-based data term, which prefers path traveling through abrupt changes in foreground probability. By using the layered graph construction, the minimization of the energy functional is achieved by finding the shortest path from the start point s to the end point t. The Dijkstra's algorithm is used to calculate the shortest path in the layered directed graph. Note that the interlayer edges are unidirectional so that the path cannot travel back to previously visited layers.

(a)   (b)

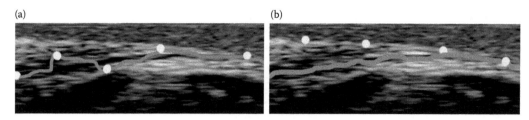

Figure 18.14 Effect of changing α and β. (a) The ratio of these two constants skewed toward adding more emphasis on the user points, thus reducing the "elastic" properties. (b) The other extreme, with the user points being bypassed in favor of the stronger edge.

Dijkstra's algorithm is working on a directed graph $G(V, E)$ to find the shortest path between two defined nodes, and the algorithm divides the nodes of the graph into two sets: visited and unvisited nodes. Once the node is marked as a visited node, it will not be checked again. The algorithm starts searching from the starting node s, assigns an initial tentative distance of zero to the starting node and infinity to all other nodes, and then calculates the tentative distances for all neighboring nodes. These tentative distances are defined as the summation of the edge weight w_i and the current distance of the beginning node of that edge. The edge weight must be nonnegative value. The algorithm will mark the node that has the minimum distance as a visited node. The algorithm will repeat the process by calculating the tentative distance for all neighboring nodes for all visited nodes and only mark the node having the minimum distance as a visited node until reaching the terminal node t. The running time of Dijkstra's algorithm is $O(|E| + |V|log|V|)$ where E is the number of edges and V is the number of nodes.

18.3   *Experimental results*

To show the effectiveness of the proposed method, we test our method for two different medical applications. The two applications use medical dataset of IVUS images that has ground truth available for quantitative comparisons, and a set of OCT images. The segmentation of images in the medical application is very challenging as it generally requires anatomical prior knowledge, as well as other expert knowledge in some cases, in order to sufficiently perform the segmentation task. This makes interactive segmentation the preferred approach to this application. Wherever appropriate, we present comparison to other interactive segmentation techniques. We also show a more generic set of images, to illustrate the versatility of our method, to highlight how it can be used for other (medical) applications.

18.3.1   *IVUS image segmentation*

To study the efficiency and efficacy of the proposed method, we apply our method to a medical image segmentation problem where expert prior knowledge in anatomy is necessary but also often subjective. Here we need to interactively identify the media–adventitia border in IVUS images where imaging artifacts are common place.

There have been many different approaches to the problem of segmenting IVUS images [28,31,41–45]. These can be broadly categorized into fully automatic methods, or methods that allow user interactions. In Luo et al. [41], the authors used contour detection and

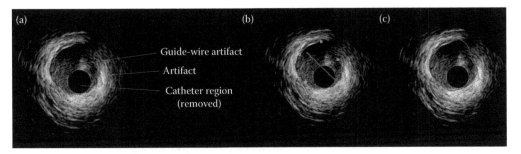

Figure 18.15 Overview of an IVUS image, and segmentation by the proposed method. (a) Original IVUS image. (b) User input. (c) Segmentation result.

tracing with smoothness constraint and circular dynamic programming optimization to segment lumen border. It assumes homogeneity of the lumen region and high contrast between lumen and artery wall. Katouzian et al. [42] applied complex brushlet transform and constructed magnitudes-phase histograms of coefficients that contain distinct peaks corresponding to lumen and nonlumen regions. The lumen region is then segmented based on K-means classification and a parametric deformable model. Homogeneity of the lumen region is critical to the success of the method. Methods based on region growing, for example, Brathwaite et al. [44], also suffers from such limitations, since artifacts and irregularities are very common in IVUS images. Particularly for media–adventitia border, the region inside the border is nonuniform as seen in Figure 18.15. Calcification in arterial wall leads to acoustic shadowing and high reflectance, as well as catheter and guild wire occlusion and artifacts. Stent placed against internal wall also produces strong features and acoustic shadows that break homogeneity. Incorporating user prior knowledge into segmentation hence is often necessary and has been shown to be an effective approach. For instance, Essa et al. [31] incorporated a shape prior into graph-cut construction to regularize segmentation of media–adventitia border. However, these approaches generally require significant amount of training data and model retraining is often necessary in order to adapt to new dataset. In Sonka et al. [43], dynamic programming was used to incorporate edge information with a rudimentary prior. This required manual initialization but set the way for other more advanced techniques for incorporating priors. The work in Takagi et al. [45] carried out border detection on the envelope data before the scan conversion. The authors applied spatio temporal filters to highlight the lumen, based on the assumption that the blood speckles have higher spatial and temporal variations than arterial wall, followed by a graph-searching method similar to Sonka et al. [43]. However, image features introduced by acoustic shadow or metallic stent would seriously undermine the assumption.

User initialization is an alternative approach to transfer expert knowledge into segmentation (e.g., [5,16–20,46]). However, most user interactions are limited to either boundary-based landmark placement or strokes, indicating foreground and background regions. We adapt the approach of combining two different types of user interactions, that is boundary based and region based, to segment media–adventitia border in IVUS. The user points are treated as soft constraint, instead of hard constraint in most interactive segmentation methods. We show that this soft user constraint allows effective combination of boundary- and region-based features. The method is evaluated on an IVUS dataset with manually labeled ground truth and compared against state-of-the-art techniques.

(a)

(b)

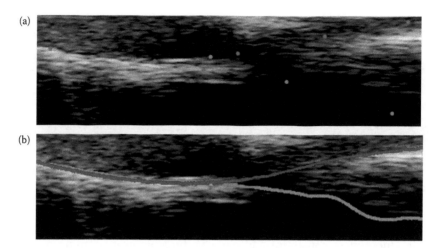

Figure 18.16 Effectiveness in imposing user prior knowledge. As in the natural image segmentation, the user can select different edges by the use of user points. In this case, it can be seen that there are two possibilities for the media–adventitia border in the image. By placing a couple of points, the user can steer the segmentation along the path they desire.

Figure 18.16 illustrates the benefit of using user interaction to effectively influence the segmentation result. Through simple user input, the expert knowledge of the user can be put into place, whilst being augmented by the automatic process. Figure 18.17 provides several examples of IVUS images (the ground truth of media–adventitia layer can be seen in green). Figure 18.18 shows further examples of IVUS image segmentation using single method approach and our proposed full method.

18.3.2   OCT image segmentation

We also compared our proposed method to other methods in OCT images. OCT is another catheter-based modality used in cardiology. In these images, we are segmenting the lumenal border rather than the media–adventitia border, which was targeted in IVUS. We chose this as OCT has far lower penetrance than IVUS images, but yields a much higher resolution view of the lumenal border. This makes it favorable for assessing stent placement and other surface lesions. Comparative examples are given in Figure 18.19, and a further comparison between the single method and the proposed full method is shown in Figure 18.20.

18.3.3   Quantitative results

In order to evaluate the results, we used a set of 248 IVUS images with ground truth. They were taken from pull backs on seven different patients. The ground truth labeling was obtained through manual labeling of the border of interest. These were then segmented using the proposed method, which was compared to the method using only the edge detection and not the background/foreground weighting (single method) [20] and star graph-cut (both with single and multiple seed points) [18]. Grab Cut segmentation was not used for the quantitative analysis, because as can be seen from Figure 18.21 it performs very poorly in this application. The quantitative analysis was also carried out on the results obtained from the OCT data. In this case, we were segmenting the lumenal edge, which

Star graph-cut [18]	Seeded star GC [18]	Single method [20]	Proposed method

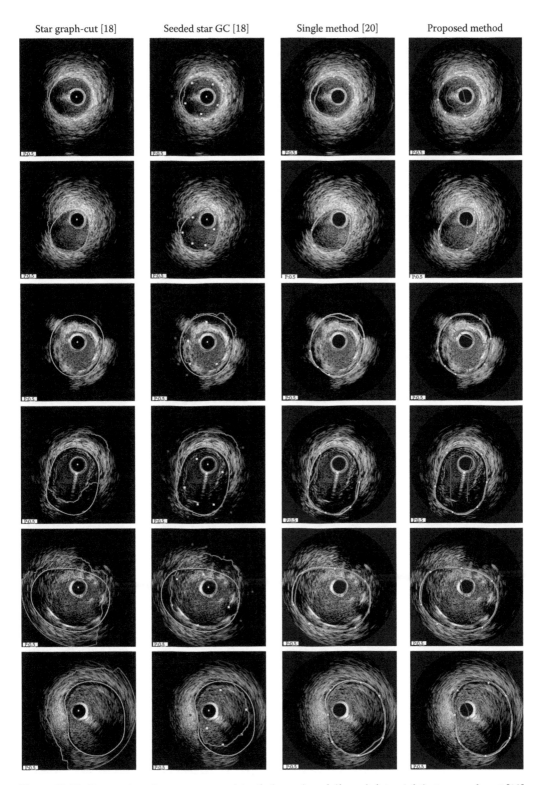

Figure 18.17 Comparison between ground truth (green) and (from left to right) star graph-cut [18], seeded star graph-cut [18], single method [20], proposed method (red). Note that the user control points used remain the same for both the single and proposed methods.

Single method   Proposed method   Single method   Proposed method

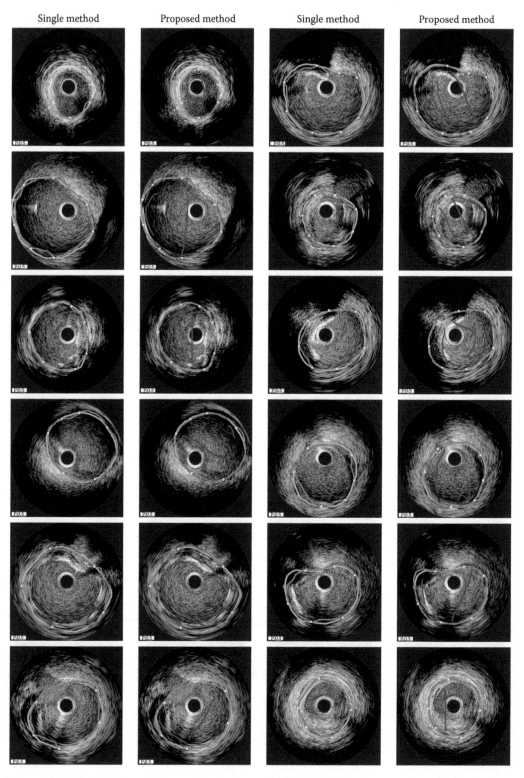

Figure 18.18 Comparison between the single method [20] and our proposed method (red). The ground truth is in shown in green. Note that the user control points used remain the same for both methods.

Star graph-cut [18]	Seeded star GC [18]	Single method [20]	Proposed method

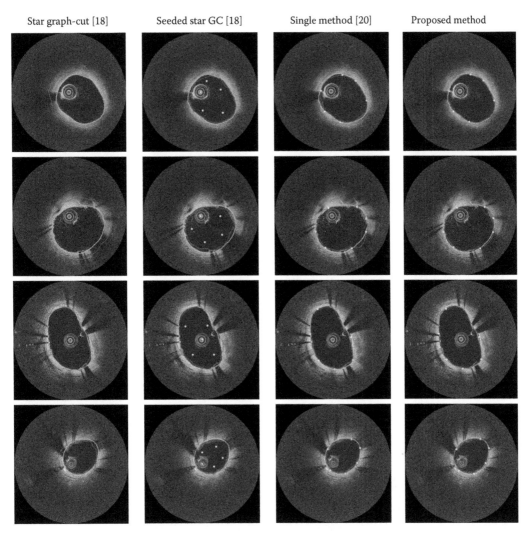

Figure 18.19 Comparison between ground truth (green) and (from left to right) star graph-cut, seeded star graph-cut, single method (no regional constraints), and proposed method (red) on OCT images to segment the lumen border.

is quite well defined and regular, so all methods saw an improvement in accuracy. The results were obtained from a similar number of images as before (280) from seven different pull-backs.

The quantitative comparison is based on a number of metrics, including Hausdorff distance, area overlap ratio, specificity, sensitivity, and accuracy. Table 18.1 shows the quantitative results obtained from the IVUS data, and Table 18.2 shows the OCT data. The star graph-cut method performed reasonably well with both foreground and background labeling. The implicit shape prior in star graph construction proved useful constraint in segmenting media–adventitia border that conforms well to this shape constraint. Comparable performance was achieved for the proposed method without regional support. However, the full proposed method outperformed the rest. Several typical segmentation results are shown in Figure 18.17.

Single method   Proposed method   Single method   Proposed method

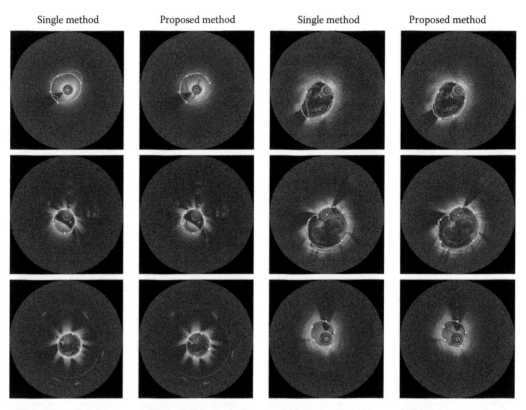

Figure 18.20 Comparison between the single method [20] and our proposed method (red) on OCT images. The ground truth is shown in green. Note that the user control points used remain the same for both methods.

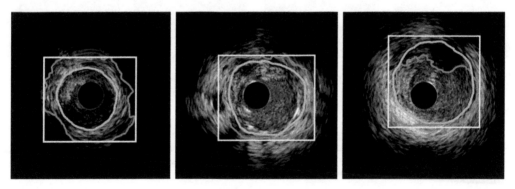

Figure 18.21 Typical Grab Cut segmentation results (red) on IVUS images. Ground truth is shown in green. It can be clearly seen that the obtained results are considerably out from the ground truth.

To study the robustness of the proposed method, we carried out an initialization dependency test. We tested our method with 15 user points as initialization. We then randomly remove one user point each time for testing until we only have two points left for initialization. The overall results using five different metrics are shown in Figure 18.22. The proposed method achieved good performance with just six user points. Considering

Table 18.1 Quantitative comparison of the IVUS dataset

Method		HD	AOR	Spec	Sens	Acc
Star graph-cut	Mean	60.57	81.22	89.22	89.86	89.29
	STD	15.64	1.00	12.00	1.00	6.52
Star graph-cut with F/B labeling	Mean	43.81	86.05	90.39	**93.99**	92.17
	STD	23.89	9.00	9.00	5.00	5.65
Single method w/o F/B labeling	Mean	46.28	69.34	84.92	89.43	88.12
	STD	9.73	9.24	5.82	10.53	8.76
Proposed method with F/B labeling	Mean	**33.57**	**89.93**	**94.21**	93.14	**94.41**
	STD	5.35	9.16	3.88	5.37	7.67

Note: HD: Hausdorff distance (pixels); AOR: Area overlap ratio (%); Spec: Specificity (%); Sens: Sensitivity (%), Acc: Accuracy (%). Bold font indicates best performance.

Table 18.2 Quantitative comparison of the OCT dataset

Method		HD	AOR	Spec	Sens	Acc
Star graph-cut	Mean	21.55	91.75	98.09	96.73	97.41
	STD	16.07	5.36	1.61	3.99	2.80
Single method w/o F/B labeling	Mean	21.47	91.66	98.01	97.11	97.56
	STD	14.94	8.21	2.32	4.25	3.28
Proposed method with F/B labeling	Mean	**20.97**	**92.31**	**98.66**	**97.92**	**98.29**
	STD	15.84	4.99	1.76	3.60	2.68

Note: HD: Hausdorff distance (pixels); AOR: Area overlap ratio (%); Spec: Specificity (%); Sens: Sensitivity (%), Acc: Accuracy (%). Bold font indicates best performance.

in actual application where user input is far more experienced than this random process, even less points may be needed.

18.3.4   Further results

In order to demonstrate the versatility of the proposed method, we carried out segmentation of examples from other medical imaging modalities, as well as generic real world images. We believe that our method could equally be used in many other types of medical image analysis, as its ability to segment open as well as closed curves effectively gives it a great deal of versatility. By showing the results of segmentation of a series of real-world images, we can further show the versatility and robustness of this method. Using sample images from other studies, we show examples of how various features can be segmented out of medical images (see Figure 18.23).

The proposed method was also evaluated using the Berkeley Image Database [47]. This dataset contains images of various types. The methods were used to perform a selection/segmentation based on features in the image that would be a realistic segmentation to be carried out (e.g., object selection, horizon selection, etc.) The results from the proposed method were then compared to other available methods, namely $s - t$ graph-cut

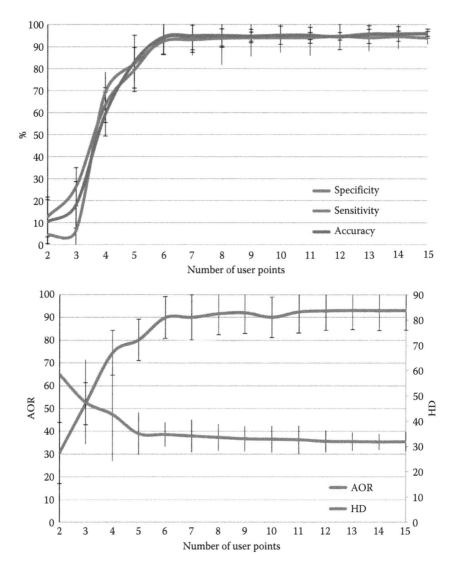

Figure 18.22 Initialization dependency test. This test was carried out using the IVUS data. The number of user points placed on the image was increased, and the effect of this on the observed metrics was recorded. It can be seen that only after a very few number of user points have been added, the accuracy reaches a plateau, which is an indication of good automation.

[15], seeded star graph-cut [18], Grab Cut [16], and layered graph search with only point-based interaction [20]. A selection of open and closed curve segmentations were used to demonstrate and compare the results.

The proposed method showed a very favorable segmentation performance compared to the methods we tested it against. The combination of a background/foreground separation, combined with the edge-based approach, gave the method a very robust segmentation, being able to segment an object of interest from an image where other (single methodology based) techniques found difficult to handle, for example if colors were closely

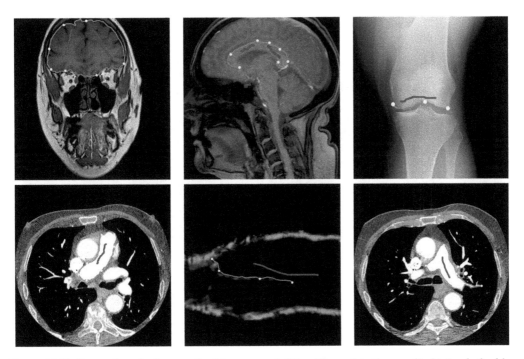

Figure 18.23 Examples of other medical image modalities. The red is the result obtained, the blue lines and the yellow circles the region selection and control points added, respectively.

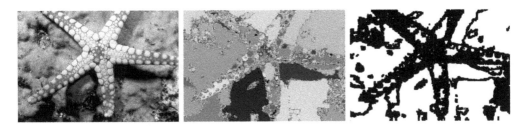

Figure 18.24 The use of superpixel segmentation of real-world images to identify graph nodes. From left to right, initial image, superpixel segmentation, binary representation of graph nodes.

related to background, or if there were many conflicting edges. This method utilizes super-pixels to speed up the segmentation in the same manner as with the medical images. However, do to the nature of real-world images, the increase in speed is more significant (as there are more distinct regions that can be segmented out using the presegmentation step as shown in Figure 18.24).

The advantage in being able to perform with open or closed curves is shown in some of the images, for example dividing the image on the horizon or segmenting figures that extend to the edge of the image. Figure 18.25 provides several comparative results in segmenting images of humans from complex backgrounds.

Figure 18.26 demonstrates the advantages of the inclusion of regional data into the algorithm, in comparison to Windheuser et al. [20]. In some cases, where there are edges other than those required, without the regional selection, the segmentation can lose

Graph-cut [15]   Seeded star graph-cut [18]   Grab Cut [16]   Proposed method

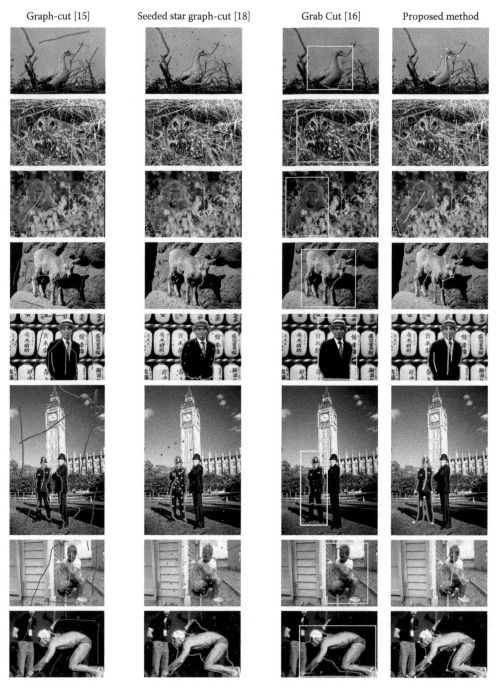

Figure 18.25 Segmenting human from complex scenes. From left: Original image, graph-cut [15], seeded star graph-cut [18], Grab Cut [16], and the proposed method. Red curve shows the segmentation result, blue for the background strokes, green for foreground strokes, and yellow for star point and the initial window of the Grab Cut.

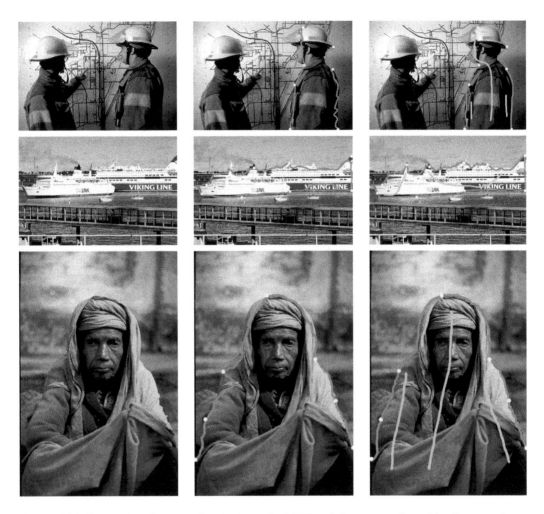

Figure 18.26 Comparison between the single method [20] and the proposed combined approach.

accuracy. By selecting the region specificity, in most cases, these edges can be ignored without the requirement for more user points, which would increase the complexity of the graph.

18.4 Conclusion

We presented an interactive segmentation technique that combines boundary- and region-based object representations. We used this method to segment two sets of medical images (IVUS and OCT). We adopted a layered graph representation to simplify computation, and a superpixel method to improve segmentation speed and efficiency. The proposed method was compared against a number of recent methods, and the standard graph-cut techniques, showing improved versatility and better results. Where other methods had difficulty with certain image types, the combined approach was able to segment the desired information. We also show our method being used to segment different medical images, using open and closed objects, as well as generic real-world images. This we believe shows how versatile the method is, and how easily it could be used for other applications.

Acknowledgment

We would like to thank Dr. Dave Smith from Swansea Morriston Hospital and Dr. James Cotton from the Royal Wolverhampton NHS Trust for providing the IVUS and OCT datasets and their expertise in establishing the ground truth. This research is funded by NISCHR. J. Jones is a recipient of EPSRC Doctoral Training Grant.2.5pc]Q4

References

1. F. Zhao and X. Xie, An overview of interactive medical image segmentation, *Annals of the BMVA*, vol. 7, pp. 1–22, 2013.
2. E. Essa, X. Xie, I. Sazonov, and P. Nithiarasu, Automatic IVUS media–adventitia border extraction using double interface graph cut segmentation, *IEEE International Conference on Image Processing*, pp. 69–72, 2011.
3. L. J. Reese, Intelligent paint: Region-based interactive image segmentation, Masters Thesis, Department of Computer Science, Brigham Young University, 1999.
4. E. N. Mortensen and W. A. Barrett, Interactive segmentation with intelligent scissors, *Graphical Models and Image Processing*, vol. 60, no. 5, pp. 349–384, 1998.
5. A. X. Falco, J. K. Udupa, S. Samarasekera, S. Sharma, B. Elliot Hirsch, and R. de A. Lotufo, User-steered image segmentation paradigms: Live wire and live lane, *Graphical Models and Image Processing*, vol. 60, no. 4, pp. 233–260, 1998.
6. K. Humnabadkar, S. Singh, D. Ghosh, and P.K. Bora, Unsupervised active contour model for biological image segmentation and analysis, In *Instrumentation and Measurement Technology Conference (I2MTC) Proceedings, 2014 IEEE International*, pp. 1443–1448, 2014.
7. X. Li, X. Wang, and Y. Dai, Robust global minimization of active contour model for multi-object medical image segmentation, In *Instrumentation and Measurement Technology Conference (I2MTC) Proceedings, 2014 IEEE International*, pp. 1443–1448, 2014.
8. X. Xie and M. Mirmehdi, Magnetostatic field for the active contour model: A study in convergence, In *Proceedings of the 17th British Machine Vision Conference*, pp. 127–136, 2008.
9. X. Xie and M. Mirmehdi, Magnetostatic active contour mode, In *IEEE Transactions on Pattern Analysis and Machine Intelligence (T-PAMI)*, pp. 632–646, 2008.
10. L. Cohen and I. Cohen, Finite-element methods for active contour models and balloons for 2-D and 3-D images, *IEEE Transactions on Pattern Analysis and Machine Intelligence*, vol. 15, no. 11, pp. 1131–1147, 1993.
11. V. Caselles, R. Kimmel, and G. Sapiro, Geodesic active contour, *International Journal of Computer Vision*, vol. 22, no. 1, pp. 61–79, 1997.
12. C. Xu and J. Prince, Generalized gradient vector flow external forces for active contours, *Signal Processing*, vol. 71, no. 2, pp. 131–139, 1998.
13. N. Paragios, O. Mellina-Gottardo, and V. Ramesh, Gradient vector flow geometric active contours, *IEEE Transactions on Pattern Analysis and Machine Intelligence*, vol. 26, no. 3, pp. 402–407, 2004.
14. A. Jalba, M. Wilkinson, and J. Roerdink, CPM: A deformable model for shape recovery and segmentation based on charged particles, *IEEE Transactions on Pattern Analysis and Machine Intelligence*, vol. 26, no. 10, pp. 1320–1335, 2004.
15. Y. Y. Boykov and M.-P. Jolly, Interactive graph cuts for optimal boundary and region segmentation of objects in n-d images, *International Conference on Computer Vision*, vol. 1, pp. 105–112, 2001.
16. A. Blake C. Rother, and V. Kolmogorov, Grabcut: Interactive foreground extraction using iterated graph cuts, *ACM Transactions on Graphics*, vol. 23, no. 3, pp. 309–314, 2004.

17. A. K. Sinop and L. Grady, A seeded image segmentation framework unifying graph cuts and random walker which yields a new algorithm, *International Conference on Computer Vision*, pp. 1–8, 2007.
18. O. Veksler, Star shape prior for graph-cut image segmentation, In *ECCV*, pp. 454–467, 2008.
19. L. D. Cohen and R. Kimmel, Global minimum for active contour models: A minimal path approach, *International Journal of Computer Vision*, vol. 24, no. 1, pp. 57–78, 1997.
20. T. Windheuser, T. Schoenemann, and D. Cremers, Beyond connecting the dots: A polynomial-time algorithm for segmentation and boundary estimation with imprecise user input, *International Conference on Computer Vision*, pp. 717–722, 2009.
21. H. Zhang, E. Essa, and X. Xie, Graph based segmentation with minimal user interaction, In *Proceedings of IEEE International Conference on Image Processing*, pp. 4074–4078, 2011.
22. Y. Li, J. Sun, C.-K. Tang, and H.-Y. Shum, Lazy snapping, *ACM Transactions on Graphics*, vol. 23, no. 3, pp. 303–308, 2004.
23. D. Freedman and T. Zhang, Interactive graph cut based segmentation with shape priors, *IEEE Conference on Computer Vision and Pattern Recognition*, pp. 755–762, 2005.
24. J. Malcolm, Y. Rathi, and A. Tannenbaum, Graph cut segmentation with nonlinear shape priors, *IEEE International Conference on Image Processing*, pp. 365–368, 2007.
25. N. Vu and B. S. Manjunath, Shape prior segmentation of multiple objects with graph cuts, *IEEE Conference on Computer Vision and Pattern Recognition*, pp. 1–8, 2008.
26. V. Gulshan, C. Rother, A. Criminisi, A. Blake, and A. Zisserman, Geodesic star convexity for interactive image segmentation, *IEEE Conference on Computer Vision and Pattern Recognition*, pp. 3129–3136, 2010.
27. O. Duchenne, J.-Y. Audibert, R. Keriven, J. Ponce, and F. Segonne, Segmentation by transduction, *IEEE Conference on Computer Vision and Pattern Recognition*, pp. 1–8, 2008.
28. A. Katouzian, E. D. Angelini, S. G. Carlier, J. S. Suri, N. Navab, and A. F. Laine, A state-of-the-art review on segmentation algorithms in intravascular ultrasound (IVUS) images, *IEEE Transactions on Information Technology in Biomedicine*, vol. 16, no. 5, pp. 823–834, 2012.
29. M. C. Moraes and S. S. Furuie, An automatic media–adventitia border segmentation approach for IVUS images, *Computing in Cardiology*, pp. 389–392, 2010.
30. L. S. Atahnasiou, C. V. Bourantas, G. A. Rigas, and T. P. Exarchos, Fully automated calcium detection using optical coherence tomography, In *Engineering in Medicine and Biology Society (EMBC), 2013 35th Annual International Conference of the IEEE*, pp. 1430–1433, 2013.
31. E. Essa, X. Xie, I. Sazonov, P. Nithiarasu, and D. Smith, Shape prior model for media–adventitia border segmentation in IVUS using graph cut, *LNCS, Medical Computer Vision. Recognition Techniques and Applications in Medical Imaging*, vol. 7766, pp. 114–123, 2013.
32. K.-P. Tung, W.-Z. Shi, R. De Silva, and E. Edwards, Automatical vessel wall detection in intravascular coronary OCT, In *Biomedical Imaging: From Nano to Macro, 2011 IEEE International Symposium on*, pp. 610–613, 2011.
33. M. Holzer, F. Schulz, and D. Wagner, Engineering multilevel overlay graphs for shortest-path queries, *Journal of Experimental Algorithmics*, vol. 13, no. 5, pp. 2.5–2.26, 2009.
34. D. Wagner and T. Willhalm, Geometric speed-up techniques for finding shortest paths in large sparse graphs, *European Symposium on Algorithms (ESA)*, vol. 2832, pp. 776–787, 2003.
35. B. Fulkerson, A. Vedaldi, and S. Soatto, Class segmentation and object localization with superpixel neighborhoods, *International Conference on Computer Vision*, pp. 670–677, 2009.
36. J. Shi and J. Malik, Normalized cuts and image segmentation, *IEEE Transactions on Pattern Analysis and Machine Intelligence*, vol. 22, no. 8, pp. 888–905, 2000.
37. A. P. Moore, S. J. D. Prince, and J. Warrell, Lattice cut—Constructing superpixels using layer constraints, *IEEE Conference on Computer Vision and Pattern Recognition*, pp. 2117–2124, 2010.
38. D. Comaniciu and P. Meer, Mean shift: A robust approach toward feature space analysis, *T-PAMI*, vol. 24, no. 5, pp. 603–619, 2002.
39. L. Vincent and P. Soille, Watersheds in digital spaces: An efficient algorithm based on immersion simulations, *IEEE Transactions on Pattern Analysis and Machine Intelligence*, vol. 13, no. 6, pp. 583–598, 1991.

40. D. Comaniciu, V. Ramesh, and P. Meer, Real-time tracking of non-rigid objects using mean shift, *IEEE Conference on Computer Vision and Pattern Recognition*, pp. 142–149, 2000.

41. Z. Luo, Y. Wang, and W. Wang, Estimating coronary artery lumen area with optimization-based contour detection, *IEEE Transactions on Medical Imaging*, vol. 22, no. 4, pp. 564–566, 2003.

42. A. Katouzian, E. D. Angelini, B. Sturm, and A. F. Laine, Automatic detection of luminal borders in IVUS images by magnitude-phase histograms of complex brushlet coefficients, *International Conference of the IEEE Engineering in Medicine and Biology Society*, pp. 3072–3076, 2010.

43. M. Sonka, X. Zhang, M. Siebes, M. S. Bissing, S. C. DeJong, S. M. Collins, and C. R. McKay, Segmentation of intravascular ultrasound images: A knowledge-based approach, *T-MI*, vol. 14, no. 4, pp. 719–732, 1995.

44. P. A Brathwaite, K. B. Chandran, D. D. McPherson, and E. L Dove, Lumen detection in human IVUS images using region-growing, In *Computers in Cardiology*, pp. 37–40, 1996.

45. A. Takagi, K. Hibi, X. Zhang, T. J. Teo, H. N. Bonneau, P. G. Yock, and P. J. Fitzgerald, Automated contour detection for high frequency intravascular ultrasound imaging: A technique with blood noise reduction for edge enhancement, In *Ultrasound Medical Biology*, 2000, pp. 1033–1041, 2000.

46. Y. Boykov and M.-P. Jolly, Interactive organ segmentation using graph cuts, In *MICCAI*, pp. 276–286, 2000.

47. D. Martin, C. Fowlkes, D. Tal, and J. Malik, A database of human segmented natural images and its application to evaluating segmentation algorithms and measuring ecological statistics, In *Proceedings of the 8th International Conference on Computer Vision*, vol. 2, pp. 416–423, 2001.

chapter nineteen

Local statistical models for ultrasound image segmentation

Djamal Boukerroui

Contents

Abstract

Ultrasound images are very noisy, with poor contrast and the attenuation of the acoustic wave in the depth of the observed medium leads to strong inhomogeneities in the image. Segmentation methods using global image statistics are known to give unsatisfactory results on such data. In the last decade, there has been a reinvestigation of the use of local statistics by the image segmentation community in a variational framework. These studies show improved performance of local models on images with strong intensity inhomogeneities.

Thus local segmentation models have become very popular. Locality is generally defined by means of an isotropic spatial kernel. Very little work, however, has been carried out to address the problem of the choice of the local kernel's scale (or bandwidth). We investigate the problem of the estimation of a pixel-dependent and pixel-independent local scale in the context of local parametric region segmentation models. Two main strategies will be presented. The first one is statistical and is based on a bias-variance trade-off principle. The second one is a variational approach and we believe to be more generic. Therefore, it may also profit alternative image processing problems. All contributions are demonstrated on synthetic and realistic simulations of ultrasound images with intensity inhomogeneities of a variable strength.

19.1   Introduction

In medical imaging, the ultrasonic wave is modeled as a progressive plane mechanical wave. When this wave encounters an interface between two tissues with different acoustic characteristics, a part of the incident wave is reflected (specular echoes) in the direction of the probe. Along with these specular echoes, backscattered echoes are added by the microscopic structure of the medium. Backscattering is the origin of the speckle phenomenon, which characterizes ultrasound imaging with a granular appearance. The speckle is a multiplicative noise, strongly correlated and more importantly, with non-Gaussian statistics. These characteristics differ greatly from the traditional assumption of white additive Gaussian noise, often taken in ultrasound image segmentation, which leads to limited effectiveness of such methods. Thus, several researchers have studied the statistics of the envelope image of the received echo signal in order to derive processing algorithms specific to ultrasonic data [44,45]. Several distribution families have been proposed in the literature: specific models such as the Rayleigh [14], Rice [58], Nakagami [53], K-distribution [25,53,54], and more general models such as the Homodyne K-distribution [20] and the RIIG [22,23]. Notice the large variability of the proposed models, which is due to both the strong dependence of the observed statistics on the density of scatters, and on to their spatial distribution (uniform or random) in the analyzed tissue [58]. All these models are valid only for the envelope of the received echo signal (i.e., before interpolation, log-compression, and time-gain-compensation). Thus, the direct use of such models on ultrasound images acquired under clinical conditions is questionable [55,64].

Image segmentation in general is an ill-posed problem in the sense of Hadamard and difficult to solve. A large variety of algorithms have been developed over the last few decades. This problem is especially difficult when the data to be processed are medical in nature. The literature on ultrasound image segmentation is abundant and the performances of the proposed techniques are highly dependent on the quality of data [45]. Ultrasound data are very noisy, with poor contrast, and often presents missing boundaries of the object of interest due to problems of specular reflection, shadows, signal dropout, and attenuation. As a consequence, conventional intensity gradient-based methods have had limited success on typical clinical images [45]. Solutions using the phase information, theoretically invariant to image contrast, are successfully used in Belaid et al. [5] and Mulet-Parada and Noble [42]. Note also that segmentation methods based on global statistical models, regardless of the used framework, fail on this type of data, mainly because of the attenuation problem. Adaptive solutions robust to attenuation were first introduced within the Bayesian framework with a Markov random field prior [2,9]. Local image statistics were used for the estimation of the segmentation model's parameters.

The introduction of the level set method [47] as a general framework for segmentation has overcome many limitations of traditional image segmentation techniques; they have become very popular and are widely used in segmentation [41,46]. The level set framework provides an elegant approach to handle the topological changes and the estimation of geometric properties of the evolving interface. Furthermore, it allows the integration of the extensive existing literature on region-based image segmentation [18]. Indeed, the use of statistical models in region-based image segmentation has a long tradition. Their introduction in active contour segmentation methods, mostly within the level set framework, have led to a considerable improvement not only in efficiency and robustness to noise, but also in overcoming the initialization problem, thus resulting in automatic segmentation methods. Pioneering works were mostly based on parametric models that used global image statistics (see, e.g., Chan and Vese [15], Chesnaud et al. [17], Cremers et al. [18], Lecellier et al. [33], and Mitiche and Ben Ayed [41]). Nonparametric criteria then appeared [3,28,31,39,40,49,63]. These models are, however, bound to the global statistical homogeneity assumption of all image regions. As a result, they cannot deal with intensity inhomogeneities, which is almost unavoidable in real images.

Probably one of the earliest solution to the above problem was given by the piecewise smooth model of Mumford and Shah [43], as it can tolerate smooth variations within regions. Therefore it offers more flexibility by relaxing the homogeneity constraint of regions. The first solutions of this model in the context of active contours are complex as they require solving a system of partial differential equations to obtain the approximation functions. An effective solution is to search for a representation of the approximation functions in a set of basis functions, not necessarily smooth, as originally proposed in Vazquez et al. [56,57]. This formulation has reappeared (perhaps independently) in Mahmoodi and Sharif [38] and more recently in Chen et al. [16]. An alternative solution has emerged from the recent introduction of local parametric statistical models. Brox and Cremers [12] showed that the minimization of the piecewise smooth Mumford–Shah functional is equivalent to a first-order approximation of a Bayesian a posteriori maximization based on local Gaussian distributions. The link is a consequence of the fact that local region models are not bounded by the strong assumption of identically distributed pixel intensities. Since then, there has been a reinvestigation of the use of local statistical models by the image segmentation community within the variational framework. In this context, most of the models are parametric [6,19,21,35–37,51,59]. A comprehensive formalization of generic local segmentation models is proposed in Lankton and Tannenbaum [32], with examples of local energies derived from global ones.

A second class of recent solutions includes nonlocal models, which are based on patch comparisons (see Jung et al. [27], and references therein). The idea is to use all local information around a given pixel as an observation vector. This representation was initially used in texture synthesis algorithms, and then it became very popular after the introduction of the nonlocal means denoising algorithm [13].

All of the above examples demonstrate that methods that use local image statistics have the ability to capture boundaries of inhomogeneous objects. Local region-based segmentation models are found, however, to be more sensitive to noise than global ones. If the size of the local window is not appropriate, such models may also be more sensitive to initialization. This brings out several problems that need to be addressed, such as how do we choose between global and local methods to segment a given image? How can global and local image statistics be combined effectively in one model? And finally, is it possible to define an "optimal" (global or pixel dependent) local scale for the estimation of image statistics?

Although local segmentation models have become very popular, to our knowledge, very few contributions have attempted to answer the above open issues. Works on the joint use of global and local statistics are addressed in Bresson and Chan [11] and Wang et al. [60] and automatic pixel-dependent scale selection strategies have been investigated by Piovano and Papadopoulo [50]. The method is ad hoc but has the advantage of being generic.

In this chapter, we investigate the problem of a pixel-dependent and -independent scale estimation for local parametric region models within the level set framework. Two different estimation strategies will be presented.

The first one is statistical in nature and is based on a bias-variance trade-off. Two pixel dependent estimation methods will be presented within this context. In the first method, the optimal scale is defined "in the sense of the mean-square error minimization of a Local Polynomials Approximation (LPA) of the observed image conditional on the current segmentation" [61,62]. The approach is based on the intersection of confidence intervals (ICI) algorithm, which finds the optimal LPA estimate of the image. The underlying model supposes an additive Gaussian white noise. The second one is an ICI generic approach for the class of parametric noise models. The approach is driven by a bias-variance trade-off for the local estimation of the segmentation model parameter, conditional on the current segmentation map [6].

The second strategy is variational. Therefore, it is not limited to parametric noise models. It can be applied to nonparametric ones with little effort, and again, two methods will be presented. We first tackle the problem of the estimation of a single scale (i.e., pixel independent) [7]. Then, we study the pixel-dependent scale selection problem. The main idea is to define at every image location the local kernel as a convex combination of a set of predefined kernels, with different spatial sizes. All four methods will be demonstrated with two parametric noise models: the local Gaussian model of Brox and Cremers [12] and the local Rayleigh model of Boukerroui [6].

19.2   *Segmentation model*

Let $I : \Omega \to \mathbb{R}^+$ denotes a given observed image and $\mathcal{C}$ be a closed contour represented as the zero level set of a signed distance function ϕ, that is, $\mathcal{C} = \{\mathbf{x} \mid \phi(\mathbf{x}) = 0, \ \mathbf{x} \in \Omega\}$. The interior Ω_i and the exterior Ω_e of $\mathcal{C}$ are defined by a smooth approximation of the Heaviside function respectively by $H_i(\phi) = H_\epsilon(\phi)$ and $H_o(\phi) = 1 - H_\epsilon(\phi)$ [15]. Image intensities are supposed to be independent realization of random variables with a certain probability density function (PDF) $p(I, \theta)$. We seek the partition of Ω that maximizes the likelihood function of the observed data. Given the independence assumption, this leads to the minimization of the following energy function:

$$E(\phi) = - \sum_{r \in \{i,o\}} \int_{\Omega_r} \log p(I(\mathbf{x}), \theta_r) \mathrm{d}\mathbf{x} + \lambda \int_\Omega \delta(\phi) |\nabla \phi| \mathrm{d}\mathbf{x}, \qquad (19.1)$$

where the first two terms are data fidelity terms and the last one is a curve length regularization term. The latter controls the smoothness of the solution with a positive penalty weight λ. The parameters of the underlying probabilistic model, θ_r, are generally estimated via the maximum likelihood method and under the assumption that all the observed pixels in the image domain Ω_r are independent and identically distributed (iid) observations.

In global active contour methods, only two global domains are used, Ω_i for the inside and Ω_e for the outside pixels. Therefore the hypothesis of identically distributed observations is generally false for ultrasound images because of the presence of strong intensity inhomogeneities due to attenuation and other factors. However, the assumption remains true if the estimate is made locally in a neighboring region, $\mathcal{V}(\mathbf{x})$, centered around each pixel location, $\mathbf{x}$, in Ω. By doing so, it relaxes the hypothesis of iid observations on the whole domain Ω_r. The hypothesis is assumed to hold only locally at every image location. Thus, the estimates $\widehat{\theta}_r(\mathbf{x})$ become pixel dependent.

The local region can be defined by any given spatial kernel $K(\cdot)$. In this work, a Gaussian kernel with a standard deviation σ_s is used, as its differentiability with respect to σ_s is required in the variational approach. This choice is also motivated by the presence of fast implementations (see e.g., Getreuer [24]). Also, we will consider two particular parametric noise distributions with ML parameter estimation:

- *Rayleigh model*: When the observed image intensity, $I(\mathbf{x})$, is assumed to follow a Rayleigh pdf with a parameter $\theta = \sigma^2$. The data term in Equation 19.1 is given by:

$$E_R(\phi) = \sum_{r \in \{i,o\}} \int_{\Omega_r} \left[\frac{I(\mathbf{x})^2}{2\sigma_r^2(\mathbf{x})} + \log(\sigma_r^2(\mathbf{x})) \right] d\mathbf{x} \tag{19.2}$$

$$\text{and} \quad \widehat{\sigma_r^2}(\mathbf{x}) = \frac{\int_{\Omega_r} K(\mathbf{x} - \mathbf{y})I(\mathbf{y})^2 d\mathbf{y}}{2 \int_{\Omega_r} K(\mathbf{x} - \mathbf{y}) d\mathbf{y}}. \tag{19.3}$$

- *Gaussian model*: In this case, $\theta = [\mu, \sigma^2]^T$. The data term in Equation 19.1 is as follows:

$$E_G(\phi) = \sum_{r \in \{i,o\}} \int_{\Omega_r} \left[\frac{(I(\mathbf{x}) - \mu_r(\mathbf{x}))^2}{\sigma_r^2(\mathbf{x})} + \log(\sigma_r^2(\mathbf{x})) \right] d\mathbf{x} \tag{19.4}$$

$$\text{with} \quad \widehat{\mu}_r(\mathbf{x}) = \frac{\int_{\Omega_r} K(\mathbf{x} - \mathbf{y})I(\mathbf{y}) d\mathbf{y}}{\int_{\Omega_r} K(\mathbf{x} - \mathbf{y}) d\mathbf{y}} \tag{19.5}$$

$$\text{and} \quad \widehat{\sigma_r^2}(\mathbf{x}) = \frac{\int_{\Omega_r} K(\mathbf{x} - \mathbf{y})I(\mathbf{y})^2 d\mathbf{y}}{\int_{\Omega_r} K(\mathbf{x} - \mathbf{y}) d\mathbf{y}} - \widehat{\mu}_r(\mathbf{x})^2. \tag{19.6}$$

The minimization of Equation 19.1 is generally performed using gradient decent techniques. The gradient is obtained by shape derivatives tools or by the derivation of the Euler–Lagrange equation using the Gâteaux derivative tool. The gradients of the global Gaussian and Rayleigh models can be found respectively in Chan and Vese [15], Lecellier et al. [33], and Mitiche and Ben Ayed [41] and in Lecellier et al. [33], Mitiche and Ben Ayed [41], and Sarti et al. [52]. The corresponding gradients for the local models can be found respectively in Boukerroui [6] and Brox and Cremers [12]. The gradient of the length term may be found in Chan and Vese [15], Mitiche and Ben Ayed [41], and Sarti et al. [52].

19.3   Spatial scale selection strategies

19.3.1   Problem position

Local region-based segmentation models are surely a better alternative to global ones in the presence of intensity inhomogeneities. Such models however may be more sensitive to initialization if the chosen local spatial scale is not appropriate. A decrease of robustness to noise is also observed when small scales are used. The choice of the scale of the spatial kernel defining locality is therefore crucial in local segmentation models. Indeed, if a given image to be segmented presents homogenous regions, then larger scales are preferred in order to increase the capture range of the active contour and to have a better estimate of the probabilistic model. When the image presents strong intensity inhomogeneities, smaller scales are preferred. Furthermore, the "optimal" scale may also depend on the adopted choice of the noise model. In this section, several selection strategies are presented.

19.3.2   Evolution speed threshold based approach

Piovano and Papadopoulo [50] defined the local scale at every image location as "the smallest one inducing an evolution speed superior to a given threshold" ϵ. The idea is to find the most salient scale to make the contour locally evolve.

$$\sigma_s^*(\mathbf{x}) = \min_{\sigma_s \in \mathbf{h}} \{\sigma_s : |\partial_t \phi(\mathbf{x})| > \epsilon\} \tag{19.7}$$

where the search is limited to a finite set of ordered scale values $\mathbf{h} = \{h_1 < h_2 < \ldots < h_J\}$. Thus, at each iteration of the level set evolution, the optimal scale is found for every image pixel along the zero level set function, by increasing $\sigma_s(\mathbf{x})$ from the minimum h_1 to the maximum h_J, until the absolute value of the evolution speed is superior to ϵ. It is unclear how to set the positive constant ϵ.

19.3.3   Bias-variance trade-off based approaches

The scale selection problem is widely studied in regression or in nonparametric density estimation where the problem to be solved is often formulated as a bias-variance trade-off. However, very little work exists in image processing. Among the pioneering works, we have Boykov et al. [10] and Katkovnik [29]. Katkovnik applied this formulation to image denoising. His contributions are summarized in a monograph [30]. The two subsequent contributions are inspired by his work.

19.3.3.1   LPA-ICI rule

In the context of image denoising, Katkovnik [29] proposed a local polynomial approximation (LPA) algorithm with an adaptive mechanism based on a bias-variance trade-off to optimize the size of the local spatial window. Formally the selection algorithm is based on the intersection of confidence invervals (ICI) rule, first proposed by Lepskii [34]. The ICI rules aims at searching for the largest local window size (minimizing variance) where the LPA fits well the observed data (minimizing bias). Specifically, let for each $h \in \mathbf{h}$, $\widehat{I}_h(\mathbf{x})$ the image local estimate obtained by the LPA at that scale and $Q_i = Q(h = h_i)$ the corresponding $1 - \alpha$ Confidence intervals (CIs) given by Katkovnik et al. [30]:

$$Q(h) = \left[\widehat{I}_h(\mathbf{x}) - \Gamma \cdot \widehat{\sigma}_{\widehat{I}_h}(\mathbf{x}, h) \, , \, \widehat{I}_h(\mathbf{x}) + \Gamma \cdot \widehat{\sigma}_{\widehat{I}_h}(\mathbf{x}, h)\right], \tag{19.8}$$

where $\widehat{\sigma}_{\widetilde{I}_{h}}(\mathbf{x}, h)$ is a local estimation of the noise standard deviation of the denoised image and $\Gamma = \beta + u_{1-\alpha/2}$ where β is a constant depending of the polynomial order of the LPA and u_{α} is the αth percentile of the standard Gaussian distribution $\mathcal{N}(0, 1)$. As the variance is a decreasing function of h and the bias is an increasing function, there is necessarily a scale for which the intersection of two successive CIs is zero. This contradicts the assumption that all $Q(h_i)$ should have at least one common value. That would be the true unknown image value. Therefore, the ICI method defines the optimal scale at every image location as:

$$\sigma_s^*(\mathbf{x}) = h^* = \max_{k \in 1...J} \left\{ h_k : \bigcap_{i=1}^{k} Q(h_i) \neq \emptyset \right\}. \tag{19.9}$$

The LPA-ICI rule for image segmentation: In order to adapt the LPA-ICI rule to image segmentation we estimate the optimal scale conditional on the current segmentation. Consequently, the LPA estimate does not use the whole neighborhood $\mathcal{V}(\mathbf{x})$, but its intersection with the current image partition, that is, in the neighborhood defined by $\mathcal{V}(\mathbf{x}) \cap \Omega_i$ if the pixel belongs to Ω_i or $\mathcal{V}(\mathbf{x}) \cap \Omega_0$ if the pixel belongs to Ω_0. To summarize, the search for the optimal scale is "in the sense of the Mean-Square Error minimization of a LPA of the observed image conditional on the current segmentation". A few implementation details, given in Section 19.3.3.3, are also necessary to make this work.

19.3.3.2 ICI rule

The scale selection presented in the previous section is valid only where the underlying LPA hypothesis holds. Specifically, an additive white noise model. An alternative that avoids this limitation is presented here. The idea is to choose the largest scale that gives the best estimate of the segmentation model parameters. The approach is generic and can be applied to any parametric pdf. For the sake of clarity, we detail the development for the Rayleigh case only and we give the main results for the Gaussian case.

The Rayleigh case: It can be shown that the ML estimator of σ^2 for the Rayleigh model is *efficient*. It is therefore unbiased and has the lowest possible variance defined by the Cramer-Rao bound. It is also asymptotically Gaussian as it is a ML estimator. Formally, when $n \to \infty$, we have $\widehat{\sigma}^2 \to \mathcal{N}(\sigma^2, \sigma^4/n)$ where $n = \int_{\Omega_r} d\mathbf{x}$ in our context. Therefore, we can estimate a Confidence Interval on σ^2 using[*]

$$P\left(\sigma^2 \in \left[\frac{\widehat{\sigma^2}}{1 + \frac{u_{1-\alpha/2}}{\sqrt{n}}}, \frac{\widehat{\sigma^2}}{1 - \frac{u_{1-\alpha/2}}{\sqrt{n}}} \right] \right) \simeq 1 - \alpha. \tag{19.10}$$

Equivalently, the CIs for the local parameter $\sigma_r^2(\mathbf{x})$ are given by Equation 19.10 with

$$\widehat{\sigma^2} = \widehat{\sigma_r^2}(\mathbf{x}) \quad \text{and} \quad n = \frac{\left(\int_\Omega H(\phi) K(\mathbf{x} - \xi) d\xi \right)^2}{\int_\Omega (H(\phi) K(\mathbf{x} - \xi))^2 d\xi}.$$

---

[*] Actually an exact CI can be built using $2n\frac{\widehat{\sigma^2}}{\sigma^2} \sim \chi_{2n}^2$. Here our intention is to show a generic approach that uses the properties of the ML estimator.

Therefore in an ideal situation, where the observed data is identically distributed, the bigger n is, the better is the estimates of σ^2. Bear in mind that the hypothesis of identically distributed data in the local window will become less and less valid as the scale of the kernel K grows and will lead to an increasingly biased estimations. This means that there exists a bias-variance balance that gives the ideal scale. In a same manner as in the LPA-ICI strategy, we can make use of the ICI algorithm to search for the largest local window (minimizing variance) that gives us the best estimate of σ^2 (minimizing bias).

The Gaussian case: When the observed image intensities $I(\mathbf{x})$ are supposed to follow local Gaussian distributions [12], we can base the scale estimation on the CIs of the local means. Recall that if $X \sim \mathcal{N}(\mu, \sigma^2)$ and given an iid sample of size n then

$$P\left(\mu \in \left[\overline{X} - \frac{S}{\sqrt{n}}t_{n-1,1-\alpha/2}, \quad \overline{X} + \frac{S}{\sqrt{n}}t_{n-1,1-\alpha/2}\right]\right) = 1 - \alpha. \tag{19.11}$$

where S^2 is the unbiased estimate of the variance and $t_{n,\alpha}$ is the αth percentile of a Student's t-distribution of n degrees of freedom [48]. Thus, Equation 19.11 gives us a set of CIs that can be utilized in an ICI algorithm in order to select the best scale for the estimation of the local means. Note that Equation 19.11 is exact $\forall$ n. By use of the central limit theorem, Equation 19.11 can be used as an approximation of the CIs by replacing Student's percentiles by the Gaussian one in the general non Gaussian case.

19.3.3.3 Implementation details

We used a narrow band level set implementation. The above ICI-based algorithms are used to estimate the best spatial kernel at every pixel location along the contour. Note, however, that the ICI rule will produce two scale values, $h_i^*(\mathbf{x})$ and $h_o^*(\mathbf{x})$ corresponding to the inside region Ω_i and the outside region Ω_o respectively. A postprocessing consisting of a median filtering, as suggested in Katkovnik et al. [30], followed by a smoothing operation are performed on the inside and outside narrow bands separately. During the first iterations, only one scale is used for the estimation of the segmentation model parameters. We have defined it as the maximum scale in the narrow band along the normal to the curve $\mathcal{C}$ (see Figure 19.1). In the final iterations, meaning once convergence is almost reached, we

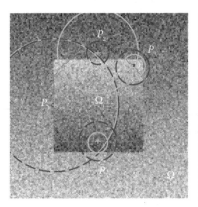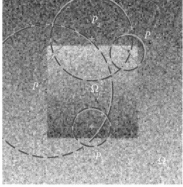

Figure 19.1 Illustration of the bias-variance scale selection approach on a synthetic image; four pairs of points P_1 to P_4 are shown in the narrow band of the current segmentation $\mathcal{C}$ (red curve). Green + are in Ω_i; blue • are in Ω_o. The circles indicate the size of the kernel: Estimated (left); used by the segmentation algorithm (right). This experiment illustrates why a maximum operation is need in locations where the actual segmentation is not the correct one (see P_2, P_3, and P_4).

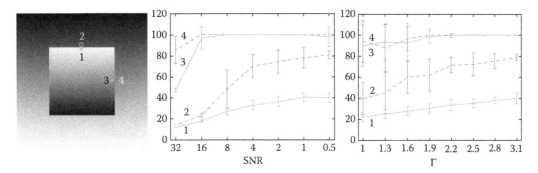

Figure 19.2 Influence of the noise level and the control parameter Γ on the estimation of the local scales. The plots, at four typical image locations, shows the average value of the estimated scales conditional on the ideal segmentation. The error bars are drawn from 20 repeated experiments. Left: 128×128 test image with a SNR=32dB; Middle: h^* function of the image SNR for $\Gamma = 2.2$; Right: h^* function of Γ for a SNR=4dB. In this experiment, values of h^* represent $3\sigma_s$ in pixels (i.e. half kernel size in pixels).

ran a few iterations by replacing the maximum by an average filtering and then by using directly the estimated scales: $h_i^*(\mathbf{x})$ for the inside energy term and $h_o^*(\mathbf{x})$ for the outside energy term.

The key parameter in all the above bias-variance methods is α. The higher α is set, the tighter are the estimated CIs and smaller the selected scales are. α has a precise probabilistic interpretation; therefore, it is easy to set, and for a large class of images. Observe that for the LPA-ICI approach, setting α is equivalent to setting Γ (see Equation 19.8). The interested reader is also referred to Boukerroui [6], Yang and Boukerroui [61,62], where this work appeared for the first time.

19.3.3.4   Illustrative example

Explanatory examples are given in order to better illustrate the bias-variance based scale estimation approach. We only show results of the LPA-ICI algorithm. Figure 19.1 shows results of the scale selection on typical image locations of a synthetic image with strong intensity inhomogeneities. Figure 19.2 summarizes the results of an experiment to study the influence of the control parameter Γ and the image SNR on the LPA-ICI scale estimation algorithm. As expected, we observe that h^* is proportional to Γ and is inversely proportional to the SNR and the degree of inhomogeneity of the image. Additionally, the experiment highlights that the estimated scales are also dependent on the type of inhomogeneity. Notice, for example, the difference between points "1" and "3"; In contrast to image point "1", the symmetry of the inhomogeneity in the vicinity of "3" suggests a zero bias for an isotropic neighborhood; which leads into larger scale estimation and, therefore, reducing the variance. A segmentation example is shown in Figure 19.3.

19.3.4   Variational approaches

The extension of the above estimation theory to the nonparametric case is not trivial. It is also difficult to built a method that estimates a single scale for the whole image. Variational tools are more flexible in this context. The hypothesis that the kernel is a differentiable function with respect to its scaling parameter is of course required. Needless to mention that this is not a serious limitation. However, we will show that extra regularization terms

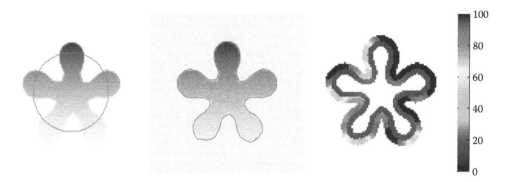

Figure 19.3 From left to right: noise-free image with initialization. Noisy image with the the result of the LPA-ICI level segmentation algorithm with a Gaussian noise model. LPA-ICI estimated kernel size of the final contour. Image size 128×128.

are needed in order to obtain meaningful solutions. A single scale estimation and a pixel dependent scale methods will be presented.

19.3.4.1 Single scale case

We take a straightforward approach in order to propose a pixel independent dynamic scale selection by defining the optimal scale as the one minimizing the cost function (Equation 19.1). In other words, that is the scale minimizing Equation 19.2 in the Rayleigh case and Equation 19.4 for the Gaussian model. Given an initial guess σ_s^0, the minimum is computed using the steepest gradient descent according to

$$\sigma_s^{t+1} = \sigma_s^t - dt \frac{\partial E}{\partial \sigma_s}. \tag{19.12}$$

Prior on σ_s: A closer look at the minimization problem reveals that a trivial solution is obtained for $\sigma_s = 0$. Indeed, the smaller the local kernel is, the better is the fit of the probabilistic model to the observed image intensities, and the lower is the energy function. It is therefore necessary to constrain the minimization problem. One way of doing this is to add a penalty term to the energy function. We may suggest such penalty by adding a cost in the sense of the minimum description length (MDL). When $\sigma_s = 0$, the spatial kernel is a Dirac function and the probabilistic model requires $|\Omega|$ parameters to be estimated (i.e., one at every pixel location). When σ_s increases the model becomes simpler. Indeed, although $\widehat{\theta}$ is estimated at every image pixel $\mathbf{x}$, the function $\widehat{\theta}(\mathbf{x})$ will become increasingly smoother. Its description will therefore require less code and is inversely proportional to σ_s^2. Thus we can define a penalty in the form of

$$E_{MDL}(\sigma_s) = \gamma \frac{|\Omega|}{\sigma_s^2}, \tag{19.13}$$

where γ is a positive control parameter. The minimization of this prior favors larger values of σ_s. Such a prior, however, does not have a probabilistic interpretation as $\exp(-\frac{a}{\sigma_s^2})$ does not define a pdf. The following function

$$f(\sigma_s) = \frac{2\alpha}{\sqrt{\pi}\sigma_s^2} \exp\left(-\frac{\alpha^2}{\sigma_s^2}\right) \tag{19.14}$$

(a) (b)

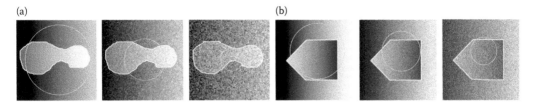

Figure 19.4 Illustrative segmentation results on two synthetic images with intensity inhomogeneities. Results are shown for 3 different initializations and for an additive Gaussian noise with SNR $\in$ [40, 20, 10] dB. Image sizes: 85×88 (a); 256×256 (b).

is however a pdf with a non existing mean and a mode at $\sigma_s = \alpha$. We can use the above PDF as a prior model of σ_s. By doing so, it leads us to the following prior energy term:

$$E_p(\sigma_s) = \gamma |\Omega| \left(\frac{\alpha^2}{\sigma_s^2} + \log(\sigma_s^2) \right). \tag{19.15}$$

The gradients with respect to σ_s of the above prior terms are easy to calculate. The analytical expressions of the gradients of the data terms are given in Appendices 19A.1 and 19A.2 respectively for the Rayleigh and the Gaussian models. The use of a Gaussian spatial kernel allows a separable implementations as its derivative with respect to σ_s also has a separable implementation.

Illustrative examples: We did not observe a major difference between the two proposed priors on σ_s in our experiments. $E_p(\sigma_s)$ has the advantage of having a Bayesian interpretation. The MDL prior is, however, simpler as only one parameter has to be set. The results shown below are for the Gaussian noise model with the MDL prior with $\gamma = 20$. The initial contours are drawn in cyan curves and the final segmentation results are shown in yellow on the images.

The segmentation of two synthetic images with a combination of: three initializations, four noise levels (SNR $\in$ [40 20 15 10] dB) and two to three initial values of σ_s^0 are analyzed. In all combinations, the correct segmentation is obtained (see Figure 19.4). Notice the difference in the nature of intensity inhomogeneity between the two images. The degradation field of image (b) is nonsmooth over the whole image. Therefore, a method such in Li et al. [36] will fail. Figure 19.5 shows the estimated kernel scale values, σ_s, function of the segmentation iterations for this experiment. Different colors correspond to different noise levels and different curves correspond to different initializations. As expected, the final σ_s is inversely proportional to the SNR of the image. Observe that different curve initializations lead to different paths of σ_s over iterations (see Figure 19.5b). Observe also that the optimal scale depends not only on the severity of the degradation field but also on the image and objects sizes. Finally, notice that only about 10 iterations are needed to have a good estimation of σ_s for both images and in all combinations.

19.3.4.2 Convex combination of kernels

Here, we are interested in the estimation of a pixel-dependent scale estimation. One may adopt a similar variational approach as the one we have proposed above. An example in the context of image denoising is given in Azzabou et al. [4]. Doing so, however, may have a serious drawback because the estimated local scales is a real valued positive function of $\mathbf{x}$. Therefore, the use of the estimated local scales for the estimation of the model parameters θ at every image pixel and possibly at every iteration will probably be computationally very

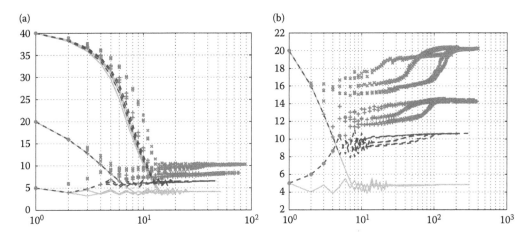

Figure 19.5 Evolution of the estimated σ_s function of segmentation iterations for the experiments on the image shown in (a) and (b). Different colors correspond to different noise levels. The final σ_s is inversely proportional to the image SNR.

heavy. One way to overcome this difficulty is to project the solution on a set of predefined discrete scale values. This brings out the alternative, which we believe is a better idea, of the projection of the local kernel on a set of predefined kernels.

Problem Formulation: Given a finite set of kernels $\mathcal{K} = \{K_{h_i} : i = 1...J\}$ with increasing spatial scales h_i, we can define the local kernel by the following convex combination:

$$K(\mathbf{x}) = \sum_{i=1}^{J} \alpha_i K_{h_i}(\mathbf{x}), \tag{19.16}$$

where $\alpha_i \geq 0$ and $\sum_{i=1}^{J} \alpha_i = 1$. Using the above definition of K, Equation 19.3 giving the parameter for the local Rayleigh model can be written as

$$\widehat{\sigma}_r^2(\mathbf{x}) = \frac{(K * I^2)_{\Omega_r}(\mathbf{x})}{2(K * \mathbb{1})_{\Omega_r}(\mathbf{x})} = \frac{\sum_{i=1}^{J} \alpha_i(K_{h_i} * I^2)_{\Omega_r}(\mathbf{x})}{2\sum_{i=1}^{J} \alpha_i(K_{h_i} * \mathbb{1})_{\Omega_r}(\mathbf{x})} = \frac{\alpha^T \mathbf{g}_{I^2}(\mathbf{x})}{2\alpha^T \mathbf{g}_{\mathbb{1}}(\mathbf{x})}, \tag{19.17}$$

where we have defined the following convolution operator

$$(f * g)_{\Omega_r}(\mathbf{x}) = \int_{\Omega_r} f(\mathbf{x} - \mathbf{y})g(\mathbf{y})\mathrm{d}\mathbf{y}. \tag{19.18}$$

Here, $\mathbb{1}(\mathbf{x}) = 1, \forall \mathbf{x} \in \Omega$ is the indicator function of Ω and the last equality is a compact vector notation. Now, we can define a pixel-dependent local scale of the kernel by allowing the coefficient α_i to be spatially variable. More precisely, we have defined a spatially adaptive local kernel as the kernel's shape changes with position. The advantage of the above formulation is that the model parameters $\theta(\mathbf{x})$, as illustrated above for the Rayleigh model, can be estimated efficiently as all the needed convolutions are pixel independent. Thus, they can be computed once. The price we pay is an increase of the complexity of the optimization problem as now we have to estimate a vector of unknowns, $\boldsymbol{\alpha}$, at every image location $\mathbf{x}$. Indeed, the full optimization problem to solve is the following:

minimization of Equation 19.1 with respect to $\phi(\mathbf{x})$ and $\boldsymbol{\alpha}(\mathbf{x})$ and under the constraints $\alpha_i(\mathbf{x}) \geq 0$ and $\sum_{i=1}^{J} \alpha_i(\mathbf{x}) = 1, \forall \mathbf{x} \in \Omega$.

To solve the above, we alternate between the minimization over $\phi(\mathbf{x})$ and $\boldsymbol{\alpha}(\mathbf{x})$. We will focus on the latter as it is the main novelty. The problem is a nonlinear constrained optimization problem. In the following, we will present two algorithms to solve it in our context. Both methods make use of the prior information that the optimal spatial scale is a smooth function of $\mathbf{x}$. Therefore, the coefficients $\alpha_i(\mathbf{x})$ should also be smooth functions of $\mathbf{x}$.

Case J > 2: In the general situation where the set of predefined kernels contains more than two kernels, solving the nonlinear minimization problem for all $\mathbf{x} \in \Omega$ is too costly. Furthermore, the restriction of the solution to the narrow band region is not sufficient enough to produce a practical algorithm. The only way to substantially reduce the computation load is by solving the problem at a very limited number of image positions. Then, we make use of the smoothness hypothesis of $\alpha_i(\mathbf{x})$ in order to obtain a solution at every image location. Practically, we select a set of image locations by uniformly sampling the zero level set, that is, the current curve $\mathcal{C}(\mathbf{x})$, to get a set of candidate points $\mathcal{X} = \{\mathbf{x}_k : k = 1 \dots n_{\mathcal{X}}\}$. In order to obtain a robust estimation of $\boldsymbol{\alpha}(\mathbf{x}_k)$, we assume that all image pixels in a small neighborhood $\mathcal{N}_{\mathbf{x}_k}$ around $\mathbf{x}_k$ have the same solution $\boldsymbol{\alpha}(\mathbf{x}_k)$. The size of the neighborhood is chosen to be inversely proportional to $n_{\mathcal{X}}$. Formally we can write $\boldsymbol{\alpha}(\mathbf{x}) = \boldsymbol{\alpha}(\mathbf{x}_k), \forall \mathbf{x} \in \mathcal{N}_{\mathbf{x}_k}$. In this way, the optimal vector of coefficients $\boldsymbol{\alpha}(\mathbf{x}_k)$ is dependent on the observed image data and on the current image partition at all image pixels in $\mathcal{N}_{\mathbf{x}_k}$. This is equivalent to searching for a piecewise constant solution along the curve $\mathcal{C}$. Every subproblem at image location $\mathbf{x}_k$ is solved using an interior-point based solver. Practically, we used the MATLAB `fmincon` function to which we provided an analytical expression of the gradient. In a second step, a solution is obtained for all pixels in the narrow band region using a zero order interpolator, followed by a spatial Gaussian smoothing for regularization. It is important to highlight that both operations in the second step preserve the convexity constraint of $\boldsymbol{\alpha}$.

Case J = 2: In the particular case of a convex combination of two kernels, Equation 19.16 may be simplified as:

$$K(\mathbf{x}) = (1 - \alpha)K_l(\mathbf{x}) + \alpha K_g(\mathbf{x}), \text{ with } \alpha \in [0,1], \tag{19.19}$$

where we have denoted by $K_l(\mathbf{x})$ the kernel with the small scale and by $K_g(\mathbf{x})$ the one with a larger scale. Equation 19.19 may also be written in the form of $K(\mathbf{x}) = K_l(\mathbf{x}) + \alpha(K_g(\mathbf{x}) - K_l(\mathbf{x}))$. The optimization problem becomes simpler because $\alpha(\mathbf{x})$ is a scalar image and the constraints are reduced to upper and lower bounds. The problem can be converted to an unconstrained one by defining α via a function that takes values in $[0,1]$. Doing so, and following [1], we define α via a sigmoid function:

$$\alpha(\mathbf{x}) = \text{sgm}(\eta(\mathbf{x})) = \frac{1}{1 + e^{-\eta(\mathbf{x})}}, \ \eta \in \mathbb{R}. \tag{19.20}$$

The adaptation of $\alpha(\mathbf{x})$ can then be obtained using the steepest gradient descent according to:

$$\eta^{t+1} = \eta^t - dt \frac{\partial E}{\partial \eta}. \tag{19.21}$$

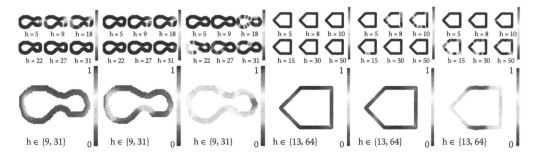

Figure 19.6 First line $J = 6$. Second line $J = 2$. Coefficients of the convex combination of kernels, $\alpha_i(\mathbf{x})$ (for J = 6) and $\alpha(\mathbf{x})$ (for J = 2) corresponding to the images shown in Figure 19.4. Here, the values of h are the standard deviation of the Gaussian kernels used in the combination.

The analytical expressions of the gradient of the data terms for the Rayleigh model is given in Appendix 19B. The corresponding gradient for the Gaussian case can be derived in the same manner without difficulty. Practically we alternate between one gradient descent step on α and one on ϕ for all pixels in the narrow band region. A spatial Gaussian smoothing of $\alpha(\mathbf{x})$ is applied for regularization. This is equivalent to adding a quadratic cost function on the spatial gradient of $\alpha(\mathbf{x})$ to the energy function given in Equation 19.1. Specifically a term given by $\int_{\Omega} |\nabla \alpha(\mathbf{x})|^2 d\mathbf{x}$.

Prior on α: Here too, and for the same reasons as in the single-scale approach, a trivial solution is obtained for small kernel sizes. It is therefore necessary to constrain the minimization problem on α. The good performances of the MDL prior, used previously in the single scale approach, are in favor of its adaptation [7]. Thus, reworking Equation 19.13 for the case of a convex combination of kernels will lead to the following prior term:

$$E_{MDL}(h_1, \ldots, h_n) = \gamma \int_{\Omega} \sum_{i=1}^{J} \frac{\alpha_i(\mathbf{x})}{h_i^2(\mathbf{x})} d\mathbf{x}. \tag{19.22}$$

The minimization of this prior favors larger kernels.

Illustrative Results: We tested the convex combination of kernels on the same set of test images as for the single scale approach (see Figure 19.4). We run experiments for $J = 6$ and $J = 2$. In both settings, the approach succeeded to segment correctly the two images, for all combinations (4 noise levels times 3 initializations). Figure 19.6 shows the estimated coefficients of the combination $\alpha_i(\mathbf{x})$ (in the case of $J = 6$) and the $\alpha(\mathbf{x})$ maps in the narrow bands of the final contours, corresponding to the images shown in Figure 19.4. Observe, as expected, that the contribution of larger kernels is inversely proportional to the SNR of the images.

19.4   Experimental results

We have already presented illustrative results of the different scale selection strategies in the previous sections. Here, we will demonstrate the usefulness of the proposed methods and quantify the performance of the segmentations. To this end, we chose to use realistic US simulations for testing. We used the simulation program Field-II [26], to synthesize phantom data with known ground truth. A linear scan of a first phantom (PH1) was done

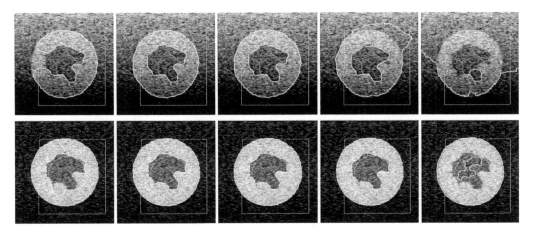

Figure 19.7 Illustrative segmentation results of the Rayleigh model without scale selection on a simulated US image. From left to right $h = 20, 30, 40, 70, 200$.

with a 290 elements transducer using 64 active elements. The scatterers in the phantom were randomly distributed within the phantom of $80 \times 80 \times 15$ mm cube size. One hundred and twenty-eight lines were simulated at 5 MHz. The second phantom (PH2) of size $100 \times 100 \times 15$ mm cube was placed at 10 mm depth from the transducer surface, and was scanned with a 7 MHz 128 elements phased array transducer. The images consist of 128 lines with 0.7 degrees between lines. Hanning apodization in transmit and receive was used in all experiments. Two scatterers amplitudes with three levels of tissue attenuations were simulated for both phantoms. We also used several dB ranges for the envelope logarithmic compression to simulate different image contrasts. A total of 60 images were simulated and used for testing. The final reconstructed envelope images were sampled and interpolated to 256×256 pixels.

In all our experiments, the kernel $K_h(\mathbf{x})$ is a 2D Gaussian kernel with a standard deviation h. The initial contours are drawn in cyan curves and the final segmentation results are shown in yellow on the images. For the bias-variance approaches, only results of the ICI method will be shown with $\alpha = 0.05$ and a set of predefined scales $\mathbf{h} = \{5, 10, 15, 20, 25, 30, 35, 40, 45, 50, 60, 70, 80\}$. For the variational strategies, the MDL prior parameter is set to 20 except for the 2 scales convex combination method where a value of 1 is used. In the case of $J = 6$, the set of predefined kernels is set to $\mathcal{K} = \{5, 10, 20, 25, 30, 35\}\%$ of the image size. For $J = 2$, $\mathcal{K} = \{8, 30\}\%$ of the image size. Segmentation algorithms are run with four different curve initializations. The results of the two noise models will be presented.

Figure 19.7 shows results of the single scale local Rayleigh model on the same image with the same initialization for different values of h (from left to right $h = 20, 30, 40, 70$, and 200). Equivalent results (not shown) are obtained when a Gaussian noise model is assumed [12]. Good segmentations are only obtained when an appropriate value of h is specified. We can clearly observe that the segmentation algorithm converges to a local minimum when the kernel is small. Furthermore, when very large kernels are used, the obtained partition is meaningless either because of the presence of intensity inhomogeneities (first line) or a binary partition is not sufficient and a multiple phase level set method should be used (second line).

Figure 19.8 shows a selection of five segmentation results of the local Rayleigh model for each of the five presented scale selection methods. Almost all selection strategies were

(a)

(b)

(c)

(d)

(e)

(f)

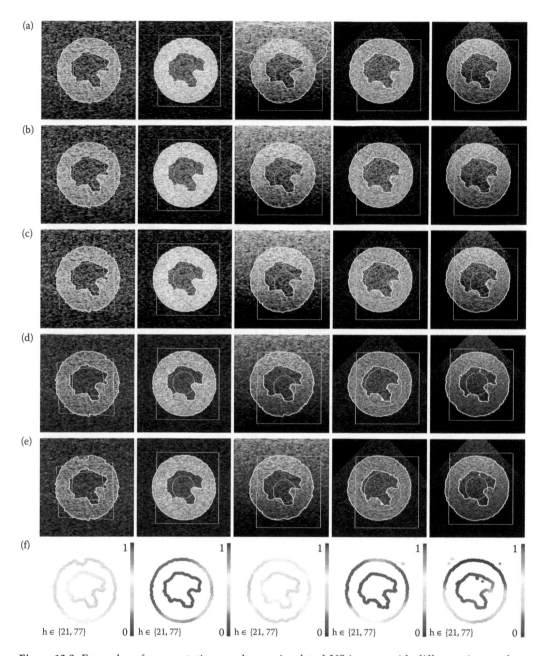

h ∈ {21, 77}   h ∈ {21, 77}   h ∈ {21, 77}   h ∈ {21, 77}   h ∈ {21, 77}

Figure 19.8 Examples of segmentation results on simulated US images with different tissues characteristics, attenuation level and log compression parameters. All results are obtained with the local Rayleigh model with an automatic scale selection: (a) [50] with $\epsilon = 0.5$; (b) ICI selection with $\alpha = 0.05$; (c) variational single scale with: from left to right $\sigma_s^0 = 20, 30, 40, 70, 200$. (d) Convex combination of six scales; (e) Convex combination of two scales. (f) image map of $\alpha(\mathbf{x})$ for the final contour of the results shown in (e).

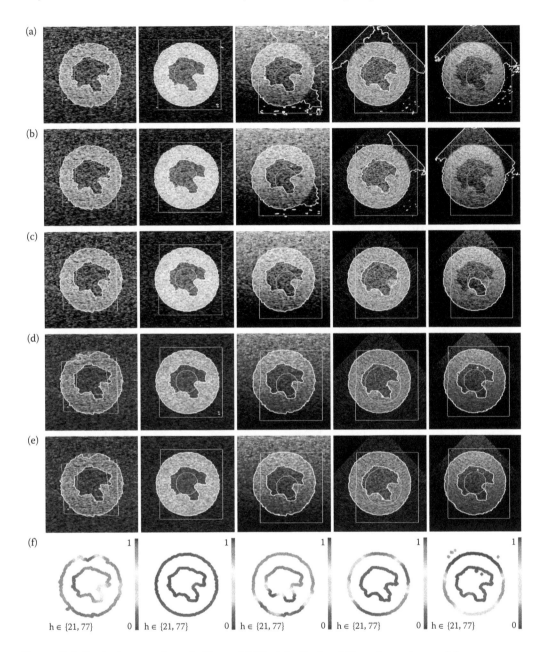

Figure 19.9 Equivalent results as in Figure 19.8 but for the local Gaussian noise model.

able to estimate appropriate scales in order to obtained acceptable results. Piovano and Papadopoulo's method failed on one image. Equivalent results are shown when a local Gaussian noise model is assumed in Figure 19.9. The analysis of this last figure suggests a superiority of the variational strategy on the bias-variance one. This is probably because the assumed noise model does not explain the observed data. The last row of the two figures shows the estimated map images of the coefficient of the 2 scales convex combination. Red

Table 19.1 Statistics of the DSC and the MAD measures of 240 (60 images × 4 initializations) segmentations of the local Rayleigh model

	DSC×100						MAD (in pixels)					
	min	Q_1	Q_2	Q_3	max	IQR	min	Q_1	Q_2	Q_3	max	IQR
Ad'hoc, $\epsilon = 0.5$	62.4	93.6	95.9	96.2	96.5	2.6	1.11	1.21	1.31	1.90	24.27	0.69
ICI, $\alpha = .05$	68.2	95.5	96.1	96.2	96.5	0.7	1.09	1.29	1.36	1.47	21.54	0.17
VSS, $\sigma_s^0 = 10$	69.2	95.6	95.9	96.1	96.7	0.5	1.13	1.32	1.45	1.60	9.30	0.28
VSS, $\sigma_s^0 = 40$	69.5	95.5	95.8	96.0	96.7	0.5	1.13	1.33	1.48	1.63	9.24	0.30
VSS, $\sigma_s^0 = 70$	69.4	95.6	95.8	96.1	96.7	0.5	1.13	1.33	1.48	1.63	9.32	0.30
VSS, $\sigma_s^0 = 200$	68.3	95.3	95.8	96.0	96.7	0.7	1.13	1.39	1.51	1.72	20.11	0.33
CCK, J = 6	78.1	95.2	95.6	95.9	96.3	0.7	1.24	1.41	1.55	1.77	10.92	0.36
CCK, J = 2	69.9	95.2	95.6	95.9	96.4	0.7	1.21	1.42	1.55	1.77	16.96	0.35

Note: Five scale selection. VSS, variational single scale; CCS, convex combination of scales.

color means the larger-scale contribution is higher. The comparison of the obtained maps between the two noise models is very informative. We observe that the selected optimal scale is also noise model dependent.

The quantitative evaluation of the proposed algorithms compared to ground truth is summarized in Table 19.1. It shows statistics of the dice similarity coefficient (DSC) $(S, S_{ideal}) = 2\frac{|S \cap S_{ideal}|}{|S| + |S_{ideal}|}$ and the mean absolute distance (MAD) of segmentation results of the 60 simulated images with four different initializations ($60 \times 4 = 240$ results). The closer the DSC and the MAD values are to 1 and 0 respectively, the better is the segmentation. The table shows the minimum, the three quartiles, the maximum and the interquartile range (IQR) of the measurements. Similarly to the results shown in Figure 19.8, five-scale selection algorithms are compared. The quantitative evaluation suggests that the performances of the variational approaches are slightly better on this data. The worst method being the ad hoc one.

19.5   Conclusion

We investigated the problem scale selection for local active contours. Two main methodologies were presented. The first one is based on a bias-variance trade-off. Then we approached the problem in a straightforward manner using variational tools. Four methods in total were detailed and illustrated on simple synthetic images in order to illustrate the benefit of scale selection when the observed data are inhomogeneous. Although our experiments suggest that the performances of the variational approaches are slightly better, It is still unclear what method should be used for a given segmentation problem. We may, however, advise to use the bias-variance strategy when a correct parametric noise model is available and the variational method otherwise.

Acknowledgment

The author thanks Dr Izumi Otani and Dr Timor Kadir for comments and English proofreading.

19A.1 Gradients for the single-scale approach

19A.1.1 Rayleigh model

The derivative of the objective function (19.2) with respect to σ_s is given by:

$$\frac{\partial E_R}{\partial \sigma_s} = \sum_{r \in \{i,o\}} \int_{\Omega_r} \left(\frac{1}{\sigma_r^2(\mathbf{x})} - \frac{I(\mathbf{x})^2}{2\sigma_r^4(\mathbf{x})} \right) \frac{\partial \sigma_r^2(\mathbf{x})}{\partial \sigma_s} d\mathbf{x} \tag{19A.1}$$

with $\qquad \dfrac{\partial \sigma_r^2(\mathbf{x})}{\partial \sigma_s} = \dfrac{(K' * I^2)_{\Omega_r}(\mathbf{x})}{2(K * \mathbb{1})_{\Omega_r}(\mathbf{x})} - \dfrac{(K' * \mathbb{1})_{\Omega_r}(\mathbf{x})}{(K * \mathbb{1})_{\Omega_r}(\mathbf{x})} \sigma_r^2(\mathbf{x}). \tag{19A.2}$

where we have used the previously defined convolution operator given in Equation 19.18. The function $\mathbb{1}(\mathbf{x}) = 1, \forall \mathbf{x} \in \Omega$ and K' is the derivative of the spatial kernel with respect to σ_s. For the Gaussian kernel, we have

$$K(\mathbf{x}) = \exp \left(-\frac{\|\mathbf{x}\|_2^2}{2\sigma_s^2} \right) \quad \text{and} \quad K'(\mathbf{x}) = \frac{\|\mathbf{x}\|_2^2}{\sigma_s^3} \exp \left(-\frac{\|\mathbf{x}\|_2^2}{2\sigma_s^2} \right). \tag{19A.3}$$

19A.1.2 Gaussian model

The derivative of the objective function Equation 19.4 with respect to σ_s is as follow:

$$\frac{\partial E_G}{\partial \sigma_s} = \sum_{r \in \{i,o\}} \int_{\Omega_r} -2 \frac{(I(\mathbf{x}) - \mu_r(\mathbf{x}))}{\sigma_r^2(\mathbf{x})} \frac{\partial \mu_r(\mathbf{x})}{\partial \sigma_s} d\mathbf{x}$$

$$+ \sum_{r \in \{i,o\}} \int_{\Omega_r} \frac{1}{\sigma_r^2(\mathbf{x})} \left(1 - \frac{(I(\mathbf{x}) - \mu_r(\mathbf{x}))^2}{\sigma_r^2(\mathbf{x})} \right) \frac{\partial \sigma_r^2(\mathbf{x})}{\partial \sigma_s} \tag{19A.4}$$

with

$$\frac{\partial \mu_r(\mathbf{x})}{\partial \sigma_s} = \frac{(K' * I)_{\Omega_r}(\mathbf{x})}{(K * \mathbb{1})_{\Omega_r}(\mathbf{x})} - \frac{(K' * \mathbb{1})_{\Omega_r}(\mathbf{x})}{(K * \mathbb{1})_{\Omega_r}(\mathbf{x})} \mu_r(\mathbf{x}), \tag{19A.5}$$

$$\frac{\partial \sigma_r^2(\mathbf{x})}{\partial \sigma_s} = \frac{(K' * I^2)_{\Omega_r}(\mathbf{x})}{(K * \mathbb{1})_{\Omega_r}(\mathbf{x})} - \frac{(K' * \mathbb{1})_{\Omega_r}(\mathbf{x})}{(K * \mathbb{1})_{\Omega_r}(\mathbf{x})} \frac{(K * I^2)_{\Omega_r}(\mathbf{x})}{(K * \mathbb{1})_{\Omega_r}(\mathbf{x})} - 2\mu_r(\mathbf{x}) \frac{\partial \mu_r(\mathbf{x})}{\partial \sigma_s}. \tag{19A.6}$$

19B.1 Gradient for the convex combination of kernels approach

In the case of a Rayleigh model, the derivative of the objective function Equation 19.2 with respect to $\eta(\mathbf{x})$ is given by

$$\frac{\partial E_R}{\partial \eta} = \sum_{r \in \{i,o\}} \frac{1}{\sigma_r^2(\mathbf{x})} \left(1 - \frac{I(\mathbf{x})^2}{2\sigma_r^2(\mathbf{x})} \right) \frac{\partial \sigma_r^2(\mathbf{x})}{\partial \alpha} \frac{\partial \alpha(\mathbf{x})}{\partial \eta}, \tag{19B.1}$$

where the remaining partial derivatives are given with the help of Equation 19.18 as:

$$\frac{\partial \sigma_r^2(\mathbf{x})}{\partial \alpha} = \frac{((K_g - K_l) * I^2)_{\Omega_r}(\mathbf{x}) - 2((K_g - K_l) * \mathbb{1})_{\Omega_r}(\mathbf{x})\sigma_r^2(\mathbf{x})}{2(K_l * \mathbb{1})_{\Omega_r}(\mathbf{x}) + 2\alpha((K_g - K_l) * \mathbb{1})_{\Omega_r}(\mathbf{x})} \tag{19B.2}$$

$$\frac{\partial \alpha(\mathbf{x})}{\partial \eta} = \alpha^2(\mathbf{x})e^{-\eta(\mathbf{x})}. \tag{19B.3}$$

References

1. J. Arenas-Garcia, A. Figueiras-Vidal, and A. Sayed, Mean-square performance of a convex combination of two adaptive filters, *IEEE Transactions on Signal Processing*, vol. 54, no. 3, pp. 1078–1090, 2006.
2. E. Ashton and K. Parker, Multiple resolution Bayesian segmentation of ultrasound images, *Ultrasonic Imaging*, vol. 17, no. 2, pp. 291–304, 1995.
3. G. Aubert, M. Barlaud, O. D. Faugeras, and S. Jehan-Besson, Image segmentation using active contours: Calculus of variations or shape gradients? *SIAM Journal of Applied Mathematics*, vol. 63, no. 6, pp. 2128–2154, 2003.
4. N. Azzabou, N. Paragios, F. Guichard, and F. Cao, Variable bandwidth image denoising using image-based noise models, in *CVPR*, IEEE Computer Society, 2007, pp. 1–7.
5. A. Belaid, D. Boukerroui, Y. Maingourd, and J.-F. Lerallut, Phase-based level set segmentation of ultrasound images, *IEEE Transactions on Information Technology in Biomedicine*, vol. 15, no. 1, pp. 138–147, 2011.
6. D. Boukerroui, A local Rayleigh model with spatial scale selection for ultrasound image segmentation, in *British Machine Vision Conference*, R. Bowden, J. Collomosse, and K. Mikolajczyk, Eds., Surrey, UK, Sep. 2012, pp. 84–84.
7. D. Boukerroui, Optimal spatial scale for local region-based active contours, in *IEEE International Conference on Image Processing*, IEEE, 2014, pp. 4393–4397.
8. D. Boukerroui, O. Basset, A. Baskurt, and A. Noble, Segmentation of echocardiographic data. Multiresolution 2D and 3D algorithm based on gray level statistics, in *MICCAI*. Cambridge, UK: Springer-Verlag, 1999, pp. 516–524.
9. D. Boukerroui, A. Baskurt, A. Noble, and O. Basset, Segmentation of ultrasound images— Multiresolution 2D and 3D algorithm based on global and local statistics, *Pattern Recognition Letters*, vol. 24, pp. 779–790, 2003.
10. Y. Boykov, O. Veksler, and R. Zabih, A variable window approach to early vision, *IEEE Transactions on.Pattern Analysis and Machine Intelligence*, vol. 20, no. 12, pp. 1283–1294, 1998.
11. X. Bresson and T. F. Chan, Non-local unsupervised variational image segmentation models, UCLA C.A.M. Report, Tech. Rep. 08-67, 2008.
12. T. Brox and D. Cremers, On local region models and a statistical interpretation of the piecewise smooth Mumford-Shah functional, *International Journal Computer Vision*, vol. 84, no. 2, pp. 184–193, 2009.
13. A. Buades, B. Coll, and J. M. Morel, A review of image denoising algorithms, with a new one, *Multiscal Modeling and Simulation*, vol. 4, no. 2, pp. 490–530, 2005.
14. C. B. Burckhardt, Speckle in ultrasound B-mode scans, *IEEE Transactions on Sonics and Ultrasound*, vol. 25, no. 1, pp. 1–6, 1978.
15. T. Chan and L. Vese, Active contours without edges, *IEEE Transactions on Image Processing*, vol. 10, no. 2, pp. 266–277, 2001.
16. C. Chen, J. Leng, and G. Xu, A general framework of piecewise-polynomial Mumford–Shah model for image segmentation, UCLA C.A.M. Report, Tech. Rep. 13-50, Sep. 2013.
17. C. Chesnaud, P. Réfrégier, and V. Boulet, Statistical region snake-based segmentation adapted to different physical noise models, *IEEE Transactions on Pattern Analysis and Machine Intelligence*, vol. 21, no. 11, pp. 1145–1157, 1999.

18. D. Cremers, M. Rousson, and R. Deriche, A review of statistical approaches to level set segmentation: Integrating color, texture, motion and shape, *International Journal of Computer Vision*, vol. 72, no. 2, pp. 195–215, 2007.
19. C. Darolti, A. Mertins, C. Bodensteiner, and U. G. Hofmann, Local region descriptors for active contours evolution, *IEEE Transactions on Image Processing*, vol. 17, no. 12, pp. 2275–2288, 2008.
20. V. Dutt and J. Greenleaf, Ultrasound echo envelope analysis using a homodyned K-distribution signal model, *Ultrasonic Imaging*, vol. 16, pp. 265–287, 1994.
21. N. El-Zehiry and A. Elmaghraby, A graph cut based active contour without edges with relaxed homogeneity constraint, in *International Conference on Pattern Recognition*, 2008, pp. 1–4.
22. T. Eltoft, The Rician inverse Gaussian distribution: A new model for non-Rayleigh signal amplitude statistics, *IEEE Transactions on Image Processing*, vol. 14, no. 11, pp. 1722–1735, 2005.
23. T. Eltoft, Modeling the amplitude statistics of ultrasonic images, *IEEE Transactions on Medical Imaging*, vol. 25, no. 2, pp. 229–240, 2006.
24. P. Getreuer, A survey of Gaussian convolution algorithms, *Image Processing On Line*, vol. 2013, pp. 276–300, 2013.
25. E. Jakeman, K-distributed noise, *Journal of Optics A: Pure and Applied Optics*, vol. 1, pp. 784–789, 1999.
26. J. A. Jensen, Field: A program for simulating ultrasound systems, *Medical Biology and Engineering Computation*, vol. 34, no. Supplement 1, Part 1, pp. 351–353, 1996.
27. M. Jung, G. Peyré, and L. D. Cohen, Nonlocal active contours, *SIAM Journal of Imaging Sciences*, vol. 5, no. 3, pp. 1022–1054, 2012.
28. T. Kadir and M. Brady, Unsupervised non-parametric region segmentation using level sets, in *IEEE International Conference on Computer Vision*, vol. 2, pp. 1267–1274, 2003.
29. V. Katkovnik, A new method for varying adaptive bandwidth selection, *IEEE Transactions on Signal Processing*, vol. 47, no. 9, pp. 2567–2571, 1999.
30. V. Katkovnik, K. Egiazarian, and J. Astola, *Local Approximation Techniques in Signal and Image Processing*. Washington: International Society for Optical Engineering, 2006.
31. J. Kim, J. Fisher, A. Yezzi, M. Çetin, and A. Willsky, A nonparametric statistical method for image segmentation using information theory and curve evolution, *IEEE Transactions on Image Processing*, vol. 14, pp. 1486–1502, 2005.
32. S. Lankton and A. Tannenbaum, Localizing region-based active contours, *IEEE Transactions on Image Processing*, vol. 17, no. 11, pp. 2029–2039, 2008.
33. F. Lecellier, J. Fadili, S. Jehan-Besson, G. Aubert, M. Revenu, and E. Saloux, Region-based active contours with exponential family observations, *Journal of Mathematical Image Vision*, vol. 36, no. 1, pp. 28–45, 2010.
34. O. Lepskii, On a problem of adaptive estimation in Gaussian white noise, *Theory of Probability and Its Applications*, vol. 35, no. 3, pp. 454–466, 1990.
35. C. Li, C.-Y. Kao, J. C. Gore, and Z. Ding, Minimization of region-scalable fitting energy for image segmentation, *IEEE Transactions on Image Processing*, vol. 17, no. 10, pp. 1940–1949, 2008.
36. C. Li, R. Huang, Z. Ding, J. C. Gatenby, and D. N. Metaxas, A level set method for image segmentation in the presence of intensity inhomogeneities with application to MRI, *IEEE Transactions on Image Processing*, vol. 20, no. 7, pp. 2007–2016, 2011.
37. J. Liu and H. Zhang, Image segmentation using a local GMM in a variational framework, *Journal of Mathematical Image Vision*, pp. 1–16, 2013.
38. S. Mahmoodi and B. Sharif, Contour evolution scheme for variational image segmentation and smoothing, *IET Image Processing*, vol. 1, no. 3, pp. 287–294, 2007.
39. P. Martin, P. Réfrégier, F. Galland, and F. Guerault, Nonparametric statistical snake based on the minimum stochastic complexity, *IEEE Transactions on Image Processing*, vol. 15, no. 9, pp. 2762–2770, 2006.
40. O. Michailovich, Y. Rathi, and A. Tannenbaum, Image segmentation using active contours driven by the Bhattacharyya gradient flow, *IEEE Transactions on Image Processing*, vol. 16, no. 11, pp. 2787–2801, 2007.

41. A. Mitiche and I. Ben Ayed, *Variational and Level Set Methods in Image Segmentation*, Springer Topics in Signal Processing series. Berlin: Springer, 2010.

42. M. Mulet-Parada and J. Noble, 2D+T acoustic boundary detection in echocardiography, *Medical Image Analysis*, vol. 4, no. 1, pp. 21–30, 2000.

43. D. Mumford and J. Shah, Boundary detection by minimizing functionals, in *Proc. of IEEE Conference on Computating and Visual Pattern Recognition (CVPR)*, 1985.

44. S. Nadarajah, Statistical distributions of potential interest in ultrasound speckle analysis, *Physical and Medical Biology*, vol. 52, pp. 213–227, 2007.

45. A. Noble and D. Boukerroui, Ultrasound image segmentation: A survey, *IEEE Transactions on Medical Imaging*, vol. 25, no. 8, pp. 987–1010, 2006.

46. S. Osher and N. Paragois, *Geometric Level Set Methods in Imaging Vision and Graphics*. Berlin: Springer Verlag, 2003.

47. S. Osher and J. A. Sethian, Fronts propagating with curvature-dependent speed: Algorithms based on Hamilton–Jacobi formulations, *Journal of Computational Physics*, vol. 79, no. 1, pp. 12–49, 1988.

48. A. Papoulis and S. U. Pillai, *Probability, Random Variables and Stochastic Processes*, 4th edn. New York: McGraw-Hill Science/Engineering/Math, 2001.

49. G. Peyre, J. Fadili, and J. Rabin, Wasserstein active contours, in *IEEE International Conference on Image Processing*, 2012, pp. 2541–2544.

50. J. Piovano and T. Papadopoulo, Local statistic based region segmentation with automatic scale selection, in *European Conference on Computer Vision*, Marseille, France, 2008, pp. 486–499.

51. J. Piovano, M. Rousson, and T. Papadopoulo, Efficient segmentation of piecewise smooth images, in *Scale Space and Variational Methods in Computer Vision*, Lecture Notes in Computer Science series, F. Sgallari, A. Murli, and N. Paragios, Eds. Berlin: Springer Berlin Heidelberg, 2007, vol. 4485, pp. 709–720.

52. A. Sarti, C. Corsi, E. Mazzini, and C. Lamberti, Maximum likelihood segmentation of ultrasound images with Rayleigh distribution, *IEEE Transactions on Ultrasonics, Ferroelectrics, and Frequency Control*, vol. 52, no. 6, pp. 947–960, 2005.

53. P. M. Shankar, V. A. Dumane, T. George, C. W. Piccoli, J. M. Reid, F. Forsberg, and B. B. Goldberg, Classification of breast masses in ultrasonic B scans using Nakagami and K-distributions, *Physical and Medical Biology*, vol. 48, no. 14, pp. 2229–2240, 2003.

54. P. Shankar, J. Reid, H. Ortega, C. Piccoli, and B. Goldberg, Use of non-Rayleigh statistics for the identification of tumors in ultrasonic B-scans of the breast, *IEEE Transactions on Medical Imaging*, vol. 12, no. 4, pp. 687–692, 1993.

55. Z. Tao, H. Tagare, and J. Beaty, Evaluation of four probability distribution models for speckle in clinical cardiac ultrasound images, *IEEE Transactions on Medical Imaging*, vol. 25, no. 11, pp. 1483–1491, 2006.

56. C. Vazquez, A.-R. Mansouri, and A. Mitiche, Approximation of images by basis functions for multiple region segmentation with level sets, in *IEEE International Conference on Image Processing*, vol. 1, 2004, pp. 549–552.

57. C. Vazquez, A. Mitiche, and R. Laganiere, Joint multiregion segmentation and parametric estimation of image motion by basis function representation and level set evolution, *IEEE Transactions on Pattern Analysis and Machine Intelligence*, vol. 28, no. 5, pp. 782–793, 2006.

58. R. F. Wagner, S. W. Smith, J. M. Sandrik, and H. Lopez, Statistics of speckle in ultrasound B-scans, *IEEE Transactions on Sonics and Ultrasonics*, vol. 30, no. 3, pp. 156–163, 1983.

59. L. Wang, L. He, A. Mishra, and C. Li, Active contours driven by local Gaussian distribution fitting energy, *Signal Processing*, vol. 89, pp. 2435–2447, 2009.

60. L. Wang, C. Li, Q. Sun, D. Xia, and C.-Y. Kao, Active contours driven by local and global intensity fitting energy with application to brain MR image segmentation, *Computations in Medical Image Graphics*, vol. 33, no. 7, pp. 520–531, 2009.

61. Q. Yang and D. Boukerroui, Optimal spatial adaptation for local region-based active contours: An intersection of confidence intervals approach, in *VISIGRAPP*, Algarve, Portugal, March 2011, pp. 87–93.

62. Q. Yang and D. Boukerroui, Ultrasound image segmentation using local statistics with an adaptive scale selection, in *IEEE International Symposium on Biomedical Imaging*, Barcelona, Spain, May 2012, pp. 1096–1099.
63. H. Zhang, Y. Chen, and J. Shi, Nonparametric image segmentation using Rényi's statistical dependence measure, *Journal of Mathematical Image Vision*, vol. 44, no. 3, pp. 330–340, 2012.
64. Y. Zhu, X. Papademetris, A. J. Sinusas, and J. S. Duncan, A coupled deformable model for tracking myocardial borders from real-time echocardiography using an incompressibility constraint, *Medical Image Analysis*, vol. 14, no. 3, 2010.

chapter twenty

Image segmentation with physical noise models

Daniel Tenbrinck and Xiaoyi Jiang

Contents

Abstract

Image segmentation algorithms typically (often implicitly) assume that the image is perturbed by additive Gaussian noise. However, this is not the case in many real-life applications. While image noise plays an inferior role for segmentation of natural images, it

becomes crucial for example, biomedical images. In particular, physical noise modeling is indispensable for segmentation in the case
of lower signal-to-noise ratio. Image segmentation under consideration of physical noise models has received relatively little attention
only. In this chapter, we discuss typical noise models encountered in
biomedical imaging. Additionally, the related algorithmic development, including explicit and implicit physical noise consideration, is
briefly reviewed and exemplarily presented by some recent works
from our own research.

20.1   *Introduction*

One common problem for biomedical imaging is the omnipresence of physical noise perturbations, which are induced by the image acquisition process and thus strongly depend
on the respective imaging modality. While image noise plays an inferior role for segmentation of natural images, it becomes crucial for biomedical images. In particular, the lower
the signal-to-noise ratio (SNR) the more important is the consideration of physical noise
modeling for segmentation. The left image in Figure 20.1 fortifies this fact by an example of $H_2^{15}O$ PET data. Since the half-life of this substance is very short (≈ 2 min), only
few events are detected during image acquisition and thus the reconstructed images have
a very low SNR. This noise phenomenon can be modeled as a Poisson random process.
Another example is diagnostic ultrasound imaging as shown in Figure 20.1b, where the
noise characteristic can be typically described by a statistical model of multiplicative noise.

A majority of works from the vast image segmentation literature typically (often
implicitly) assumes that the given image is perturbed by additive Gaussian noise. However, there are many real-life applications, such as in biomedical imaging, in which other
types of noise occur. In general, they have a very different impact on the data, thus
making physical noise modeling necessary to achieve satisfactory segmentation results in
biomedical imaging. Image segmentation under consideration of physical noise models
has received relatively little attention only. In this paper we discuss various aspects of this

(a)   (b)

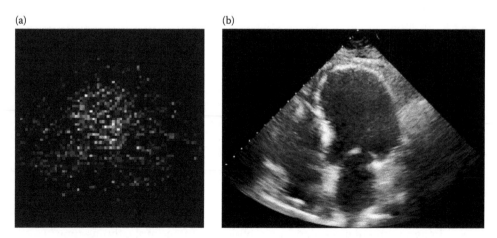

Figure 20.1 (a) Thoracic cross-section of reconstructed $H_2^{15}O$ PET data with a low signal-to-noise
ratio due to the measurement of very few decay events. (b) Medical ultrasound image showing the
left ventricle of a human heart.

topic. The related algorithmic development is exemplarily presented by some recent works from our own research and a discussion of further important works in this field.

The rest of the paper is organized as follows. We start with a formal definition of the segmentation problem in Section 20.2. Several popular noise models are summarized in Section 20.3. In Section 20.4 we provide a brief overview of segmentation methods that are designed for dealing with physical noise models. Then, two segmentation approaches are exemplarily discussed in the next two sections: a general segmentation framework in Section 20.5 which incorporates explicitly physical noise models into a variational segmentation formulation and an alternative solution based on minimal surface problems in Section 20.6 which aims to handle physical noise without explicitly modeling it. Finally, some concluding remarks are given in Section 20.7.

20.2   Region-based segmentation problem

The general task of region-based segmentation is to obtain a partition $\mathcal{P}_m(\Omega)$ of the image domain Ω into pairwise disjoint regions Ω_i for $i = 1, \ldots, m$,

$$\mathcal{P}_m(\Omega) \in \left\{ (\Omega_1, \ldots, \Omega_m) : \Omega = \bigcup_{i=1}^{m} \Omega_i \text{ and } \Omega_i \cap \Omega_j = \emptyset \text{ for all } i \neq j \right\} \tag{20.1}$$

The finite number of separate regions $m \geq 2$ corresponds to the number of expected semantic compartments in the data, for example, the separation of cell nuclei from the rest of a microscopic image ($m = 2$), or the delineation of organs, bones, and background regions in a CT scan ($m = 3$). The partitioning of Ω in Equation 20.1 is not arbitrary but should fulfill the following properties:

- Each region $\Omega_1, \ldots, \Omega_m$ should consist of pixels that can be reasonably grouped according to a suitable feature of the image f. Simultaneously, these regions should be easy to differentiate according to the chosen image feature.
- The respective interiors of image regions should have a simple geometry without holes or gaps. Boundaries of image regions should be smooth but also accurate with respect to the chosen image feature.

The majority of segmentation approaches in the literature utilize image features based on the signal intensity, for example, the partition of Ω into regions with homogeneous grayscale values [1–5]. Typically, these approaches aim to minimize the signal variance in the respective regions. However, there also exist segmentation methods based on the feature of motion or texture [6].

20.3   Physical noise modeling

We summarize five typical physical noise models from the literature in this section and discuss their applicability for biomedical image segmentation. In addition, parametrized families can be defined with noise models commonly encountered in image acquisition systems as special cases, for instance, the exponential families in Lecellier et al. [2] and Chesnaud et al. [7]. Figure 20.2 exemplarily shows the impact of these noise models on a one-dimensional ground truth signal. As can be observed, their respective impact on the signal differs substantially. This fact gives a clear indication of the need of physical noise

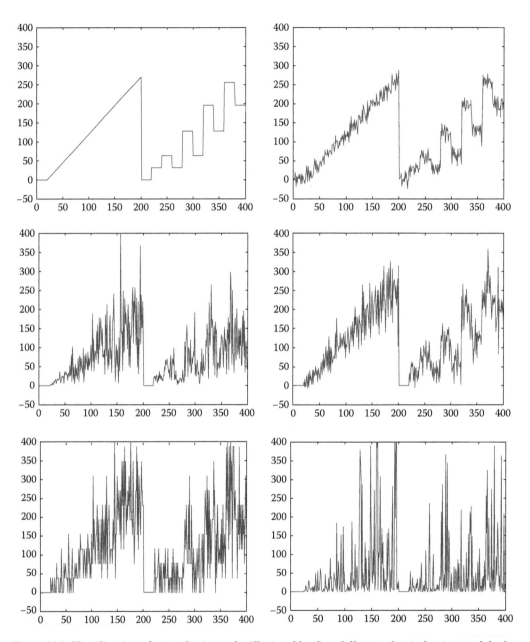

Figure 20.2 Visualization of perturbations of a 1D signal by five different physical noise models that typically occur in computer vision applications and in particular in biomedical imaging. From top to bottom and left to right: exact signal, additive Gaussian noise (Equation 20.2, $\sigma = 5$), Rayleigh noise (Equation 20.3, $\sigma = 0.5$), multiplicative speckle noise (Equation 20.5, $\sigma = 3$, $\gamma = 1$), Poisson noise (Equation 20.6, $s = 5$), and Gamma noise (Equation 20.8, $\alpha = 0.3$).

modeling and developing segmentation algorithms capable of dealing with such noise models in order to achieve satisfactory segmentation results in biomedical imaging.

20.3.1   Additive Gaussian noise model

One of the most commonly used noise models in computer vision is the additive Gaussian noise model:

$$f = u + \eta, \qquad \eta \sim \mathcal{N}(0, \sigma^2) \tag{20.2}$$

where η is a normally distributed random variable with expectation 0 and variance σ^2. Clearly, this kind of noise is signal-independent and has a global noise distribution.

Numerous segmentation methods including the Mumford–Shah [4] or Chan–Vese model [1] are based on this noise model (see Section 20.4). These segmentation methods are successful on a large class of images, since additive Gaussian noise is the most common form of noise in computer vision applications. Note that conventional images consist of positive integers due to the image quantization process. On the other hand, the perturbed signal f in Equation 20.2 can take any real value (cf. Figure 20.2). Therefore, the Gaussian additive noise model might not be optimal even for conventional images. In general, an investigation of other noise models is highly desired, in particular in biomedical imaging.

20.3.2   Rayleigh noise model

Speckle noise is a noise model known to follow a Rayleigh distribution. Here the data are modeled in a signal-dependent manner,

$$f = u\eta \tag{20.3}$$

where η is a Rayleigh distributed random variable with the probability density function

$$p(\eta) = \frac{\eta}{\sigma^2} e^{-\frac{\eta^2}{2\sigma^2}} \tag{20.4}$$

This noise model is assumed to be appropriate for ultrasound B-mode images in the presence of a large number of randomly located scatters [8].

When working with ultrasound images, the magnitude image typically has a large dynamic range. Therefore, the standard is to log-compress the image to produce an image suitable for display, resulting in a doubly exponential distribution that has the form of a Fisher–Tippett distribution [9]. This distribution is a suitable model for fully formed speckle in log-compressed in-phase/quadrature images.

20.3.3   Multiplicative speckle noise model

The next noise model is similarly multiplicative and signal-dependent. Using the notation from above, the image perturbation with multiplicative speckle noise can be described by

$$f = u + u^{\frac{\gamma}{2}} \eta, \qquad \eta \sim \mathcal{N}(0, \sigma^2) \tag{20.5}$$

The fixed parameter $\gamma \geq 0$ determines the signal-dependence of the noise variance and typical values in the literature are $\gamma \in \{1, 2\}$ [10,11]. Note that for $\gamma = 0$ one obtains the case of additive Gaussian noise as already discussed above. Obviously, for $\gamma > 0$ the induced noise model is signal-dependent and perturbations on the image are amplified depending on the image intensity (cf. Figure 20.2).

One possible application of this noise model is medical ultrasound imaging. In particular, for $\gamma = 1$ one obtains the Loupas noise model [10], which is related to the Rayleigh noise in the following way [12]. The displayed images from ultrasound devices have, among others, the property of logarithmic compression. The analytic study of log-compressed Rayleigh signals in medical ultrasound has been addressed for example in Dutt and Greenleaf [13]. Loupas et al. [10] shows that the linear relationship between the mean and the standard deviation valid for Rayleigh-distributed speckle no longer holds for general log-compressed ultrasound images. Experimental measurements indicate that the noise of displayed ultrasonic images can be modeled as signal-dependent speckle noise with $\gamma = 1$ (see Tenbrinck [14] and references therein).

20.3.4   Poisson noise model

Another interesting noise model for biomedical image segmentation is Poisson noise or the so-called photon counting noise. This type of noise is also signal-dependent and appears in different biomedical applications, for example in fluorescence microscopy [15] or positron emission tomography [16]. For Poisson noise one has to consider the following image generation process for natural numbers $k \in \mathbb{N}$:

$$f \sim \text{Poisson}(u), \quad \text{with} \quad p(f = k \mid u = \lambda) = \frac{\lambda^k}{k!}e^{-\lambda} \tag{20.6}$$

Notably, the resulting random variables are positive integers and the associated probability distribution is especially challenging for a low parameter $\lambda \in \mathbb{R}^+$ in Equation 20.6. For numerical experiments, one may rescale the image intensities of f by dividing it with $s > 0$, apply Poisson noise according to Equation 20.6, and subsequently rescale the images back.

20.3.5   Gamma noise model

The last noise model to discuss is the Gamma noise model, which is described by a shape parameter α and a scale parameter β with $\alpha, \beta > 0$. Typically, the scale parameter β can be rewritten in terms of the unbiased signal intensity u. Thus, for a fixed shape parameter α, the observed noisy image f is modeled by

$$f = \eta(u) \tag{20.7}$$

with the probability density function [17]

$$p(\eta) = \begin{cases} \frac{\alpha^\alpha}{u^\alpha \Gamma(\alpha)}\eta^{\alpha-1}e^{-\frac{\alpha\eta}{u}}, & \text{if } u > 0 \\ 0, & \text{otherwise} \end{cases} \tag{20.8}$$

where Γ is the Gamma function. Next to its possible application in biomedical imaging, this model has been used to represent speckle in synthetic aperture radar (SAR) [18]. Typically, this noise model is assumed for strong perturbations of data by speckle noise.

In addition to the popular noise models discussed above, a few others have also been studied in the literature. As soon as SAR images become more complex (e.g., with textures or strong reflectors), the Gamma noise model may be not sufficient. Different noise models have thus been taken into account to deal with such images (see Galland et al. [19] for a discussion). In particular, the Fisher model has been studied in that work. Another example is the Weibull model, which has been investigated in Ayed et al. [20] for a wide variety of image types (radar, sonar, etc.).

20.4 Brief overview of segmentation methods considering physical noise models

In this section, we discuss various segmentation methods that consider certain physical noise models. It turns out that variational segmentation models dominate this field. This is not surprising as this class of methods have been successfully applied to many segmentation tasks in the past and have become a standard tool in recent literature. Furthermore, their respective mathematical theory, that is, the calculus of variations and its related fields, is well understood and allows for important conclusions, for example, existence and uniqueness of respective minimizers. Note that for the sake of brevity, we restrain ourselves from giving details about the numerical realization of the discussed methods but rather focus on the conceptual idea of considering physical noise models in each segmentation method.

20.4.1 Classical variational segmentation methods

We begin by reviewing classical segmentation formulations that have inspired most of the works presented in the course of this paper and build the base for many applied methods in biomedical imaging today. First, we discuss the well-known Mumford–Shah segmentation model [4]:

$$E_{MS}(u, \Gamma) = \int_{\Omega} (u - f)^2 + \mu \int_{\Omega \backslash \Gamma} |\nabla u|^2 + \beta \mathcal{H}^{d-1}(\Gamma) \tag{20.9}$$

which estimates a piecewise-smooth approximation $u \colon \Omega \to \mathbb{R}$ to the given image $f \colon \Omega \to \mathbb{R}$ and a suitable segmentation contour $\Gamma \subset \Omega$. In particular, this model enforces the segmentation contour Γ to partition the image domain Ω in a way such that the approximation u to f is smooth within each region $\Omega_i \subset \Omega, i = 1, \ldots, m$, while discontinuities are allowed at the location of the segmentation contour Γ. In addition, this segmentation model favors smaller contour length as represented by the $(d - 1)$-dimensional Hausdorff measure $\mathcal{H}^{d-1}(\Gamma)$. In practice, it is however difficult to minimize this functional due to its nonconvexity and the nonfixed boundary conditions during evolution of the contour Γ.

Alternative methods have been proposed to simplify or modify the Mumford–Shah functional. The influential Chan–Vese segmentation model [1] assumes a piecewise constant approximation u. The related energy functional for a two-phase segmentation problem is given by

$$E_{CV}(c_1, c_2, \Gamma) = \lambda_1 \int_{\Omega_1} (f - c_1)^2 + \lambda_2 \int_{\Omega_2} (f - c_2)^2 + \beta \mathcal{H}^{d-1}(\Gamma) \tag{20.10}$$

For images with intensity inhomogeneities, that is, nonconstant signal intensities in semantic image regions, the Chan–Vese model does not work well. In order to overcome this difficulty, Chan and Vese [1] proposed another method, which aims at expressing the intensities inside and outside the contour as piecewise smooth functions instead of constants [21]. Additional methods for dealing with intensity inhomogeneities include the region-scalable fitting model [22], which uses a local intensity fitting (two spatially varying fitting functions f_1 and f_2 for approximating the local image intensities on both sides of the contour) instead of the smooth function or constant approximation, and its modified versions [23]. In another work [24], the image inhomogeneity is modeled in the following way. An image u is decomposed into $f = u + v + \eta$, where u is piecewise-constant and v is smooth, thus capturing global intensity inhomogeneities caused by a variety of reasons, and η denotes additive Gaussian noise as given in Equation 20.2. An alternative multiplicative model $f = u \cdot v \cdot \eta$ is also addressed. A similar approach using additive noise $u = u \cdot v + \eta$ is considered in Liu et al. [25].

All the segmentation methods mentioned before have in common that they are designed to work well on natural images perturbed by additive Gaussian noise. This is induced by the standard choice of data fidelity: a quadratic distance, also known as L^2 fidelity term (cf. Equations 20.9 and 20.10). As we will see in the next section, this quadratic term is a natural choice for additive Gaussian noise from a statistical point of view.

In the context of modeling physical noise in the process of segmentation, the valid question arises if one could perform a preprocessing step to denoise the image and subsequently apply standard methods for image segmentation on the approximated data. In general, this approach is especially tempting if one aims to use denoising techniques based on filter operations since this reduces the mathematical complexity of the whole segmentation task at hand tremendously. However, as has been reported in Diaz et al. [26], denoising in a preprocessing step may lead to image artifacts, which compromise segmentation results. Additionally, small image details might be oversmoothed by the denoising step and thus their information gets lost. Depending on the application, this might be a critical criterion, for example, for the detection of small tumors in biomedical imaging. Therefore, it is not wise to decouple the denoising step from the segmentation step, as both parts give valuable information that can be mutually exploited. It is clear that the segmentation process benefits from the denoising step as misleading perturbations are eliminated. On the other hand, the segmentation step can partition the image domain into regions with different noise characteristics. A global denoising approach for all these regions might not be valid and give suboptimal results. For this reason, many works try to incorporate physical noise models directly into segmentation approaches and optimize both problems in an interleaved manner (cf. Sawatzky et al. [5] and references therein).

20.4.2   *Maximum-a-posteriori estimation*

A common trick to deal with noise perturbations is to model the data from a statistical point of view. Given noisy data f, one is interested in the (unknown) unbiased data u. In this setting, the pixels of f are assumed to be independent and identically distributed random variables. In order to have a good estimation for u, one aims to maximize the conditional probability $p(u|f)$, that is, observing the random events induced by f under the unknown conditions given by u. Since it is difficult to work directly with this term, the famous Bayes' theorem is used:

$$p(u|f) = \frac{p(f|u)p(u)}{p(f)} \tag{20.11}$$

By applying the negative logarithm to Equation 20.11, one derives a maximum a posteriori estimator (MAP) as follows (neglecting constant terms),

$$-\log p(u|f) = -\log p(f|u) - \log p(u) \tag{20.12}$$

Note that the a-priori probabilities $p(f|u)$ and $p(u)$ in Equation 20.12 are usually easier to handle than the a posteriori probability on the left side itself. Assuming an explicit noise model (cf. the models in Section 20.3), one is able to compute the probability $p(f|u)$ and derive a feasible data fidelity term for performing segmentation as $D(f,u) = -\log p(f | u)$ [5,17,27,28] (see also Section 20.5). In the following, we give some examples for these terms.

For the signal-independent additive Gaussian noise the data fidelity term is easily derived [5],

$$D(f,u) = \frac{1}{2\sigma^2} (u - f)^2 \tag{20.13}$$

that is, the commonly used L^2 data fidelity term, which is the canonical choice of fidelity in many segmentation formulations, for example, in the Mumford–Shah [4] or Chan–Vese model [1] (cf. also Equations 20.9 and 20.10). These segmentation methods are successful on a large class of images, since additive Gaussian noise is the most common form of noise in computer vision applications.

The data fidelity term for the Rayleigh noise model can be found in Tenbrinck et al. [29]:

$$D(f,u) = -\log \left(\frac{f}{\sigma^2 u^2} \right) + \frac{f^2}{2\sigma^2 u^2} \tag{20.14}$$

The Loupas noise model [10] results in the data fidelity term [5]

$$D(f,u) = \frac{1}{2\sigma^2} \frac{(u - f)^2}{u} + \frac{\log u}{2} \tag{20.15}$$

Due to the multiplicative nature of the Loupas noise model, one has to deal with a more complicated data fidelity term in Equation 20.15 and hence with more challenges in the minimization computation compared to additive Gaussian noise.

For the Poisson noise model, the data fidelity term becomes the so-called Kullback–Leibler (KL) divergence [16,30] (also known as cross entropy or I-divergence) between two nonnegative measures f and u, that is,

$$D(f,u) = u - f \log u \tag{20.16}$$

A significant difference between the KL and the L^2 fidelity in Equation 20.13 is the nonlinearity in the KL functional, again leading to complications in the minimization process.

For the Gamma noise model the data fidelity term reads as the following [17]:

$$D(f,u) = \log u + \frac{f}{u} \tag{20.17}$$

However, using this data, fidelity term leads to non-convex functionals to be minimized. For this reason variations of the maximum-likelihood term in Equation 20.17 are discussed in Steidl and Teuber [28] and a relationship to the KL fidelity in Equation 20.16 is investigated.

20.4.3   Segmentation methods explicitly modeling non-Gaussian noise

It has been shown above that in the Bayesian inference paradigm the data fidelity term (negative log-likelihood for the a posteriori probability density) is simply the popular L^2 norm Equation 20.13. For the Poisson noise model, the data fidelity term becomes the KL divergence Equation 20.16. Based on this fact, several works have replaced the L^2 by the KL fidelity term to obtain an energy functional that is capable of dealing with Poisson-distorted data. In Lee and Le [27], this leads to a straightforward extension of the Chan–Vese model:

$$E(c_1, c_2, \Gamma) = \lambda_1 \int_{\Omega_1} (c_1 - f \log c_1) + \lambda_2 \int_{\Omega_2} (c_2 - f \log c_2) + \beta \mathcal{H}^{d-1}(\Gamma) \tag{20.18}$$

Similarly, this replacement is done in Chen and He [31] using the region-scalable fitting model [22]. Another variant is proposed in Chen et al. [32], where the data term $(f - f_i)^2$, $i = 1, 2$, in Li et al. [22] is replaced by the Kullback–Leibler divergence between f and the fitting function f_i. The recent work [33] is based on the energy functional

$$E(u) = \int_{\Omega} |\nabla u| + \mu \int_{\Omega} |\nabla u|^2 + \lambda \int_{\Omega} (\mathcal{A}u - f \log \mathcal{A}u) \tag{20.19}$$

Note that the blurring operator $\mathcal{A}$ is included to deal with blurred images (it is set to the identity operator in case of no blur). This functional is adopted from Cai et al. [34], only the last term $(\mathcal{A}u - f)^2$ is replaced by $\mathcal{A}u - f \log \mathcal{A}u$, in the same logic as Equation 20.16. The authors referenced the denoising work [28], which argues theoretically and experimentally that the term $\int_{\Omega} (\mathcal{A}u - f \log \mathcal{A}u)$ is also suitable for handling multiplicative Gamma noise. Thus, the proposed energy functional in Equation 20.19 is expected to work well with both Poisson and Gamma noise.

There are a few other works that are devoted to a single noise model. Intended for processing ultrasound images a maximum likelihood approach is applied in Sarti et al. [35]. The Rayleigh noise model is assumed to obtain an appropriate energy functional to be optimized. Another ultrasound-related work [9] is based on the Fisher–Tippett distribution. For synthetic aperture radar (SAR) image segmentation, an earlier work [36] used the Gamma noise model to formulate a segmentation optimality measure based on the minimum description length (MDL) principle and proposed a heuristic method that consists in simple operations like region merging. Generally, it can only achieve a suboptimal solution to the MDL criterion optimization problem. Later, this approach has been extended to deal with the Fisher noise model [19]. The Gamma noise model is used also by the maximum likelihood approach proposed in Ayed et al. [18] for SAR image segmentation. In Ayed et al. [20], a variational level set segmentation method is presented using the Weibull noise model.

Note that the limitation to a single noise model is mostly attributed to the applications in mind. From a methodological point of view, methods like in Sarti et al. [35] and Galland et al. [36] can be elaborated for other noise models as well. Indeed, the work in

Galland et al. [37] presents such an extension from the Gamma noise [36] to others such as Rayleigh, Poisson, and Bernoulli. A maximum likelihood formulation for segmentation explicitly considering physical noise models is proposed in Chesnaud et al. [7] with a polygonal snake implementation. Arbitrary noise models can be incorporated into this segmentation model and the authors particularly studied an exponential family, which included the Gaussian, Gamma, Rayleigh, Bernoulli, and Poisson noise models. Later, this work was extended to a level set implementation in Martin et al. [3]. A general segmentation framework is proposed in Sawatzky et al. [5], which allows to perform physical noise modeling for different image regions independently and at the same time flexibly incorporate a priori knowledge about the expected unperturbed image (see Section 20.5 for details). In particular, one important special case of this framework is an extended formulation of the popular Chan–Vese segmentation model, which can handle arbitrary noise models. To perform this extension, it suffices to exchange the L^2 distance functions in Equation 20.10 by general negative log-likelihood functions:

$$E(c_1, c_2, \Gamma) = -\lambda_1 \int_{\Omega_1} \log p_1(f \mid c_1) - \lambda_2 \int_{\Omega_2} \log p_2(f \mid c_2) + \beta \mathcal{H}^{d-1}(\Gamma) \qquad (20.20)$$

While all methods discussed so far are based on low-level features such as intensity information, the approach proposed in Lecellier et al. [2] is unique in the sense that it is based on shape descriptors as a higher-order feature.

20.4.4 Segmentation methods dealing implicitly with non-Gaussian noise

The segmentation models discussed above make fixed assumptions on the image degradation process (noise model) and incorporate these explicitly into the segmentation procedure, for example, by means of Bayesian modeling. Although this approach is typical in the literature, there exist several arguments against explicit noise modeling. First, modeling noise characteristics demands deep insight in the physical processes of image acquisition, for example, photon counting during radioactive decay in positron emission tomography [16]. Another technical problem is to prove the well-posedness of derived segmentation formulations based on Bayesian modeling because very often the deduced data fidelity terms turn out to be mathematically challenging, for example, see Sawatzky et al. [5]. Furthermore, it is often not clear if a proposed noise model is suitable for an application at hand and the used imaging technology [14,41,42]. Finally, researchers in computer vision are regularly faced with the problem of dealing with data for which the image acquisition process and/or the subsequent postprocessing steps, for example, filtering and transformations, are not fully known and thus cannot be modeled. This is in particular true for commercial imaging systems in biomedical imaging. For the reasons discussed above, the question arises how to perform robust image segmentation in the presence of image noise without explicit assumptions on the underlying physical principles.

The MDL-based segmentation algorithm [36] based on Gamma noise model has been extended to handle the case of a priori unknown noise models [38,39]. The intensity distribution is modeled by a piecewise constant step function. The parameters of this step function (number of steps, locations of step changes) are integrated into the MDL criterion so that they are simultaneously determined during the segmentation process. The remaining parameter (height for each step) is estimated in the maximum likelihood sense given the other parameters. Another recent attempt in this direction is reported in Tenbrinck and

Table 20.1 Segmentation methods for dealing with physical noise models

Segmentation method	Noise models	Explicit noise modeling
Chesnaud et al. 1999 [7]	General	Yes
Galland et al. 2003 [36]	Gamma	Yes
Martin et al. 2004 [3]	General	Yes
Ayed et al. 2005 [18]	Gamma	Yes
Galland et al. 2005 [37]	General	Yes
Sarti et al. 2005 [35]	Rayleigh	Yes
Ayed et al. 2006 [20]	Weibull	Yes
Slabaugh et al. 2006 [9]	Fisher–Tippett	Yes
Galland et al. 2009 [19]	Fisher	Yes
Lecellier et al. 2010 [2]	General	Yes
Lee and Le 2011 [27]	Poisson	Yes
Chen and He 2013 [31]	Poisson	Yes
Sawatzky et al. 2013 [5]	General	Yes
Chan et al. 2014 [33]	Poisson, Gamma	Yes
Chen et al. 2014 [32]	Poisson	Yes
Delyon et al. 2006 [38,39]	General	No
Tenbrinck and Jiang 2015 [40]	General	No

Jiang [40]. In this work, the segmentation task is formulated as a minimal surface problem for an unknown threshold t. This threshold is meant to partition the data optimally with respect to the intensity distributions in the image. Since it is based on the image histogram only, this partition step makes no explicit assumptions on the underlying noise models and thus can deal with arbitrary perturbations. We will present more details of this method in Section 20.6.

Image segmentation under consideration of physical noise models has received relatively little attention only. The methods discussed above can be grouped based on the criterion of explicit or implicit noise modeling. As can be clearly seen in Table 20.1, a majority of the proposed methods is based on explicit noise modeling. In the next two sections, each group will be exemplarily illustrated using the general segmentation framework for various noise models [5] and the computation of minimum surface solutions [40], respectively.

20.5 A general framework for explicit physical noise modeling in segmentation

In this section, we exemplarily discuss a general framework recently proposed in Sawatzky et al. [5], which is designed to explicitly incorporate different noise models into the process of image segmentation. For the sake of simplicity, we restrict the discussion to two-phase segmentation problems in the following, that is, the case $m = 2$ in Equation 20.1. In general, these problems require a partition $\mathcal{P}_2(\Omega)$ of the image domain into a background region $\Omega_1 \subset \Omega$ and a target region $\Omega_2 \subset \Omega$.

The main idea in Sawatzky et al. [5] is to simultaneously estimate $u \colon \Omega \to \mathbb{R}$ from the noisy observed image f by the means of Bayesian modeling in the process of segmentation. In order to allow for a separate modeling of target and background regions, an indicator function $\chi\colon \Omega \to \{0,1\}$ is used to represent the noise-free image u as a sum of two smooth functions $u_1, u_2\colon \Omega \to \mathbb{R}$, which are only considered in their respective region Ω_1 and Ω_2, that is,

$$u = \chi u_1 + (1 - \chi)u_2, \quad \text{with} \quad \chi(x) = \begin{cases} 1, & \text{for } x \in \Omega_1 \\ 0, & \text{else} \end{cases} \tag{20.21}$$

In this way discontinuities of u, that is, the edge set Γ, are induced by the indicator function, that is, at the edge set of the respective regions defined by χ. It is clear that the indicator function χ already represents the wanted partition of Ω. The globally smooth functions u_1 and u_2 have to fulfill certain requirements with respect to f to be meaningful for segmentation, that is,

$$u_i \mathrel{\hat{=}} \begin{cases} \text{denoised approximation of } f \text{ in } \Omega_i \\ \text{appropriate extension in } \Omega \backslash \Omega_i \end{cases} \tag{20.22}$$

In order to perform physical noise modeling, one can reformulate the task of image segmentation as a Bayesian inference problem. For the sake of brevity, we refrain to give a proper introduction of the needed probability spaces and densities here, but use a less rigorous notation to summarize the main idea in Sawatzky et al. [5]. Here, image intensities are modeled as observed random variables and one tries to maximize the probability of a partition $\mathcal{P}_2(\Omega)$ of the image domain given the observed random variables induced by the image f, that is, by computing a maximum a posteriori probability (MAP) estimation $p(\mathcal{P}_2(\Omega) \,|\, f)$ (cf. Section 20.4). Since we also aim to restore an approximation u of the original noise-free image, one has to maximize a modified a posteriori probability density

$$p(u, \mathcal{P}_2(\Omega) \,|\, f) \propto p(\mathcal{P}_2(\Omega))\, p(u \,|\, \mathcal{P}_2(\Omega))\, p(f \,|\, u, \mathcal{P}_2(\Omega)) \tag{20.23}$$

By using Bayes' theorem, one gains the possibility to separate geometric properties of the partition of Ω (first term) from image-based features (second and third term). In addition, the densities on the right-hand side of Equation 20.23 are often easier to be modeled than the a posteriori probability density $p(u, \mathcal{P}_2(\Omega) \,|\, f)$ itself.

20.5.1 Geometric prior

In order to characterize the a priori probability density $p(\mathcal{P}_2(\Omega))$ for the geometric term in Equation 20.23, one might consider a geometric prior, which favors the smallness of the region boundary $\Gamma = (\partial\Omega_1 \cup \partial\Omega_2)/\partial\Omega$ in the $(d-1)$-dimensional Hausdorff measure $\mathcal{H}^{d-1}$, that is,

$$p(\mathcal{P}_2(\Omega)) \propto e^{-\beta\, \mathcal{H}^{d-1}(\Gamma)}, \qquad \beta > 0 \tag{20.24}$$

20.5.2 Image prior

To characterize the image-based density $p(u \,|\, \mathcal{P}_2(\Omega))$ in Equation 20.23, one may assume that the functions u_1 and u_2 in Equation 20.23 are uncorrelated to each other and independent with respect to the partition $\mathcal{P}_2(\Omega)$. This is a valid assumption, as one is interested in a partition that exactly separates the image regions with different behavior. Due to the composition of u by the functions u_1 and u_2 in Equation 20.23 and the pairwise disjoint partition of Ω by Ω_1 and Ω_2, one obtains simplified expressions of the form

$$p(u \,|\, \mathcal{P}_2(\Omega)) = p(u_1 \,|\, \Omega_1)\, p(u_2 \,|\, \Omega_2)$$

These densities $p(u_i \mid \Omega_i), i = 1, 2$, can be further reduced to a priori probability density functions $p(u_i)$. The most frequently used a priori densities, in analogy to statistical mechanics, are Gibbs functions [43] of the form

$$p(u_i) \propto e^{-\alpha_i R_i(u_i)}, \qquad \alpha_i > 0 \tag{20.25}$$

where R_i is a nonnegative (and usually convex) energy functional. Typical examples for R_i are the H^1 seminorm regularization as used in the Mumford–Shah model [4], the Fisher information regularization as used in Burger et al. [44], or the enforcement of piecewise constant functions as in the Chan–Vese method [1]. For further details on these image priors we refer to Sawatzky et al. [5].

20.5.3 Data fidelity

To characterize the densities $p(f \mid u_i, \Omega_i), i = 1, 2$, in Equation 20.23, one commonly assumes (in a discrete setting) that each value of f describes a realization of a random variable and all random variables are pairwise independent and identically distributed within the same corresponding region Ω_i. Due to the pairwise disjoint partition of Ω by Ω_1 and Ω_2 (as in the case of the image prior), one can replace the densities $p(f \mid u_i, \Omega_i)$ by a joint a posteriori probability $p_i(f \mid u_i)$ and hence one obtains simplified expressions of the form

$$p(f \mid u, \mathcal{P}_2(\Omega)) = p_i(f \mid u_1) \, p_i(f \mid u_2) \tag{20.26}$$

One can think of the probability in Equation 20.26 as the likelihood for observing the random events induced by f under the unknown conditions given by the approximation u. Naturally, one wants to maximize this likelihood with respect to u to determine a good estimation from a statistical point of view. For more details on likelihood functions, we refer to Grimmett and Welsh [45].

20.5.4 Variational segmentation model

In order to compute a MAP estimation for Equation 20.23 it is beneficial to replace the respective terms by the derived densities in Equations 20.24 through 20.26 and minimize the negative logarithm of the resulting product. Defining $D_i(f, u_i) = -\log p_i(f \mid u_i)$, $i = 1, 2$, as data fidelity terms, one is able to perform segmentation by minimizing the following functional:

$$E(u_1, u_2, \chi) = \int_{\Omega} \left[\chi D_1(f, u_1) + (1 - \chi) D_2(f, u_2) \right]$$

$$+ \alpha_1 R_1(u_1) + \alpha_2 R_2(u_2) + \beta \mathcal{H}^{d-1}(\Gamma) \tag{20.27}$$

The regularization functionals R_1 and R_2 can also be used to incorporate a priori knowledge about the expected unperturbed signals u_1 and u_2.

The main advantage of the region-based segmentation framework Equation 20.27 is the ability to handle the information, that is, the occurring type of noise and the desired smoothness conditions, in each region Ω_i of the image domain Ω separately. For example, it is possible to choose different smoothing functionals R_i, if regions of different characteristics are expected. Moreover, the proposed framework is a direct generalization of the Chan–Vese segmentation model and the region-based version of the Mumford–Shah segmentation model to non-Gaussian noise problems. An extensive analysis of the segmentation model and in particular the existence of respective minimizers for the associated optimization problem in Equation 20.27 can be found in Sawatzky et al. [5] together with details on its numerical realization.

20.5.5 Application to noise models

The variational segmentation model can be specialized (instanced) to specific noise models. For this purpose, one has to choose the appropriate probability densities $D_i(f, u_i) = -\log p_i(f \mid u_i)$, $i = 1, 2$, in Equation 20.27. Section 20.3 summarizes these terms for the noise models presented there. That fact reflects the general nature of the approach from Sawatzky et al. [5]. One important special case of this framework is an extended formulation of the popular Chan–Vese segmentation model, which can handle arbitrary noise models. To perform this extension, it suffices to exchange the L^2 distance functions in Equation 20.10 by general negative log-likelihood functions, see Equation 20.20. This extension of the Chan–Vese segmentation method to non-Gaussian noise models is easy to implement and allows to be used in a wide range of applications in which piecewise constant approximations can be expected. Note that for certain noise models, for example, Poisson noise, the formulation in Equation 20.20 coincides with other works already discussed in Section 20.4.

20.5.6 Impact of physical noise modeling on image segmentation

The segmentation framework described above assumes an explicit noise modeling. In this context, the question naturally arises to which extent the appropriate noise modeling influences the segmentation performance. In Tenbrinck et al. [29], a study is presented to answer this question based on echocardiography segmentation. Since the intention was to concentrate on the influence of noise models on high-level segmentation results, the framework Equation 20.27 is reduced to a Chan–Vese-like [1] energy functional $E(u_1, u_2, \chi)$ based on the formulation Equation 20.20 (discarding the regularization terms R_1 and R_2), which assumes constant approximations c_1 and c_2 in regions Ω_1 and Ω_2, respectively,

$$E(u_1, u_2, \chi) = \int_\Omega \left[\chi D_1(f, u_1) + (1 - \chi) D_2(f, u_2) \right] + \beta \mathcal{H}^{d-1}(\Gamma) \qquad (20.28)$$

In order to incorporate both low-level and high-level information in a unified framework, the energy functional in Equation 20.28 is extended to include a shape prior energy $R_{sh}()$,

$$E(u_1, u_2, \chi, \chi_{sh}) = \int_\Omega \left[\chi D_1(f, u_1) + (1 - \chi) D_2(f, u_2) \right] + \beta \mathcal{H}^{d-1}(\Gamma)$$

$$+ \gamma R_{sh}(\chi_{sh}) + \frac{\delta}{2} \|\chi - \chi_{sh}\|^2 \qquad (20.29)$$

The shape prior is based on the central-normalized Legendre moments as proposed in Foulonneau et al. [46] (see Tenbrinck et al. [29] for details). In addition, a L^2 similarity distance between the image region-driven segmentation χ and the shape space-driven segmentation χ_{sh} is added since it is desired to ensure $\chi = \chi_{sh}$ in case of convergence.

Datasets from echocardiography-containing images of the left ventricle of the human heart from different acquisition angles, that is, apical two-chamber and four-chamber views, of the human myocardium were used, which were manually segmented by two experts. Figure 20.3 illustrates one representative result. Figure 20.3b–d demonstrate the typical observations for this noise model with different parameter settings. (It was not possible to find a good parameter setting for the case of additive Gaussian noise.) Using the Rayleigh or Loupas noise model leads to reasonable results as can be seen in Figure 20.3e–f.

The segmentation performance is measured using the Dice index, which compares two given segmentations A and B by $D(A, B) = \frac{2|A \cap B|}{|A|+|B|}$, which is normalized between 0 (no similarity) and 1 (exact match). The Dice indices of segmentation results on a test set of eight images are presented in Table 20.2. For each test image, the table also lists the interobserver variability between the two physicians and the average similarity between the automatically segmented images and the two observers. Not surprisingly, the segmentation with the additive Gaussian noise model failed on all test images. The cases of Rayleigh and Loupas noise model lead to significantly better results (see Table 20.2). It can be observed that the model of Loupas has an average Dice index of 0.87 and thus is more suitable for high-level segmentation of ultrasound B-mode images than the Rayleigh modeling, which has an average segmentation performance of 0.78 on the eight test images.

In a particular context (ultrasound segmentation, using a reduced version of framework Equation 20.27 with integrated shape prior) the study reported in Tenbrinck et al. [29] clearly shows that correct physical noise modeling is of high importance for the computation of accurate segmentation results. It can be expected that the same conclusion can be made in general.

20.6   *Minimal surface solution for arbitrary noise models*

In contrast to the segmentation framework discussed in Section 20.5 the approach proposed in Tenbrinck and Jiang [40] does not depend on explicit noise modeling. This work is motivated by observations on the popular Chan–Vese segmentation model [1]. The energy functional of the Chan–Vese model is non-convex and its solution thus crucially depends on the initialization of the segmentation contour. Indeed, for each choice of the three parameters and the initialization, one has to deal with a different set of local minima. This makes it difficult to achieve satisfactory segmentation results on different images, which is undesirable in practical applications. Another interesting observation can be made when looking at the data fidelity of the Chan–Vese segmentation method with respect to noise perturbations of the image. The data fidelity term gets minimal if all intensity values are clustered according to the class mean values of the respective regions. In particular, for two fixed constants c_1 and c_2 (constant approximation of the noisy image f in Ω_1 and Ω_2) the Chan–Vese energy gets minimal if the data is partitioned according to a natural threshold $t_{CV} = (c_1 + c_2)/2$. This is, however, appropriate for the case of natural images perturbed by additive Gaussian noise only. The situation in presence of signal-dependent noise is different and the optimal threshold cannot be t_{CV} in this case (see Sawatzky et al. [5] for details). Thus, for certain imaging applications with non-Gaussian noise models, for example, biomedical imaging, the Chan–Vese model is not suitable. To overcome these drawbacks the work, Tenbrinck and Jiang [40] proposes a convex segmentation model based on solving minimum surface problems, which allows the computation of a global (unique) minimizer.

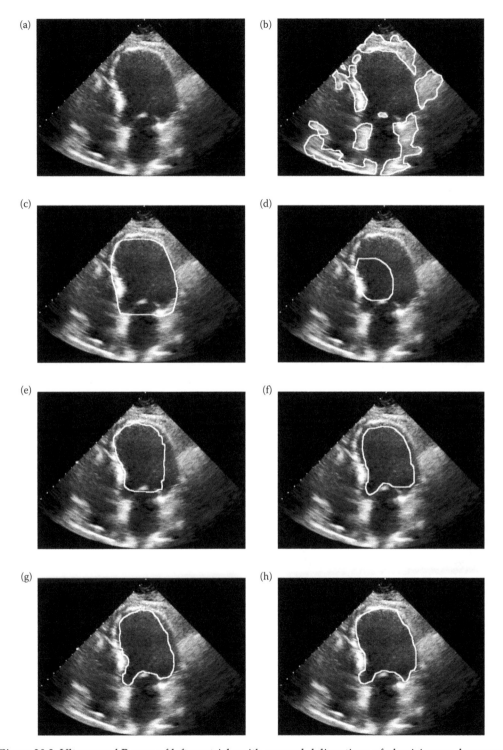

Figure 20.3 Ultrasound B-scan of left ventricle with manual delineations of physicians and segmentation results. (a) B-scan of LV, (b) Gaussian noise, (c) Gaussian noise, (d) Gaussian noise, (e) Rayleigh noise, (f) Loupas noise, (g) 1st physician, (h) 2nd physician.

Table 20.2 Dice index values for comparison with manual segmentation

Dataset	1	2	3	4	5	6	7	8
Observer variability	0.9228	0.9354	0.9034	0.9310	0.9151	0.9246	0.9391	0.8435
Gaussian noise	0.3444	0.4470	0.3306	0.3595	0.3439	0.4754	0.2953	0.3689
Rayleigh noise	0.8123	**0.7838**	0.7539	0.8017	0.7999	0.7693	0.7689	0.7368
Loupas noise	**0.8245**	0.7559	**0.9106**	**0.8891**	**0.9030**	**0.8862**	**0.8855**	**0.8942**

20.6.1 Minimal surface problem

In the well-known minimal surface problem in the calculus of variations [4,47–49] one wants to partition the image domain $\Omega \subset \mathbb{R}^n$ for any fixed $t \in \mathbb{R}$ by finding a subset $\Sigma \subset \Omega$ that has a finite perimeter and simultaneously minimizes the following energy:

$$E(\Sigma) = P(\Sigma, \Omega) + \frac{1}{\beta} \int_\Sigma t - f(x)\, \mathrm{d}x \qquad (20.30)$$

for which $P(\Sigma, \Omega)$ denotes the perimeter of Σ in Ω and $\beta > 0$ is a regularization parameter controlling the smoothness of this perimeter. Note that the constant t in Equation 20.30 represents a threshold, which separates the data f with respect to the partition induced by the subset Σ, that is, disregarding the term $P(\Sigma, \Omega)$ an optimal subset Σ would contain all points $x \in \Omega$ with $f(x) > t$.

Following Sawatzky et al. [5] and Caselles et al. [47], the perimeter of Σ in Ω is given by the total variation of its characteristic function $\chi \colon \Omega \to \{0, 1\}$. Note that χ already represents a partition of the image domain Ω in the sense of (20.1), that is,

$$\chi(x) = \begin{cases} 1, & \text{for } x \in \Sigma =: \Omega_1 \\ 0, & \text{for } x \in \Omega/\Sigma =: \Omega_2 \end{cases} \qquad (20.31)$$

Utilizing the idea in Caselles et al. [47] and Chan et al. [50], one can use the characteristic function χ to reformulate the minimal surface problem in Equation 20.30 and obtain the following equivalent optimization problem for image segmentation:

Find a minimizer $\chi \in BV(\Omega; \{0, 1\})$ of the functional

$$E(\chi) = \int_\Omega \chi(x)(t - f(x))\, \mathrm{d}x + \beta\, |\chi|_{BV} \qquad (20.32)$$

for which $BV(\Omega; \{0, 1\})$ is the Banach space of functions of bounded variation with values 0 and 1, $|\cdot|_{BV}$ is the total variation seminorm given by

$$|u|_{BV(\Omega)} = \sup_{\|v\|_\infty \leq 1} \left\{ \int_\Omega u(x)\, \mathrm{div}\, v(x)\, \mathrm{d}x : v \in C_0^\infty(\Omega; \mathbb{R}^n) \right\} \qquad (20.33)$$

and $\beta > 0$ is a regularization parameter controlling the smoothness of the edge set of χ and hence the smoothness of the partition. Note that the regularization term in Equation 20.32

is equivalent to the $(d-1)$-dimensional Hausdorff measure of the segmentation contour Γ in Equation 20.27.

20.6.2 Threshold-based segmentation with unique global minimizers

A rather simple variational segmentation method based on the minimal surface problem (20.30) is proposed in Tenbrinck and Jiang [40]. The problem of nonconvexity is overcome by using a two-stage approach, in which the denoising step is completely decoupled from the actual segmentation step. In particular, the relationship to a strictly convex denoising problem is utilized to guarantee the existence of a unique optimal segmentation result.

It can be shown that there exist minimizers for the minimal surface problem Equation 20.32 [40]. The following strategy is applied to guarantee the existence of a unique global minimizer (up to a Lebesgue-negligible set). Castelles et al. [47] described a particularly interesting relationship between the minimal surface problem Equation 20.32 and the strictly convex Rudin–Osher–Fatemi (ROF) total variation denoising model in Rudin et al. [51] based on the coarea formula

$$|u|_{BV} = \int\limits_{-\infty}^{\infty} P(\{x \in \Omega : u(x) > t\}, \Omega)\, dt \qquad (20.34)$$

that is, the total variation seminorm in Equation 20.33 of a function $u \in BV(\Omega)$ is the integral over all perimeters of its level sets. This relationship enables the unification of image segmentation and denoising tasks into a global minimization framework according to the following fundamental result from Caselles et al. [47].

Proposition 20.1: Segmentation by solving ROF denoising problem

Let $\beta > 0$ be a fixed parameter, $f \in L^2(\Omega)$, and $\hat{u}$ the unique solution of the ROF denoising functional,

$$\min_{u \in BV(\Omega)} \frac{1}{2} \int\limits_{\Omega} (u-f)^2\, dx + \beta\, |u|_{BV(\Omega)} \qquad (20.35)$$

Then, for almost every $t \in \mathbb{R}$, the indicator function

$$\hat{\chi}(x) = \begin{cases} 1, & \text{if } \hat{u}(x) > t \\ 0, & \text{else,} \end{cases} \qquad (20.36)$$

is a solution of the minimal surface problem

$$\min_{\chi \in BV(\Omega; \{0,1\})} \int\limits_{\Omega} \chi(x)\, (t-f)\, dx + \beta\, |\chi|_{BV(\Omega)} \qquad (20.37)$$

In particular, for all t but a countable set, the solution of Equation 20.37 is even unique.

Proposition 20.1 enables to determine a global minimum of the segmentation problem Equation 20.32 uniquely by solving an associated denoising problem. This idea has the advantage that for a fixed regularization parameter $\beta > 0$ there exist no local minima

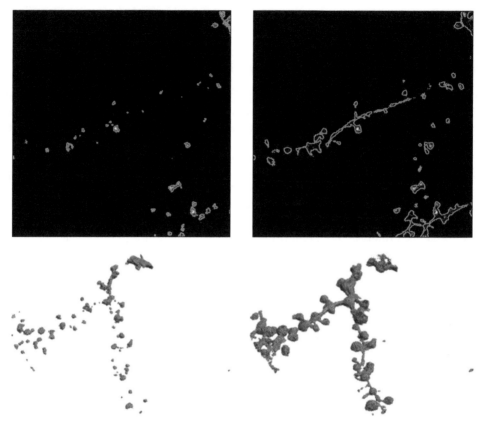

Figure 20.4 *Top:* Segmentation results of the Chan–Vese segmentation method and the minimum surface solution. *Bottom:* Rendering of the segmentation results.

and there is no need of any initialization. This overcomes especially the drawbacks of the Chan–Vese method as discussed before. Even more, it is well known that the level sets of a solution of the total variation denoising problem Equation 20.35 are themselves minimal surfaces [48]. This fact is very important and useful as it means that by minimization of Equation 20.35 one gets the whole set of minimal surface solutions of Equation 20.37 at once and the only problem left to solve is the determination of a proper threshold for segmentation. Finally, this approach has the advantage that there exists only one effective parameter β.

The thresholding step Equation 20.36 can be performed independently of the total variation denoising step. Note that an automatic estimation of a threshold t in the case of non-Gaussian noise has not been investigated so far. However, the choice of an optimal threshold is crucial for dealing implicitly with physical noise models. In Tenbrinck and Jiang [40], several thresholding methods [52] have been studied for this scenario. Since thresholding operations can be performed for even huge data in real-time nowadays, it is possible to determine the best threshold interactively by the user, for example, by shifting a slider. By this approach, one can determine the best threshold for each image and thus compute satisfactory segmentation results easily. Especially in biomedical imaging, semi-automatic methods are preferred by physicians and biologists, as they give more control to the trained expert.

20.6.3 Application: Confocal microscopy of small animal dendrites

Among others, the approach above has been applied in Tenbrinck and Jiang [40] to segment 3D volume data ($512 \times 512 \times 40$ voxels) of small animal neurons acquired by confocal microscopy. The main task is to separate the signal of the imaged dendrites and spines from the background voxels and thus to delineate the connected tree structure. Since a fluorescent tracer has been injected before the image acquisition process and the image acquisition time is relatively low, the data has a very low contrast and one can assume that it is perturbed by Poisson noise [15].

Figure 20.4 shows the segmentation results of the Chan–Vese segmentation method and the minimum surface solution for an exemplary slice of the volume data. The Chan–Vese method only segments the very bright regions of the data that correspond to anatomical structures with a high uptake of fluorescent tracer. Consequently, the main branch of the illustrated dendrite is not segmented due to the low contrast. The rendering (three-dimensional visualization) allows another view to the segmentation results. The Chan–Vese segmentation method fails to segment the 3D structure of the dendrites. The minimum surface solution with an automatically determined threshold is able to segment even the small spine necks connecting the spines to the dendrites.

20.7 Conclusions

In many real-life applications, for example, in biomedical imaging, physical noise modeling is indispensable to achieve reasonable segmentation result. In this chapter, we have discussed various aspects of image segmentation under consideration of physical noise models. In addition to the various noise models, we have briefly reviewed the related algorithmic development and exemplarily presented some recent works from our own research.

Despite of the vast literature on image segmentation, segmentation based on physical noise models has received relatively little attention only. In particular, methods without explicit noise modeling are still very rare. Also, the published methods have typically been tested on synthetic images and a small number of real images. Generally, it still lacks a large-scale real testing and performance comparison. Solutions toward improvement with regard to several factors (parameter selection, stability, computational efficiency, etc.) are needed in future to make the algorithms mature for real applications.

Acknowledgments

The authors would like to thank Jörg Stypmann from the University Hospital of Münster for his expertise in echocardiography, providing ultrasound images, and the manual segmentations. Furthermore, the authors thank the GIP Cyceron Caen for providing the fluorescence microscopy images of small animal neurons. Finally, the authors thank Martin Burger and Alex Sawatzky from the University of Münster for the insightful discussions on variational segmentation problems. This work was supported by the Deutsche Forschungsgemeinschaft (DFG), SFB 656 MoBil, Münster, Germany (project B3). D. Tenbrinck is supported by the ERC via Grant EU FP7 – ERC Consolidator Grant 615216 LifeInverse.

References

1. T. Chan and L. Vese, Active contours without edges, *IEEE Transactions on Image Processing*, vol. 10, no. 2, pp. 266–277, 2001.
2. F. Lecellier, J. Fadili, S. Jehan-Besson, G. Aubert, M. Revenu, and E. Saloux, Region-based active contours with exponential family observations, *Journal of Mathematical Imaging and Vision*, vol. 36, no. 1, pp. 28–45, 2010.
3. P. Martin, P. Réfrégier, F. Goudail, and F. Guérault, Influence of the noise model on level set active contour segmentation, *IEEE Transactions on Pattern Analysis and Machine Intelligence*, vol. 26, no. 6, pp. 799–803, 2004.
4. D. Mumford and J. Shah, Optimal approximations by piecewise smooth functions and associated variational problems, *Communications on Pure and Applied Mathematics*, vol. 42, no. 5, pp. 577–685, 1989.
5. A. Sawatzky, D. Tenbrinck, X. Jiang, and M. Burger, A variational framework for region-based segmentation incorporating physical noise models, *Journal of Mathematical Imaging and Vision*, vol. 47, no. 3, pp. 179–209, 2013.
6. D. Cremers, M. Rousson, and R. Deriche, A review of statistical approaches to level set segmentation: Integrating color, texture, motion and shape, *International Journal of Computer Vision*, vol. 72, no. 2, pp. 195–215, 2007.
7. C. Chesnaud, P. Réfrégier, and V. Boulet, Statistical region snake-based segmentation adapted to different physical noise models, *IEEE Transactions on Pattern Analysis and Machine Intelligence*, vol. 21, no. 11, pp. 1145–1157, 1999.
8. R. F. Wagner, S. W. Smith, J. M. Sandrik, and H. Lopez, Statistics of speckle in ultrasound B-scans, *IEEE Transactions on Sonics and Ultrasonics*, vol. 30, no. 3, pp. 156–163, 1983.
9. G. Slabaugh, G. Unal, T. Fang, and M. Wels, Ultrasound-specific segmentation via decorrelation and statistical region-based active contours, in *Proceedings of CVPR*, 2006, pp. 45–53.
10. T. Loupas, W. McDicken, and P. Allan, An adaptive weighted median filter for speckle suppression in medical ultrasonic images, *IEEE Transactions on Circuits and Systems*, vol. 36, no. 1, pp. 129–135, 1989.
11. L. Rudin, P.-L. Lions, and S. Osher, *Geometric Level Set Methods in Imaging, Vision, and Graphics*. Berlin: Springer, 2003, ch. Multiplicative Denoising and Deblurring: Theory and Algorithms, pp. 103–119.
12. K. Krissian, R. Kikinis, C. Westin, and K. G. Vosburgh, Speckle-constrained filtering of ultrasound images, in *Proceedings of CVPR*, 2005, pp. 547–552.
13. V. Dutt and J. F. Greenleaf, Adaptive speckle reduction filter for log-compressed B-scan images, *IEEE Transactions on Medical Imaging*, vol. 15, no. 6, pp. 802–813, 1996.
14. D. Tenbrinck, Variational methods for medical ultrasound imaging, Ph.D. dissertation, University of Muenster, 2013.
15. S. Hell, Toward fluorescence nanoscopy, *Nature Biotechnology*, vol. 21, no. 11, pp. 1347–1355, 2003.
16. Y. Vardi, L. Shepp, and L. Kaufman, A statistical model for positron emission tomography, *Journal of American Statistical Association*, vol. 80, pp. 8–20, 1985.
17. G. Aubert and J.-F. Aujol, A variational approach to removing multiplicative noise, *SIAM Journal on Applied Mathematics*, vol. 68, no. 4, pp. 925–946, 2008.
18. I. B. Ayed, A. Mitiche, and Z. Belhadj, Multiregion level-set partitioning of synthetic aperture radar images, *IEEE Transactions on Pattern Analysis and Machine Intelligence*, vol. 27, no. 5, pp. 793–800, 2005.
19. F. Galland, J. Nicolas, H. Sportouche, M. Roche, F. Tupin, and P. Réfrégier, Unsupervised synthetic aperture radar image segmentation using Fisher distributions, *IEEE Transactions on Geoscience and Remote Sensing*, vol. 47, no. 8–2, pp. 2966–2972, 2009.
20. I. B. Ayed, N. Hennane, and A. Mitiche, Unsupervised variational image segmentation/classification using a Weibull observation model, *IEEE Transactions on Image Processing*, vol. 15, no. 11, pp. 3431–3439, 2006.

21. L. A. Vese and T. F. Chan, A multiphase level set framework for image segmentation using the Mumford and Shah model, *International Journal of Computer Vision*, vol. 50, no. 3, pp. 271–293, 2002.
22. C. Li, C. Kao, J. C. Gore, and Z. Ding, Minimization of region-scalable fitting energy for image segmentation, *IEEE Trans. Image Processing*, vol. 17, no. 10, pp. 1940–1949, 2008.
23. K. Zhang, H. Song, and L. Zhang, Active contours driven by local image fitting energy, *Pattern Recognition*, vol. 43, no. 4, pp. 1199–1206, 2010.
24. T. Le and L. Vese, Additive and multiplicative piecewise-smooth segmentation models in a functional minimization approach, in *Interpolation Theory and Applications*, Contemporary Mathematics series, vol. 445, 2007, pp. 207–223.
25. F. Liu, Y. Luo, and D. Hu, Adaptive level set image segmentation using the Mumford and Shah functional, *Optical Engineering*, vol. 41, no. 12, pp. 3002–3003, 2002.
26. I. Diaz, P. Boulanger, R. Greiner, and A. Murtha, A critical review of the effect of de-noising algorithms on MRI brain tumor segmentation, in *Proceedings of the Annual International Conference of the IEEE Engineering in Medicine and Biology Society*, 2011, pp. 3934–3937.
27. Y.-T. Lee and T.M. Le, Active contour without edges for multiphase segmentations with the presence of Poisson noise, UCLA CAM, Technical Report, 11–46, 2011.
28. G. Steidl and T. Teuber, Removing multiplicative noise by Douglas-Rachford splitting methods, *Journal of Mathematical Imaging and Vision*, vol. 36, no. 2, pp. 168–184, 2010.
29. D. Tenbrinck, A. Sawatzky, X. Jiang, M. Burger, W. Haffner, P. Willems, M. Paul, and J. Stypmann, Impact of physical noise modeling on image segmentation in echocardiography, in *Proceedings of Eurographics Workshop on Visual Computing for Biology and Medicine*, 2012, pp. 33–40.
30. R. Zanella, P. Boccacci, L. Zanni, and M. Bertero, Efficient gradient projection methods for edge-preserving removal of Poisson noise, *Inverse Problems*, vol. 25, no. 4, p. 045010, 2009.
31. Q. Chen and C. He, Variational segmentation model for images with intensity inhomogeneity and Poisson noise, *EURASIP Journal on Image and Video Processing*, vol. 28, pp. 1–11, 2013.
32. D.-Q. Chen, L.-Z. Cheng, and X.-P. Du, Fast Poissonian image segmentation with a spatially adaptive kernel, *Optik*, vol. 125, no. 4, p. 15071516, 2014.
33. R. Chan, H. Yang, and T. Zeng, A two-stage image segmentation method for blurry images with Poisson or multiplicative Gamma noise, *SIAM Journal on Imaging Sciences*, vol. 7, no. 1, pp. 98–127, 2014.
34. X. Cai, R. Chan, and T. Zeng, A two-stage image segmentation method using a convex variant of the Mumford–Shah model and thresholding, *SIAM Journal on Imaging Sciences*, vol. 6, no. 1, pp. 368–390, 2013.
35. A. Sarti, C. Corsi, E. Mazzini, and C. Lamberti, Maximum likelihood segmentation of ultrasound images with Rayleigh distribution, *IEEE Transactions on Ultrasonics, Ferroelectrics, and Frequency Control*, vol. 25, no. 6, pp. 947–960, 2005.
36. F. Galland, N. Bertaux, and P. Réfrégier, Minimum description length synthetic aperture radar image segmentation, *IEEE Transactions on Image Processing*, vol. 12, no. 9, pp. 995–1006, 2003.
37. F. Galland, N. Bertaux, and P. Réfrégier, Multi-component image segmentation in homogeneous regions based on description length minimization: Application to speckle, Poisson and Bernoulli noise, *Pattern Recognition*, vol. 38, no. 11, pp. 1926–1936, 2005.
38. G. Delyon, F. Galland, and P. Réfrégier, Minimal stochastic complexity image partitioning with unknown noise model, *IEEE Transactions on Image Processing*, vol. 15, no. 10, pp. 3207–3212, 2006.
39. G. Delyon and P. Réfrégier, SAR image segmentation by stochastic complexity minimization with a nonparametric noise model, *IEEE Transactions on Geoscience and Remote Sensing*, vol. 44, no. 7–2, pp. 1954–1961, 2006.
40. D. Tenbrinck and X. Jiang, Image segmentation with arbitrary noise models by solving minimal surface problems, *Pattern Recognition*, vol. 48, no. 11, pp. 3293–3309, 2015.
41. D. Boukerroui, A local Rayleigh model with spatial scale selection for ultrasound image segmentation, in *Proceedings of the British Machine Vision Conference*, 2012, pp. 1–12.

42. Z. Tao, H. Tagare, and J. Beaty, Evaluation of four probability distribution models for speckle in clinic cardiac ultrasound images, *IEEE Transactions on Medical Imaging*, vol. 25, no. 11, pp. 1483–1491, 2006.

43. S. Geman and D. Geman, Stochastic relaxation, Gibbs distributions and the Bayesian restoration of images, *IEEE Transactions on Pattern Analysis and Machine Intelligence*, vol. 6, no. 6, pp. 721–741, 1984.

44. M. Burger, M. Franek, and C.-B. Schönlieb, Regularized regression and density estimation based on optimal transport, *Applied Mathematics Research eXpress*, 2012.

45. G. Grimmett and D. Welsh, *Probability: An Introduction*. Oxford: Oxford Science, 1986.

46. A. Foulonneau, P. Charbonnier, and F. Heitz, Multi-reference shape priors for active contours, *International Journal of Computer Vision*, vol. 81, pp. 68–81, 2009.

47. V. Caselles, A. Chambolle, and M. Novaga, The discontinuity set of solutions of the TV denoising problem and some extensions, *Multiscale Modeling and Simulation*, vol. 6, no. 3, pp. 879–894, 2007.

48. A. Chambolle, An algorithm for total variation minimization and applications, *International Journal of Computer Vision*, vol. 84, pp. 288–307, 2009.

49. D. Chopp, Computing minimal surfaces via level set curvature flow, *Journal of Computational Physics*, vol. 106, pp. 77–91, 1993.

50. T. Chan, S. Esedoglu, and M. Nikolova, Algorithms for finding global minimizers of image segmentation and denoising models, *SIAM Journal on Applied Mathematics*, vol. 66, no. 5, pp. 1632–1648, 2006.

51. L. Rudin, S. Osher, and E. Fatemi, Nonlinear total variation based noise removal algorithms, *Physica D*, vol. 60, pp. 259–268, 1992.

52. M. Sezgin and B. Sankur, Survey over image thresholding techniques and quantitative performance evaluation, *Journal of Electronic Imaging*, vol. 13, no. 1, pp. 146–165, 2004.

chapter twenty-one

A fast lung segmentation approach

Maryam El-Baz, Mohamed Abou El-Ghar, and Ayman El-Baz

Contents

Abstract

New techniques for more accurate unsupervised segmentation of lung tissues from low-dose computed tomography (LDCT) are proposed. In this chapter we describe LDCT images and desired maps of regions (lung and the other chest tissues) by a joint Markov–Gibbs random field model (GMRF) of independent image signals and interdependent region labels but focus on most accurate model identification. To better specify region borders, each empirical distribution of signals is precisely approximated by a linear combination of discrete Gaussians (LCDG) with positive and negative components. The initial segmentation based on the LCDG models is then iteratively refined using a GMRF model with analytically estimated potentials. To validate the accuracy of our algorithm, a special geometrical phantom motivated by statistical analysis of the LDCT data is designed. Experiments with both the phantom and real datasets confirm high accuracy of the proposed approach.

21.1   Introduction

Lung cancer remains the leading cause of cancer-related death in the United States. In 2006, there were approximately 174,470 new cases of lung cancer and 162,460 related deaths [1]. Early diagnosis of cancer can improve the effectiveness of treatment and increase the patient's chance of survival. Segmentation of the lung tissues is a crucial step for early detection and diagnosis of lung nodules. Accurate segmentation of lung tissues from LDCT images is a challenging problem because some lung tissues such as arteries, veins, bronchi, and bronchioles are very close to the chest tissues. Therefore, the segmentation cannot be based only on image signals but have to account also for spatial relationships between the region labels in order to preserve the details of the lung region.

In the literature, there are many techniques were developed for lung segmentation in CT images. Sluimer et al. [2] presented a survey on computer analysis of the lungs in CT scans. This survey addressed segmentation of various pulmonary structures, registration of chest scans, and their applications. Hu et al. [3], proposed an optimal gray level threshold-ing technique, which is used to select a threshold value based on the unique characteristics of the dataset. A segmentation-by-registration scheme was proposed by Sluimer et al. [4] for automated segmentation of the pathological lung in CT. For more on lung segmentation techniques, refer, for example, to the survey by Sluimer et al. [2].

In this chapter, we describe LDCT images and desired maps of regions (lung and the other chest tissues) by a joint Markov–Gibbs random field model (GMRF) of independent image signals and interdependent region labels but focus on most accurate model identifi-cation. To better specify region borders, each empirical distribution of signals is precisely approximated by a linear combination of discrete Gaussians (LCDG) with positive and neg-ative components. Approximation of an empirical relative frequency distribution of scalar data with a particular probability density function is widely used in pattern recognition and image processing, for example, for data clustering or image segmentation [5,6]. The basic problem is to accurately approximate, to within the data range, not only the peaks, or modes of the probability density function for the measurements but also its behavior between the peaks. This is most essential for a precise data classification because borders between data classes are usually formed by intersecting tails of the class distributions.

21.2 Joint Markov–Gibbs model of LDCT lung images

Let $\mathbf{R} = \{(i,j) : 1 \le i \le I, 1 \le j \le J\}$ denote a finite arithmetic grid supporting grayscale LDCT images $\mathbf{g} : \mathbf{R} \to \mathbf{Q}$ and their region maps $\mathbf{m} : \mathbf{R} \to \mathbf{X}$. Here, $\mathbf{Q} = \{0, \dots, Q-1\}$ and $\mathbf{X} = \{1, \dots, X\}$ are the sets of gray levels and region labels, respectively, where Q is the number of gray levels and X is the number of image classes to separate by segmentation.

The GMRF model of images to segment is given by a joint probability distribution of LDCT images and desired region maps $P(\mathbf{g}, \mathbf{m}) = P(\mathbf{m})P(\mathbf{g}|\mathbf{m})$. Here, $P(\mathbf{m})$ is an uncondi-tional distribution of maps and $P(\mathbf{g}|\mathbf{m})$ is a conditional distribution of images, given a map. The Bayesian MAP estimate of the map, in this work, we focus on accurate identification of the spatial interaction between the lung pixels ($P(\mathbf{m})$) and the intensity distribution for the lung tissues ($P(\mathbf{g}|\mathbf{m})$) as shown in Figure 21.1. Given the image $\mathbf{g}$, $\mathbf{m}^* = \arg\max_{\mathbf{m}} L(\mathbf{g}, \mathbf{m})$ maximizes the log-likelihood function:

$$L(\mathbf{g}, \mathbf{m}) = \log P(\mathbf{g}|\mathbf{m}) + \log P(\mathbf{m}) \tag{21.1}$$

21.2.1 Spatial interaction model of LDCT images

Generic Markov–Gibbs model of region maps [7] that account for only pairwise interac-tions between each region label and its neighbors have generally an arbitrary interaction structure and arbitrary Gibbs potentials identified from image data. For simplicity, we restrict the interactions to the nearest pixel 8-neighborhood and assume, by symmetry considerations, that the interactions are independent of relative region orientation, are the same for all classes, and depend only on intra- or inter-region position of each pixel pair

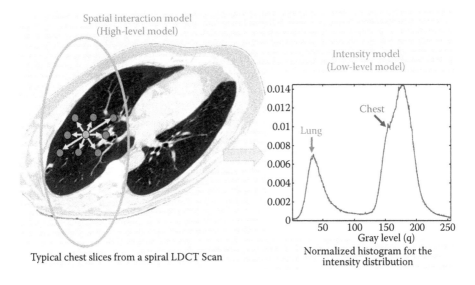

Figure 21.1 Illustration of joint Markov–Gibbs model of LDCT lung images.

(i.e., whether the labels are equal or not). Under these restrictions, the model is similar to the conventional autobinomial ones [7] and differs only in that the potentials are not related to a predefined function and have analytical estimates.

The symmetric label interactions are twofold: the closest horizontal-vertical (hv) and the slightly more distant left-right-diagonal ones (lr), and the potentials of each type are bivalued because only coincidence or difference of the labels are taken into account. Let $\mathbf{V}_a = \{V_a(x, \chi) = V_{a,\text{eq}} \text{ if } x = \chi \text{ and } V_a(x, \chi) = V_{a,\text{ne}} \text{ if } x \neq \chi : x, \chi \in \mathbf{X}\}$ denote bivalued Gibbs potentials describing symmetric pairwise interactions of type $a \in \mathbf{A} = \{\text{hv, lr}\}$ between the region labels. Let $\mathbf{N}_{\text{hv}} = \{(1, 0), (0, 1)\}$ and $\mathbf{N}_{\text{lr}} = \{(-1, 1), (1, 1)\}$ be subsets of interpixel offsets for the vertical-horizontal and left-right-diagonal interacting pixel pairs, respectively. Then the Gibbs probability distribution (GPD) of region maps is as follows:

$$P(\mathbf{m}) \propto \exp\left(\sum_{(i,j) \in \mathbf{R}} \sum_{a \in \mathbf{A}} \sum_{(\xi, \eta) \in \mathbf{N}_a} V_a(m_{i,j}, m_{i+\xi, j+\eta}) \right) \tag{21.2}$$

To identify the MGRF model described in Equation 21.2, we have to estimate the Gibbs potential $\mathbf{V}$. In this chapter, we introduce a new analytical maximum likelihood estimation for the Gibbs potentials (the mathematical proof for this new estimator is shown in the supplementary material).

$$V_{a,\text{eq}} = \frac{X^2}{X-1} \left(f_a'(\mathbf{m}) - \frac{1}{X} \right) \quad and \quad V_{a,\text{ne}} = \frac{X^2}{X-1} \left(f_a''(\mathbf{m}) - 1 + \frac{1}{X} \right) \tag{21.3}$$

where $f_a'(\mathbf{m})$ and $f_a''(\mathbf{m})$ denote the relative frequency of the equal and nonequal pairs of the labels in all the equivalent pixel pairs $\{((i, j), (i + \xi, j + \eta)) : (i, j) \in \mathbf{R}; (i + \xi, j + \eta) \in \mathbf{R}; (\xi, \eta) \in \mathbf{N}_a\}$, respectively.

21.2.2   Intensity model of LDCT lung images

Let q; $q \in \mathbf{Q} = \{0, 1, \ldots, Q - 1\}$, denote the Q-ary gray level. The discrete Gaussian (DG) is defined as the probability distribution $\Psi_\theta = (\psi(q|\theta) : q \in \mathbf{Q})$ on $\mathbf{Q}$ such that $\psi(q|\theta) = \Phi_\theta(q + 0.5) - \Phi_\theta(q - 0.5)$ for $q = 1, \ldots, Q - 2$, $\psi(0|\theta) = \Phi_\theta(0.5)$, $\psi(Q - 1|\theta) = 1 - \Phi_\theta(Q - 1.5)$ where $\Phi_\theta(q)$ is the cumulative Gaussian probability function with a shorthand notation $\theta = (\mu, \sigma^2)$ for its mean, μ, and variance, σ^2.

We assume the number K of dominant modes, that is, regions, objects, or classes of interest in a given LDCT images, is already known. In contrast to a conventional mixture of Gaussians and/or other simple distributions, one per region, we closely approximate the empirical gray level distribution for LDCT images with an LCDG having C_p positive and C_n negative components such that $C_p \geq K$:

$$p_{\mathbf{w}, \Theta}(q) = \sum_{r=1}^{C_p} w_{p,r} \psi(q|\theta_{p,r}) - \sum_{l=1}^{C_n} w_{n,l} \psi(q|\theta_{n,l}) \tag{21.4}$$

under the obvious restrictions on the weights $\mathbf{w} = [w_{p,.}, w_{n,.}]$: all the weights are nonnegative and

$$\sum_{r=1}^{C_p} w_{p,r} - \sum_{l=1}^{C_n} w_{n,l} = 1 \tag{21.5}$$

To identify the LCDG model including the numbers of its positive and negative components, we modify the expectation-maximization (EM) algorithm to deal with the LCDG.

First the numbers $C_p - K$, C_n and parameters $\mathbf{w}$, Θ (weights, means, and variances) of the positive and negative DG components are estimated with a sequential EM-based initializing algorithm. The goal is to produce a close initial LCDG approximation of the empirical distribution. Then under the fixed C_p and C_n, all other model parameters are refined with an EM algorithm that modifies the conventional one in Schlesinger and Hlavac [8] to account for the components with alternating signs.

21.2.2.1   Sequential EM-based initialization

Sequential EM-based initialization forms an LCDG approximation of a given empirical marginal gray level distribution using the conventional EM-algorithm [8] adapted to the DGs. At the first stage, the empirical distribution is represented with a mixture of K-positive DGs, each dominant mode being roughly approximated with a single DG. At the second stage, deviations of the empirical distribution from the dominant K-component mixture are modeled with other, "subordinate" components of the LCDG. The resulting initial LCDG has K-dominant weights, say, $w_{p,1}, \ldots, w_{p,K}$ such that $\sum_{r=1}^{K} w_{p,r} = 1$, and a number of subordinate weights of smaller values such that $\sum_{r=K+1}^{C_p} w_{p,r} - \sum_{l=1}^{C_n} w_{n,l} = 0$.

The subordinate components are determined as follows. The positive and negative deviations of the empirical distribution from the dominant mixture are separated and scaled up to form two new "empirical distributions." The same conventional EM algorithm is iteratively exploited to find the subordinate mixtures of positive or negative DGs that approximate best the scaled-up positive or negative deviations, respectively. The sizes $C_p - K$ and C_n of these mixtures are found by sequential minimization of the total absolute error between each scaled-up deviation and its mixture model by the number of the components. Then the obtained positive and negative subordinate models are scaled down and then added to the dominant mixture yielding the initial LCDG model of the size $C = C_p + C_n$.

21.2.2.2 Modified EM algorithm for LCDG

Modified EM algorithm for LCDG maximizes the log-likelihood of the empirical data by the model parameters assuming statistically independent signals:

$$L(\mathbf{w}, \Theta) = \sum_{q \in \mathbf{Q}} f(q) \log p_{\mathbf{w}, \Theta}(q) \tag{21.6}$$

A local maximum of the log-likelihood in Equation 21.6 is given with the EM process extending the one in Schlesinger and Hlavac [8] onto alternating signs of the components. Let $p_{\mathbf{w},\Theta}^{[m]}(q) = \sum_{r=1}^{C_p} w_{p,r}^{[m]} \psi(q|\theta_{p,r}^{[m]}) - \sum_{l=1}^{C_n} w_{n,l}^{[m]} \psi(q|\theta_{n,l}^{[m]})$ denote the current LCDG at iteration m. Relative contributions of each signal $q \in \mathbf{Q}$ to each positive and negative DG at iteration m are specified by the respective conditional weights

$$\pi_p^{[m]}(r|q) = \frac{w_{p,r}^{[m]} \psi(q|\theta_{p,r}^{[m]})}{p_{\mathbf{w},\Theta}^{[m]}(q)}; \quad \pi_n^{[m]}(l|q) = \frac{w_{n,l}^{[m]} \psi(q|\theta_{n,l}^{[m]})}{p_{\mathbf{w},\Theta}^{[m]}(q)} \tag{21.7}$$

such that the following constraints hold:

$$\sum_{r=1}^{C_p} \pi_p^{[m]}(r|q) - \sum_{l=1}^{C_n} \pi_n^{[m]}(l|q) = 1; \quad q = 0, \ldots, Q-1 \tag{21.8}$$

The following two steps iterate until the log-likelihood changes become small:

E–step[m+1]: Find the weights of Equation 21.7 under the fixed parameters $\mathbf{w}^{[m]}$, $\Theta^{[m]}$ from the previous iteration m, and

M–step[m+1]: Find conditional MLEs $\mathbf{w}^{[m+1]}$, $\Theta^{[m+1]}$ by maximizing $L(\mathbf{w}, \Theta)$ under the fixed weights of Equation 21.7.

Considerations closely similar to those in Schlesinger and Hlavac [8] show this process converges to a local log-likelihood maximum. Let the log-likelihood of Equation 21.6 be rewritten in the equivalent form with the constraints of Equation 21.8 as unit factors:

$$L(\mathbf{w}^{[m]}, \Theta^{[m]}) = \sum_{q=0}^{Q} f(q) \left[\sum_{r=1}^{C_p} \pi_p^{[m]}(r|q) \log p^{[m]}(q) - \sum_{l=1}^{C_n} \pi_n^{[m]}(l|q) \log p^{[m]}(q) \right] \tag{21.9}$$

Let the terms $\log p^{[m]}(q)$ in the first and second brackets be replaced with the equal terms $\log w_{p,r}^{[m]} + \log \psi(q|\theta_{p,r}^{[m]}) - \log \pi_p^{[m]}(r|q)$ and $\log w_{n,l}^{[m]} + \log \psi(q|\theta_{n,l}^{[m]}) - \log \pi_n^{[m]}(l|q)$, respectively, which follow from Equation 21.7. At the E-step, the conditional Lagrange maximization of the log-likelihood of Equation 21.9 under the Q restrictions of Equation 21.8 results just in the weights $\pi_p^{[m+1]}(r|q)$ and $\pi_n^{[m+1]}(l|q)$ of Equation 21.7 for all $r = 1, \ldots, C_p$; $l = 1, \ldots, C_n$; and $q \in \mathbf{Q}$. At the M-step, the DG weights $w_{p,r}^{[m+1]} = \sum_{q \in \mathbf{Q}} f(q) \pi_p^{[m+1]}(r|q)$ and $w_{n,l}^{[m+1]} = \sum_{q \in \mathbf{Q}} f(q) \pi_n^{[m+1]}(l|q)$ follow from the conditional Lagrange maximization of the log-likelihood in Equation 21.9 under the restriction of Equation 21.5 and the fixed conditional weights of Equation 21.7. Under these latter, the conventional MLEs of the parameters of each DG stem from maximizing the log-likelihood after each difference of the cumulative Gaussians is replaced with its close approximation with the Gaussian density (below "c" stands for "p" or "n," respectively):

$$\mu_{c,r}^{[m+1]} = \frac{1}{w_{c,r}^{[m+1]}} \sum_{q \in \mathbf{Q}} q \cdot f(q) \pi_c^{[m+1]}(r|q)$$

$$(\sigma_{c,r}^{[m+1]})^2 = \frac{1}{w_{c,r}^{[m+1]}} \sum_{q \in \mathbf{Q}} \left(q - \mu_{c,i}^{[m+1]}\right)^2 \cdot f(q) \pi_c^{[m+1]}(r|q)$$

This modified EM algorithm is valid until the weights $\mathbf{w}$ are strictly positive. The iterations should be terminated when the log-likelihood of Equation 21.6 does not change or begins to decrease due to accumulation of rounding errors.

The final mixed LCDG model $p_C(q)$ is partitioned into the K LCDG-submodels $P_{[k]} = [p(q|k) : q \in \mathbf{Q}]$, one per class $k = 1, \ldots, K$, by associating the subordinate DGs with the dominant terms so that the misclassification rate is minimal.

The whole iterative segmentation process is as follows:

- *Initialization*: Find an initial map by the pixelwise Bayesian MAP classification of a given LDCT image after initial estimation of X LCDG-models of signals of each object class represented by one of the dominant modes.
- *Iterative refinement*: Refine the initial map by iterating the following two steps:
    1. Estimate the potential values for region map model using Equation 21.3.
    2. Recollect the empirical gray level densities for the current regions, reapproximate these densities, and update the map using the pixelwise Bayesian classification.

21.3   *Experimental results and validation*

Experiments were conducted with the low-dose computed tomography (LDCT) images acquired with a multidetector GE Light Speed Plus scanner (General Electric, Milwuakee, Wisconsin) with the following scanning parameters: slice thickness of 2.5 mm reconstructed every 1.5 mm, scanning pitch 1.5, pitch 1 mm, 140 kV, 100 MA, and FOV 36 cm. The size of each 3D dataset is $512 \times 512 \times 182$. The LDCT images contain two classes ($K = 2$), namely, darker lung tissues and brighter chest region. A typical LDCT slice, its empirical marginal gray level distribution $f(q)$, and the initial two-component Gaussian dominant mixture $p_2(q)$ are shown in Figure 21.2. Figure 21.3 illustrates basic stages of our sequential EM-based initialization by showing the scaled-up alternating and absolute deviations $f(q) - p_2(q)$, the best mixture model estimated for the absolute deviations (these 10 Gaussian components give the minimum approximation error), and the initial LCDG models for each class.

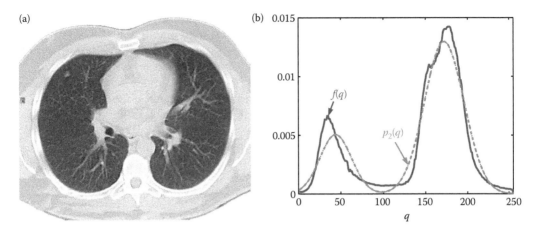

Figure 21.2 Typical LDCT scan slice (a) and deviations between the empirical distribution $f(q)$ and the dominant 2-component mixture $p_2(q)$ (b).

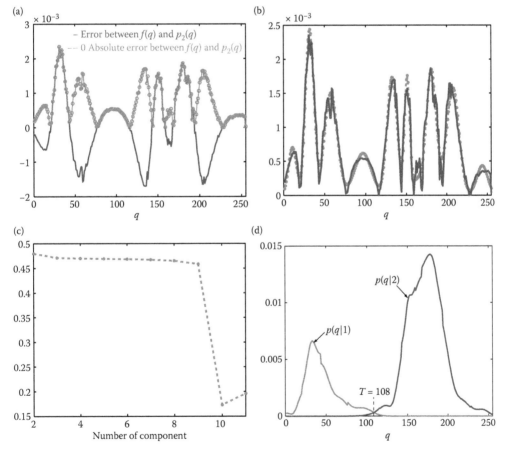

Figure 21.3 Deviations and absolute deviations between $f(q)$ and $p_3(q)$ (a), the mixture model (b) of the absolute deviations in (a), the absolute error (c) as a function of the number of Gaussians approximating the scaled-up absolute deviations in (a), and the initial estimated LCDG models for each class (d).

Figure 21.4 presents the final LCDG model after refining the initial one with the modified EM algorithm and shows successive changes of the log-likelihood at the refinement iterations. The final LCDG of each class are obtained with the best separation threshold $t = 109$. The first six refining iterations increase the log-likelihood from -5.7 to -5.2.

The region map obtained first with only the class LCDG-models is further refined using the iterative segmentation algorithm. Changes in the likelihood $L(\mathbf{g}, \mathbf{m})$ become very small after 12 iterations. For this map, the initial estimated parameters are $V_{a,\text{eq}} = -V_{a,\text{ne}} = 1.02$, and the final estimated parameters are $V_{a,\text{eq}} = -V_{a,\text{ne}} = 1.67$. The final region map produced with these parameters using the Metropolis pixelwise relaxation is shown in Figure 21.5. For comparison, Figure 21.5 presents also the initial region map, the map refined with the randomly selected potentials, segmentation obtained by MRS algorithm [9], segmentation obtained by ICM algorithm [10], and the "ground truth" segmentation done by a radiologist.

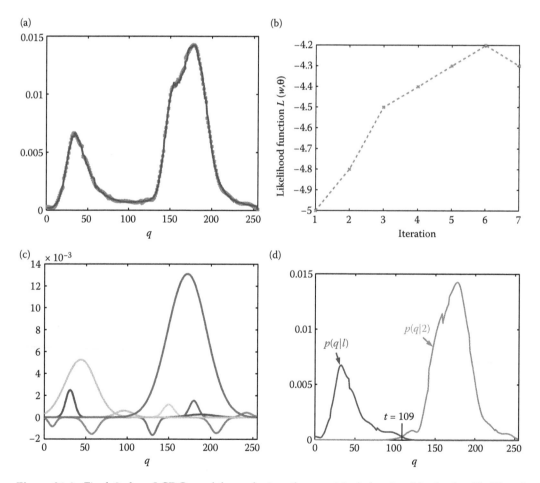

Figure 21.4 Final 3-class LCDG model overlaying the empirical density (a), the log-likelihood dynamics (b) for the refining EM-iterations, the refined model components (c), and the class LCDG-models (d).

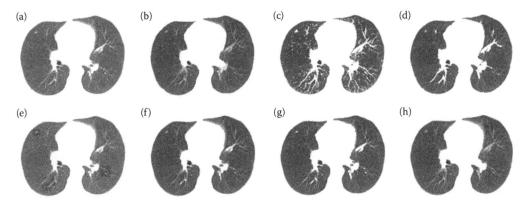

Figure 21.5 Initial (a) and final (b) segmentation by the proposed approach (the final error 1.1% comparing to the ground truth); initial (c) and final (d) segmentation using the conventional normal mixture obtained by the EM algorithm (the final error 5.1%); refined lung regions (e) obtained from (a) using the randomly chosen Gibbs potentials of the map model (the final error 1.8%); (f) best segmentation obtained by the MRS algorithm with the potential values 0.3 and three-level of resolution (error 2.3%); (g) best segmentation obtained by the ICM algorithm with the potential values 0.3 (error 2.9%), and the ground truth (h) produced by a radiologist.

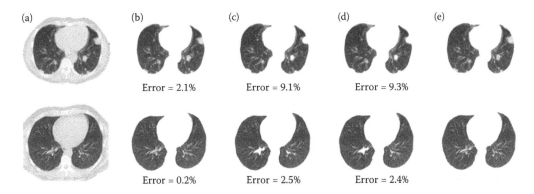

Figure 21.6 Original CT slices (a), their lung regions segmented with our approach (b), with the iterative threshold (IT) algorithm (c), with the conventional normal mixtures with positive Gaussian components only (d), and the ground truth (e) produced by a radiologist.

Figure 21.6 compares our segmentation to iterative thresholding algorithm. In contrast to this method, our segmentation does not lose abnormal lung tissues. In these and preceding experiments, the errors are evaluated with respect to the "ground truth" produced by an expert. But these prototypes may contain errors due to hand positioning instabilities during manual segmentation. In order to better measure the accuracy of our approach, we have created a geometric phantom with the same gray level distribution in regions as in the CT slices at hand. The phantom, its ideal region map, and results of our segmentation are shown in Figure 21.7. The error 0.09% between the found regions and ground truth confirms the high accuracy of the proposed segmentation techniques. For comparison, Figure 21.7 shows also the segmentation obtained with the iterative thresholding (IT) approach, the ICM algorithm [10], the MRS algorithm [9], the deformable model, which

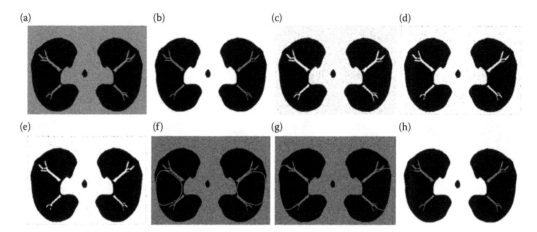

Figure 21.7 Generated phantom (a), its lung regions segmented with our approach (b; the error 0.09%), the IT approach (c; the error 5.97%), the ICM algorithm (d; the least error 2.91% obtained with the potential values 0.3); the MRS algorithm (e; the error 1.98% with the potential values 0.3 and three resolution levels), the deformable model using the traditional image gradient as an external force (f; the error 59.4%), the deformable model with the gradient vector field as an external force (g; the error 51.9%), and the ground truth (h).

Table 21.1 Accuracy of our segmentation in comparison to five conventional algorithms (IT, MRS [9], ICM [10], the gradient-based deformable model DMG [11], and the deformable model based on the gradient vector flow GVF [12])

Error, %	Segmentation algorithm					
	Our	IT	MRS	ICM	DMG	GVF
Minimum	**0.1**	2.81	1.90	2.03	10.1	4.10
Maximum	**2.15**	21.9	9.80	17.1	29.1	18.2
Mean	**0.32**	10.9	5.10	9.80	15.1	13.2
St.dev.	**0.71**	6.04	3.31	5.11	7.77	4.81

uses the tractional gradient-based external force [11], and the more advanced deformable model using the GVF [12].

The above experiments as well as additional experiments with 1820 different bimodal LDCT slices have shown that our segmentation yields much better results than several more conventional algorithms. As indicated in Table 21.1, the most accurate algorithm among these latter algorithms, namely, the MRS [9], has the larger error range of 1.9%–9.8% the mean error of 5.1% with respect to the ground truth. Our segmentation has the notably smaller error range of 0.1%–2.15% and its mean error of 0.32% is more than 15 times less.

21.4   Conclusions

Our experiments show that the proposed accurate identification of the Markov–Gibbs random field model demonstrates promising results in segmenting the lung region from LDCT images. The main difference with respect to more conventional schemes is in the use of precise LCDG models to approximate signal distributions and analytical estimates of the MGRF parameters. The proposed segmentation techniques include (i) the accurate sequential initialization to form a starting LCDG model, (ii) the modified EM algorithm for refining the starting model, and (iii) the iterative map refinement using the identified conditional MGRF model. Our present implementation on C++ programming language on the Intel dual processor (3 GHz each) with 8 GB memory and 1.5 TB hard drive with RAID technology takes about 596 s for processing 182 LDCT slices of size 512×512 pixels each, that is, about 3.27 s per slice.

References

1. American Cancer Society: Cancer Facts and Figures, 2006.
2. I. Sluimer, A. Schilham, M. Prokop, and B. van Ginneken, Computer analysis of computed tomography scans of the lung: A survey, *IEEE TMI*, vol. 25, no. 4, pp. 385–405, 2006.
3. S. Hu, E. A. Hoffman, and J. Reinhardt, Automatic lung segmentation for accurate quantitation of volumetric x-ray CT images, *IEEE TMI*, vol. 20, no. 6, pp. 490–498, 2001.
4. I. Sluimer, Mathias Prokop, and Bram van Ginneken, Toward automated segmentation of the pathological lung in CT, *IEEE TMI*, vol. 24, no. 8, pp. 1025–1038, 2005.
5. R. O. Duda, P. E. Hart, and D. G. Stork, *Pattern Classification*, 2nd ed., Wiley: New York, 2001.
6. A. Goshtasby and W. D. O'Neill, Curve fitting by a sum of Gaussians, *CVGIP: Graphical Models and Image Processing*, vol. 56, no. 4, pp. 281–288, 1999.
7. A. El-Baz, Novel stochastic models for medical image analysis, PhD Dissertation, University of Louisville, Louisville, KY, 2006.
8. M. I. Schlesinger and V. Hlavac, *Ten Lectures on Statistical and Structural Pattern Recognition.* Dordrecht: Kluwer Academic, 2002.
9. C. Bouman and B. Liu, Multiple resolution segmentation of textured images, *IEEE Transactions on Pattern Analysis and Machine Intelligence*, vol. 13, pp. 99–113, 1991.
10. J. E. Besag, On the statistical analysis of dirty pictures, *Journal of Royal Statistical Society*, vol. B48, pp. 259–302, 1986.
11. M. Kass, A. Witkin, and D. Terzopoulos, Snakes: Active contour models, *International Journal of Computer Vision*, vol. 1, pp. 321–331, 1987.
12. C. Xu and J. L. Prince, Snakes, shapes, and gradient vector flow, *IEEE Transactions on Pattern Analysis Machine Intelligence*, vol. 7, pp. 359–369, 1998.

chapter twenty-two

Fully automatic segmentation of hip CT images via landmark detection-based atlas selection and optimal surface detection

Chengwen Chu and Guoyan Zheng

Contents

Abstract

Automatic extraction of surface models of both pelvis-32pc]Q1 and proximal femur of a hip joint from 3D CT images is an important and challenging task for computer-assisted diagnosis and planning of periacetabular osteotomy (PAO). Due to the narrowness of hip joint space, the adjacent surfaces of the acetabulum and the femoral head are hardly distinguishable from each other in the target CT images. This chapter presents a fully automatic method for segmenting hip CT images using landmark detection-based atlas selection and optimal graph search-based surface detection. The two fundamental contributions of our method are: (1) an efficient random forest (RF) regression framework is developed for a fast and accurate landmark detection from the hip CT images. The detected landmarks allow for not only a robust and accurate initialization of the atlases within the target image space but also an effective selection of a subset of atlases for a fast atlas-based segmentation; and (2) 3D graph theory-based optimal surface detection is used to refine the extraction of the surfaces of the acetabulum and the femoral head with the ultimate goal to preserve hip joint structure and to avoid penetration between the two extracted surfaces. Validation on 30 hip CT images shows that our method achieves high performance in segmenting pelvis, left proximal femur, and right proximal femur with an average accuracy of 0.56 mm, 0.61 mm, and 0.57 mm, respectively.

22.1   Introduction

Developmental dysplasia of hip (DDH) is a congenital defect that seriously affects young people nowadays. In many treatment procedures for patients with DDH, periacetabular osteotomy (PAO) recently becomes a common surgical intervention [1], aiming to improve ability of weight-bearing and stability of the diseased hip joint. To reach this goal, knowing acetabular coverage, which is defined as a ratio between the femoral head surface covered by the acetabulum and the complete femoral head surface, is important for operative planning for PAO. For this purpose, we need to extract surface models of both the pelvis and the proximal femur from hip CT images.

Automatic extraction of the surface models of both the pelvis and the proximal femur from hip CT images comprises two key steps. First, both anatomical structures have to be detected in the target volume data and second, both models need to be segmented. Furthermore, the fact that the two structures compose a hip joint should not be neglected. Otherwise, the resultant models may penetrate each other due to the narrowness of the hip joint and hence do not represent a true hip joint.

For detection, reported methods in literature address the problem either by assuming an user-supplied initialization [2–3] or by using generalized Hough transform (GHT) [4,5]. For segmentation, both multiatlas-based segmentation methods [6–8] and statistical shape model (SSM)-based segmentation methods [2–5,9,10] are proposed. Here we define an atlas as a pair of data consisting of a CT volume and its corresponding segmentation. Given a set of atlases, atlas-based segmentation methods segment a target volume by registering the atlases to the volume first, followed by a label fusion process. Multiatlas-based segmentation methods may be applicable for extraction of surface models of individual structures of the hip joint, but they cannot guarantee the preservation of the hip joint space and the prevention of the penetration of the extracted surface models. The other segmentation option is the SSM-based methods, which perform an adaption of the SSM to the target image data. Similar to atlas-based methods, conventional SSM-based methods are difficult, if not impossible, to guarantee the preservation of the hip joint structure [2–4,9]. This problem is recently addressed by introducing an articulated statistical shape model (aSSM) [5]. Another solution is to simultaneously detect both surfaces of the adjacent structures based on graph optimization theory [10]. By incorporating prior knowledge about spatial relationship in the graph optimization, the adjacent surfaces can be segmented without penetration to each other.

In this chapter, we propose a two-stage automatic hip CT segmentation method. In the first stage, we use a multiatlas-based method to segment the regions of the pelvis and the bilateral proximal femurs. An efficient random forest (RF) regression-based landmark detection method is developed to detect landmarks from the target CT images. The detected landmarks allow for not only a robust and accurate initialization of the atlases

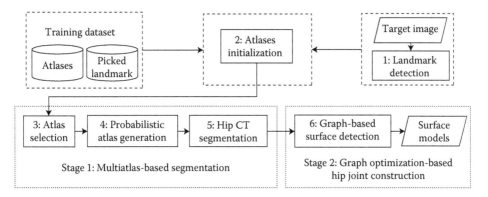

Figure 22.1 The flowchart of our proposed segmentation method.

within the target image space but also an effective selection of a subset of atlases for a fast atlas-based segmentation. In the second stage, we refine the-18.6pc]Q2 segmentation of the hip joint area using graph optimization theory-based multi surface detection [11,12], which guarantees the preservation of the hip joint space and the prevention of the penetration of the extracted surface models with a carefully constructed graph. Different from the method introduced in Kainmueller et al. [10], where the optimal surfaces are detected in the original CT image space, here we propose to first unfold the hip joint area obtained from the multiatlas-based segmentation stage using a spherical coordinate transform and then detect the surfaces of the acetabulum and the femoral head in the unfolded space. By unfolding the hip joint area using the spherical coordinate transform, we convert the problem of detection of two half-spherically shaped surfaces of the acetabulum and the femoral head in the original image space to a problem of detection of two terrain-like surfaces in the unfolded space, which can be efficiently solved using the methods presented in Li et al. [11] and Song et al. [12]. Figure 22.1 presents a schematic overview of the complete workflow of our method.

22.2 Multiatlas-based hip CT segmentation

22.2.1 Landmark detection by fast random forest regression

22.2.1.1 Basic algorithm

We have a separate RF landmark detector for each landmark. During training, in each training image, we sample a set of image volumes around the ground truth landmark position, which is known. Each sampled volume is represented by its visual feature $\mathbf{f}_i \in \mathbb{R}^{d_f}$ and the displacement $\mathbf{d}_i \in \mathbb{R}^3$ from its center to the landmark (Figure 22.2a). Let's denote all the sampled volumes in all training images as $\{P_i = (\mathbf{f}_i, \mathbf{d}_i)\}_{i=1...N}$ (Figure 22.2b). The goal is then to learn a mapping function $\phi : \mathbb{R}^{d_f} \to \mathbb{R}^3$ from the feature space to the displacement space. Principally, any regression method can be used. In this chapter, similar to Criminisi et al. [13] and Lindner et al. [14], we utilize the random forest regressors [15].

Once the regressor is trained, given a new image (Figure 22.2c), we randomly sample another set of volumes $\{P'_k = (\mathbf{f}'_k, \mathbf{c}'_k)\}_{k=1...N'}$ all over the image (or a region of interest if an initial guess of the landmark position is known), where $\mathbf{f}'_k$ and $\mathbf{c}'_k$ are the visual feature and center coordinate of the kth volume, respectively (Figure 22.2d). Through the trained regressor ϕ, we can calculate the predicted displacement $\mathbf{d}'_k = \phi(\mathbf{f}'_k)$, and then $\mathbf{d}'_k + \mathbf{c}'_k$

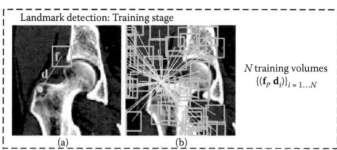

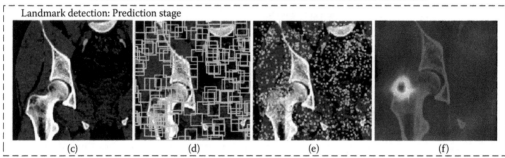

Figure 22.2 The RF training and landmark detection. Illustration on coronal slice for easy under-standing. (a) A volume sampled around the true landmark position. (b) Multiple sampled training volumes from one atlas. (c) A target image. (d) Multiple sampled test volumes over target image. (e) Each volume gives a single vote for landmark position. (f) Response volume calculated using improved fast Gaussian transform.

becomes the prediction of the landmark position by a single volume P'_k (Figure 22.2e). Note that each tree in the random forest will return a prediction. Therefore, supposing that there are t trees in the forest, we will get $N' \times t$ predictions. These individual predictions are very noisy, but when combined, they approach an accurate prediction. To this end, we consider each single vote as a small Gaussian distribution. We developed a fast probability aggregating algorithm as described below to add these distributions to get a soft probability map called response volume, which gives, for every position of the CT volume, its probability of being the landmark (Figure 22.2f).

22.2.1.2 Fast probability aggregation

As described above, $N' \times t$ predictions are produced to detect each landmark. We consider each prediction a Gaussian model $\mathcal{N} \sim (\bar{\mathbf{d}}_k, \Sigma(\mathbf{d}_k))$, where $\bar{\mathbf{d}}_k$ and $\Sigma(\mathbf{d}_k) = diag(\sigma^2_{k,x} \quad \sigma^2_{k,y} \quad \sigma^2_{k,z})$ are mean and covariance (which can be calculated from the displace-ments of the training samples that arrived at particular leaf node). All the $N' \times t$ predictions are accumulated to compute the likelihood of being a true landmark position for all M voxeles in the image. This finally yields a response volume for each landmark. Once the response volume has been obtained for each landmark, the position mode is selected as the landmark position.

The computational time of landmark prediction is mainly on multivariate Gaussian accumulation which is usually computed using

$$G(\mathbf{y}_i) = \sum_k^{N' \times t} \frac{1}{\sqrt{(2\pi)^3 |\Sigma(\mathbf{d}_k)|}} exp(-\frac{1}{2}(\mathbf{d}_{\mathbf{y}_i} - \bar{\mathbf{d}}_k)^T \Sigma(\mathbf{d}_k)^{-1}(\mathbf{d}_{\mathbf{y}_i} - \bar{\mathbf{d}}_k)) \qquad (22.1)$$

where $\mathbf{d}_{\mathbf{y}_i} = \mathbf{y}_i - \mathbf{x}_k$, $\mathbf{y}_i$ is a voxel in target image and $\mathbf{x}_k$ is the center of volume k. For all of the N_l landmarks, such calculation will result in prohibitively expensive computation time of $O(M \times N' \times t \times N_l)$ on a 3D CT image with M voxels. In this chapter, we propose to approximate Equation 22.1 by:

$$G(\mathbf{y}_i) = \sum_k^{N' \times t} W_k \cdot e^{(\|\mathbf{d}_{\mathbf{y}_i} - \bar{\mathbf{d}}_k\|^2 / h^2)} \tag{22.2}$$

Here we rewrite the Equation 22.1 by introducing a constant kernel size of h, and moving the constrains of the variance out of the exponential part by introducing a weight $W_k = 1/\sigma_{k,x}\sigma_{k,y}\sigma_{k,z}$. With such an approximation, we develop an efficient probability aggregation strategy based on the improved fast Gaussian transform (IFGT) [16] to calculate the response volumes with highly reduced time of $O((M + N' \times t) \times N_l)$.

22.2.1.3 Visual feature

As for the visual feature over the sampled subvolume, we use mean and variance of intensities in a small volume obtained by subdividing the sampled subvolume. In this chapter, we subdivide each sampled subvolume into a grid of $q \times q \times q$ blocks (see Figure 22.3 for details).

To accelerate the feature extraction within each block, we use the well-known integral image technique as introduced in Viola and Jones [17]. Details about how to compute the integral image of a quantity can be found in Viola and Jones [17]. The quantity can be the voxel intensity value or any arithmetic computation on the intensity value. The advantage of using integral image lies in the fact that once we obtain an integral image of the quantity over the complete hip CT volume, the sum of the quantity in any subvolume can be calculated quickly in constant time O(1) regardless of the size of the volume [17]. Here we assume that we already computed the integral image of the voxel intensity I and the integral image of the squared voxel intensity S of the complete hip CT volume using the technique introduced in Viola and Jones [17]. We then compute the mean $E[X]$ and the variance $Var(X)$ of the intensity value of any block (Figure 22.3, right) as:

$$\begin{cases} E[X] = (I(\mathbf{h}) - I(\mathbf{d}) - I(\mathbf{f}) - I(\mathbf{g}) + I(\mathbf{b}) + I(\mathbf{c}) + I(\mathbf{e}) - I(\mathbf{a}))/N \\ E[X^2] = (S(\mathbf{h}) - S(\mathbf{d}) - S(\mathbf{f}) - S(\mathbf{g}) + S(\mathbf{b}) + S(\mathbf{c}) + S(\mathbf{e}) - S(\mathbf{a}))/N \\ Var(X) = E[X^2] - (E[X])^2 \end{cases} \tag{22.3}$$

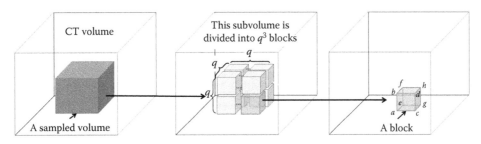

Figure 22.3 A schematic view illustrating how to compute the visual feature of a sampled subvolume for RF training and regression. *Left*: A subvolume is sampled from a hip joint CT volume. *Middle*: We subdivide the sampled subvolume into $q \times q \times q$ blocks. *Right*: For each block, we compute its mean and variance using the integral image technique.

where $\{\mathbf{a}, \ldots \mathbf{h}\} \in \mathcal{R}^3$ are the eight vertices of a block and N is the number of voxels within the block, as shown in Figure 22.3, right.

22.2.2   Atlas initialization and atlas-based segmentation

Using the detected N_l anatomical landmarks, scaled rigid registrations are performed to align all the N_A atlases to the target image space. Then we select N_s most similar atlases for the given target image. This is achieved by comparing the sum of the distance of the landmarks for all the aligned atlases after the scaled rigid registration. The selected atlases are further registered to the target image with a Markov random field (MRF) based non rigid registration [18]. We then use the selected atlases to generate probabilistic atlas (PA) for pelvis, bilateral proximal femurs, and background following the idea introduced in Chu et al. [19]. The generated PAs are further incorporated to a maximum a posteriori (MAP) estimation, which is then optimized by a graph-cut method [20] to obtain segmentation results.

22.3   Graph optimization-based hip joint surface detection

22.3.1   Problem formulation

After we extract surface models of the pelvis and femur using multiatlas-based segmentation, we expect to refine the hip joint segmentation in the second stage by separating two surfaces of the adjacent structures, that is, separating the surface of the acetabulum from the surface of the femoral head. In the CT image space, both the acetabulum and the femoral head are ball-like structures and their surfaces can be approximately represented as half-spherically shaped models. To separate these two surfaces, directly applying graph optimization-based surface detection in the CT image space as described in Kainmueller et al. [10] and Song et al. [12] would be an option. However, construction of a graph in the original CT image is not straightforward and requires finding correspondences between two adjacent surfaces obtained from a rough segmentation stage as done in Kainmueller et al. [10] and Song et al. [12], which is challenging.

   In our method, instead of performing surface detection in the original CT image space, we first define a hip joint area in the CT image based on the multiatlas-based segmentation results, and then unfold this area using a spherical coordinate transform as shown in Figure 22.4. Since the spherical coordinate transform converts a half-spherically shaped surface to a planar surface, the surfaces of the acetabulum and the femoral head can therefore be unfolded to two terrain-like surfaces with a gap (joint space) between them as shown in Figure 22.4. We reach this goal with following steps:

1. Detecting rim points of the acetabulum from segmented surface model of the pelvis using the method that we developed before [21] (Figure 22.4: 1).
2. Fitting a circle to the detected rim points, determining radius R_c and center of the circle, as well as normal to the plane where the fitted circle is located (Figure 22.4: 2).
3. Constructing a spherical coordinate system as shown in Figure 22.4: 3, taking the center of the fitted circle as the origin, the normal to the fitted circle as the fixed zenith direction, and one randomly selected direction on the plane where the fitted circle is located as the reference direction on that plane. Now, the position of a point in this coordinate system is specified by three numbers: the radial distance R of that point from the origin, its polar angle Θ measured from the zenith direction, and the azimuth

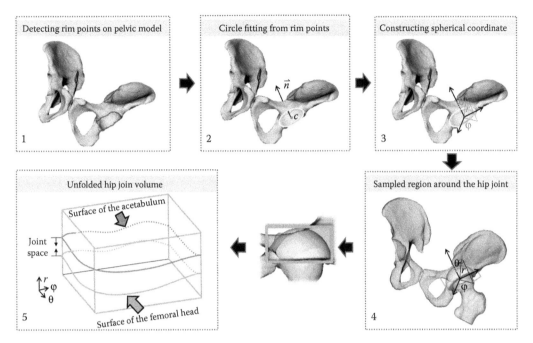

Figure 22.4 A schematic illustration of defining and unfolding a hip joint. Please see text in Section 22.3.1 for a detailed explanation.

angle Φ measured from the reference direction on the plane where the fitted circle is located.

4. Sampling points in the spherical coordinate system from the hip joint area (see Figure 22.4: 4) using a radial resolution of 0.25 mm and angular resolutions of 0.03 radians (for both polar and azimuth angles). Furthermore, we require the sampled points satisfying following conditions:

$$\begin{cases} R_c + 10 \le R \le R_c/2 \\ 0 \le \Theta \le \pi/2 \\ 0 \le \Phi \le 2\pi \end{cases} \tag{22.4}$$

5. Getting corresponding intensity values of the sampled points from the CT image, which finally forms an image volume $I(\theta, \varphi, r)$ (Figure 22.4: 5), where $0 \le r \le \left\lceil (10 + \frac{R_c}{2})/0.25 \right\rceil$, $0 \le \theta \le \lceil \pi/0.06 \rceil$ and $0 \le \varphi \le \lceil 2\pi/0.03 \rceil$. The dimension of r depends on the radius of the fitted circle while the dimensions of θ and φ are fixed. To easy the description later, here we define the dimension of r as D_r.

Figure 22.5 shows an example of the unfolded volume $I(\theta, \varphi, r)$ of a hip joint. With such an unfolded volume, graph construction and optimal multiple-surface detection will be straightforward when the graph optimization-based multiple-surface detection strategy as introduced in Li et al. [11] and Song et al. [12] is used.

(a)   (b)

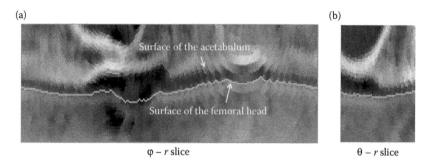

φ – r slice   θ – r slice

Figure 22.5 An example of unfolded volume $I(\theta, \varphi, r)$ of a hip joint, visualized in 2D slices. (a) A 2D φ-r slice. (b) A 2D θ-r slice. In both slices, the green line indicates the surface of the femoral head and the red line indicates the surface of the acetabulum. The gap between these two surface corresponds to the joint space of the hip.

22.3.2 Graph construction for multisurface detection

For the generated volume $I(\theta, \varphi, r)$ as shown in Figure 22.5, we assume that r is implicitly represented by a pair of (θ, φ), for example, $r = p(\theta, \varphi)$. For a fixed (θ, φ) pair, the voxel subset $\{I(\theta, \varphi, r)|0 \leq r < D_r\}$ forms a column along the r-axis and is defined as $Col(p)$. Each column has a set of neighbors and in this chapter four-neighbor system is adopted. The problem is now to find k coupled surfaces such that each surface intersects each column exactly at one voxel. In our case, we expect to detect two adjacent surfaces of a hip joint, that is, the surface of the acetabulum S_a and the surface of the femoral head S_f. To accurately detect these two surfaces using graph optimization-based approach, following geometric constraints need to be considered:

1. For each individual surface, the shape changes of this surface on two neighboring columns $Col(p)$ and $Col(q)$ are constrained by smoothness conditions. Specifically, if $Col(p)$ and $Col(q)$ are neighbored columns along the θ-axis, for each surface S (either S_a or S_f), the shape change should satisfy the constraint of $|S(p) - S(q)| = |r_p - r_q| \leq \Delta_\theta$, where $r_p = p(\theta_1, \varphi)$ and $r_q = q(\theta_2, \varphi)$ are coordinate values of the surface S (either S_a or S_f) intersecting columns $Col(p)$ and $Col(q)$, respectively. The same constraint could also be applied along the φ-axis with a smoothness parameter Δ_φ.
2. For the pair of surfaces S_a and S_f, their surface distance in the same column is constrained. For example, in column $Col(p)$, the distance between these two surface should be constrained in a specified range of $0 \leq \delta_p^l \leq (|S_a(p) - S_f(p)|) \leq \delta_p^u$. In addition, S_f requires to be located below the S_a (as shown in Figure 22.5).

To enforce above geometric constraints, three types of arcs are constructed to define a directed graph $G = \{G_a \cup G_s\}$ (see Figure 22.6 for details), where G_a and G_s are two subgraphs and each for detecting one surface of S_a and S_f, respectively. For each subgraph, we construct both intra- and intercolumn arcs. We also construct intersurface arcs between two subgraphs G_a and G_s, following the graph construction methods introduced in Li et al. [11] and Song et al. [12].

Intracolumn arcs: This type of arcs is added to ensure that the target surface intersects each column at exactly one position. In our case, along each column $p(\theta, \varphi)$, every node $V(\theta, \varphi, r)$ has a directed arc to the node immediately below it $V(\theta, \varphi, r - 1)$ with $+\infty$ weight (Figure 22.6a).

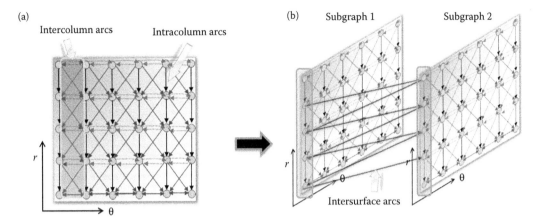

Figure 22.6 Graph construction for detecting adjacent two surfaces of a hip joint. An example is presented in 2D r-θ slice from the unfolded volume $I(\theta, \varphi, r)$. (a) Intracolumn (black arrows) and intercolumn (red and blue) arcs for each subgraph; (b) Intersurface arcs to connect two subgraphs. Please note that these two subgraphs share the same nodes as well as the same inter- and intracolumn arcs. The intersurface arcs are constructed between the corresponding two columns which have exactly the same column of voxels in the unfolded volume.

Intercolumn Arcs: This type of arc is added to constrain the shape changes of each individual surface S on neighboring columns under a four-neighborhood system. With two predefined smoothness parameters Δ_θ and Δ_φ, we construct these arcs with $+\infty$ weight along both the θ-axis and the φ-axis (Figure 22.6a). In summary, we have arcs:

$$E = \begin{cases} \{< V(\theta, \varphi, r), V(\theta + 1, \varphi, max(0, r - \Delta_\theta)) >\}\cup \\ \{< V(\theta, \varphi, r), V(\theta - 1, \varphi, max(0, r - \Delta_\theta)) >\}\cup \\ \{< V(\theta, \varphi, r), V(\theta, \varphi + 1, max(0, r - \Delta_\varphi)) >\}\cup \\ \{< V(\theta, \varphi, r), V(\theta, \varphi - 1, max(0, r - \Delta_\varphi)) >\} \end{cases} \tag{22.5}$$

To get a smooth segmentation, we further enforce soft smoothness shape compliance by adding another type of intracolumn arc (Figure 22.6a) [12]:

$$E = \begin{cases} \{< V(\theta, \varphi, r), V(\theta + 1, \varphi, r) > |r \geq 1\}\cup \\ \{< V(\theta, \varphi, r), V(\theta - 1, \varphi, r) > |r \geq 1\}\cup \\ \{< V(\theta, \varphi, r), V(\theta, \varphi + 1, r) > |r \geq 1\}\cup \\ \{< V(\theta, \varphi, r), V(\theta, \varphi - 1, r) > |r \geq 1\} \end{cases} \tag{22.6}$$

Again we construct these arcs along both the θ-axis and the φ-axis using a four-neighborhood system. The a prior shape compliance smoothness energy that assigned to these arcs are determined by a nondecreasing function $f_{p,q}(|S(p) - S(q)|)$, where $|S(p) - S(q)|$ represents the shape change (determined by the smoothness parameters Δ_θ and Δ_φ) for a surface S on neighbored columns $Col(p)$ and $Col(q)$. We select a linear function $f_{p,q}(|S(p) - S(q)|) = a(|S(p) - S(q)|) + b$, following the method introduced in Song et al. [12]. Thus, along the θ-axis, we assign a weight a to the arcs. Likewise, for the arcs along the φ-axis, we assign a similar weight for each arc.

Intersurface arcs: This type of arcs is added to constrain surface distance between S_a and S_f in each column. In our case S_f is required to be below the S_a. Thus, assuming that distance in column p between surfaces S_a and S_f ranges from δ_p^l to δ_p^u, we add the following arcs (Figure 22.6b):

$$
E_s = \begin{cases}
\{< V_a(\theta, \varphi, r), V_f(\theta, \varphi, r - \delta_p^u) > | r \geq \delta_p^u\} \cup \\
\{< V_f(\theta, \varphi, r), V_a(\theta, \varphi, r + \delta_p^l) > | r < R - \delta_p^l\} \cup \\
\{< V_a(0, 0, \delta_p^l), V_f(0, 0, 0) >\}
\end{cases}
\tag{22.7}
$$

where V_a and V_f denote the node in the corresponding column from each subgraph as shown in (Figure 22.6b). For each column p, we have a different distance range (δ_p^l, δ_p^u) that is statistically learned from a set of training data.

By adding all the arcs as described above, we establish a directed graph $G = (V, E)$, where $V = V_a \cup V_f$ and $E = E_a \cup E_f \cup E_s$. Here, V_a and V_f are node sets from each subgraph, E_a and E_f are intra- and intercolumn arcs from each subgraph, and E_s is the intersurface arcs between two subgraphs. In order to detect surfaces based on graph optimization, a new digraph $G_{st}(V \cup \{s, t\}, E \cup E_{st})$ is defined. This is achieved by adding a source node s and a sink node t as well as new edge set E_{st}, which includes the edges between nodes in the graph G and the nodes of $\{s, t\}$. Then surface detection can be solved using the minimum s-t cuts established by Kolmogorov et al. [22]. We add new edges for the edge set E_{st} following the method introduced in Li et al. [11]. The most important point here is to assign an appropriate penalty for each edge, which is also called t-link. As described in Li et al. [11], the penalty for each t-link is determined by a precomputed cost of each node. In our method, a carefully designed node cost function is calculated by considering both intensity information and a prior information. In the next section, we will introduce how such a cost function is calculated for each graph node.

22.3.3   Node cost function

Node cost function plays an important role for a successful surface detection. In our method, we first encode the boundary information to the cost function using the gradient information of each node following the method introduced in Li et al. [11]. The negative magnitude of the gradient of the volume $I(\theta, \varphi, r)$ is computed at each voxel as $c_{edge}(\theta, \varphi, r) = -|\nabla I(\theta, \varphi, r)|$. We give each node a weight as:

$$
w(\theta, \varphi, r) = \begin{cases}
c_{edge}(\theta, \varphi, r) & \text{if } z = 0 \\
c_{edge}(\theta, \varphi, r) - c_{edge}(\theta, \varphi, r - 1) & \text{otherwise}
\end{cases}
\tag{22.8}
$$

These weights are then modified by adding three types of constraints from a prior information: (1) The generated PA of the pelvis and the femur in the multiatlas-based segmentation stage. (2) Intensity histograms of surface points, which approximately indicate the intensity distribution of the points on each surface. They are statistically learned from a set of training data by extracting all the points on manually segmented surfaces from each training data. We learned two histograms, one for the acetabulum surface and the other for the femoral head surface. (3) The orientation of the gradient along the r-axis, which is determined by a sign function $Sgn(I_i(\theta, \varphi, r) - I_i(\theta, \varphi, r - 1))$, where $I_i(\theta, \varphi, r)$ is the intensity of voxel $V(\theta, \varphi, r)$.

The PA gives the probability of each voxel belonging to a specified bone region (background, pelvis, or bilateral proximal femurs). If any voxel have probability close or equal to 1 in the PA, it means that the atlases used for generating PA voted for this voxel, and thus this voxel is more likely to appear inside the bone region rather than on the surface of the bone. Considering that our purpose is to detect the surfaces of the bones, we decrease the weights for such nodes by:

$$w'(\theta, \varphi, r) = \begin{cases} w(\theta, \varphi, r) - h \cdot PA(\theta, \varphi, r), & \text{if } w(\theta, \varphi, r) > 0 \\ w(\theta, \varphi, r) + h \cdot PA(\theta, \varphi, r), & \text{if } w(\theta, \varphi, r) \leq 0 \end{cases} \tag{22.9}$$

where h is a constant value and $PA(\theta, \varphi, r)$ is the probability for a voxel $V(\theta, \varphi, r)$. For the nodes in the subgraph for detecting the surface of the acetabulum, we perform such a modification using the PA of the pelvis. Likewise, we encode information from the PA of the femur for the nodes in the other subgraph.

The intensity distribution of the bone surface points is limited in a specified range. For voxels whose intensity values are in this specified range, they are more likely to appear on the bone surfaces. We increase the weights for these nodes using the associated intensity histograms of surface points that are learned from a set of training data as described above.

$$w''(\theta, \varphi, r) = \begin{cases} w'(\theta, \varphi, r) + m \cdot Hist(I_i(\theta, \varphi, r)), & \text{if } w(\theta, \varphi, r) > 0 \\ w'(\theta, \varphi, r) - m \cdot Hist(I_i(\theta, \varphi, r)), & \text{if } w(\theta, \varphi, r) \leq 0 \end{cases} \tag{22.10}$$

where m is a constant value and $Hist(I_i(\theta, \varphi, r))$ is the corresponding value in the associated histogram for voxel $V(\theta, \varphi, r)$ which have intensity value of $I_i(\theta, \varphi, r)$. Please note that we have learned two intensity histograms, one for surface points of the acetabulum and the other for the surface points of the femoral head. When modifying the weights of nodes in each subgraph, the associated histogram is used.

As shown in Figure 22.5, for voxels on the surface of the acetabulum, since the intensity at $V(\theta, \varphi, r)$ is bigger than $V(\theta, \varphi, r - 1)$, the value of the $Sgn(I_i(\theta, \varphi, r) - I_i(\theta, \varphi, r - 1))$ should be positive and we define the orientation of these voxels as positive too. Similarly, for voxels on the surface of the femoral head, we define their orientation in r-axis as negative. Therefore, for a node in the subgraph for detecting the surface of the acetabulum, if its gradient orientation is not consistent with our definition, we set its weight to 0. For a node in the subgraph for detecting the surface of the femoral head, we perform a similar modification.

After we modify the weight for each node in the graph G_{st}, we assign penalty for each t-link based on the modified weight using the method introduced in Li et al. [11]. Our problem is then to optimally detect two surfaces from the constructed graph, which can be solved using the minimum s-t cuts algorithm [20,22].

22.4 Experiments and results

We evaluated the present method on hip CT data of 30 patients after ethical approval. The intraslice resolutions range from 0.576 to 0.744 mm while the inter-slice resolutions are 1.6 mm for all CT data. Manual segmentation of all 30 CT data were done by a trained rater. Approximately, 20 of them were selected as the training data both for the RF regression-based landmark detection and the multiatlas-based segmentation. The rest 10 datasets (20 hip joints) were used for evaluation.

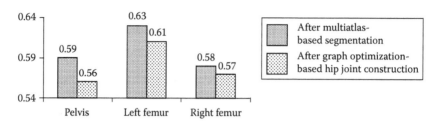

Figure 22.7 Evaluation of the segmentation performance after each stage in the present method. The average surface distance (mm) on 10 test images are shown in the figure.

As for performance evaluation, we computed two different metrics. First, surface distance (SD) between automatic segmentation and ground truth segmentation are computed after each stage of the present method. Figure 22.7 shows the average SD which was computed on the entire pelvis and femur regions. More specifically, our method achieves high performance in segmenting pelvis, left proximal femur, and right proximal femur with an average accuracy of 0.56 mm, 0.61 mm, and 0.57 mm, respectively. Furthermore, we also looked at the segmentation accuracy around the hip joint local areas which are important for our target clinical applications. The local evaluation results are shown in Table 22.1. It is observed from Figure 22.7 that the segmentation results of the two stages in the present method are quite close if we evaluate the performance in the entire regions of the pelvis and the femur. However, when we focus on the local hip joint area, one can find from Table 22.1 that the graph optimization-based surface detection improves the hip joint segmentation accuracy. Second, we also computed the Dice overlap coefficients (DOC) between automatic segmentation and ground truth segmentation. The present method achieved a mean DOC of $93.3 \pm 1.1\%$, $95.2 \pm 1.3\%$, and $95.5 \pm 0.8\%$ for pelvis, left femur, and right femur, respectively.

We checked whether the present method could preserve the hip joint space and prevent the penetration of the extracted surface models. For all the 20 hip joints that were segmented with the present method, we have consistently found that the hip joint spaces

Table 22.1 Surface distance (mm) between automatic and ground truth segmentation of the bilateral hip joints from 10 CT data

Bone	Stage	CT 1	CT 2	CT 3	CT 4	CT 5	CT 6	CT 7	CT 8	CT 9	CT 10	Average
LA	MA	0.42	0.30	0.24	0.24	0.26	0.30	0.46	0.40	0.29	0.35	0.33
	GO	0.20	0.29	0.21	0.23	0.23	0.17	0.31	0.26	0.26	0.24	0.24
LFH	MA	0.40	0.56	0.41	0.34	0.51	0.36	0.51	0.81	0.38	0.49	0.48
	GO	0.30	0.25	0.24	0.37	0.33	0.32	0.41	0.64	0.31	0.27	0.34
RA	MA	0.43	0.36	0.22	0.33	0.24	0.30	0.48	0.31	0.25	0.32	0.32
	GO	0.23	0.23	0.18	0.30	0.17	0.22	0.22	0.21	0.22	0.30	0.23
RFH	MA	0.40	0.42	0.54	0.29	0.34	0.39	0.55	0.52	0.43	0.53	0.44
	GO	0.41	0.40	0.46	0.36	0.38	0.38	0.45	0.59	0.38	0.28	0.41

Note: Results after stage I (multiatlas-based segmentation: MA) and after stage II (graph optimization-based surface detection: GO) are shown, where LA stands for the left acetabulum, LFH for the left femoral head, RA for the right acetabulum, and RFH for the right femoral head.

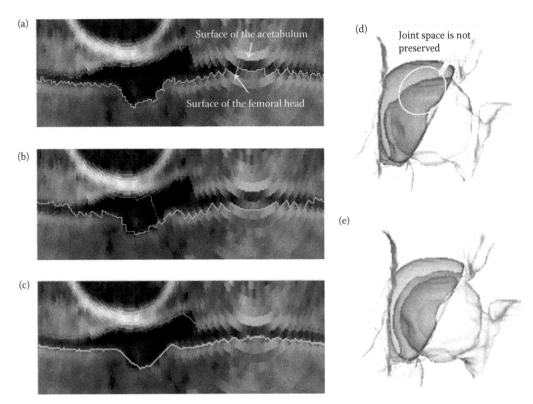

Figure 22.8 An example of segmenting a hip joint with the present method. Both 2D and 3D visualizations of results from different stages of our method are presented. (a) Ground truth. (b) Multiatlas based segmentation. (c) Graph optimization based surface detection. (d) Hip joint after multiatlas-based segmentation. (e) Reconstructed hip joint by graph optimization based surface detection.

were preserved and that there was no penetration between the extracted adjacent surface models. Figure 22.8 shows a segmentation example. From this figure, we can clearly see that the graph optimization-based surface detection stage further improve the results from the multiatlas-based segmentation.

22.5   Discussions and conclusion

The goal of the present study is to develop and validate a fully automatic hip joint segmentation approach. Our experimental results showed that the present method not only achieved a good overall segmentation accuracy for both the pelvis and the proximal femur, but also had the advantages of preservation of hip joint space and prevention of the penetration of the extracted adjacent surface models, which are prerequisite conditions to use the segmented models for computer assisted diagnosis and planning of PAO surgery.

The performance of the present method is compared with those of the state-of-the-art hip CT segmentation methods [2–5,9]. The comparison results are summarized in Table 22.2. From this table, one can see that the performace of the present method is comparable to other state-of-the-art hip CT segmentation methods [2–5,9].

Table 22.2 Comparison of the results achieved by the present method with those
reported in the literature

Method	Preserving hip joint	Average SD (mm)	Average DOC (%)
Lamecker et al. [9]	No	1.80	–
Semi et al. [4]	No	0.70	–
Kainmueller et al. [5]	Yes	0.60	–
Yokota et al. [2]	No	1.10	92.7
Yokota et al. [3]	No	0.98	–
The present method	Yes	0.58	94.7

In conclusion, we presented a fully automatic and accurate method for segmenting CT images of a hip joint. The strength of the present method lies in the combination of a multiatlas-based hip CT segmentation with a graph optimization-based multisurface detection. The present method can be extended to segment CT data of other anatomical structures.

References

1. R. Ganz, K. Klaue, T. Vinh, and J. Mast, A new periacetabular osteotomy for the treatment of hip dysplasia: Technique and preliminary results, *Clinical Orthopedics*, vol. 232, pp. 26–36, 1988.
2. F. Yokota, T. Okada, M. Takao, S. Sugano, Y. Tada, and Y. Sato, Automated segmentation of the femur and pelvis from 3D CT data of diseased hip using hierarchical statistical shape model of joint structure, in MICCAI 2009, vol. 5762, LNCS, G. Yang, D. Hawkes, D. Rueckert, A. Noble, and C. Taylor, Eds., 2009, pp. 811–818.
3. F. Yokota, T. Okada, M. Takao, S. Sugano, Y. Tada, Y. Tomiyama, and Y. Sato, Automated CT segmentation of diseased hip using hierarchical and conditional statistical shape models, in MICCAI 2013, vol. 8150, LNCS, K. Mori, I. Sakuma, Y. Sato, C. Barillot, and N. Navab, Eds., 2013, pp. 190–197.
4. H. Seim, D. Kainmueller, M. Heller, H. Lamecker, S. Zachow, and H. C. Hege, Automatic segmentation of the pelvic bones from CT data based on a statistical shape model, in *Eurographics Workshop on Visual Computing for Biomedicine*, 2008, pp. 67–78.
5. D. Kainmueller, H. Lamecker, S. Zachow, and H. C. Hege, An articulated statistical shape model for accurate hip joint segmentation, in IEEE EMBC 2009, 2009, pp. 6345–6351.
6. J. Ehrhardte, H. Handels, W. Plotz, and S. J. Poppl, Atlas-based recognition of anatomical structures and landmarks and the automatic computation of orthopedic parameters, *Methods in Informatics and Medicine*, vol. 43, pp. 391–397, 2004.
7. J. Pettersson, H. Knutsson, and M. Borga, Automatic hip bone segmentation using non-rigid registration, In: ICPR 2006, 2006.
8. X. Ying, F. Jurgen, S. Shekhar, S. Raphael, E. Craig, and C. Stuart, Automated bone segmentation from large field of view 3D MR images of the hip joint, *Physics in Medicine and Biology*, vol. 58, pp. 7375–7390, 2013.
9. H. Lamecker, M. Seeba, H. C. Hege, and P. Deuflhard, A 3D statistical shape model of the pelvic bone for segmentation, in SPIE, vol. 5370, pp. 1341–1351, 2004.
10. D. Kainmueller, H. Lamecker, S. Zachow, and H. C. Hege, Coupling deformable models for multi-object segmentation, in ISBMS, vol. 5104, pp. 69–78, 2008.
11. K. Li, X. Wu, D. Chen, and M. Sonka, Optimal surface segmentation in volumetric images—A graph-theoretic approach, *IEEE Transactions on Pattern Analysis and Machine Intelligence*, vol. 28, pp. 119–134, 2006.

12. Q. Song, X. Wu, Y. Liu, M. Smith, J. Buatti, and M. Sonka, Optimal graph search segmentation using arc-weighted graph for simultaneous surface detection of bladder and prostate, in MICCAI 2009, vol. 5762, LNCS, 2009, pp. 827–835.

13. A. Criminisi, J. Shotton, D. Robertson, and E. Konukoglu, Regression forests for efficient anatomy detection and localization in CT studies, in MICCAI 2011, vol. 6533, LNCS, B. Menze, G. Langs, Z. Tu, and A. Criminisi, Eds., 2011, pp. 106–117.

14. C. Lindner, S. Thiagarajah, and J. M. Wilkinson, arcOGEN Consortium, G. Wallis, and T. F. Cootes, Fully automatic segmentation of the proximal femur using random forest regression voting, *IEEE TMI*, vol. 32, pp. 1462–1472, 2013.

15. L. Breiman, Random forests, *Machine Learning*, vol. 45 , pp. 5–32, 2001.

16. C. Yang, R. Duraiswami, and L. Davis, Efficient kernel machines using the improved fast gauss transform. *Advances in Neural Information Processing Systems*, vol. 17, pp. 1561–1568, 2005.

17. P. Viola and M. Jones, Rapid object detection using a boosted cascade of simple features, in CVPR 2001, vol. I, pp. 511–518, 2001.

18. B. Glocker, M. Komodakis, G. Tziritas, N. Navab, and N. Paragios, Dense image registration through mrfs and efficient linear programming, *Medical Image Analysis*, vol. 12, pp. 731–741, 2008.

19. C. Chu, M. Oda, T. Kitasaka, K. Misawa, M. Fujiwara, Y. Hayashi, Y. Nimura, D. Rueckert, and K. Mori, Multi-organ segmentation based on spatially-divided probabilistic atlas from 3D abdominal CT images, in MICCAI 2013, vol. 8150, LNCS, K. Mori, I. Sakuma, Y. Sato, C. Barillot, and N. Navab, Eds., 2013, pp. 165–172.

20. Y. Boykov, O. Veksler, and R. Zabih, Fast approximate energy minimization via graph cuts, *IEEE PAMI*, vol. 23, pp. 1222–1239, 2001.

21. L. Liu, T. Ecker, S. Schumann, K. Siebenrock, L. Nolte, and G. Zheng, Computer assisted planning and navigation of periacetabular osteotomy with range of motion optimization, in MICCAI 2014, vol. part II, LNCS 8674, P. Golland et al., eds. Berlin, Springer, 2014, pp. 643–650.

22. V. Kolmogorov and R. Zabih, What energy functions can be minimized via graph cuts? *IEEE Transactions on PAMI*, vol. 26, pp. 147–159, 2004.

Index